Physeal Injury Other Than Fracture

Hamlet A. Peterson

Physeal Injury Other Than Fracture

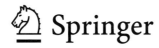 Springer

Hamlet A. Peterson, MD, MS
Emeritus Consultant
Department of Orthopedic
Surgery and Emeritus Chair
Mayo Clinic Division of Pediatric Orthopedic Surgery
Emeritus Professor of Orthopedics
Mayo Medical School
Mayo Clinic College of Medicine
200 First St. SW
Rochester, Minnesota 55905
USA
peterson.hamlet@mayo.edu

ISBN 978-3-642-22562-8   e-ISBN 978-3-642-22563-5
DOI 10.1007/978-3-642-22563-5
Springer Heidelberg Dordrecht London New York

Library of Congress Control Number: 2011940864

© Mayo Foundation for Medical Education and Research 2012

This work is subject to copyright. All rights are reserved, whether the whole or part of the material is concerned, specifically the rights of translation, reprinting, reuse of illustrations, recitation, broadcasting, reproduction on microfilm or in any other way, and storage in data banks. Permission requests should be directed to Scientific Publications, Plummer 10, Mayo Clinic, 200 First Street SW, Rochester, MN 55905, USA.

The use of general descriptive names, registered names, trademarks, etc. in this publication does not imply, even in the absence of a specific statement, that such names are exempt from the relevant protective laws and regulations and therefore free for general use.

Product liability: The publishers cannot guarantee the accuracy of any information about dosage and application contained in this book. In every individual case the user must check such information by consulting the relevant literature.

Printed on acid-free paper

Springer is part of Springer Science+Business Media (www.springer.com)

To my wife, Suzanne, my parents Hamlet E. and Thelma, my children, Erik, Heidi, and Nils, and my siblings, Helen and Luther, who all in their own special way made my life full, making this book possible.

Introduction

This book is a sequel to my previous book "Epiphyseal Growth Plate Fractures (Springer, Heidelberg, 2007, 914pp). Although physeal injuries other than fracture combined are far less common than fractures, they cause similar morbidity. This book is an expression of, and a testament to, the breadth of pediatric orthopedics.

It was my intention to include the material in this book in my first book, Epiphyseal Growth Plate Fractures. However, as that book became larger and larger, and as the years of research and writing continued to pass, it became obvious that if all the material of both subjects was included in one book, the book would never be finished. The most expeditious way to proceed was to divide the material into two books: "Fractures" and "Injuries other than Fracture".

As with Epiphyseal Growth Plate Fractures, the case material presented here is predominantly from patients for whom I cared, supplemented with cases from my Mayo Clinic colleagues, and a few sent to me for review and comments but were never seen at Mayo. Credit for these latter cases is given to the referring physician, when appropriate. Most cases were referred in some stage of complication. When possible, I have gathered preceding data, to determine whether a different course of action could have prevented the complication. In all cases I have attempted to determine the best treatment as well as the treatment used and its outcome. The greatest impediment to advancing the science of growth plate injuries is the paucity of long term follow-up. Thus, where possible, illustrative cases have been chosen in which long follow-up was available. The information found herein will be of most value to the pediatric orthopedist, pediatrician, and pediatric radiologist.

Preface

The subspecialty of Pediatric Orthopedics is distinguished from adult orthopedics in many ways. The most prominent difference is the presence of growth plates (physes). Once the growth plates close the patient physically becomes an adult. Growth disturbance of long bones is a common major clinical issue for pediatric orthopedics. Physes of epiphyses are the sole providers of longitudinal bone growth. Since physes of apophyses provide no longitudinal growth, apophyseal injuries are not included in this text.

Physes may be injured in many ways, the most common of which is fracture. This textbook is an overview of injuries to the epiphyseal growth plate *other than* fracture. Most non-fracture injuries of epiphyseal physes sufficient to cause diminution of growth have two similar characteristics: roentgenographically normal physes at the time of injury and physeal abnormality noted weeks, months, or years later. Injuries which meet these criteria are described in the following chapters:

1. Vascular
2. Disuse
3. Infection
4. Tumor
5. Metabolic
6. Neural
7. Cold (frostbite)
8. Heat (burn)
9. Electrical
10. Compression
11. Distraction
12. Stress
13. Irradiation
14. Light Waves
15. Sound Waves
16. Shock Waves
17. Atmospheric Pressure
18. Oxygen
19. Developmental
20. Surgical
21. Unknown

The number of patients sustaining growth arrest from each of these conditions is low. Even combined, their numbers do not equal physeal injuries due to fracture. However, in most of these conditions, premature growth arrest is the most common serious complication. In many, the precise pathogenesis of the physeal impairment is obscure, speculative, or unknown. Grouping these conditions together may help to better understand them and hopefully help to prevent the harmful effects from occurring, or at least to anticipate them and thereby mitigate their harmful effects.

Many conditions resulting in physeal arrest could be appropriately recorded in one of several chapters. A prime example is poliomyelitis, an infection involving the nervous system. It could therefore be reported in Chap. 3, Infection, or Chap. 6, Neural. However, compelling evidence suggests that growth arrest in patients with poliomyelitis is due to disuse, and it is therefore reported in Chap. 2, Disuse. In most cases where a condition could be reported in more than one chapter, I have attempted to explain my reason for its location.

These injuries are extremely varied in nature. The basic insulting event may be located in a primary field of medicine far from pediatric orthopedics. Thus, although I have diligently searched the literature by computer and by reviewing reference lists in published articles, I doubt that the literature search is complete in any of the chapters. An attempt has been made to include all pertinent references in the English literature through December, 2007. Some articles in languages other than English are included, for example, a foreign language article with an English abstract which contains relevant information. In addition, some pertinent articles published after 2007 which came to my attention are included.

The rationale for the order of the chapters needs to be explained. Chapter 1 describes the vascular anatomy of the physis and vascular injuries resulting in growth arrest. Actually, many of the insults documented in subsequent chapters may primarily damage the vascularity to the physis, which thereby secondarily affects the physis, rather than damaging the physis directly. Chapters 2–13 describe injuries of the physis that are fairly well documented and accepted. Chapters 14–18 describe insults that occur due to advanced technology in modern life. Growth arrest from these insults are extremely rare and some have been found only in animals. However, since these modalities have damaged physes in animals, they could conceivably damage physes in humans. Developmental, Surgical, and Unknown causes are placed last.

Many of these injuries are iatrogenic; i.e., induced by the action of a physician. All of the conditions result in damage to selected or random physes. Conditions which affect the growth of all physis simultaneously, such as genetic disorders, skeletal dysplasias, cranial tumors which cause system wide endocrine abnormalities, etc., are not "injuries" in the sense discussed here and are not included.

Most children with physeal injuries other than fracture are treated and followed by physicians other than pediatric orthopedists. However, the management of the physeal abnormalities caused by these injuries is often similar to those caused by fracture, which is likewise greatly enhanced by their early detection. Pediatric orthopedists therefore need to be in close contact with all physicians who care for these patients. Early treatment of physeal arrest, including bar excision of affected physes in selected cases and surgical arrest of contralateral physes, should lessen the need for bone lengthening and shortening operations, arthrodesis, and amputation.

No other book or comprehensive source focuses on physeal injuries other than fracture. Several journal articles [1–8] and book chapters [9, 10] describe a few or several of these injuries, but none of these sources includes all of the conditions within this book.

Hamlet A. Peterson

References

1. Ahstrom Jr JP (1965) Epiphyseal injuries of the extremities. Surg Clin North Am 1:119–134
2. Caffey J (1970) Traumatic cupping of the metaphyses of growing bones. Am J Roentgenol 108:451–460
3. Kao SCS, Smith WL (1997) Skeletal injuries in the pediatric patient. Radiol Clin North Am 35(3):727–746
4. Kumar R, Madewell JE, Swischuk LE (1987) The normal and abnormal growth plate. Radiol Clin North Am 25:1133–1153
5. Poznanski AK (1978) Annual oration. Diagnostic clues in the growing ends of bone. J Can Assoc Radiol 29:7–21
6. Rogers LF, Poznanski AK (1994) Imaging of epiphyseal injuries. Radiology 191(2):297–308
7. Siegling JA (1937) Lesions of the epiphyseal cartilages about the knee. Surg Clin North Am 17:373–379
8. Siffert RS (1966) The growth plate and its affections. J Bone Joint Surg 48A:546–563
9. Ogden JA (2000) Injury to the growth mechanisms. In: Ogden JA (ed) Skeletal injury in the child, 3rd edn. Springer, New York, chapter 6, pp 147–208
10. Peterson HA (2001) Physeal injuries and growth arrest. In: Beaty JH, Kasser JR (eds) Rockwood and Wilkins fractures in children, 5th edn. Lippincott Williams & Wilkins, Philadelphia, chapter 5, pp 91–138

Acknowledgements

The genesis of this book began many years ago while encountering a wide variety of interesting patient problems. The collection of data from these patients and periodic publishing of related articles, supplemented by a review of the literature, forms the basis of the book. In this regard I am indebted to Mayo Clinic, and in particular to its related Departments of Orthopedic Surgery, Pediatric and Adolescent Medicine, and Radiology, Media Support Services, the Section of Scientific Publications, The Mayo Clinic Library, the Legal Department, and the Emeritus Staff Center. Also, the liberal Mayo Clinic travel policy allowed me to attend frequent meetings, symposia, and seminars to keep abreast of ongoing developments in all aspects of pediatric orthopedics.

Nearly the entirety of my 30-year career at Mayo was spent with pediatric orthopedic colleagues Drs. Tony Bianco and Rudi Klassen. For 19 of those years we saw patients in the same clinic area and operated in adjacent operating rooms on the same days. This sharing of patient experiences, trials, tribulations, successes, and failures, and their counsel and friendship have been invaluable not only for accumulating the cases in this book, but also for my professional development and insight into the material presented herein. In more recent years this was supplemented by wise counsel and patient follow-up information from pediatric orthopedic colleagues Drs. Bill Shaughnessy and Tony Stans, and from all the adult orthopedic staff who kept me informed about our former patients.

For a book of this magnitude an enormous amount of skilled support was required. I would like to thank my wife, Suzanne, who cheerfully typed the entire manuscript and its frequent revisions. Her diligence and patience is greatly appreciated. Special thanks to secretaries Kathy Grutzmacher and Delores Moore who procured and assembled patient histories and roentgenographs. I am particularly indebted to David Factor, the medical illustrator who rendered the drawings and was so patient with my multiple suggestions and requests. The professionalism of all the folks in Media Support Services, where roentgenographs were copied and graphs designed, was superb. I thank Ms. Gabriele Schröder, and the staff of Springer for their skill and imagination in creating a product of high standard and quality.

Because of the specialized nature of some of the chapter topics, individuals with special expertise reviewed and edited a number of chapters. A special thank you is given to each of these experts:

Chapter 1. Vascular

Stephan W. Carmichael, Ph.D. Emeritus Chair, Department of Anatomy, Mayo Clinic, Rochester, Minnesota; Emeritus Professor of Anatomy, College of Medicine, Mayo Clinic.

Thomas L. Schmidt, M.D., Emeritus Professor, Department of Orthopaedic Surgery, University of Missouri at Kansas City, School of Medicine, and the Rex and Lillian Diveley Emeritus Professor of Pediatric Orthopaedic Surgery, the Children's Mercy Hospital, Kansas City, MO.

Erik J. Peterson, M.D., Associate Professor of Medicine, Division of Rheumatology, University of Minnesota Medical School, Minneapolis, MN.

Chapter 2. Disuse

Kathleen H. Rhodes, M.D., Emeritus Chair, Division of Pediatric Infectious Disease, Mayo Clinic, Rochester, Minnesota; Emeritus Professor of Pediatric Infectious Disease, College of Medicine, Mayo Clinic.

Erik J. Peterson, M.D., Associate Professor of Medicine, Division of Rheumatology, University of Minnesota Medical School, Minneapolis, MN.

Chapter 3. Infection

Kathleen H. Rhodes, M.D., Emeritus Chair, Division of Pediatric Infectious Disease, Mayo Clinic, Rochester, Minnesota; Emeritus Professor of Pediatric Infectious Disease, College of Medicine, Mayo Clinic.

Chapter 4. Tumor

Franklin H. Sim, M.D., Chair, Division of Musculoskeletal Oncology, Mayo Clinic, Rochester, Minnesota; Professor of Orthopedic Surgery, College of Medicine, Mayo Clinic.

Chapter 5. Metabolic and Chapter 6. Neural

Erik J. Peterson, M.D., Associate Professor of Medicine, Division of Rheumatology, University of Minnesota Medical School, Minneapolis, MN.

Chapter 13. Irradiation

Paula J. Schomberg, M.D., Chair, Department of Radiation Oncology, Mayo Clinic, Rochester, Minnesota; Professor of Radiation Oncology, College of Medicine, Mayo Clinic.

Chapter 14. Light Waves, Chapter 15. Sound Waves, Chapter 16. Shock Waves, Chapter 17. Atmospheric Pressure, and Chapter 18. Oxygen

Richard J. Vetter, Ph.D., Emeritus Chief Safety Officer, Mayo Clinic, Rochester, Minnesota; Emeritus Professor of Biophysics and Radiation Safety, College of Medicine.

Finally, I pay tribute to all previous authors of various aspects of physeal injuries other than fracture who labored to publish their observations so that we might learn to better care for pediatric patients. In particular, I salute my mentors and colleagues in the Department of Orthopedics at Mayo Clinic who were instrumental in my development, and for fostering in me a desire to share my experience and knowledge with others.

Despite all of this help, this book would never have reached completion with the support and encouragement of my wife, Suzanne, who was constant and relentless in urging me to stay the course and finish the race.

To all, I owe immense gratitude.

Hamlet A. Peterson

Contents

1 Vascular Deficiency 1
    1.1 Introduction 1
    1.2 Vascular Anatomy of the Physis 1
        1.2.1 Epiphyseal Arteries 2
        1.2.2 Metaphyseal and Intramedullary Arteries 4
        1.2.3 Periosteal Arteries 9
        1.2.4 Normal Physeal Growth 9
        1.2.5 Normal Physiologic Physeal Closure 9
        1.2.6 Premature Physeal Closure 10
    1.3 Vascular Deficiency Due to Reduced Quantity 10
        1.3.1 Arterial Disruption 11
        1.3.2 Arterial Ligation 14
        1.3.3 Arterial Catheterization 14
        1.3.4 Arterial Injection 18
        1.3.5 Fluid Extravasation in Soft Tissues 18
        1.3.6 Interosseous Infusion 18
        1.3.7 Compartment Syndrome 18
        1.3.8 Diaphyseal Fracture 18
        1.3.9 Periosteal Stripping 27
        1.3.10 Joint Dislocation 27
        1.3.11 Extremity Traction 27
        1.3.12 Fixation Bandages 27
        1.3.13 Developmental Dislocation of the Hip 29
        1.3.14 Perthes Disease 31
        1.3.15 Transplantation of the Physis 32
    1.4 Vascular Deficiency Due to Reduced Quality 32
        1.4.1 Sickle Cell Anemia 33
        1.4.2 Thalassemia Major (Cooley's Anemia) 40
        1.4.3 Meningococcemia 40
        1.4.4 Purpura Fulminans 41
        1.4.5 Other Conditions 42
    1.5 Physeal Cupping 42
    1.6 Author's Perspective 46
    References 47

2 Disuse ... 53
- 2.1 Introduction ... 53
- 2.2 Tuberculosis ... 53
- 2.3 Poliomyelitis ... 54
- 2.4 Diaphyseal Fracture ... 57
- 2.5 Developmental Dislocation of the Hip ... 61
- 2.6 Perthes Disease ... 61
- 2.7 Osteomyelitis ... 61
- 2.8 Slipped Capital Femoral Epiphysis ... 61
- 2.9 Chemically Induced Immobilization ... 62
- 2.10 Author's Perspective ... 62
- References ... 62

3 Infection ... 65
- 3.1 Introduction ... 65
- 3.2 Metaphyseal Osteomyelitis ... 65
  - 3.2.1 The Organism ... 65
  - 3.2.2 Age of the Patient ... 66
  - 3.2.3 Pathogenesis ... 66
  - 3.2.4 Pathologic Anatomy ... 70
  - 3.2.5 The Bone Involved ... 77
  - 3.2.6 Diagnosis ... 77
  - 3.2.7 Treatment of Infection ... 77
  - 3.2.8 Treatment of Physeal Arrest ... 79
  - 3.2.9 Stimulation of Growth ... 80
  - 3.2.10 Metaphyseal-Equivalent Osteomyelitis ... 80
- 3.3 Epiphyseal Osteomyelitis ... 83
  - 3.3.1 Acute ... 83
  - 3.3.2 Subacute ... 84
  - 3.3.3 Epiphyseal Disappearance and Regeneration ... 84
- 3.4 Physeal Chondritis ... 86
- 3.5 Transphyseal Osteomyelitis ... 86
- 3.6 Subacute Osteomyelitis ... 94
- 3.7 Chronic Osteomyelitis ... 95
- 3.8 Chronic Recurrent Multifocal Osteomyelitis ... 95
- 3.9 Septic Arthritis ... 96
  - 3.9.1 Monoarticular Septic Arthritis ... 97
  - 3.9.2 Multiarticular Septic Arthritis ... 106
- 3.10 Author's Perspective ... 109
- References ... 109

4 Tumor 115

4.1 Introduction 115

4.2 Benign Bone Tumors 115
- 4.2.1 Solitary Bone Cyst 115
- 4.2.2 Aneurysmal Bone Cyst 122
- 4.2.3 Osteochondroma 125
- 4.2.4 Enchondroma 140
- 4.2.5 Chondroblastoma 141
- 4.2.6 Giant Cell Tumor 142
- 4.2.7 Langerhan's Cell Histiocytosis 142
- 4.2.8 Osteoid Osteoma and Osteoblastoma 143
- 4.2.9 Focal Fibrocartilaginous Dysplasia 144
- 4.2.10 Fibrous Dysplasia of Bone 144
- 4.2.11 Miscellaneous 145
- 4.2.12 Author's Perspective 149

4.3 Malignant Bone Tumors 151
- 4.3.1 Osteosarcoma 151
- 4.3.2 Ewing Sarcoma 158
- 4.3.3 Chondrosarcoma 159
- 4.3.4 Lymphoma of Bone 159
- 4.3.5 Author's Perspective 159

4.4 Soft Tissue Tumors 159

4.5 Tumor Induced Rickets 161

References 163

5 Metabolic 173

5.1 Introduction 173

5.2 Nutrition 173
- 5.2.1 General Nutritional Deprivation 173
- 5.2.2 Vitamin A Deficiency 174
- 5.2.3 Vitamin A Excess 174
- 5.2.4 Vitamin C Deficiency (Scurvy) 174
- 5.2.5 Vitamin D Deficiency (Rickets) 175

5.3 Endocrine 176
- 5.3.1 Slipped Capital Femoral Epiphysis (SCFE) 176

5.4 Medications 181
- 5.4.1 Aminonucleoside 181
- 5.4.2 Bisphosphonates 182
- 5.4.3 2-Butoxyethanol 182
- 5.4.4 Calcitriol 182
- 5.4.5 Corticosteroids 183
- 5.4.6 Deferoxamine 183
- 5.4.7 Etretinate 183
- 5.4.8 Isotretinon (13-cis-Retinoic Acid) 186
- 5.4.9 Papain 186

		5.4.10	^{153}Sm-Ethylenediaminetetramethylene Phosphonate (^{153}Sm-EDTMP)	186

        5.4.11   Tetracycline 186

5.5 Chemotherapy 187

5.6 Chronic Renal Failure 188

References 190

6 Neural 195

6.1 Introduction 195

6.2 Peripheral Nerve Injury 195
- 6.2.1 Peripheral Denervation 195
- 6.2.2 Brachial Plexus Palsy 196
- 6.2.3 Lumbar Sympathetic Ganglionectomy 196

6.3 Spinal Cord Injury 196
- 6.3.1 Spinal Cord Traumatic Injury 196
- 6.3.2 Spinal Cord Nontraumatic Injury 198

6.4 Brain Injury 206
- 6.4.1 Physeal Growth in Hemiplegic Patients 206
- 6.4.2 Physeal Disruption in Quadriplegic Patients 207

6.5 Congenital Insensitivity to Pain 208

References 216

7 Cold Injury (Frostbite) 219

7.1 Introduction 219

7.2 Human Involvement 219
- 7.2.1 Clinical Aspects 219
- 7.2.2 Imaging Evaluation 219
- 7.2.3 Differential Diagnosis 220
- 7.2.4 Epidemiology 220
- 7.2.5 Pathological Mechanisms 222
- 7.2.6 Management 223

7.3 Animal Research 223

7.4 Author's Perspective 223

References 223

8 Heat Injury (Burns) 225

8.1 Introduction 225

8.2 Human Involvement 225
- 8.2.1 Clinical Aspects 225
- 8.2.2 Pathological Mechanism 225
- 8.2.3 Management 226

		8.3	Animal Research	226
		8.4	Author's Perspective	227
		References		227
9	Electric Injuries			229
		9.1	Introduction	229
		9.2	Electric Current	229
			9.2.1 Clinical Aspects	229
			9.2.2 Roentgenographic Studies	229
			9.2.3 Pathological Mechanism	229
			9.2.4 Management	230
		9.3	Lightning	230
		9.4	Diathermy, Microwave	231
		9.5	Author's Perspective	231
		References		231
10	Compression			233
		10.1	Introduction	233
		10.2	Continuous Compression – Human Involvement	233
			10.2.1 Pathophysiologic Mechanism of Injury	233
			10.2.2 Continuous Active Compression	234
			10.2.3 Continuous Passive Compression	236
		10.3	Continuous Compression – Animal Research	246
			10.3.1 Pathophysiologic Mechanism of Injury	246
			10.3.2 Histologic Studies	250
			10.3.3 Amount of Compression	250
			10.3.4 Duration of Compression	250
			10.3.5 Direction of Pressure Applied	250
			10.3.6 Periosteal Tether	251
			10.3.7 Staples	251
			10.3.8 Transphyseal Threaded Screws and Pins	251
			10.3.9 Crossed Smooth Metallic Pins	252
			10.3.10 Biodegradable Screws and Crossed Pins	252
			10.3.11 Absorbable Filament	253
			10.3.12 Surgical Bone Lengthening	253
			10.3.13 Spine Fusion	253
			10.3.14 Tensioned Soft Tissue Grafts	253
			10.3.15 Compensatory Growth	253
		10.4	Acute Compression – Human Involvement	253
			10.4.1 The Concept	253
			10.4.2 The Compression Concept Challenged	256
			10.4.3 Clinical Support for the S-H Type 5 Compression Injury Concept	256

		10.4.4	Alternative Mechanisms	257

		10.4.4	Alternative Mechanisms	257
		10.4.5	Clinical Opposition to or Evidence Against the S-H Type 5 Compression Injury Concept	260
		10.4.6	New Classifications	262
	10.5	Acute Compression – Animal Research		262
		10.5.1	Animal Studies Supporting the Compression Concept	262
		10.5.2	Animal Studies Refuting the Compression Concept	262
	10.6	Author's Perspective		263
	References			264
11	Distraction			271
	11.1	Introduction		271
	11.2	Human Involvement		271
		11.2.1	The Procedure	271
		11.2.2	Results	272
	11.3	Animal Research		276
	11.4	Author's Perspective		277
	References			278
12	Stress			281
	12.1	Introduction		281
	12.2	Mechanism of Injury		281
	12.3	Evaluation		283
	12.4	Management		287
	12.5	Complications		287
	12.6	Author's Perspective		287
	References			287
13	Irradiation			289
	13.1	Introduction		289
		13.1.1	Radiation Terminology	289
		13.1.2	Radiation Effects	289
		13.1.3	Side Effects and Complications	290
	13.2	Diagnostic Irradiation		291
	13.3	Therapeutic Irradiation; Extremities		291
		13.3.1	Dose and Age Effects	296
		13.3.2	Physes Involved	296
		13.3.3	Side Effects	297
		13.3.4	Multimodality Therapy	297
		13.3.5	Management	297
		13.3.6	Slipped Epiphyses	298

| | | 13.3.7 | Osteochondroma (Exostosis) | 299 |
| | | 13.3.8 | Intentional Physeal Retardation of Extremity Physes | 304 |

13.4 Therapeutic Irradiation; Head and Neck ... 304

13.5 Therapeutic Irradiation; Trunk ... 304
- 13.5.1 Stature Loss ... 305
- 13.5.2 Spine Deformity ... 305
- 13.5.3 Etiology and Natural History of Spine Deformity ... 305
- 13.5.4 Incidence of Spine Deformity ... 310
- 13.5.5 Prophylaxis ... 310
- 13.5.6 Treatment ... 311
- 13.5.7 Osteochondroma ... 311
- 13.5.8 Correction of Spine Deformity by Irradiation ... 312

13.6 Therapeutic Irradiation; Total Body ... 312

13.7 Nuclear Irradiation ... 312

13.8 Nuclear Imaging ... 313

13.9 Experimental Irradiation; Extremities ... 313
- 13.9.1 The Effect of Radiation Dose, Fractionation and Age ... 313
- 13.9.2 The Histologic Result ... 314
- 13.9.3 Oxygen Effect ... 314
- 13.9.4 Local Hormonal Effect ... 315
- 13.9.5 Abscopal Effect ... 315
- 13.9.6 Compensatory Overgrowth ... 315
- 13.9.7 Targeted Radiotherapy ... 315
- 13.9.8 Intra-Articular Radiotherapy ... 315
- 13.9.9 Radioprotectants ... 315

13.10 Experimental Irradiation; Head, Neck and Trunk ... 315

13.11 Conclusions ... 316

13.12 Author's Perspective ... 316

References ... 316

14 Light Waves ... 325

14.1 Phototherapy ... 325

14.2 Ultraviolet ... 325

14.3 Laser ... 325
- 14.3.1 Human Involvement ... 326
- 14.3.2 Animal Research ... 328

14.4 Author's Perspective ... 328

References ... 328

15 Sound Waves ... 329

References ... 330

16	**Shock Waves**		331
	16.1 Author's Perspective		332
	References		332
17	**Atmospheric Pressure**		333
	17.1 Decreased Atmospheric Pressure		333
	17.2 Increased Atmospheric Pressure		333
	17.3 Author's Perspective		333
	References		333
18	**Oxygen**		335
	References		335
19	**Developmental**		337
	19.1 Introduction		337
	19.2 Knee		337
	19.3 Ankle		338
		19.3.1 Congenital Pseudarthrosis of the Fibula	339
		19.3.2 Acquired Pseudarthrosis of the Fibula	343
		19.3.3 Multiple Hereditary Osteochondromatosis	343
		19.3.4 Neurologic Conditions	346
		19.3.5 Scleroderma	347
		19.3.6 Tibial Relative Overgrowth Compared to the Fibula	349
	19.4 Wrist		349
	References		353
20	**Surgical**		355
	20.1 Introduction		355
	20.2 Intentional Physeal Arrest – Humans		355
		20.2.1 Physeal Arrest to Curtail Slipping of an Epiphysis (1931)	355
		20.2.2 Immediate Irreversible Physeal Arrest (1933)	359
		20.2.3 Temporary Reversible Physeal Arrest (1945)	361
	20.3 Intentional Physeal Arrest – Animal Experiments		364
		20.3.1 Resection of the Periphery of the Physis	364
		20.3.2 Osteotomy Across the Physis	364
		20.3.3 Curettement	364
		20.3.4 Burring	364
		20.3.5 Intraphyseal Drilling	364
		20.3.6 Transphyseal Drilling	365
		20.3.7 Longitudinal Smooth Metallic Pins, Wires, and Nails	366
		20.3.8 Bone Grafts Across the Physis	366
		20.3.9 Staples	366

		20.3.10	Transphyseal Threaded Metallic Screws and Pins	366
		20.3.11	Crossed Smooth Metallic Pins	366
		20.3.12	Biodegradable Pins, Screws, and Filaments	366
		20.3.13	Tensioned Soft Tissue Grafts	366
	20.4	**Unintentional Physeal Arrest – Human Involvement**		367
		20.4.1	Smooth Nails, Rods, and Prosthetic Stems	367
		20.4.2	Smooth Wires and Pins	368
		20.4.3	Threaded Pins and Screws	379
		20.4.4	Cortical Bone Grafts	379
		20.4.5	Osteotomy Across the Physis	379
		20.4.6	Drilling Across the Physis	379
	20.5	**Unintentional Physeal Arrest – Animal Involvement**		387
	References			388
21	**Unknown**			399
	21.1	Introduction		399
	21.2	Knee		399
	21.3	Ankle		399
	21.4	Knee and Ankle		408
	21.5	Hand		408
	21.6	Wrist		410
	21.7	Hip		414
	21.8	Author's Perspective		414
	References			416
Epilogue				417
Index				419

Vascular Deficiency

1.1 Introduction

Normal physiologic bone growth occurs by cellular activity in the physis, which is highly vascularized by three separate sources: the epiphyseal, metaphyseal, and perichondral ring vessels (Fig. 1.1). The effect of excessive blood flow to growing limbs is well known. The overgrowth of extremities harboring hemangiomas or arteriovenous fistulae are classic examples of this phenomenon. The effect of the converse problem, vascular deficiency, occurs far more commonly.

Vascular changes that cause a reduction or loss of nutrients and oxygen to the physis are detrimental to growth. The blood may be deficient in either *quantity* or *quality*. For the purpose of this discussion, deficiency in quantity (ischemia, oligemia) includes the mechanical or anatomic interference of the blood supply by disruption or occlusion of vessels supplying the physis (Sect. 1.3). Deficiency in quality includes conditions that consist of diminution in the amount of hemoglobin, and those that result in the slowing of blood flow (Sect. 1.4). Nutritional deprivation of the physis, whether due to reduced quantity or quality, may diminish growth or result in death of germinal and proliferating physeal cells, causing growth arrest. The anatomic abnormalities resulting from these deficiencies are dependent upon the vagaries of the vascular anatomy to the physis (Sect. 1.2).

1.2 Vascular Anatomy of the Physis

The physis is a complex structure, discoidal in form and often referred to as a "plate," i.e., the epiphyseal growth plate. Based on tissue content alone, the physis may be divided anatomically into two different components: a cartilaginous component that is defined in terms of cellular layers; germinal, proliferative, columnar, hypertrophic, and provisional calcification, each with a designated function, and a fibrous component surrounding the periphery of the plate consisting of the ossification groove of Ranvier and perichondral ring of La Croix (Fig. 1.1). Various authors have divided the cartilaginous part into three, four, or five zones. The germinal zone is also called the resting zone, the reserve zone, or the zone of small size cartilage cells. The cells are widely separated, the intercellular substance is almost amorphous, and the collagen is poorly oriented [32]. Its functions include the generation and accumulation of stem cells, the storage of nutrients, and the production of matrix. The functions of the proliferative zone are twofold: cell proliferation and matrix production [2]. When the cells in these two zones are deprived of their blood supply, they fail to function or die, and growth is slowed or stopped. The function of the columnar and hypertrophic zones includes the expansion of the cells producing increased width of the physis; i.e. "longitudinal growth".

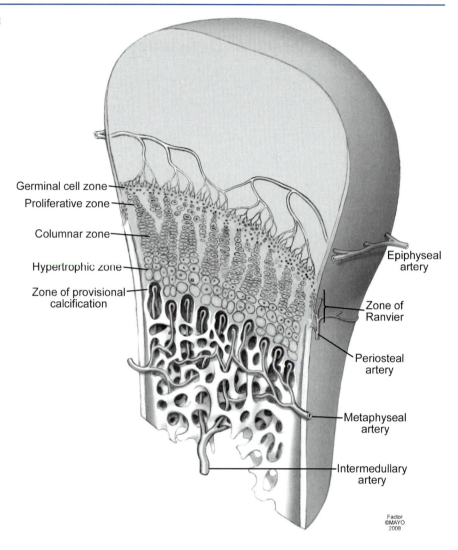

Fig. 1.1 Anatomy and blood supply of the primary physis prior to ossification of the epiphysis. The physis has been artificially expanded to detail its individual zones (From Peterson [21], with permission)

Most of the physis is avascular. All surfaces or borders of the physis, however, are amply supplied by four independent sources: epiphyseal arteries, metaphyseal arteries, the intramedullary artery, and periosteal arteries (Fig. 1.1). There are excellent anastomoses between the metaphyseal arteries and the intramedullary artery, but not between the epiphyseal arteries and the others. In late fetal and early postnatal periods the cartilaginous epiphysis contains numerous vessels, some of which cross the physis. These transphyseal vessels are derived from the epiphyseal circulation, appear venous in nature, and empty into the metaphyseal sinusoidal loops. Blood flow appears to be from epiphysis to metaphysis under normal physiologic conditions [19]. Most investigators have found no vessels passing from the metaphysis to the epiphysis (across the physis) in normal fully developed physes [2–4, 6, 8, 12, 13, 16, 23, 29–32], for example after the first 2 years of life. This generally accepted fact has recently been challenged [20, 33].

1.2.1 Epiphyseal Arteries

Usually several (2–4) arteries enter the cartilaginous epiphysis from the periphery and divide into increasing small branches in the form of an umbrella approaching the physis [23, 24] (Fig. 1.1). In early

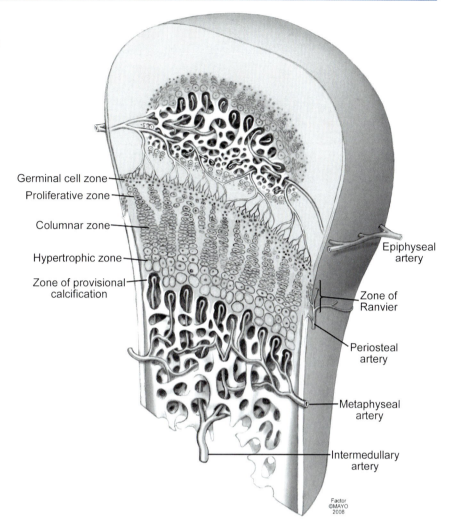

Fig. 1.2 Anatomy and blood supply of the epiphysis, and its secondary center of ossification and its physis (From Peterson [21], with permission)

development when the epiphysis is entirely cartilaginous, arteries branch into arterioles that end in small capillary loops called sinusoids between clusters of germinal cells. As the epiphysis develops it forms an osseous end-plate adjacent to the germinal cell layer. Canals in this end-plate allow capillaries to pass into the germinal zone to terminate in the matrix adjacent to the cell columns of the proliferative zone [3, 6, 13, 18, 22, 23, 31, 32]. Oxygen and nutrients pass from these capillaries through the highly hydrated cartilage by diffusion to the germinal and proliferative cells [22, 36]. No vessels pass beyond the proliferative zone [2, 31].

The secondary center of ossification (SCO) is preceded by the formation of hypertrophic chondrocytes and then by the ingrowth of vessels into the center of the epiphyseal cartilage [10] (Fig. 1.2). The pattern of vascular canals within the epiphysis changes with maturity. The most recent studies utilize MRI [1] and ultrasound [35]. In the unossified epiphysis, the vessels are mainly parallel in a longitudinal direction. After development of a SCO, the vessels converge radially toward the center [1, 29]. As the SCO forms and enlarges from its own global physis, it grows centrifugally, but more rapidly toward the physis than toward the articular surface. Concurrently, the primary germinal cell layer, formerly

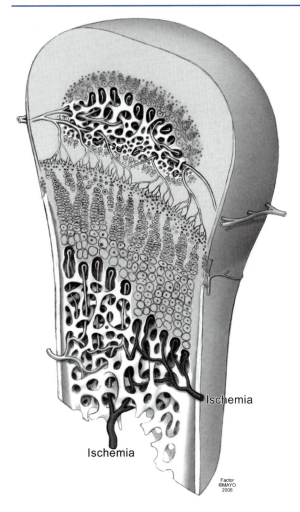

Fig. 1.3 Ischemia of the metaphysis impedes the enchondral ossification process, but not production and growth of the germinal cell, proliferative, and columnar layers of the physis. The growth plate widens and growth continues (From Peterson [21], with permission)

broad and relatively indistinguishable from epiphyseal cartilage, becomes narrower and clearly definable as an area several cells in thickness [22].

1.2.2 Metaphyseal and Intramedullary Arteries

On the metaphyseal side, the major intramedullary artery (also called the nutrient artery [5, 9, 11, 13, 16, 22, 23, 25, 30, 32, 33, 96]) divides to anastomose with metaphyseal arteries penetrating the metaphysis peripherally from the periosteum (Fig. 1.2). Together these form loops (also called juxtra-epiphyseal vessels [6, 13, 18, 27]), that penetrate into the large spaces vacated by the dying hypertrophic cells. The combined intramedullary and metaphyseal vessels nourish osteoprogenitor cells that produce bone on the cartilage matrix scaffold, called the primary spongiosa metaphyseal bone [7].

Occlusion of the intramedullary artery is not of vital importance to the physis, because the metaphyseal arteries readily supply the metaphysis [5]. Interruption of both of these vascular sources (Fig. 1.3), however, causes interference with enchondral ossification, which leads to thickening of the physis due to a combination of continuing production of cells in the germinal cell zone and enlargement of cells in the proliferative zone, without removal of hypertrophic cells [9, 14, 15, 17, 22, 23, 28, 30, 34, 42, 48, 50, 96]. As the normal uninvolved physis grows the devascularized area continues to accumulate hypertrophic cells. The widening may be a focal tongue, broad band, or mixed, and is more likely to occur when the metaphyseal insult is a single event, rather than sustained or repetitive [15]. When the vascular injury is limited to a relatively small area, widening of the physis is partial (Figs. 1.3 and 1.4a–f) [43].

After time, reconstitution of metaphyseal vascularity allows the widened portion of the physis to narrow to its original size and normal growth resumes (Fig. 1.4g, h). Any cartilage that remains in the metaphysis is gradually ossified [9, 42].

Occasionally, trauma associated with a roentgenographically minor fracture of the metaphyseal cortex, commonly found in battered infants, can result in loss of only the metaphyseal blood supply, sufficient to cause temporary widening of that part of the physis [43]. Thus, an incidental finding of physeal widening may represent a prior metaphyseal insult [15].

In summary, the influence of injury to the intramedullary and metaphyseal vessels on longitudinal physeal growth is usually temporary and negligible [11, 22, 31].

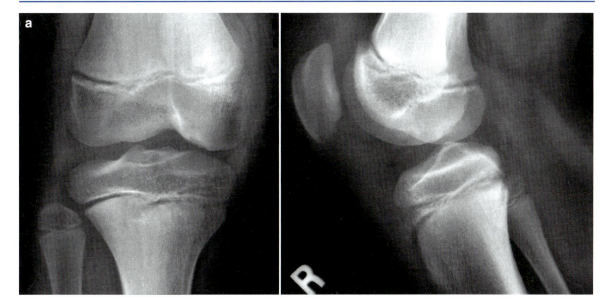

Fig. 1.4 Widening of the physis due to ischemia of the metaphyseal arteries of the proximal tibia. This 12 year 0 month old boy was kicked by another soccer player on the right knee just medial to the tibial tubercle and inferior to the joint line. There was immediate pain and he was carried from the field. (**a**) Roentgenographs were reported normal and a diagnosis of "sprain" of the knee was made. A knee immobilizer was applied and crutches given. Four days later an orthopedist noted swelling and tenderness well localized medial to the tibial tubercle. The diagnosis was "contusion, proximal right tibia". The immobilizer and crutches were continued. (**b**) Three weeks post injury, age 12 years 1 month, the pain was gone and the immobilizer and crutches had been discontinued. Examination of the knee was normal except for a smooth, raised soft tissue swelling medial to the tibial tubercle. Roentgenographs showed widening of the medial half of the right tibial physis (compare with Fig. 1.3). He was allowed to return to soccer. (**c**) Eleven weeks post injury, age 12 years 2 months, the patient noted limp and pain on the medial side of the proximal right tibia after running 5–10 min and while using a skateboard. Swelling and tenderness over the proximal medial tibia persisted. The physeal widening medially is increased. (**d**) Subperiosteal new bone is present distally on the diaphysis between (arrows) but not on the metaphysis. Activity curtailment was advised. (**e**) Twelve weeks after injury MR images confirmed widening of the medial physis. (**f**) Fourteen weeks post injury, age 12 years 3 months, the pain was less. Nontender fullness on the medial side of the proximal tibial diaphysis was receding. Discomfort in the area of the medial tibial physis occurred with valgus stress, but not with varus stress. Curtailed activities were reemphasized. (**g**) Six months post injury, age 12 years 8 months. The patient had remained relatively inactive and was asymptomatic. Knee examination was normal. The proximal tibial physis is returning to normal and the subperiosteal new bone has incorporated into the diaphysis (c ompare with **d**). (**h**) At age 14 years 6 months, 2 years 6 months post injury, the patient was normally active and asymptomatic. Roentgenographs were normal for his age. This case was previously published as a case of possible stress injury [21]. However, since the injury was acute rather than chronic and since only a portion of the physis was widened, it is a perfect example of acute ischemia of the medial metaphyseal arteries as illustrated in Fig. 1.3. Since growth proceeded normally there were no subsequent Harris growth arrest lines. This case was contributed by Dr. Thomas Schmidt, Prairie Village, Kansas (From Peterson [21], with permission)

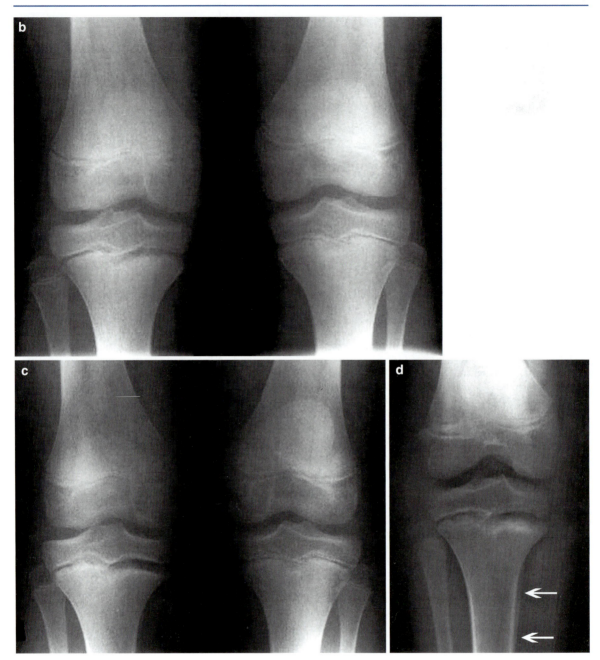

Fig. 1.4 (continued)

1.2 Vascular Anatomy of the Physis

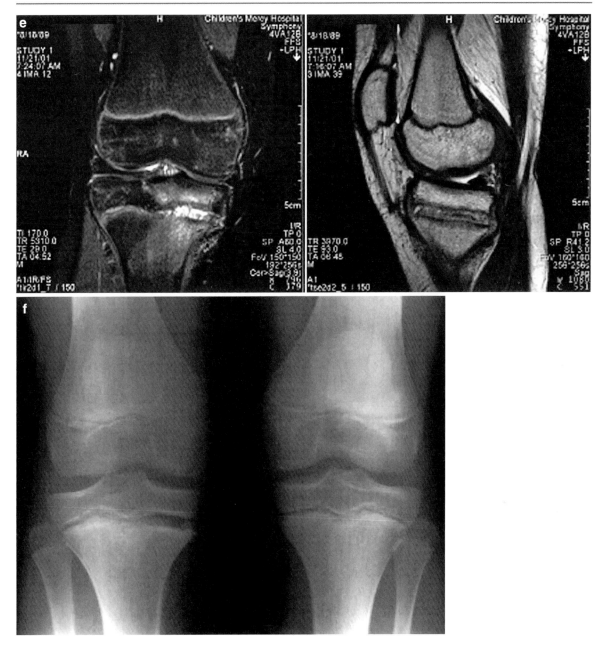

Fig. 1.4 (continued)

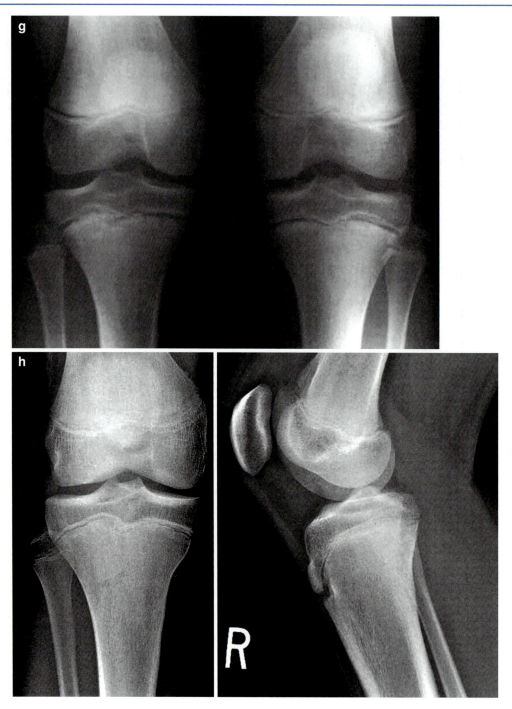

Fig. 1.4 (continued)

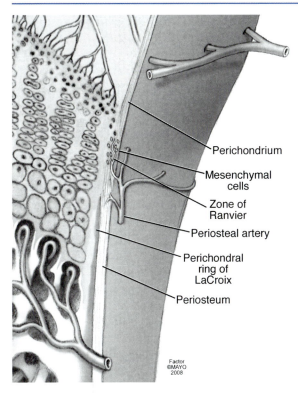

Fig. 1.5 Anatomy and blood supply of the periphery of the zone of Ranvier (From Peterson [21], with permission)

1.2.3 Periosteal Arteries

A fourth blood supply, consisting of a peripheral vascular ring, enters the surface of the outer edge of the physis circumferentially to supply the specialized zone of Ranvier and perichondrial ring of La Croix (Fig. 1.5) [13, 18]. Here, undifferentiated mesenchymal cells give rise to chondroblasts that are responsible for growth of the physis in width, termed latitudinal, peripheral, or circumferential growth [2–4, 16]. The use of the term periosteal arteries, as used here, would be more appropriately called perichondral arteries because they supply cartilage rather than bone [25, 48]. These arteries may anastomose with metaphyseal and epiphyseal vessels and participate in cupping (Sect. 1.5). In the proximal femur, there are anastomosis between metaphyseal and epiphyseal arteries on the cartilage surface, but no specific perichondral arteries [8].

1.2.4 Normal Physeal Growth

Normal longitudinal growth is a continuous process involving all layers of the physis, and occurs when cartilage is produced on the epiphyseal side at the same rate that appositional new bone is formed on the metaphyseal side [2, 3, 7, 22, 26]. Overall physeal thickness remains more or less constant throughout growth because of the exquisite balance between cartilage production and chondrocyte removal [3, 9]. The epiphyseal vessels have a nutritional role, bringing oxygen and nutrients to the germinal and proliferating layers, and therefore play the crucial role in cell production and longitudinal bone growth [1, 11, 13, 23, 27, 28, 31, 32, 48]. The function of the metaphyseal vessels is primarily enchondral ossification [28, 31].

1.2.5 Normal Physiologic Physeal Closure

The physis is a temporary structure that disappears and is replaced by bone. Physeal closure may be defined as beginning with the first mineralized bridge between the diaphysis and metaphysis, and ending with the complete disappearance of the physis and its replacement by bone and marrow [37]. Little is known concerning normal physeal closure other than anatomic observations. Longitudinal growth of the physis may be predetermined by genetics and through hormonal effects (Sect. 5.3). But if cessation of physeal activity is under hormonal control, why do various physes of the body close at different ages? [17] Could hormonal receptors be distributed differently in different physes?

At the end of skeletal growth proliferation of chondrocytes ceases. Initially, proliferating chondrocytes in the germinal and proliferating zones become "paralyzed" in terms of function, followed by orderly destruction [39], reducing their number. Chondrocytes in the columnar zone form into groups rather than columns. In the zone of hypertrophy the large vacuolated cells also decrease in number. The process of calcification encroaches from the metaphysis toward the germinal cell layer. The physis becomes progressively thinner, due to metaphyseal vascular invasion and osteogenesis. Capillary invasion from the metaphysis gradually perforates through the physis to reach the SCO. As physeal cartilage is removed, bone is laid down around the capillary tufts until bone unites the metaphysis to the epiphysis. The plate is now effectively closed, as all remains of the cartilage plate are slowly obliterated.

In large physes traces of this newly formed bone may remain as a calcified line (physeal scar) for life, visible on roentgenograms and on histologic investigation [36, 37].

In most physes normal closure begins centrally and progresses centrifugally to the periphery [9, 38, 40, 42, 48]. Growth is so slow around the time of closure that continued growth of the open physis at the periphery does not cause deformity. The arterioles in the center of the physis might be smaller, or the blood pressure lower, causing diminution of the blood supply to the center of the physis resulting in normal physeal closure. There are no reports or investigations to support these hypotheses.

1.2.6 Premature Physeal Closure

The process of premature or pathologic growth arrest, other than fracture or surgical insult, is similar to normal physiologic growth arrest, but the events which initiate it are different and in many instances not fully understood. Bone will continue to grow until maturity unless the physeal cartilage is injured, directly or indirectly. A prime example of indirect injury is interruption or disturbance of its vascular supply [11].

Physeal arrest from vascular deprivation is most frequently found in the distal femur, proximal and distal tibia, and proximal humerus. The reason for the increased incidence of arrest at these sites has not been identified. However, these physes are the largest and most rapidly growing in the body. Conceivably, the large area and fast growth may have longer or smaller arterioles in the center of the physis, resulting in less blood flowing more slowly. Finger and toe phalanges are also commonly affected in some conditions such as purpura fulminans. These are the farthest from the heart and have small arterioles and less blood pressure.

Premature physeal closure from vascular deprivation may be due to one of two causes: reduced quantity (Sect. 1.3) or reduced quality (Sect. 1.4).

1.3 Vascular Deficiency Due to Reduced Quantity

Even though the vascular supply to physeal cartilage is normally limited, chondrocytes of the germinal and proliferative zones are well adapted to low oxygen tensions and are not easily adversely affected. This explains their remarkable resilience [46, 47, 49]. However, inadequate circulation of oxygenated blood to these chondrocytes has a negative effect on their ability to grow. The critical level of oxygenated blood required by the human physis to maintain normal longitudinal growth is not known [57]. In rabbits [48, 49], total limb ischemia lasting up to 5 h caused no significant retardation of growth. Ischemia maintained for 6–7 h caused retardation of growth. Ischemia for 12 h resulted in complete growth arrest [48]. Ischemia of the epiphyseal vessels deprives the germinal and proliferative cells of nutrition; the cells become disorganized and then die (Fig. 1.6) [41, 42, 50]. The precise focus of ischemia appears to be a discrete area within and around the capillaries in the subepiphyseal bone plate cartilage canals [41, 44]. The metaphyseal vascular loops continue to invade the hypertrophic zone causing the physis to narrow. Longitudinal growth ceases in the areas affected, and if the ischemia is eccentric, angular deformity occurs. If the entire physis is affected, growth ceases completely.

Tissues other than the physis are also affected by a decrease in limb circulation. Accompanying decreased calf and thigh circumference and foot size are common [57].

Vascular deficiency due to reduced quantity occurs with arterial disruption, and with arterial occlusion which may be due to a variety of insults such as arterial ligation, compression, thrombosis, embolism, spasm, etc. The vascular deficiency associated with arterial occlusion may not seem as cataclysmic as total arterial disruption, but can be sufficient to cause slowing of growth or premature arrest. The degree and duration of the disruption or occlusion, the status of the collateral circulation, and the age of the patient at time of injury determine the m orbidity to the physis.

1.3 Vascular Deficiency Due to Reduced Quantity

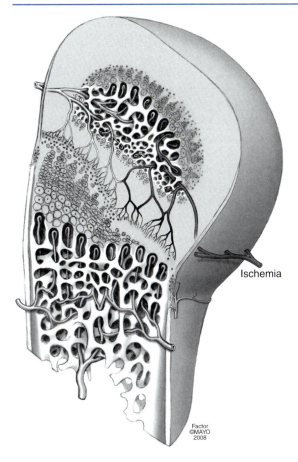

Fig. 1.6 Ischemia of the epiphyseal blood supply results in death of the germinal cells and proliferative cells, and loss of growth. The growth plate narrows. If the impairment is eccentric, angular deformity occurs (From Peterson [21], with permission)

Long term follow-up with periodic scanograms of children who have suffered arterial occlusion is essential in order to detect late limb length discrepancy. Chronic partial arterial occlusion sufficient to cause limb length discrepancy is sometimes amenable to surgical repair. Successful vascular reconstruction usually prevents the discrepancy from increasing, and on occasion may actually decrease the discrepancy due to growth in the injured limb exceeding growth in the uninjured limb [45].

1.3.1 Arterial Disruption

Arterial disruption is fairly common in children due to penetrating trauma (gunshot wounds, lacerations from knives, glass, fractures, etc.), motor vehicle accidents and surgical injuries. The arteries most commonly involved are the femoral, brachial, popliteal, radial, axillary, iliac, and tibial [52, 53]. Usually these injuries can be adequately treated and the patients are rarely followed long enough to determine the incidence of subsequent growth arrest. For example, in one series [52] of 118 children under age 15 years of age with a variety of vascular injuries, only one was found to have significant growth retardation of the injured extremity. The length of follow-up of this cohort was not specified. However, in a second study [53], limb shortening of 6–24 mm was confirmed roentgenologically in 7 of 14 patients followed an average of 36 months. Arterial reconstruction in three of these children (at 60, 60, and 66 months post injury), did not reverse their limb length disparity.

Femoral artery surgical transection with temporary vascular deficiency sufficient to cause physeal arrest has been documented [51]. When loss of femoral artery flow is acute, collateral circulation may be sufficient to save the extremity, but not all of the physes (Fig. 1.7).

Data are not available concerning which physis or physes distal to the arterial disruption will develop arrest. The size of the physis and the anatomic structure of the epiphyseal arterioles to each physis may be factors.

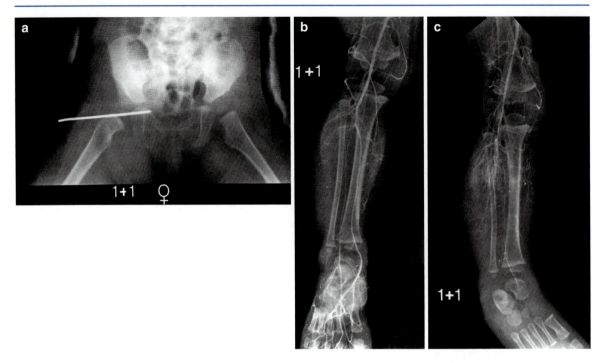

Fig. 1.7 Vascular deficiency due to femoral artery transection. An otherwise normal infant girl began walking at age 11 months, and at 12 months was noted to favor her right leg. A diagnosis of developmental dislocation of the right hip was made. At age 1 year 1 month open reduction was complicated by severance of the common femoral artery. End-to-end arterial anastomoses were performed three times by vascular surgeons, but arterial flow could not be maintained. The intima of the ends of the divided artery was noted to be damaged. After the severed ends were resected, a 3 cm segment of saphenous vein graft was inserted. The reestablished dorsal pedal pulse disappeared in 5 min. A Fogarty catheter was passed proximally and distally through the graft documenting good blood flow. After the catheter was removed and the vein was closed, the dorsal pedis pulse again disappeared. The foot was pink and had capillary refill, and vascular surgery was concluded for the day. (**a**) The reduced femoral head was fixed in the shallow acetabulum with a Steinmann pin and a 1½ spica cast was applied. (**b**) On postoperative day 1, the cast was removed, and arteriogram revealed patent distal femoral and popliteal arteries, occlusion of the anterior tibial artery in the mid-calf, and the peroneal artery in diffuse spasm. The posterior tibial artery was patent well into the foot. The thrombosed saphenous vein graft in the groin was excised, and thrombectomy of the common femoral vein was performed. There was concern that a thrombus might be present in the common peroneal tibial artery trunk. A Fogarty catheter was passed distally. No thrombus was found and flow was reestablished distally. Repeat arterial bypass graft was accomplished using an internal jugular vein. Ankle pulses were not present, but Doppler tones were. The patient was placed in the posterior half shell of the spica cast. On postoperative day 2, incomplete vascular flow to the lower leg was diagnosed as compartment syndrome. Fasciotomies were performed on the anterior and posterior compartments of the right calf. A new body cast was applied on the sixth post operative day. (**c**) On the 11th post operative day repeat arteriography showed spasm of the popliteal artery, a patent anterior tibial artery but with tiny caliber, and occlusion of the posterior tibial and peroneal arteries. Thrombectomy of the graft was repeated. A spica cast was applied on the 14th post operative day. Persistent significant reduction of arterial flow in the lower leg was noted as collateral circulation gradually developed. The Steinmann pin was removed from the hip during cast change 8 weeks postoperatively. At 16 weeks postoperatively, the final spica cast was removed, and a hip abduction orthosis was applied. During the next year, a varus deformity of the ankle gradually developed. (**d**) At age 2 years 6 months an AP roentgenogram of the ankle showed cupping at distal tibial physis and relative overgrowth of the fibula. An orthoroentgenogram showed the right leg to be 1.2 cm shorter than the left. (**e**) A tomogram confirmed premature central physeal closure (moderate cupping). At age 2 years 9 months, the normally growing distal right fibula was surgically shortened at the level of the distal metaphysis, and was internally fixed with a screw which arrested the physis. The Achilles tendon was lengthened. (**f**) At age 4 years 10 months, the right tibia was 3.6 cm shorter than the left tibia. The right hip remained reduced, but with mild coxa magna and incomplete development of the acetabulum. The patient was last seen at age 5 years 8 months. The right tibia was 4.4 cm shorter than the left. Anterior tibial and peroneal nerve function were returning, but she had no toe dorsiflexion. Without further treatment, anticipated tibial length discrepancy at maturity was estimated to be >10 cm. NOTE: This case documents premature partial closure of the distal tibial physis for no other reason than temporary vascular insufficiency. This resulted from ischemia of the epiphyseal arterioles in the center of the physis from any of a variety of causes: arterial occlusion, spasm, embolization, thrombosis, or just slow flow or low pressure. No other physis in this extremity developed similar cupping. Does this imply that the arrangement of vessels in the distal tibia were different or deficient? The diagnosis of compartment syndrome as described in (**b**) is compatible with the clinical findings, but does not further elucidate the exact cause of the eventual cupping (From Peterson [51], with permission)

1.3 Vascular Deficiency Due to Reduced Quantity

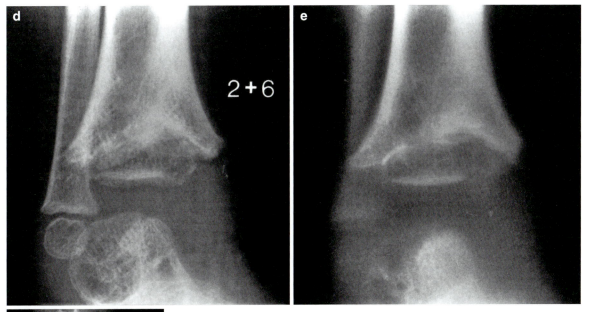

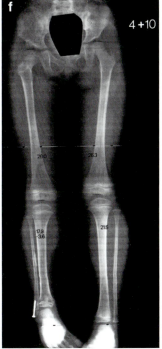

Fig. 1.7 (continued)

1.3.2 Arterial Ligation

Ligation of the subclavian artery, either following trauma or intentionally performed for a Blalock-Taussig anastomosis during cardiac bypass with extracorporal circulation, causes diminution in longitudinal growth of long bones of the arm and in muscle thickness, but not of periosteal appositional bone growth [54, 55]. The occurrence, type, and severity of the changes cannot be predicted in an individual case, probably due to differences in collateral circulation among the patients [54].

1.3.3 Arterial Catheterization

Cardiac angiography, frequently done in infants and children, is usually performed by catheterization through the femoral or brachial artery. Diminished blood flow due to vessel trauma from frequent catheter manipulation and change, is exacerbated by congestive heart failure, low cardiac output, dehydration, infection, polycythemia, hypoxia, and acidosis [52]. Post catheterization restoration of normal artery patency may be difficult to achieve in a small child. Some degree of thrombosis occurs after arterial repair, or restrictive perivascular fibrosis produces a narrowing effect on the lumen of the artery [57, 66]. Arterial thrombosis after catheterization of the femoral artery occurred in 28% of 56 young patients in one study [66]. One direct arteriovenous fistula following catheterization also resulted in associated limb shortening [66]. These data emphasize the need for meticulous arteriotomy repair.

The incidence of post catheterization growth arrest is variable and dependent on length of follow-up. Mild leg length discrepancy of 0.5–3 cm was present in 6 of 42 (14%) patients on one series [61]. In another study [57], of 28 children studied 1 year or more after femoral catheterization, 24 (86%) had a decrease of peripheral pulses and/or decrease of oscillometry associated with shortening of "over 0.3 cm", and ten had differences of more than 8 mm, occurring primarily in the tibiae. Significant inequality (>3 cm) in the length of the lower

Fig. 1.8 Marked physeal cupping secondary to vascular deficiency due to femoral artery cannulation. This male was born at 28 weeks gestation due to premature separation of the placenta. Shortly after birth a femoral venous or arterial line infiltrated causing vascular obstruction, swelling and discoloration of the leg, and subsequently skin loss and joint contractures of the lower leg and toes. The patient was hospitalized 4 months. At age 1 year 7 months the mother brought the child to our Plastic Surgery department because the right leg was larger than the left and had brawny edema with hyperpigmentation, a scar complex over the gastrocnemius muscle, atrophy of the gastrocnemius mass, and restricted foot dorsiflexion. (**a**) A scanogram showed moderate cupping of the proximal right tibial physis and enlarged irregular soft tissue outlines of the right lower extremity. The right tibia was 7 mm shorter than the left. Plastic Surgery recommended no treatment at that time and referred the patient to Pediatric Orthopedics. The mother was interested in only the plastic surgery opinion and did not keep the orthopedic appointment. (**b**) The mother returned with the child when he was 6 years 3 month old because she noted increasing leg length and foot size inequality, and inability to touch the right heel to the floor. The right tibia was now 3.5 cm shorter, and the femur 0.9 cm longer than the left. (**c**) The cupping was now marked. The articular irregularity was causing joint incongruity. Mild relative overgrowth of the proximal fibula is present. (**d**) A CT scan showed a small bar of long duration and cupping of both the physis and the articular surface. (**e**) Transverse CT scans confirmed an open physis and metaphysis surrounding the epiphysis proximally (**A, B**), and a relatively small bar at the tip of the cupping (**C**). (**f**) A reconstructed CT scan confirmed severe articular surface irregularity and circumferential cupping, was not just medial and lateral as visualized on (**d**). (**g**) At age 6 years 6 months the bar was excised and cranioplast inserted. The titanium break off wires were inserted 31 mm apart. (**h**) At age 8 years 0 months the metal markers are 46 mm apart, the right tibia 2.6 mm shorter and the right femur 0.5 cm longer than the left. Since the bar excision, the right tibia has grown more than the left, resulting in correction of the fibular relative overgrowth. The right femoral overgrowth is also less (compare with **b**). The tibial length difference continued to decrease (to 2.1 cm at age 8 years 6 months, following which it began to increase). Subsequently a recurrent bar formed and at age 9 years 3 months a second bar excision was performed. The previously inserted metal markers were left undisturbed. The knee joint incongruity has increased and is accompanied by mild loss of motion. (**i**) By age 11 years 2 months the patient was experiencing mild right knee pain with use. A scanogram showed the right tibia 4.3 cm shorter than the left. Serial scanograms since the first bar excision showed a gradual increase in the distance between the metal markers; from 31 mm (**g**) to 38, 46, 50, 51, 58, 63, 67, and 72 mm at present (*arrows*). This documents rapid growth after both bar excisions, followed by gradual slowing of growth thereafter. Note: This is a case of cupping progressing from moderate to marked after first discovery. The length of the right tibia will never catch up to the left and the patient will become a candidate for right tibial lengthening with or without left femoral and tibial physeal arrests, in the future. The proximal tibial articular surface incongruity will eventually require major surgery, and possibly improvement in length discrepancy could be made at that time

extremities is fortunately an uncommon complication of cardiac catheterization (Fig. 1.8) [64].

Careful assessment must be made of peripheral circulation post catheterization. Persistent absence of pulses more than 3 h following catheterization indicate thrombosis rather than arterial spasm [66]. In the lower extremity, early arteriography and operative intervention of post catheterization occlusion of vessels is recommended to prevent growth arrest [60]. In the upper extremity, operative intervention is rarely done since differences in bone and extremity length are less critical [60].

Data that help determine which physis or physes distal to the occlusion will develop arrest do not exist. Typically only large physes, such as the distal femoral and the proximal and distal tibial have been affected. This observation suggests that predisposition to arrest depends primarily upon the size or the anatomic structure of the arterioles of each physis.

Treatment of established occlusion by a bypass graft can result in decrease or correction in the leg length discrepancy [58, 63, 65]. Surgical repair of the occlusion should be considered only for those with a sufficient life expectancy [58].

Umbilical artery catheters have been noted to form arterial thrombi in 95% of infants. In some cases, thrombosis fragments have embolized into iliac and femoral vessels [59]. These thrombi, however, have little long-term effect on lower extremity growth. The activation of fibrinolytic systems and recruitment of collateral arterial channels combine to ensure extremity blood flow and physeal growth [59].

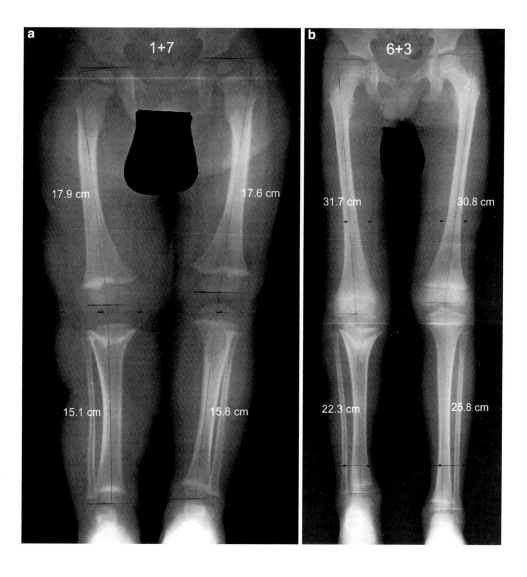

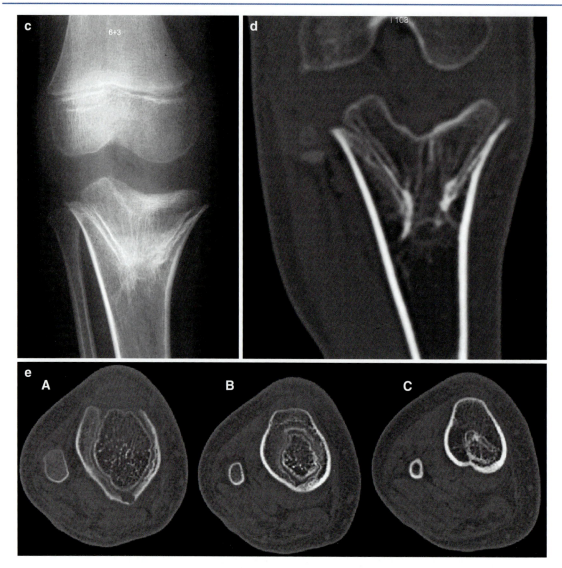

Fig. 1.8 (continued)

1.3 Vascular Deficiency Due to Reduced Quantity

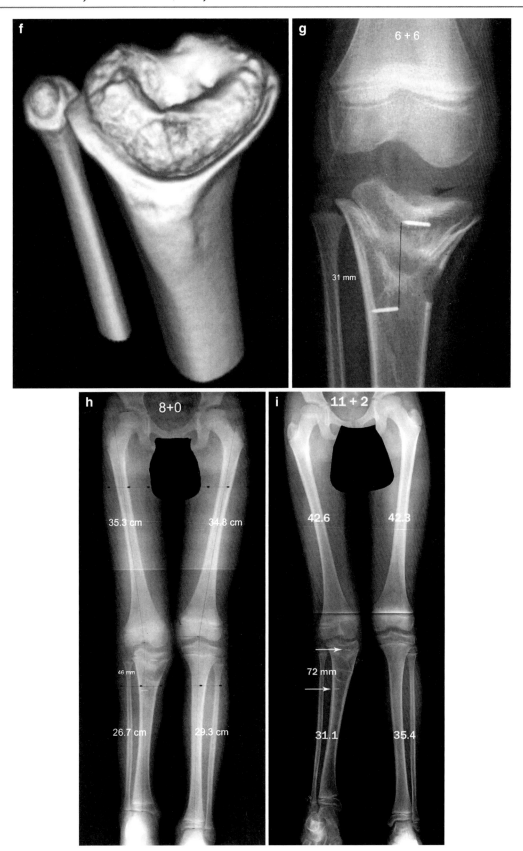

Fig. 1.8 (continued)

1.3.4 Arterial Injection

Simple arterial percutaneous needle injection, with subsequent intraluminal thrombosis or extraluminal occlusion, has also resulted in diminished limb growth [53, 62].

1.3.5 Fluid Extravasation in Soft Tissues

Faulty venous needle or catheter placement can result in fluid extravasation into soft tissue. Resulting compression of or damage to the peripheral periosteal or epiphyseal vessels may be sufficient to cause partial physeal arrest (Fig. 1.6). Continued growth of the uninvolved portion of the physis produces angular deformity. This phenomenon has been reported only at the ankle involving the distal tibial physis [67–69]. There is no standard treatment for the acute stage of this injury [69].

1.3.6 Interosseous Infusion

Interosseous infusion of fluids are sometimes used in critical care and emergency room settings when standard intravenous routes are not available. The tibial and distal femoral metaphyses are the most common sites for this procedure. Animal [70] and clinical [71] research indicates there is no adverse effect on growth when the trocar is properly placed in the metaphysis and when the concentration of drug, and the volume, rate, and pressure of the fluid infused are within reasonable guidelines.

However, improper needle placement or dislodgement has resulted in fluid extravasation into the soft tissue, resulting in compartment syndrome [72–74], which could theoretically adversely affect growth of the involved physis. None of the reported children who developed compartment syndrome secondary to interosseous infusion have been followed long enough to observe growth arrest.

1.3.7 Compartment Syndrome

Soft tissue swelling within confined fascial or skin compartments is usually due to trauma or infection. On occasion this soft tissue swelling can impair circulation sufficient to cause ischemia of the physis and Volkmann's contracture. Early fasciotomy will allow resumption of more normal blood flow in most cases. If cases are followed long enough, some may be accompanied by growth arrest distal to the compression (Figs. 1.7b and 1.14) [75–78].

1.3.8 Diaphyseal Fracture

Leg length discrepancy is one of the most common consequences of lower extremity diaphyseal fractures in children [83]. Blount may have been the first to voice concern for fracture-induced physeal arrest. In 1955 [80] he observed that "following a fracture in an older child, the overall development of the bone will be accelerated, so that the epiphyseal closure takes place a few months prematurely", resulting ultimately in a bone shorter than its contralateral counterpart. This statement, however, did not recognize the relationship of fracture to limb ischemia, in which premature physeal closure may be the result of decreased blood supply due to shunting of the vascular supply to the healing fracture [79, 93]. Later, however, Blount [81] (1960) reported a case of significant tibial shortening that occurred following treatment of a fractured femur in a spica cast. He attributed the growth arrest to "ischemic necrosis" of the tibial physes.

Occasionally, physeal arrest occurs following fracture of the diaphysis well away from the physis. The physes of the distal femur and proximal and distal tibia are particularly vulnerable, possibly because of their complex geometry [9]. When the femoral diaphysis is fractured, the physes in jeopardy of arrest are always distal to the fracture (Fig. 1.9). The arrest may occur in only one or in any combination of the three major distal physes (distal femur, proximal and distal tibia). The physis of the anterior tibial tubercle may be particularly prone to premature arrest [82, 88, 91, 95], even in the absence of documented trauma directly to the tubercle or a traction pin near the tubercle. Diminished blood flow or disuse, or peculiar vascular anatomy of the tubercle may be possible explanations.

When the tibial diaphysis is fractured, however, arrest may occur proximal to the tibial fracture, in the distal femur or in the proximal tibia, as well as in the distal tibia (Fig. 1.10) [86, 88, 89, 93]. Although

1.3 Vascular Deficiency Due to Reduced Quantity

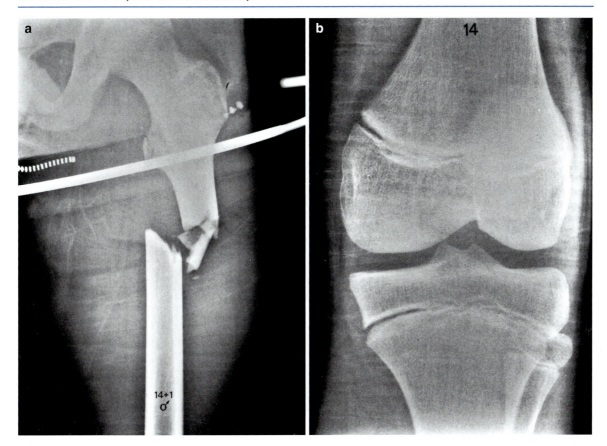

Fig. 1.9 Premature arrest of the proximal and distal tibia physes associated with a femoral diaphyseal fracture. This 14 year 1 month old boy injured his left femur when his motorcycle struck a car. (**a**) The fracture of the proximal left femoral shaft fracture is comminuted. (**b**) The physes of the knee are normal. (**c**) The physes of the ankle are normal. (**d**) A Steinmann pin was placed in the proximal left tibial metaphysis, well distal to the physis. Skeletal traction was continued 6 weeks followed by a spica cast for another 5½ weeks. Crutches with non-weight bearing to progressive weight bearing were used until 5½ months from time of fracture, at which time motion in all joints was normal. (**e**) One year from time of fracture, age 15 years 1 month, the growth arrest lines of both distal femora (*arrows*) showed equal growth from the time of fracture. On the right knee (*left*) all physes were open and accompanied with growth arrest lines. On the left knee (*right*) the proximal tibial physis was closed and there was no growth arrest line. The left fibula extended proximally more than the right (relative overgrowth). A scanogram showed the left femur 5 mm, and the left tibia 17 mm shorter than the right. (**f**) A lateral view at the same time as (**e**) showed closure of the proximal tibial physis. The skeletal pin tract (*arrow*) was well away from the physis, and the proximal tibial physeal closure is complete rather than just anterior as might be seen with an apophyseal closure due to a traction pin. (**g**) The left distal tibial physis (*right*) was also closed and had no growth arrest line. The right distal tibial physis (*left*) is open and has growth arrest lines. At age 15 years 7 months the limb length discrepancy had reached 2.9 cm, and surgical physeal arrest was performed on the right distal femur, proximal and distal tibia, and left proximal fibula. (**h**) At age 16 years 6 months, 2 years 5 months post injury, the patient was normally active and asymptomatic. All knee physes were closed. The femoral length discrepancy was unchanged at 5 mm. Since the distal left femoral physis growth post fracture was equal to the right, the femoral discrepancy had to be due to either length difference prior to the fracture, or shortening at the fracture site. The tibial length discrepancy had increased 2 mm (total 26 mm), probably due to the delay between the preoperative scanogram and the operative arrest. The growth arrest line (*arrows*) had not changed appreciably from (**e**). (**i**) The right ankle (*left*) showed the growth arrest line (*arrows*) and documents the growth between the time of fracture and surgical arrest which is greater than on (**g**). The 26 mm tibial length discrepancy is the sum of the growth of the right proximal and distal tibial physes prior to surgical arrest. The patient was given a ½" heel and sole wedge which was increased to 1 in. at age 21 years. He was followed in several departments of the clinic through age 28 years with no mention of skeletal complaint. Note: There is no way of knowing if the early physeal closures were due to initial vascular deficiency, to disuse (Chap. 2), or to both. This case is included here because the duration of disuse was modest and typical for this type of treatment. The only way to prevent the tibial length discrepancy would have been to surgically arrest the normal right tibial physes at the time of injury. Since the incidence of closure of physes distal to a fracture is unknown (and is undoubtedly extremely low), this is not indicated. The eventual surgical physeal arrests on the right leg prevented the discrepancy from increasing. Since all tibial physes were then closed, the ultimate discrepancy without surgical closure on the right cannot be determined. The value of presenting this case is to (*1*) document the possibility of physeal closure of both the proximal and distal tibial physis, but without that of the distal femur, and (*2*) to emphasize the need for close follow-up

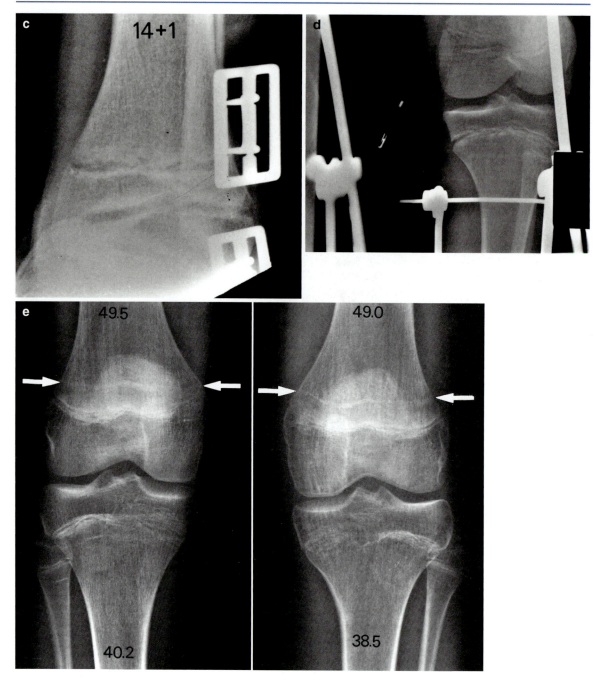

Fig. 1.9 (continued)

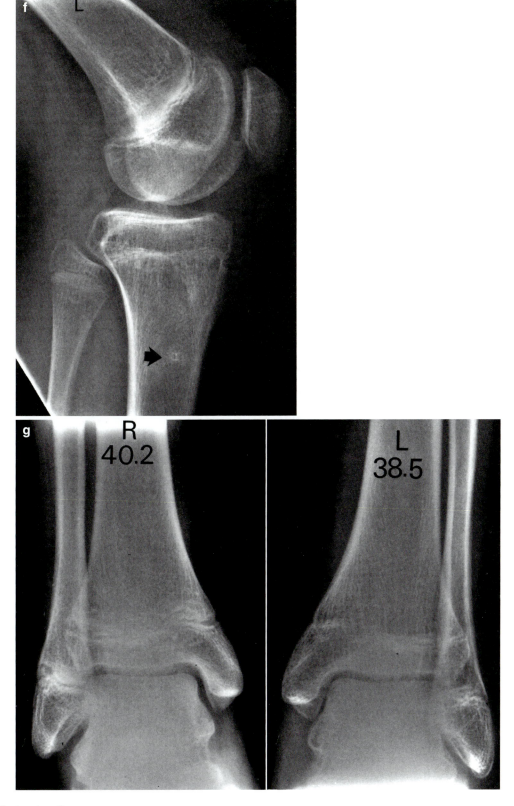

Fig. 1.9 (continued)

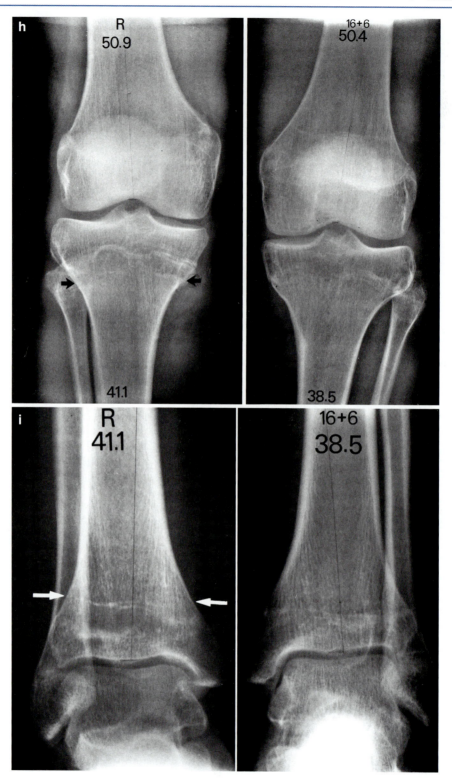

Fig. 1.9 (continued)

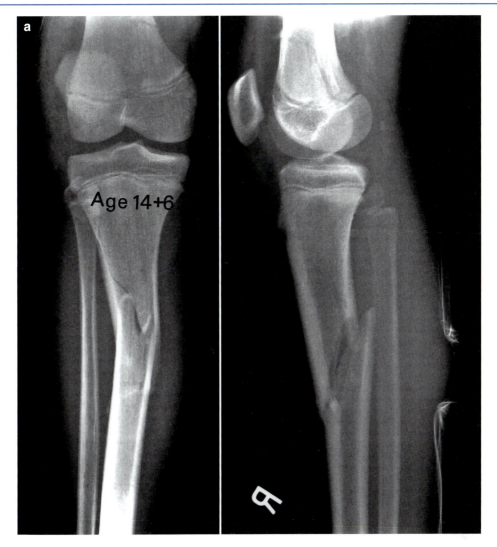

Fig. 1.10 Fracture of the tibial diaphysis with premature closure of the proximal and distal tibial physes. This male was 14 years 6 months old when he injured his right leg in a motorcycle accident. (**a**) Fractures of the right tibial diaphysis, the proximal fibular physis (Peterson type 3), and distal femoral physis (Peterson type 5) are present. The proximal tibial physis was roentgenographically normal. Treatment was by cast "until healed", duration unrecorded. (**b**) Two months post injury the fractures were healing well. Bone rarefaction was present on the metaphyseal side of both the distal femoral and proximal tibial physes (compare with **a**). A leg length discrepancy slowly developed over the next 2 years. (**c**) At age 16 years 10 months the right popliteal crease was lower than the left, causing pelvic tilt and mild lumbar scoliosis. The patient was wearing a ¾ in. lift on the shoe of the right heel. (**d**) Scanogram showed the right tibia 3 cm and the right femur 2.3 cm shorter than the left. All physes were closed. (**e**) The left femur was shortened 5 cm. The shoe lift was discontinued. The patient played high school football his junior and senior years. (**f**) At age 18 years 9 months he was normally active and asymptomatic. The relative height of the popliteal creases remained unchanged, lower on the right. The pelvis was level, and the scoliosis was much improved. A scanogram showed the right leg 2 mm longer than the left (the right femur was 3.2 cm longer and the right tibia 3.0 mm shorter than the left). (**g**) The femoral shortening was healed. All metal was removed. Note: This patient had three fractures, the most significant of which was the tibial diaphysis. The cause of the rarefaction of bone on the metaphyseal side of both the distal femur and proximal tibia metaphyses (**b**) is unknown, but most likely was vascular related and associated with the subsequent premature arrest. Since the eventual relative shortening of the tibia was greater than that of the femur, it can be concluded that both the proximal and distal tibial physes arrested early. The distal femoral premature arrest was possibly related to the undisplaced distal femoral physeal fracture (From Peterson [93], with permission)

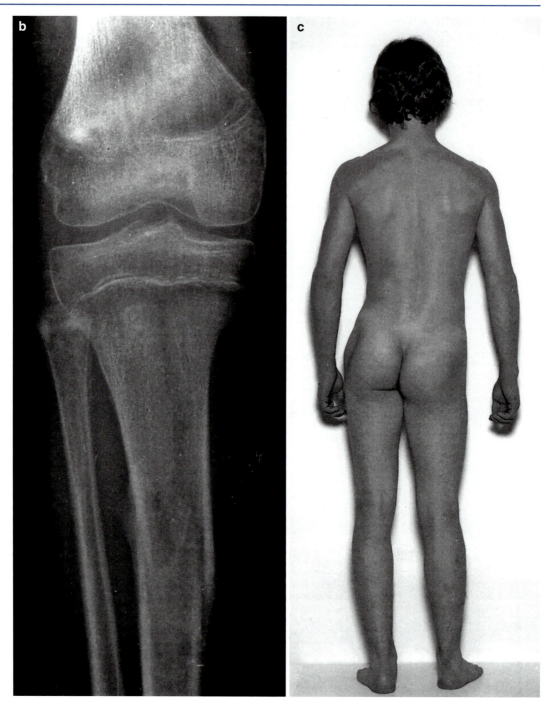

Fig. 1.10 (continued)

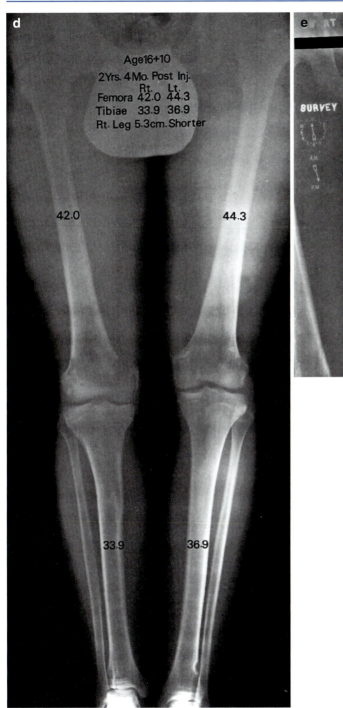

Fig. 1.10 (continued)

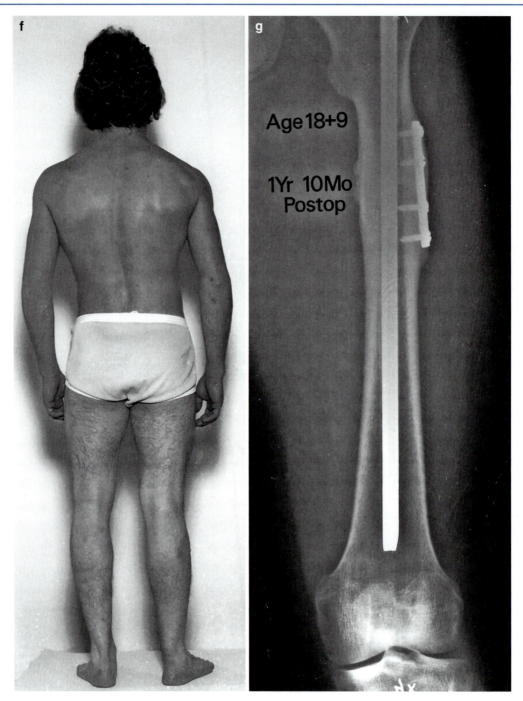

Fig. 1.10 (continued)

the arrest is usually total, it can be eccentric resulting in angular deformity, combined with loss of length [83, 88]. In a rare instance following tibial fracture with documented circulation compromise [85], a growth discrepancy of 2 cm 2 years after fracture with angular deformity of the distal tibia, was followed by gradual full correction of angular deformity and improvement in length discrepancy. Since no distal tibial physeal bar occurred, this slow down of growth followed by recovery was attributed to temporary vascular impairment with subsequent resumption of normal blood flow to the physis.

Physes exhibiting diaphyseal fracture-induced premature closure are usually large, i.e., the distal femur, proximal and distal tibia (Table 1.1). Except for the closure of two proximal fibulae [87, 94], and one distal ulna [92], premature closures of other small physis, such as the metatarsals, metacarpals, or phalanges, have not been recorded. This is contrary to the closure due to vascular deficiency due to decreased quality discussed in Sect. 1.4.

The incidence of physeal closure following diaphyseal fracture is very low. In one series [84, 89] of 354 tibial diaphyseal fractures in children between the ages of 12 and 15 years, 7 (2%) developed premature physeal closure. Recognition of the physeal arrest typically occurs 6 months [79] to 36 months [86] following fracture, with an average of 22 months in one series [86]. Physeal arrest appears to occur only in children 10 years or older (Table 1.1). Physeal cupping (Sect. 1.5) is rarely mentioned.

Concerning femoral neck fractures, it is well accepted that accurate reduction and early hip joint decompression, in an attempt to preserve vascularity to the femoral head, minimizes premature closure of the proximal femoral physis [90].

In summary, it appears that in some patients diaphyseal fracture hastens normal physeal closure, possibly precipitated through a process of fracture-induced vascular deprivation of the physis. All adolescents with diaphyseal fractures of lower extremity long bones should be monitored until they have stopped growing, because of risk of developing limb length discrepancy as a consequence of premature closure of one or more physes [89].

1.3.9 Periosteal Stripping

Stripping of the periosteum of the metaphysis near a physis, as may occur with fractures or surgery, disrupts the metaphyseal and sometimes the intramedullary blood supply. Enchondral ossification is interfered with, and coupled with continuing normal production of germinal cartilage cells, the physis widens (Figs. 1.3 and 1.4). Since the epiphyseal blood supply remains intact there is no reduction of longitudinal growth [96]. There may be an initial increase in blood flow to the epiphyseal vessels which produces a slight growth stimulating effect on the germinal cell layer. This is only temporary, following which normal longitudinal growth resumes (Fig. 1.4) [96].

1.3.10 Joint Dislocation

Isolated joint dislocation without fracture occurs occasionally in children. One patient developed ischemic necrosis leading to premature growth arrest and a shortened metacarpal [97]. The possibility of vascular damage must be considered in the immature patient, since the epiphyseal and physeal circulation may be compromised by either the dislocation or the surgical exposure for reduction [97].

1.3.11 Extremity Traction

Traction of an extremity produces a variable degree of spasm in both main and collateral arteries [99]. Excessive traction (force) in the treatment of fractures may initiate diffuse arterial spasm [88]. Prolonged traction (duration) can also be detrimental to the physis due to diminished orthostatic vascular pressure. Traction resulting in skin and soft tissue loss may cause circulatory impairment sufficient to produce closure of distal physes years later (Fig. 1.11) [98].

1.3.12 Fixation Bandages

Measurable vasoconstriction in the vessels of the hand occurs when the upper extremities of healthy human subjects are immobilized in a plaster cast [100]. Although no physeal arrests have been attributed to the short-term use of a cast alone, a cast could accentuate a coexisting vascular compromise or contain soft tissue swelling simulating a compartment syndrome. The cast, along with the position of the extremity, has been implicated as the cause of distal femoral physeal closure in cases of developmental dislocation of the hip and Perthes disease (see following sections). Growth arrest resulting from disuse due to the long-term use of a cast is documented in Chap. 2.

Table 1.1 Femoral and tibial diaphyseal fractures with subsequent physeal arrest

Year	Author[a]	Age at Fx (Year+Month)	Gender	Fracture Site[b]	Treatment[c]	Duration of Treatment	Length of Follow-up (Mo)	Site of Closure[d]	Amount of Limb Shortening (cm)
1964	Morton [88]	11	F	Tibia	Pins & Cast	3 months	33	Prox Tibia	2.5
		13	M	Femur, Tibia	Pins & Cast	2 months	21	Prox Tibia	3.75
1978	Hunter [87]	11	F	Femur	Tx	1 month	18	Dist Femur	5
					Cast	5½ months		Prox & Dist Tibia	
								Prox Fibula	
1978	Poznanski [94]		F	Femur			24	Dist Femur	
								Prox & Dist Tibia	
1981	Peterson [93]	14	M	Tibia	Cast	2 months	51	Dist Femur Prox & Dist Tibia	5.3
		12	M	Tibia	Cast		20	Prox Tibia	2.6
1984	Pappas [91]		M	Femur	Tx		24	Prox Tibia	0.7
					Cast				
1989	Hresko [86]	12+0	F	Femur	Femoral Tx	3 weeks	24	Prox Tib	
						–[e]			
		11+9	F	Femur	Femoral Tx	4 weeks	19	Prox Tib	
					Cast	–[e]			
		10+10	F	Femur	Tibial Tx	2 weeks	24	Prox Tib	
					Cast	–[e]			
		10+0	M	Femur	Cast	–[e]	12	Dist Femur	
		12+6	M	Tibia	Cast	–[e]	16	Dist Femur	
		11+0	F	Tibia	Cast	–[e]	24	Prox Tib	
		11+0	M	Femur	Cast	–[e]	36	Prox Tib	
1990	Beals [79]	14	M	Femur	Femoral Tx	6 weeks	72	Dist Femur	4.5
					Cast	–		Prox Tibia	
		11+10	F	Femur	Hip Spica Cast Brace	5 weeks	22	Prox Tibia	6.0
						–			
		11+3	M	Femur[f] Tibia[f]	Tibial Tx (Prox & Dist)	–	21	Distal Femur	8.8
						–		Prox & Dist Tibia	
2000	Navascúes [89]	12	M	Tibia	Cast	–	30	Dist Femur	0.8
		15	M	Tibia	Pins & Cast	–	23	Prox & Dist Tibia	1.4
		15	M	Tibia	Cast	–	25	Dist Femur	2.8
		15	M	Tibia	Tx & Cast	–	42	Dist Femur	2.8
		13	M	Tibia	Ex Fix	–	35	Dist Femur	2.0
								Prox & Dist Tibia	1.0
		15	M	Tibia	Cast	–	15	Dist Femur	0.4
								Prox & Dist Tibia	1.0
		15	M	Tibia	Cast	–	18	Dist Femur	1.3
								Prox & Dist Tibia	1.1

Note: Since all the patients were 11 years old or older, and the follow-up incomplete in some, the amount of limb relative shortening is mostly mild to modest. Since the duration of treatment is relatively short in most cases, the premature physeal arrest is more likely due to vascular insufficiency at the time of fracture than to disuse (Chap. 2)

[a]Most articles have more than one author. See references
[b]Tibia fractures were always accompanied by fibula fracture
[c]Pins & Cast=pins to secure the bone fragments in the cast. *Tx* skeletal pin traction, *Ex Fix* External Fixation
[d]The physis or physes which develop arrest were always on the ipsilateral limb
[e]All cases in this series wore a cast "6 weeks to 3 months"
[f]This case had compound fractures of the mid femur and tibia

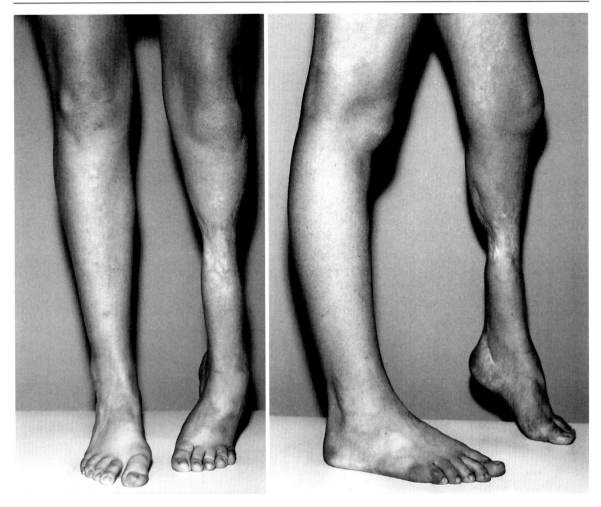

Fig 1.11 A left femoral shaft fracture at age 3½ years in this girl was treated by Bryant's skin traction for 1½ weeks when it was changed to distal femoral skeletal traction (Kirschner wire) because of "muscle spasms and darkness of the lateral side of the foot". Total traction time was 6 weeks. At 15 years 3 months there is relative tibial shortening and a smaller foot secondary to vascular deficiency. A scanogram at the time of the photograph showed 3.7 cm relative shortening of the left tibia and equal lengths of the femora

1.3.13 Developmental Dislocation of the Hip

Growth disturbance of the proximal femur in developmental dislocation of the hip (DDH) may be multifactorial, but is commonly felt to be caused by ischemia secondary to treatment [101, 103, 108]. The proximal femoral physis is particularly vulnerable because the epiphyseal artery is intraarticular [9]. Ischemia of the physis can occur with or without involvement of the epiphysis [103]. A high hip dislocation, and surgery after the age of 24 months, are associated with a higher rate of growth disturbances of the femoral head [104].

Impairment of blood flow through the epiphysial arteries may occur from increased intraarticular joint fluid pressure. Examples of causative influences include transient synovitis of the hip, and hip positioning during casting. Injection experiments on cadavers have shown that in the "frog" position, the profunda femoris and medial and lateral circumflex arteries fail to fill

[105]. Fixation of an extremity in plaster casts "causes considerable vasoconstriction." [100] Hind leg immobilization of 2½ month old rats retarded longitudinal growth by 2 weeks [102]. Growth resumed, but did not catch up. The combination of the frog position and cast immobilization may therefore produce marked diminution of blood flow to the lower extremities. Traction of the femur may produce arterial spasm [99], which could also be a factor in some cases of DDH.

There is a strong correlation between the initial degree of vascular insufficiency and subsequent radiographic changes such as a crescent-shaped epiphysis, medial bowing of the femoral neck (a shorter and more concave curve between the lesser trochanter and femoral head [the lateral portion of Shenton's line]) and premature physeal closure [103]. Premature closure of the primary physis results in relative overgrowth of the greater trochanter, a short femoral neck, and relative shortening of the femur (Fig. 1.12). If the femoral head is also deformed, incongruity between the femoral head and acetabulum leads to early osteoarthritis of the hip joint [103].

The incidence of proximal femoral premature physeal closure in DDH depends on several factors, most notably the method of treatment and the length of follow-up. In one study of 1,500 cases [101] followed 5 years, only 35 (3%) developed "vascular disorders". These children were treated by abduction pillows, abduction splints, plaster casts, and skin traction followed by casts for an unspecified period. In this study the incidence of vascular impairment was the same for both genders, and there was no relationship between the age at the start of treatment (before or after age 6 months) and vascular impairment. In another study [106] of 68 patients followed "until after maturity", 33 (49%) developed partial or complete proximal femoral closure. These children wore a full spica cast with the hips in abduction for a minimum of 3 months, followed by another spica cast or leg abduction casts "until the development of the hips was felt to be satisfactory". In each child the physeal arrest could be observed within 6 months after the end of the initial cast treatment. It is difficult to determine whether the growth arrest in these children was due to initial acute vascular deficiency or to prolonged disuse (Sect. 2.4).

Treatment of the residual deformities will depend on the nature and degree of the proximal femoral and hip joint changes, but includes physeal arrest or distal transfer of the greater trochanter, physeal arrest of the contralateral normal femur, and osteotomies of the proximal femur or pelvis, in various combinations [103,

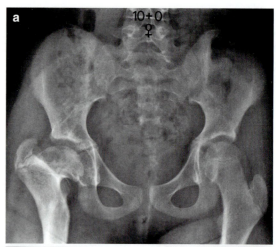

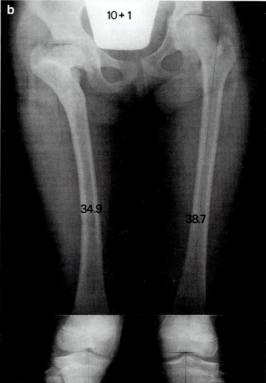

Fig. 1.12 Dislocation of the right hip was found in this girl at 2 months of age. Treatment was traction followed by a hip spica cast. Subsequent avascular necrosis of the femoral head healed well, but coxa vara was treated by valgus rotation osteotomy. (**a**) At age 10 years 0 months there was femoral neck shortening, relative overgrowth of the greater trochanter, and a healed proximal femoral osteotomy. The femoral head size and shape is fairly normal indicating that permanent arrest occurred in the primary physis (the growth plate) and not the secondary physis (the epiphysis) (Fig. 1.13). (**b**) A scanogram showed the right femur 3.8 cm shorter and the right tibia 0.4 mm longer than the left for a total discrepancy of 3.4 cm. Subsequent surgery included a right proximal femoral derotation osteotomy at age 10 years 1 month and physeal arrest of the left distal femur at age 11 years 4 months

107]. If these methods are employed early, the leg length discrepancy should not progress to an amount that would require shortening of the contralateral normal femur. Femoral lengthening of the involved femur may place additional pressure on an already abnormal hip and should be avoided.

The cause and the result of vascular insufficiency of the proximal femoral physis in DDH is similar to, if not identical with, that of Perthes' disease [103].

1.3.14 Perthes Disease

Juvenile idiopathic necrosis of the femoral head (Perthes disease) usually occurs in children between 3 and 10 years of age, and results from temporary loss of vascularity to the secondary center of ossification. Depending on the severity and duration of the avascularity, the physis of both the secondary center of ossification (the secondary physis) and the primary physis may resume growth or cease growth (Fig. 1.13). Permanent cessation of growth of the primary physis results in a short femoral neck, relative overgrowth of the greater trochanter and relative femoral shortening (similar to DDH as shown in Fig. 1.12).

Premature arrest of the primary physis occurred in 23% (100 of 930 hips) in one series [111], 25% (20 of 80) hips in another [117], and 64% (16 of 25 hips) in another [115]. Closure of the primary physis may be complete, central, or peripheral and the area varies considerably [111, 115].

The precise cause of avascular necrosis of both the epiphysis and the physis is unknown. It is more likely a result of reduced arterial blood flow than a result of venous congestion [113]. Keret et al. [117] noted that the epiphyseal arterioles and venules supplying the physis are "progressively vulnerable", and advanced the hypothesis that the primary problem of diminished growth in coxa plana originates on the epiphyseal side. Ponseti et al. [121] studied the physeal cartilage histologically. They were not able to determine if the abnormalities were primary or secondary to the ischemia.

Many possible causes for the vascular deficiency in Perthes disease have been proposed. Impairment of the blood supply from the lateral epiphyseal arteries may occur from intraarticular joint fluid pressure, for example following transient synovitis of the hip, or by other mechanical means. The lateral ascending cervical branch of the lateral circumflex femoral artery (also called the lateral epiphyseal artery) can be compressed as it passes through the joint capsule in the narrow space between the femoral neck and greater trochanter [8, 109]. This impairment may be exacerbated by acetabular retroversion [114], or hyperabduction therapy [9], such as the application of a spica or Petrie cast. Other proposed theories include: (a) disturbance of large arteries especially the obturator, possibly due to heredity, [119] (b) abnormal pressure on the physis, (c) the ischemia of prolonged treatment [110, 111], (as described in Sect. 2.6), and (d) failure of revascularization and repair of the deformed avascular epiphysis [116]. Recent advances in ultrasound [112], MRI [115, 118], and scintigraphy [120] may help clarify this issue in the future.

Perthes disease usually occurs in mid-childhood and since the proximal femur accounts for the least amount of growth of the four lower extremity major physes, leg length discrepancy is usually mild. Management of the leg length discrepancy consists of a shoe lift, or properly timed epiphyseodesis of the contralateral distal femur if necessary.

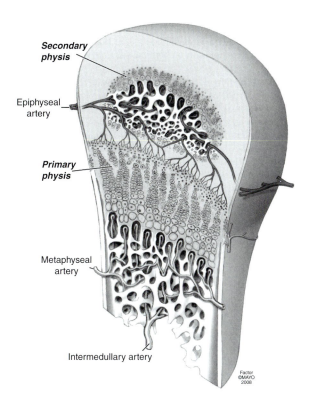

Fig. 1.13 Epiphyseal arteries supply both the secondary physis of the secondary ossification center, and primary physis of the primary ossification center. Ischemia resulting in arrest may occur in either the primary or secondary physis or both

1.3.15 Transplantation of the Physis

Autotransplantation (the transfer of tissue from one part to another in the same body) of the head of the proximal fibula in immature rabbits resulted in consistent extensive necrosis of the center of the physis (cupping, Sect. 1.5) [122]. This is mostly likely due to vascular deficiency of the epiphysis, even with vascular anastomoses of the graft.

1.4 Vascular Deficiency Due to Reduced Quality

Necrosis of the germinal and proliferative zones may also occur in conditions associated with increased blood viscosity, producing decreased blood flow, capillary stasis, thrombosis, and tissue anoxia. Sludging of blood deprives the physis of its nutrition, resulting in growth arrest. When this anemia is confined to the central portion of the physis, cupping occurs (Sect. 1.5). Arrest due to reduced quality is found in many conditions and can be found in multiple random physes in more than one extremity in the same patient (Fig. 1.14), as well as in small physes of the hands and feet. This differs from vascular deficiency due to reduced quantity (Sect. 1.3) that typically affects only the large physes of the involved extremity.

Most information concerning disorders of reduced blood flow quality has been obtained from observation of patients with the conditions described below. Animal studies support this pathogenetic theory. Rats exposed to 2-butoxyethanol produced hemolytic anemia and disseminated vascular thrombosis which resulted in

Fig. 1.14 A 2 year old boy had meningococcemia complicated by ischemia and compartment syndrome of the lower extremities. Fasciotomies and debridement of necrotic tissue resulted in complete loss of the anterior and lateral compartments of both lower legs. Extensive split thickness skin grafting was followed by heel cord lengthenings and soft tissue flaps to cover both patellae. Three toes on the left foot were amputated. At the time of active infection no bone abnormalities were noted. The diagnosis of purpura fulminans was not mentioned in referral data. (**a**) Age 7 years 0 months; skin scarring, soft tissue atrophy of the legs, and right ankle varus. (**b**) Scanogram shows abnormal distal tibial physes and right ankle valgus. The right leg is 2 mm longer than the left. All hip and knee physes are normal. (**c**) Standing AP of ankles shows bilateral moderate cupping, eccentric on the right causing varus deformity. (**d**) Bilateral distal tibial MRI (rendering technique [21]). Right tibial bar (on *Top*) measures 19%, left tibial bar (on *Bottom*) measures 23%. (**e**) Bilateral bar excisions were performed at age 7 years 0 months. The bars were exposed from the periphery, excised and filled with cranioplast. The break off titanium markers are 9 mm apart on the right, and 12 mm on the left. At the conclusion of surgery it was estimated that the remaining amount of physeal tissue was 60% bilaterally. Three months later a latissimus dorsi musculocutaneous free tissue flap graft was applied to the lateral side of the right leg to improve chances for success of a future corrective osteotomy. (**f**) Eight months post bar excision, 6 months post soft tissue graft (age 7 years 10 months) the right ankle varus was more noticeable. (**g**) At age 7 years 10 months an opening wedge osteotomy of the distal right tibia using iliac crest bone was accompanied by repeat bilateral heel cord lengthenings. The physis is open. (**h**) At age 8 years 6 months the distance between the metal markers was 25 mm on the right, 21 mm on the left. Varus tilt of the talus was 15° on the right, 11° on the left. (**i**) A recurrent bar on the left was excised and filled with cranioplast. (**j**) At age 10 year 0 months both distal tibial physes were open and the metal markers in both tibiae were 34 mm apart. There is mild varus of the right proximal tibia and its physis is now indistinct (compare with the left proximal tibia and with **b**). (**k**) Lateral view of the right knee (*left*) confirms a third physeal bar in the anterior proximal tibia with mild genu recurvatum. Left knee (*right*) for comparison. (**l**) An anterior bar is confirmed on MRI. (**m**) An MRI projection technique [21] confirms a small anterolateral bar. (**n**) Computer analysis documented the bar to be 4% of the physis. (**o**) The bar was excised and the cavity filled with cranioplast. The titanium vascular clip markers are 19 mm apart on both the AP (*left*) & lateral routine roentgenographs (*right*). (**p**) Scanogram 1 year later, age 11 years 0 months. The proximal tibial physis appears normal, the titanium markers are 28 mm apart, and the varus is improved. (**q**) On a lateral roentgenogram the anterior tilt of the tibial joint surface has improved from 18° (Fig. 1.14o) to a normal 3°. The metal markers are 31 mm apart. The 3 mm length variance between the AP scanogram (**p**) and this routine lateral view is due to a shorter focal distance and divergence of x-rays on the routine lateral view. (**r**) At age 11 years 11 months the patient was normally active. The markers in the distal tibiae were 45 mm apart on the right and 42 mm on the left. Recurrent physeal bars of the proximal right and distal left tibiae were excised at age 13 years 0 months. Surgical arrest of the distal left femoral physis was performed at age 15 years 6 months. (**s**) At age 18 years 0 months he was an active high school junior delivering papers by bicycle and working up to 10 h a day in a warehouse on Saturdays. There is mild clinical genu varum with normal gait. The recumbent scanogram shows a 2.1 cm leg length discrepancy which had not changed in the previous 2 years. The physis of the right proximal tibia had grown 37 mm, the right distal tibia 50 mm, and the left distal tibia 38 mm since initial bar excisions (**e** and **o**). His care was transferred to an adult orthopedist who elected to further observe the genu varum. Note: This patient developed three physeal bars first noted 5–9 years following acute and serious systemic meningococcemia resulting in three bar excisions and three reexcisions, all of which added measurable and worthwhile length. At the time of the multiple bar excisions no sign of active or latent osseous infection was found clinically or roentgenographically (From Peterson [142], with permission and further follow-up)

1.4 Vascular Deficiency Due to Reduced Quality

growth plate infarction and partial or complete physeal growth arrest [124]. Interestingly, venous stasis produced by ligation of various veins in dogs, did not alter growth [123].

1.4.1 Sickle Cell Anemia

Sickle cell anemia is a familial, chronic, haemolytic anemia observed in carriers of hemoglobin S. Under conditions of hypoxia the red blood cells of these patients change from round bi-concave discs to elongated crescentic ellipses, called sickle cells [128, 129]. Sickling of the red cells results in increased blood viscosity, leading to reduced tissue blood flow, erythrocyte entrapment in small vessels, stasis, vessel blockade, thromboembolic infarcts, and local tissue necrosis [131]. Thrombi comprising sickled cells form in many tissues, including bone, and as it relates to this discussion, in terminal epiphyseal arterioles.

Large physes, such as in the femur, tibia and vertebrae, are often affected. Vertebrae are particularly prone to central physeal arrest due to this vascular sludging. The resulting biconcave deformity resembles that found in certain lower vertebrates with larger notochordal remnants, thus the term "fish vertebra deformity" [125, 126, 129, 132]. This vertebral deformity seen in sickle-cell disease in children is caused by central physeal ischemia, rather than a similar deformity seen in osteoporotic adults with compression of bone.

In younger children with sickle-cell anemia, finger phalanges [128] and metacarpals [14] are also frequently involved. Younger children with sickle cell anemia also have a high susceptibility to salmonella osteomyelitis [126], but physeal infarcts resulting in cupping (Sect. 1.5) occur in sickle cell anemia even without an accompanying osteomyelitis [127].

Bone marrow and skeletal scintigrams have been found helpful in finding the location and distribution

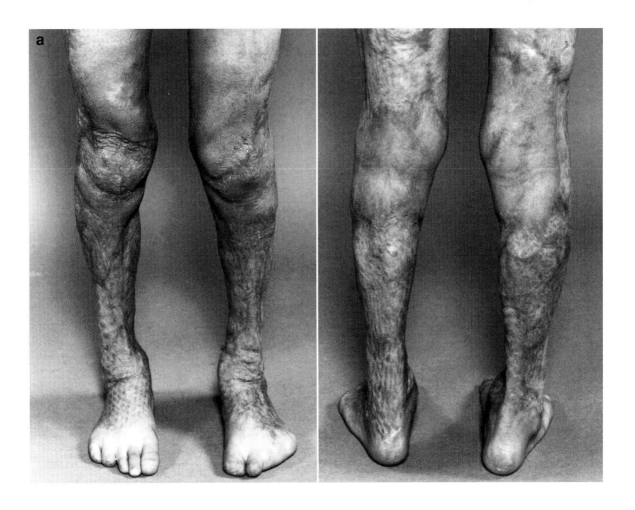

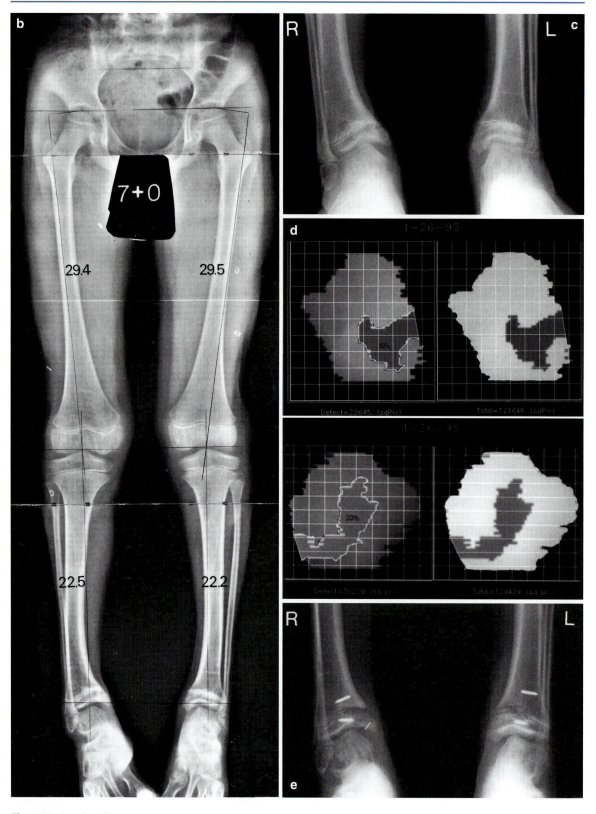

Fig. 1.14 (continued)

1.4 Vascular Deficiency Due to Reduced Quality

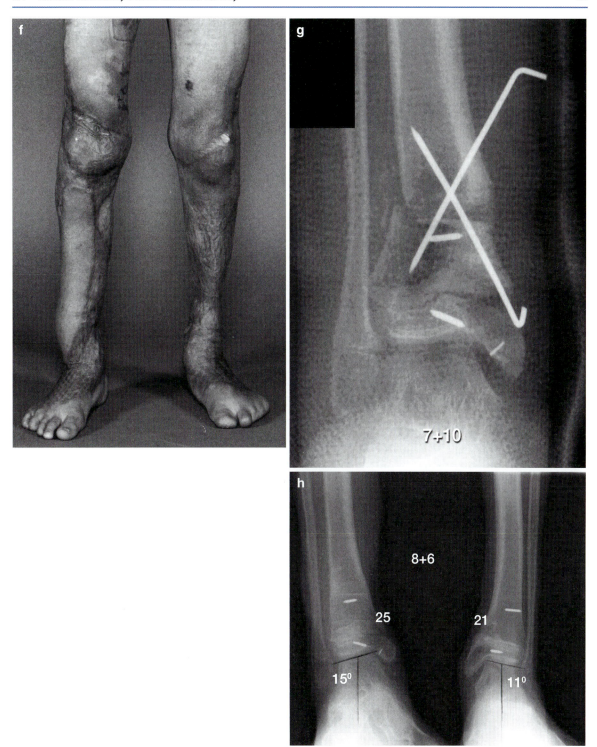

Fig. 1.14 (continued)

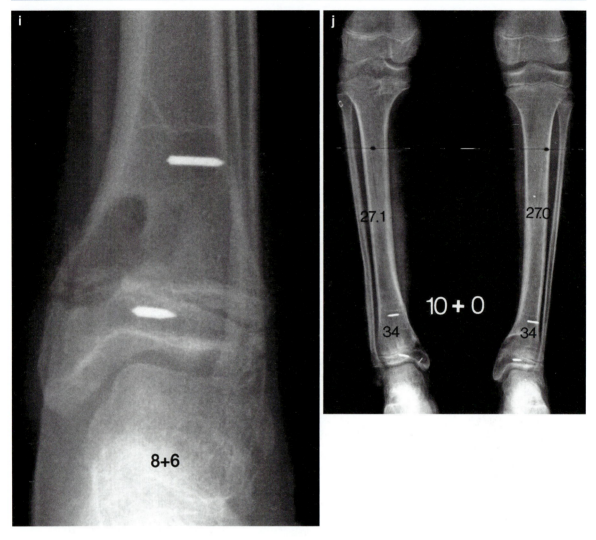

Fig. 1.14 (continued)

1.4 Vascular Deficiency Due to Reduced Quality

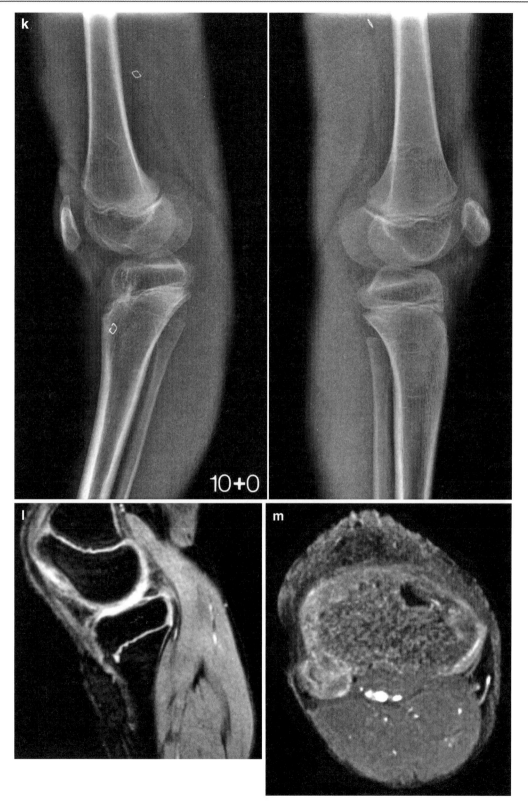

Fig. 1.14 (continued)

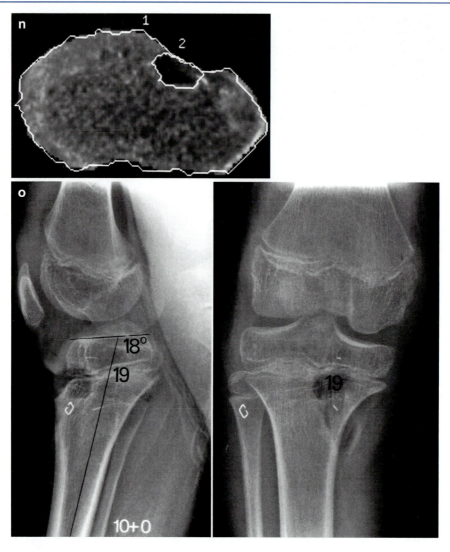

Fig. 1.14 (continued)

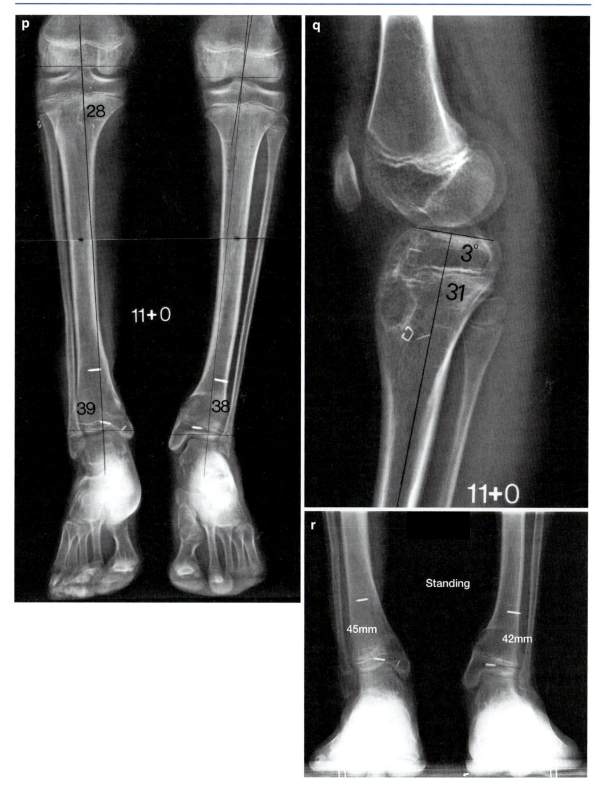

Fig. 1.14 (continued)

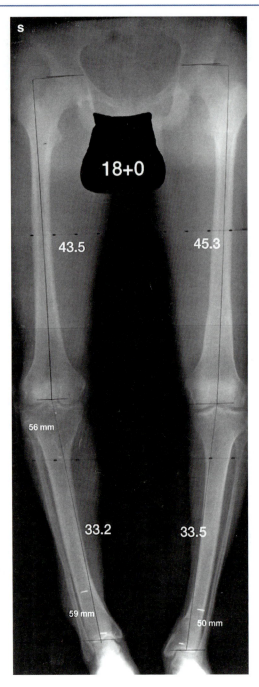

Fig. 1.14 (continued)

of bone infarcts in sickle cell disease [130], but have not been used to identify early or late physeal arrest. Sickle cell anemia has no known cure. Close follow-up with early detection of physeal arrest may allow earlier treatment, mitigating eventual bone deformities [129].

1.4.2 Thalassemia Major (Cooley's Anemia)

Premature arrest of isolated physes has been reported in patients with thalassemia [133], a familial hypochromic anemia occurring mostly in children of Mediterranean parents. Eleven of 79 (14%) patients had physeal arrest; 12 proximal humeri in 9 patients, 5 distal femora in 3 patients. Humeral and femoral involvement in the same patient occurred once. All arrests were noted only in the second decade of life; never in the first decade. The initial area of fusion involved only a segment of the physis, never complete fusion. All cases progressed to complete early arrest resulting in relative shortening of the involved bone. The cause of the arrests was not identified, but genetic abnormality is not likely since no affected siblings were reported among the eleven affected patients. Vascular coagulopathy is a possible cause.

1.4.3 Meningococcemia

The gram-negative diplococcus *Neisseria meningitidis* inhabits the superior respiratory tract in humans and can spread hematogenously. The toxin produced by these bacteria causes hypotension and acute vascular injury. Meningococcal septicemia is a life threatening illness associated with disseminated intravascular coagulation (DIC) resulting in diffuse vasculitis, hemorrhage, and thrombosis in any organ system, including the skeleton. Children who survive are often left with long-term sequelae including physeal arrest resulting in bone length inequality and angular deformity. This vascular deficiency involving the physeal circulation may take several years to adversely affect bone growth and become manifest (Fig. 1.14) [134–141, 143–145].

Although disseminated meningococcemia is a generalized inflammatory process, most authors believe that the subsequent physeal arrest is due to small vessel thrombi associated with DIC, rather than to direct infection or septic embolization [136, 138,

141, 146, 147]. Speculation that the arrests are the result of septic embolization leading to septic arthritis or osteomyelitis [141], has not been verified. Since no abscess forms, this entity is reported here rather than in the chapter on infection. In all reported cases no microbiological or histologic evidence of active or latent infection has been found at the site of physeal damage, either at the time of original illness or at the time of discovery or treatment of physeal abnormality [136, 141, 146]. The fact that over half of the subsequent physeal arrests occur under areas of cutaneous scarring [135], introduces a second possible explanation supporting a prolonged vascular deficiency as the cause of arrest. The cutaneous scarring itself is also most likely due to vascular deficiency.

In each patient one or several physes may be involved (Fig. 1.14). The response of the physis is dependent on the current rate of growth, but can be identified as early as 3–4 months after the acute episode [134, 136, 139]. The precise location of physeal plate destruction can be peripheral (with angular deformity), central (with cupping, Sect. 1.5), or complete (with relative shortening) [134, 135, 140, 144]. One study [134] of 11 patients found 7 peripheral bars, 3 central bars, and 3 complete closures. Premature closure sites occur apparently at random. Large physes such as the proximal and distal femur [134–138, 141, 143, 149], proximal and distal tibia [134–138, 140, 143, 147, 149], proximal humerus [135, 138, 143], are more commonly involved than smaller physes such as the distal fibula [134, 135, 144] the distal ulna [135], the distal radius, [135] and the finger phalanges [141]. In most cases with tibial involvement the fibula continues to grow normally. The axial skeleton is usually spared [134, 136, 139].

Recent improvements in treating Neisseria sepsis have resulted in decreased mortality rates, and corresponding higher rates of adverse sequelae [134]. Patients with significant skin lesions requiring debridement, and patients who have amputations, are at high risk of subsequent growth arrests and should be followed appropriately [135]. Treatment of physeal arrest by bar excision has been suggested [139, 148], and recorded [138, 141], but no long term results have been given. Reestablished growth by bar excision is present in three physes in Fig. 1.14.

Cardiogenic shock associated with extensive necrotic purpura (purple patches on the skin and mucous membranes due to subcutaneous extravasation of blood), is classically described as purpura fulminans, and is sometimes associated with meningococcal septicemia. In one recent series [147] of 46 cases of meningococcemia, 26 had purpura fulminans, and 15 of them died, representing a mortality of 33% for those with meningococcemia and of 58% for those with purpura fulminans.

1.4.4 Purpura Fulminans

Purpura fulminans (PF), a rapidly spreading hemorrhage in skin, is a disseminated intravascular coagulopathy (DIC) resulting in occlusion of end arteries by platelets and fibrin thrombi. Purpura fulminans typically occurs 1–4 weeks following benign infectious disease, such as streptococcal and H influenza infections, or viral syndromes such as varicella (chicken pox), rubella (measles), scarlatina (scarlet fever), and viral gastroenteritis. By contrast, when PF occurs as a sequella of meningococcemia, it occurs early, usually on the day of onset of infection [136, 149, 152].

The etiology of PF is thought to be an antigen-antibody reaction, mediated through the generalized Schwartzman reaction [136]. This requires an initial or sensitizing exposure to an antigen, usually endotoxin, followed by a second eliciting exposure of the same antigen approximately 24 h later. The antigen-antibody reaction triggers the formation of intravascular coagulation and prevents the reticulo-endothelial system from clearing the activated coagulation products from the circulation. The severity of the reaction depends on the amount of endotoxin in the eliciting and further exposures. In addition to the vaso-occlusion secondary to DIC, there may be an inflammatory response to the meningococcus itself [138]. The resulting coagulation products within capillaries produce hemorrhage and thrombosis. Skin and muscle necrosis is often accompanied by damage to kidney, adrenal glands, lungs, brain and gastrointestinal tract. This can result in dry gangrene of extremities, as well as organ failure. Initially joints may be unaffected

[148], a marked difference from septic arthritis. Auto or surgical amputation of fingers, toes, and more proximal extremity parts is common. The mortality rate of 50% is secondary to renal damage [136] or multiple organ failure [155]. Those who survive are often subjected to auto- or surgical amputation of the distal ends of limbs [150].

In recent years progress in medical treatment has resulted in decreased mortality, and a corresponding increase in orthopedic complications [147, 154]. Roentgenographic physeal abnormalities are first noted approximately 1 year after the onset of the disorder [152]. Physeal arrest often occurs in physes proximal to the soft tissue limb damage, or involves physes where no soft tissue damage exists [151]. The most distal physis proximal to the amputation is the one most likely to show physeal arrest [149, 152, 153]. Ischemic damage to physes is in the central portion, which is not supplied by collateral vessels [148, 154]. The resulting bar is cup-shaped (Sect. 1.5). The abnormalities created by the damaged physis may be sufficiently severe to consider surgical amputation [154].

Purpura fulminans may represent a hyperaggressive form of meningococcemia. Most authors do not provide criteria or definitions that separate or join these two conditions. They are presented here as separate entities because, (1) one can occur without the other, (2) they are often described separately in the literature, (3) there may be a difference in the time of onset, and (4) a variety of bacteria and viruses may cause PF, but only meningococci cause meningococcemia.

1.4.5 Other Conditions

Other conditions in which diminished blood flow may cause reduced growth are prolonged regional body immobilization and limb disuse (Chap. 2), osteomyelitis and septic arthritis (Chap. 3), tumors (Chap. 4) metabolic diseases such as scurvy, rickets, and collagen vascular disorders (Chap. 5). Physeal arrest following freezing (Chap. 7) and burns (Chap. 8), and irradiation (Chap. 13) could also be explained on the basis of arteriolar damage or intravascular thrombosis.

1.5 Physeal Cupping

The normal physis is more or less a flat disk. Normal growth cessation (see Sect. 1.2) first occurs typically in the central portion of the physis [9, 38, 40, 42, 48]. Growth is so slow at this time that no deformity of the physis occurs. Prior to the onset of normal physeal closure abnormal vascular deficiency may also cause growth to cease centrally (Fig. 1.15). As growth continues peripherally, a curved, actually dome-shaped, deformity of the physis (Fig. 1.16) may occur. This has been called metaphyseal cupping, peaking, tenting, or a cone-shaped or ball-in-socket epiphysis [9, 14, 17, 126, 141, 147, 156–160]. Cupping is the hallmark of temporary or partial central vascular deprivation due to either reduced quantity or quality, and occurs with many types of insults to the physis.

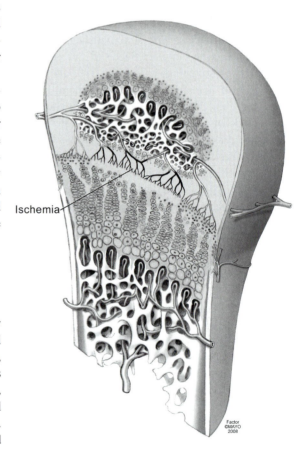

Fig. 1.15 Ischemia of the center of the physis results in death of the central germinal cells

1.5 Physeal Cupping

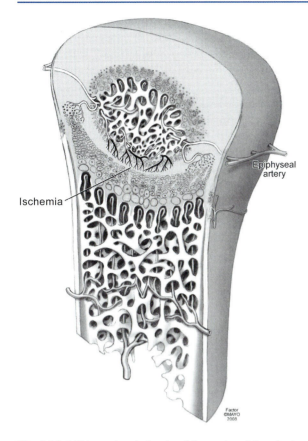

Fig. 1.16 Mild cupping: ischemia of the center of the physis with continued growth peripherally

The converse of cupping, loss of peripheral physeal growth circumferentially with growth persisting centrally (producing an inverted cup), has never been described or illustrated.

The etiology and pathogenesis of cupping is due to the unique anatomical vascular distribution to the physis. The tenuous vascular supply to the central portion of the growth plate makes it particularly vulnerable (Fig. 1.15) [9, 48, 122, 141]. The periphery of the physis has the richest blood supply, being nourished directly by periosteal vessels with collaterals from epiphyseal and metaphyseal arteries [48]. Trueta and Morgan [32], while discussing the epiphyseal vascular pattern, state "the vascular pattern is similar throughout the periphery of the epiphysis." Does this imply a difference in blood supply between the periphery and the center of the physis?

Cupping has been depicted in line drawings as occurring in varieties [14, 127], but has never been classified. Basically, the area, severity, and duration of central ischemia will determine the degree of cupping. Therefore, the following classification of cupping is offered (Fig. 1.17). *Mild cupping* is a curved physis with no identifiable bar (Fig. 13.2c). The articular surface is normal. It has the possibility to correct spontaneously if the insult is mild and promptly reversed [122], but is likely to progress to "moderate." *Moderate*

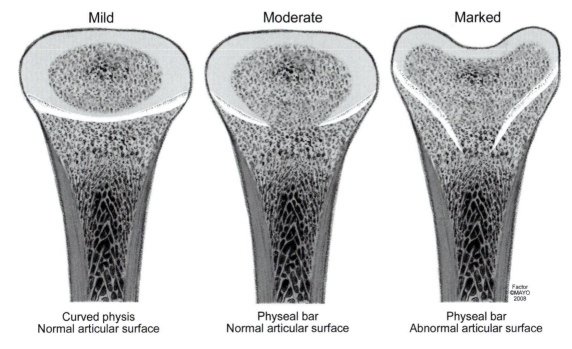

Fig. 1.17 Classification of cupping

cupping is a curved physis with a central bar and with a normal articular surface (Fig. 1.18). The secondary center of ossification may be less well developed than its contralateral counterpart (Fig. 1.8a). This cup has no possibility to resolve spontaneously and will progress to either prompt complete physeal arrest without articular deformity or to marked cupping. *Marked cupping* has a central bar with significant physeal deformity, and epiphyseal articular deformity (Figs. 1.17 and 1.8).

Cupping is invariably accompanied by relative bone shortening. Retardation of bone growth corresponds with the degree and duration of cupping. Eccentric cupping can result in angular deformity (Fig. 1.14c) [159]. Marked cupping predisposes to loss of joint motion (Fig. 1.6h) [158].

Cone-shaped epiphyses commonly occur in finger and toe phalanges, and appear roentgenographically similar to mild cupping (Fig. 1.19a). They are found in up to 13% of normal children with female predominance (2.3–1). Cone-shaped epiphyses are typically regarded as normal variants of growth, but animal experiments suggest the cause is a circulatory disturbance of the physis [157]. Cone-shaped epiphyses are asymptomatic and usually mature normally (Fig. 1.19b).

Although cupping that occurs with vascular deficiency due to reduced quantity is always distal to the vascular disruption, any distal physis may be affected. For example, femoral artery obstruction may result in cupping of the distal femur, proximal tibia (Fig. 1.8), or distal tibia (Fig. 1.7), or in all three [160], but not

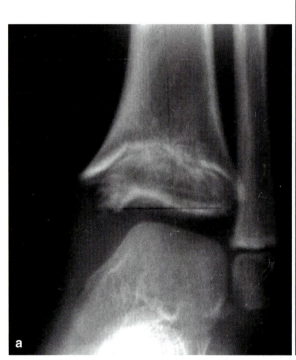

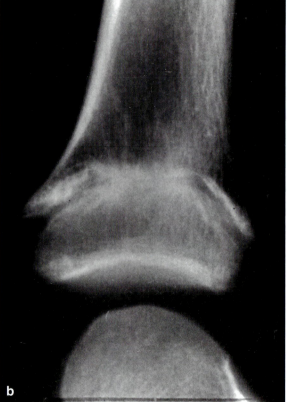

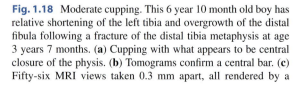

Fig. 1.18 Moderate cupping. This 6 year 10 month old boy has relative shortening of the left tibia and overgrowth of the distal fibula following a fracture of the distal tibia metaphysis at age 3 years 7 months. (**a**) Cupping with what appears to be central closure of the physis. (**b**) Tomograms confirm a central bar. (**c**) Fifty-six MRI views taken 0.3 mm apart, all rendered by a technician. (**d**). Rendered cut 50 (posterior aspect of ankle) shows a curved physis with normal articular surface consistent with mild cupping. (**e**) Rendered cut 60 (center portion of ankle) shows a bar with normal articular surface consistent with moderate cupping (From Peterson [21], with permission)

1.5 Physeal Cupping

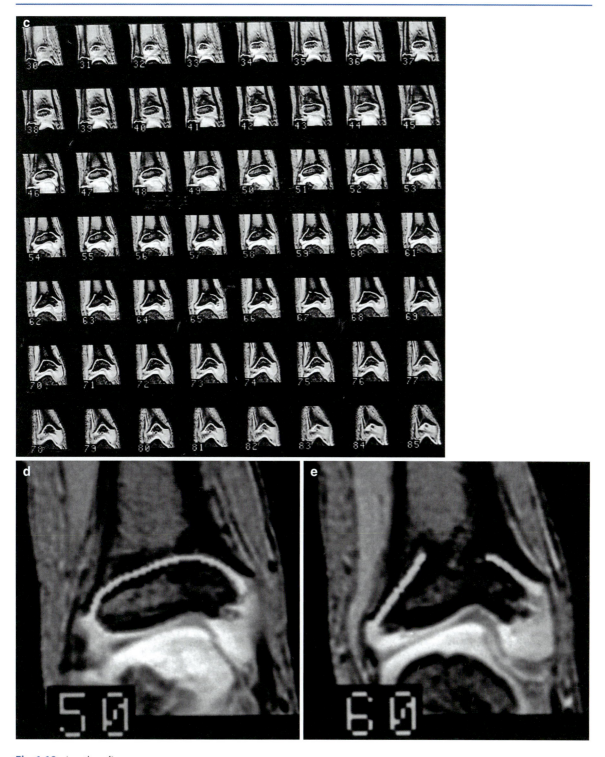

Fig. 1.18 (continued)

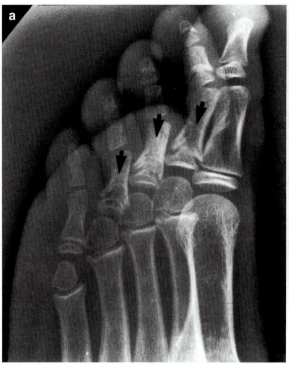
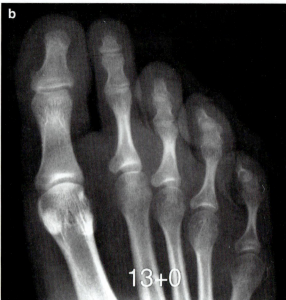

Fig. 1.19 Cone-shaped phalanges in a 6 year 2 month old female. (**a**) Oblique view of the right forefoot shows cone-shaped proximal phalangeal physes of the middle three toes (*arrows*). Compare with the physes of the great and fifth toes. (**b**) At age 13 years 0 months all physes are closed and all phalanges are normal (From Peterson [21], with permission)

in the fibula or foot metatarsals or phalanges. This can only be explained on an anatomic basis, such as the large size of these physes or a structural difference of the vascular anatomy of the affected physis as compared with an unaffected physis. The prime suspected causes would be smaller or fewer epiphyseal vessels in the area adjacent to the center of the involved larger physes.

Cupping has been noted to occur following femoral artery transection (Fig. 1.7) [51], femoral artery cannulation (Fig. 1.8), [56, 62] and transplantation of the head of the fibula [122], as well as in may conditions when vascular deficiency is due to reduced quality of blood flow (Sect. 1.4). In addition to the vascular causes described in this chapter, cupping occurs with a variety of metabolic conditions such as Rickets, copper deficiency, diphosphonate therapy, hypervitaminosis A, and scurvy, as well as in poliomyelitis, tuberculosis of the hip, osteomyelitis, frostbite, and irradiation, described elsewhere in this book, and in some congenital syndromes not described in this book.

1.6 Author's Perspective

It seems inappropriate to call the intramedullary artery the "nutrient" artery when it is well accepted that the function of the intramedullary artery is ossification of the existing scaffold, whereas the epiphyseal vessels supply nutrition to the germinal and proliferating zones.

Knowledge of normal physeal vascularity is essential to understand vascular processes that result in abnormal physeal growth. The severity of skeletal abnormalities appear long after acute vascular episodes, do not necessarily correlate with the severity of the initial clinical insult. Although the late skeletal changes in all of these conditions are presently not preventable, closer orthopedic follow-up could minimize the late sequelae, particularly early treatment of physeal bars. Occult bars found on bone scans or MRI performed on children recovering from vascular insults should be investigated and followed roentgenographically. The success rate for excision of bars due to vascular insults is unknown, but positive results are possible (Figs. 1.8g–h and 1.14e–s). The musculoskeletal growth and development of these children requires long-term orthopedic management.

References

Vascular Anatomy of the Physis

1. Barnewolt CE, Shapiro F, Jaramillo D (1997) Normal gadolinium enhanced MR images of the developing appendular skeleton: part 1. Cartilaginous epiphysis and physis. AJR Am J Roentgenol 169(1):183–189
2. Brighton CT (1974) Clinical problems in epiphyseal plate growth and development. AAOS Instruct Course Lect Chapter 7, pp 105–122
3. Brighton CL (1978) Structure and function of the growth plate. Clin Orthop 136:22–32
4. Brighton CT (1984) The growth plate. Orthop Clin North Am 15:571–595
5. Brookes M (1957) Femoral growth after occlusion of the principal nutrient canal in day old rabbits. J Bone Joint Surg Br 39B:563–571
6. Brookes M, Landon DH (1964) The juxta-epiphyseal vessels in the long bones of fetal rats. J Bone Joint Surg Br 46B:336–345
7. Cameron DA (1961) Erosion of the epiphysis of the rat tibia by capillaries. J Bone Joint Surg Br 43B:590–594
8. Chung SMK (1976) The arterial supply of the developing proximal end of the human femur. J Bone Joint Surg Am 58A(7):961–970
9. Eklund K, Jarmillo D (2001) Imaging of growth disturbance in children. Radiol Clin North Am 39(4):823–841
10. Floyd WE III, Zaleske DJ, Schiller AL, Trahan C, Mankin HJ (1987) Vascular events associated with the appearance of the secondary center of ossification in the murine distal femoral epiphysis. J Bone Joint Surg Am 69A:185–190
11. Haas SL (1917) The relationship of the blood supply to the longitudinal growth of bone. Am J Orthop Surg 15(157–171): 305–316
12. Harris HA (1929) The vascular supply of bone, with special reference to the epiphyseal cartilage. J Anat 64:1–4
13. Irving MH (1964) The blood supply of the growth cartilage of growing rats. J Anat Lond 98(4):631–639
14. Kumar R, Madewell JE, Swischuck LE (1987) The normal and abnormal growth plate. Radiol Clin North Am 25: 1133–1153
15. Laor T, Hartman AL, Jaramillo D (1997) Local physeal widening on MR imaging: an incidental finding suggesting prior metaphyseal injury. Pediatr Radiol 27(8):654–662
16. Lewis OJ (1956) The blood supply of developing long bones with special reference to the metaphyses. J Bone Joint Surg Br 38B:928–933
17. Menelaus M (1981) Opening and closing the growth plate. Aust NZ J Surg 51(6):518–527
18. Morgan JD (1959) Blood supply of growing rabbit's tibia. J Bone Joint Surg Br 41B:185–203
19. Ogden JA (1979) Pediatric osteomyelitis and septic arthritis: the pathology of neonatal disease. Yale J Biol Med 52(5): 423–445
20. Oni OAA (1999) The microvascular anatomy of the physis as revealed by osteomedullography and correlated histology. Orthopedics 22(2):239–241
21. Peterson HA (2007) Epiphyseal growth plate fractures. Springer, Heidelberg, p 914
22. Siffert RS (1966) The growth plate and its affections. J Bone Joint Surg Am 48A:546–563
23. Spira E, Farin I (1967) The vascular supply to the epiphyseal plate under normal and pathologic conditions. Acta Orthop Scand 38:1–22
24. Teot L, Gilbert A, Amichot G, Berniére J, Pous JG, Carlioz A (1984) Epiphyseal vascularization during growth: the upper limb. Ann Chir Main 3(3):237–244
25. Tilling G (1958) The vascular anatomy of long bones; a radiological and histological study. Acta Radiol Suppl 161:1–101
26. Tomita Y, Tsai T, Steyers C, Ogden L, Jupiter JB, Kutz JE (1986) The role of the epiphyseal and metaphyseal vessels on longitudinal growth in the dog. J Hand Surg Am 11A:375–382
27. Trueta J (1959) The blood supply adjacent to the epiphyseal plate and its influence on growth (abstr). J Bone Joint Surg 41B:206
28. Trueta J (1958) The influence of growth on the sequelae of bone and joint injuries (abstr). J Bone Joint Surg 40B:154
29. Trueta J (1957) The normal vascular anatomy of the human femoral head during growth. J Bone Joint Surg Br 39B: 358–394
30. Trueta J (1963) The role of the vessels in osteogenesis. J Bone Joint Surg 45B:402–418
31. Trueta J, Little K (1960) The vascular contribution to osteogenesis. II. Studies with the electron microscope. J Bone Joint Surg Br 42B:367–376
32. Trueta J, Morgan JD (1960) The vascular contribution to osteogenesis. I. Studies by the injection method. J Bone Joint Surg Br 42B:97–109
33. Wirth T, Syed Ali MM, Rauer C, Sub D, Griss P, Syed Ali S (1996) The blood supply in the growth plate: a microangiographic study in sheep. J Bone Joint Surg Br [abstr] 78B(suppl):77–78
34. Young MH (1963) Changes in the growth cartilage resulting from ischaemic necrosis of the metaphysis. J Pathol Bacteriol 85:481–488
35. Yousefzadeh DK, Doerger K, Sullivan C (2008) The blood supply of early, late, and nonossifying cartilage: preliminary gray-scale and Doppler assessment and their implications. Pediatr Radiol 38(2):146–158

Normal Physiologic Physeal Closure

36. Eeg-Larsen N (1956) An experimental study on growth and glycolysis in the epiphyseal cartilage of rats. Acta Physiol Scand 38(suppl 128):1–77
37. Haines RW (1975) The histology of epiphyseal union in mammals. J Anat 120:1–25
38. Harcke HT, Synder M, Caro PA, Bowen JR (1992) Growth plate of the normal knee: evaluation with MR imaging. Radiology 183:119–123

39. Roach HI, Clarke NMP (1999) Cell paralysis as an intermediate stage in the programmed cell death of epiphyseal chondrocytes during development. J Bone Miner Res 14(8): 1367–1378
40. Sasaki T, Ishibashi Y, Okamura Y, Toh S, Sasaki T (2002) MRI evaluation of growth plate closure rate and pattern in the normal knee joint. J Knee Surg 15(2):72–76

Vascular Deficiency Due to Reduced Quantity

41. Brashear HR Jr (1963) Epiphyseal avascular necrosis and its relation to longitudinal bone growth. J Bone Joint Surg Am 45A:1423–1438
42. Jaramillo D, Laor T, Jaleske DJ (1993) Indirect trauma to the growth plate: results of MRI imaging after epiphyseal and metaphyseal injury in rabbits. Radiology 183:171–178
43. Kleinman PK, Marks SC Jr, Spevak MF, Belanger PL, Richmond JM (1991) Extrusion of the growth plate cartilage into the metaphysis: a sign of healing fracture in abused infants. AJR 156:775–779
44. Ogden JA (1990) Transphyseal linear ossification striations of the distal radius and ulna. Skeletal Radiol 19:173–180
45. Pinkerton JA Jr, Davidson KK, Wood WG (1985) Femorotibial vein bypass in a child. J Vasc Surg 2(5):735–738
46. Rajpurohit R, Koch CJ, Tao Z, Teixeira CM, Shapiro IM (1996) Adaptation of chondrocytes to low oxygen tension: relationship between hypoxia and cellular metabolism. J Cell Physiol 168:424–432
47. Shapiro IM, Mansfield KD, Evans SM, Lord EM, Koch CJ (1997) Chondrocytes in the endochondrol growth plate cartilage are not hypoxic. Am J Physiol 272(Cell Physiol. 41):C1134–C1143
48. Stark RH, Matloub HS, Sanger JR, Cohen EG, Lynch K (1987) Warm ischemic damage to the epiphyseal growth plate: a rabbit model. J Hand Surg Am 12A:54–61
49. Troupp H (1961) Nervous and vascular influence on longitudinal growth of bone. An experimental study on rabbits. Acta Orthop Scand Suppl 51:1–78
50. Trueta J, Amato VP (1960) The vascular contribution to osteogenesis. III. Changes in the growth cartilage caused by experimentally induced ischemia. J Bone Joint Surg Br 42B:571–587

Arterial Disruption

51. Peterson HA (1993) Premature physeal arrest of the distal tibia associated with temporary arterial insufficiency. Case report. J Pediatr Orthop 13:672–675
52. Shaker IJ, White JJ, Signer RD, Golladay ES, Haller JA (1976) Special problems of vascular injuries in children. J Trauma 16(11):863–867
53. Whitehouse WM Jr, Coran AG, Stanley JC, Kuhns LR, Weintraub WH, Fry WJ (1976) Pediatric vascular trauma: manifestations, management, and sequelae of extremity arterial injury in patients undergoing surgical treatment. Arch Surg 111:1269–1275

Arterial Ligation

54. Currarino G, Engle MA (1965) The effects of ligation of the subclavian artery of the bones and soft tissues of the arms. J Pediatr 67(5):808–811
55. Harris AM, Segel N, Bishop JM (1964) Blalock-Taussig anastomosis for tetralogy of fallot. A ten-to-fifteen year follow-up. Br Heart J 26:266–273

Arterial Catheterization

56. Bassett III FH (1968) Short leg may follow long catheter. Medical World News, October 25, 1968
57. Bassett FH III, Lincoln CR, King TD, Canent RV Jr (1968) Inequality in the size of the lower extremity following cardiac catheterization. South Med J 61(100):1013–1017
58. Bloom JD, Mozersky DJ, Buckley CJ, Hagood CO Jr (1974) Defective limb growth as a complication of catheterization of the femoral artery. Surg Gynecol Obstet 138(4): 524–526
59. Boros SJ, Nystrom JF, Thompson TR, Reynolds JW, Williams HJ (1975) Leg growth following umbilical artery catheter-associated thrombus formation: a 4-year follow-up. J Pediatr 87(10):973–976
60. Ehrenfeld WK (1976) Pediatric vascular trauma (discussion). Arch Surg 111:1274
61. Flanigan DP, Keifer TJ, Schuler JJ, Ryan TJ, Castronuovo JJ (1983) Experience with iatrogenic pediatric vascular injuries. Ann Surg 198(4):430–439
62. Macnicol MF, Anagnostopoulos J (2000) Arrest of the growth plate after arterial cannulation in infancy. J Bone Joint Surg Br 82B:172–175
63. Richardson JD, Fallat M, Nagaraji HS, Groff DB, Flint LM (1981) Arterial injuries in children. Arch Surg 116: 685–690
64. Rosenthal A, Anderson M, Thomson SJ, Pappas AM, Fyler DC (1972) Superficial femoral artery catheterization. Effect on extremity length. Am J Dis Child 124:240–242
65. Walter PK, Hoffman W (2000) Diminished epiphyseal growth following iatrogenic vascular trauma. Eur J Vasc Endovasc Surg 20:214–216
66. White JJ, Talbert JL, Haller JA Jr (1968) Peripheral arterial injuries in infants and children. Ann Surg 167(5):757–765

Fluid Extravasation in Soft Tissues

67. Sampera I Jr, Fixsen JA, Hill RA (1994) Injuries to the physis by extravasation. A rare cause of growth plate arrest. J Bone Joint Surg Br 76B:278–280
68. Sampera I Jr, Fixsen JA, Hill RA (1993) Partial physeal arrest after severe extravasation injuries. Mapfre Medicina 4(Suppl II):272
69. Wada A, Fujii T, Takamura K, Yanagida H, Matsuura A, Katayama A (2003) Physeal arrest of the ankle secondary to extravasation in a neonata and its treatment by the Gruea operation: a modern application of an old technique. J Pediatr Orthop 12B:129–132

Interosseous Infusion

70. Bielski RJ, Bassett GS, Fideler B, Tolo V (1993) Interosseous infusions: effects on the immature physis: an experimental model in rabbits. J Pediatr Orthop 13(4):511–515
71. Claudet I, Baunin C, Laporte-Turpin E, Marcoux MO, Grouteau E, Cahuzac JB (2003) Long-term effects on tibial growth after interosseous infusion: a prospective, radiographic analysis. Pediatr Emerg Care 19(6):397–401
72. Burke T, Kehl D (1993) Interosseous infusion in infants. Case report of a complication. J Bone Joint Surg Am 75A(3):428–429
73. Galpin R, Kronick JB, Willis RB, Frewen TC (1991) Bilateral lower extremity compartment syndromes secondary to interosseous fluid resuscitation. Case report. J Pediatr Orthop 11(6):773–776
74. Ribeiro JA, Price CT, Knapp DR Jr (1993) Compartment syndrome of the lower extremity after interosseous infusion of fluid. A report of two cases. J Bone Joint Surg Am 75A(3):430–433

Compartment Syndrome

75. Caouette-Laberge L, Bortoluzzi P, Egerszegi EP, Marton D (1992) Neonatal Volkman's ischemic contracture of the forearm: a report of five cases. Plast Reconstr Surg 90(4):621–628
76. Engel J, Heim M, Tsur H (1982) Late complications of neonatal Volkmann's ischaemia. Hand 14(2):162–163
77. Hernandez H Jr, Peterson HA (1986) Fracture of the distal radial physis complicated by compartment syndrome and premautre physeal closure. Case report. J Petiatr Orthop 6:627–630
78. Tsujino A, Hooper G (1997) Neonatal compression ischaemia of the forearm. J Hand Surg Br 22B(5):612–614

Diaphyseal Fracture

79. Beals RK (1990) Premature physeal closure of the physis following diaphyseal fractures. J Pediatr Orthop 10:717–720
80. Blount WP (1955) Fractures in children. Williams and Wilkins, Baltimore, p 132
81. Blount WP (1960) Unequal leg length. Instructional course lectures, 17th edn. CV Mosby Co, St. Louis, pp 218–245
82. Bowler JR, Mubarak SJ, Wenger DR (1990) Tibial physeal closure and genu recurvatum after femoral fracture: occurrence without a tibial traction pin. J Pediatr Orthop 10(5):653–657
83. Chapchal G (1979) Late complication of fractures in children. Reconstr Surg Traumatol 17:130–138
84. Gonzalez-Lopez JL (2000) Letter to the editors. Incidence of physeal arrest following diaphyseal fractures. J Pediatr Orthop 20:826
85. Herring JA, Birch J (1987) (Discussion): Whither the bar. Instructional case. J Pediatr Orthop 7:722–725
86. Hresko MT, Kasser JR (1989) Physeal arrest about the knee associated with non-physeal fractures in the lower extremity. J Bone Joint Surg Am 71A:698–703
87. Hunter LY, Hensinger RN (1989) Premature monomelic growth arrest following fracture of the femoral shaft. J Bone Joint Surg Am 71A:698–703
88. Morton KS, Starr DE (1964) Closure of the anterior portion of the upper tibial epiphysis as a complication of tibial shaft fracture. J Bone Joint Surg Am 46A:570–574
89. Navasués JA, Gonzales-Lopez JL, Lopez-Valverde S, Soleto J, Rodriguéz-Durantez JA, Garcia-Trovijano JL (2000) Premature physeal closure after tibial diaphyseal fractures in adolescents. J Pediatr Orthop 20(2):193–196
90. Ng DP, Cole WG (1996) The effect of early hip decompression on the frequency of avascular necrosis in children with fractures of the neck of the femur. Injury 27(6):419–421
91. Pappas AM, Anas P, Toczylowski HM (1984) Asymmetrical arrest of the proximal tibial physis and genu recurvatum deformity. J Bone Joint Surg Am 66A:575–581
92. Paul AS, Kay PR, Haines JF (1992) Distal ulnar growth plate arrest following a diaphyseal fracture. J R Coll Surg Edinb 37:347–348
93. Peterson HA, Burkhart SS (1981) Compression injury of the epiphyseal growth plate: fact or fiction? J Pediatr Orthop 1:377–384
94. Poznanski AK (1978) Diagnostic clues in the growing ends of bones. Annual Oration. J Can Assoc Radiol 29:7–21
95. Shively JL (1990) Genu recurvatum after femoral fracture. Contemp Orthop 21(6):577–580

Periosteal Stripping

96. Yabley RH, Harris WR (1965) The effect of shaft fractures and periosteal stripping on the vascular supply to the epiphyseal plates. J Bone Joint Surg Am 47A:551–566

Joint Dislocation

97. Light TR, Ogden JA (1988) Complex dislocation of the index metacarpal joint in children. J Pediatr Orthop 8(3):300–305

Extremity Traction

98. Ahstrom JP (1965) Epiphyseal injuries of the lower extremity. Surg Clin North Am 1:119–134
99. Mustard WT, Simons EH (1954) Experimental arterial spasm in the lower extremities produced by traction. J Bone Joint Surg 36A:503–510

Fixation Bandages

100. Hultén O (1951) The influence of a fixation bandage on the peripheral blood vessels and the circulation. Acta Chir Scand 101:151–154

Developmental Dislocation of the Hip

101. Bensahel H, Csukonyi Z, Huguenin P (1988) Vascular disorders of the proximal femur following treatment for congenital hip dislocation. Arch Orthop Trauma Surg 107(6):372–376
102. Chen MM, Jee WS, Ke HZ, Lin BY, Li QN, Li XJ (1992) Adaptation of cancellous bone to aging and immobilization in growing rats. Anat Rec 234(3):317–334
103. Keret D, MacEwen GD (1991) Growth disturbance of the proximal part of the femur after treatment for congenital dislocation of the hip. J Bone Joint Surg Am 73A(3):410–423
104. Morcuende JA, Meyer MD, Dolan LA, Weinstein SL (1997) Long-term outcome after open reduction through an arteromedial approach for congenital dislocation of the hip. J Bone Joint Surg Am 79A:810–817
105. Nicholson JT, Kapell HP, Matteri FA (1954) Regional stress arteriography of the hip; a preliminary report. J Bone Joint Surg Am 36A:503–510
106. O'Brien T, Millis MB, Griffin PP (1986) The early identification and classification of growth disturbance of the proximal end of the femur. J Bone Joint Surg Am 68A:970–980
107. Porat S, Robin GC, Howard CB (1994) Cure of the limp in children with congenital dislocation of the hip and ischaemic necrosis. Fifteen cases treated by trochanteric transfer and contralateral epiphysiodesis. J Bone Joint Surg Br 76B(3):463–467
108. Salter RB, Kostuik J, Dallas S (1969) Avascular necrosis of the femoral head as a complication of treatment of congenital dislocation of the hip in children. A clinical and experimental investigation. Can J Surg 12:44–61

Perthes Disease

109. Atsumi T, Yamano K, Muraki M, Yoshihara S, Kajihara T (2000) The blood supply of the lateral epiphyseal arteries in Perthes' disease. J Bone Joint Surg Br 82B:392–398
110. Barnes JM (1980) Premature epiphyseal closure in Perthes' disease. J Bone Joint Surg Br 62B:432–437
111. Bowen RJ, Schreiber FC, Foster BK, Wein BK (1982) Premature femoral neck physeal closure in Perthes' disease. Clin Orthop 171:24–29
112. Doria AS, Guarniero R, Cunha FG, Modena M, DeGodoy RM Jr, Luzo C, Neto RB, Molnar LJ, Cerri GG (2002) Contrast-enhanced power Doppler sonography: assessment of revascularization flow in Legg-Calve-Perthes' disease. Ultrasound Med Biol 28(2):171–182
113. Dustman HO (1996) Etiology and pathology of epiphyseal necrosis in children as exemplified with the hip [German]. Zeitschrift fur Orthopadie und ihre Grenzgebiete 134(5):407–412
114. Eijer H (2007) Towards a better understanding of Legg-Calve-Perthes' disease: acetabular retroversion may cause abnormal loading of dorsal femoral head-neck junction with restricted blood supply to the femoral epiphysis. Med Hypotheses 68(5):995–997
115. Jaramillo D, Kasser JR, Villegas-Medina OL, Gaary E, Zurakowski D (1995) Cartilaginous abnormalities and growth disturbances in Legg-Calve-Perthes disease: evaluation with MR imaging. Radiology 197:767–773
116. Joseph B, Mulpuri K (2001) Varghese: Perthes' disease in the adolescent. J Bone Joint Surg Br 83B(5):715–720
117. Keret D, Harrison MHM, Clarke NMP, Hall DF (1984) Coxa plana – the fate of the physis. J Bone Joint Surg Am 66A:870–877
118. Lamar S, Dorgeret S, Khairouri A, Mazda K, Billet PY, Bacheville E, Bloch J, Pennecot GF, Hassan M, Sebag GH (2002) Femoral head vascularization in Legg-Calve-Perthes disease: comparison of dynamic gadolinium-enhanced subtraction MRI with bone scintigraphy. Pediatr Radiol 32(8):580–585
119. McNutt W (1962) Inherited vascular pattern of the femoral head and neck as a predisposing factor to Legg-Calve-Perthes disease. Tex Rep Biol Med 20(4):525–531
120. Oshima H, Mizutani H, Ohba S (2002) Gray-scale and Gray-scale and Doppler ultrasound imaging features of vascular canals in human femoral condyles Acta Radiol 43(2):217–220
121. Ponseti IV, Maynard JA, Weinstein SL, Ippolito EG, Pous JG (1983) Legg-Calvé-Perthes disease: histochemical and ultrastructural observations of the epiphyseal cartilage and physis. J Bone Joint Surg Am 65A:797–807

Transplantation of the Physis

122. Heikel HV (1960–1961) Experimental epiphyseal transplantation. Acta Orthop Scand 30:1–19

Vascular Deficiency Due to Reduced Quality

123. Keck SW, Kelly PJ (1965) The effect of venus stasis on intraosseous pressure and longitudinal bone growth in dogs. J Bone Joint Surg Am 47A:539–544
124. Nyska M, Shabat S, Long PN, Howard C, Ezov N, Levin-Harris T, Mittelman M, Redich M, Yedgar S, Nyska A (2005) Disseminated thrombosis-induced growth plate necrosis in rat: a unique model for growth plate arrest. J Pediatr Orthop 25:346–350

Sickle-Cell Anemia

125. Barton CJ, Cockshott WP (1962) Bone changes in hemoglobin SC disease. Am J Roentgenol Radium Ther Nucl Med 88:523–532
126. Bennett OM, Namnyak SK (1990) Bone and joint manifestations of sickle cell anemia. J Bone Joint Surg Br 72B:494–499
127. Bohrer SP (1974) Growth disturbance of the distal femur following sickle cell bone infarcts and/or osteomyelitis. Clin Radiol 25:221–235
128. Cockshott WP (1963) Dactylitis and growth disorders. Br J Radiol 36:19–25
129. Golding JSR (1956) The bone changes in sickle cell anemia. Ann R Coll Surg Engl 19:296–315

130. Kim SK, Miller JN (2002) Natural history and distribution of bone and marrow infarction in sickle hemoglobinopathies. J Nucl Med 43:896–900
131. Onuba O (1993) Bone disorders in sickle-cell disease. Int Orthop 17(6):397–399
132. Reynolds J (1966) A re-evaluation of the "fish vertebra" sign in sickle cell hemoglobinopathy. Am J Roentgenol Radium Ther Nucl Med 97:693–707

Thalassemia Major (Cooley's Anemia)

133. Currarino G, Erlandson ME (1964) Premature fusion of epiphyses in Cooley's anemia. Radiology 83:656–664

Meningococcemia

134. Appel M, Pauleto AC, Cunha LAM (2002) Osteochondral sequelae of meningococcemia: radiographic aspects. J Pediatr Orthop 22:511–516
135. Bache CE, Torode IP (2006) Orthopaedic sequelae of meningiococeal septicemia. J Pediatr Orthop 26(1):135–139
136. Barre PS, Thompson GH, Morrison SC (1985) Late skeletal deformities following meningococcal sepsis and disseminated intravascular coagulation: case report. J Pediatr Orthop 5:584–588
137. Fernández F, Pueyo I, Jiménez JR, Vigil E (1981) Guzmán: epiphyseal changes in children after severe meningococcic sepsis. AJR Am J Roentgenol 136:1236–1238
138. Grogan DP, Love SM, Ogden JA, Miller EA, Johnson LO (1989) Chondro-osseous growth abnormalities after meningococcemia: a clinical and histopathological study. J Bone Joint Surg Am 71A(6):920–928
139. Kruse RW, Tassanawipas A, Bowen JR (1991) Orthopedic sequelae of meningococcemia. Orthopedics 14(2):174–178
140. O'Sullivan ME, Fogarty EE (1990) Distal tibial arrest: a complication of meningococcal septicemia. Case report. J Pediatr Orthop 10:549–550
141. Patriquin HB, Trias A, Jecquier S, Marton D (1981) Late sequelae of infantile meningococcemia in growing bones in children. Radiology 141(1):77–82
142. Peterson HA (2001) Physeal injuries and growth arrest. In: Beaty JN, Kasser JR (eds) Rockwood and Wilkins' fractures in children, 5th edn. Lippincott, Williams and Wilkins, Philadelphia, Chapter 5
143. Robinow M, Johnson F, Nanagas MT, Mesghali H (1983) Skeletal lesions following meningococcemia and disseminated intravascular coagulation. Am J Dis Child 137:279–281
144. Santos E, Boavida JE, Barroso A, Seabra J, Carmona de Mota H (1989) Late osteoarticular lesions following meningococcemia with disseminated intravascular coagulation. Pediatr Radiol 19:199–202
145. Soulen MC, Miller WT Jr (1990) Ten-year old boy with a limp. Invest Radiol 25(3):299–301
146. Watson CHC, Asworth MA (1983) Growth disturbance and meningococcal sepsis: report of two cases. J Bone Joint Surg Am 65A:1181–1183
147. Wyssa B, Le Coultre C, Kaelin A (1992) Orthopaedic and surgical complications of meningococcemia. J Pediatr Orthop B 1:73–77

Purpura Fulminans

148. Acheson LS (1986) Disturbances of bone growth in a child who survived septic shock. J Fam Pract 23(4):321–329
149. Genoff MC, Hoffer MM, Achauer B, Formosa P (1992) Extremity amputations in meningococcemia induced purpura fulminans. Plast Reconstr Surg 89:878–881
150. Jacobsen ST, Crawford AH (1984) Amputation following meningococcemia. A sequela to purpura fulminans. Clin Orthop Relat Res 185:214–219
151. Krajbich JI (1998) Lower limb deficiencies and amputations in children. J Am Acad Orthop Surg 6:358–366
152. Nogi J (1989) Physeal arrest in purpura fulminans: a report of three cases. J Bone Joint Surg Am 71A:929–931
153. Rodgers WB, Kennedy JG, Hergreuter CA, Kasser JR (2000) Massive subperiosteal hemorrhage and femoral shaft osteonecrosis: a complication of tissue plasminogen activator therapy for purpura fulminans. Am J Orthop 29(4):315–319
154. Schaller RT Jr, Schaller JF (1986) Surgical management of life-threatening and disfiguring sequelae of fulminant meningococcemia. Am J Surg 151:553–556
155. Sheridan RL, Briggs SE, Remensnyder JP, Tompkins RG (1996) Management strategy in purpura fulminans with multiple organ failure in children. Burns 22(1):53–56

Cupping

156. Caffey J (1970) Traumatic cupping of the metaphyses of growing bones. AJR Am J Roentgenol 108:451–460
157. Inoue H (1987) Cone-shaped epiphyses in the phalanges of the hand – a statistical and experimental study [*Japanese*]. J Japanese Orthop Assn 61(4):939–410
158. Kumar SJ, Forlin E, Guille JT (1992) Epiphyseometaphyseal cupping of the distal femur with knee-flexion contracture. Orthop Rev 21(1):67–70
159. Matthiesen DE (1957) Premature growth arrest of the knee epiphyses. Am J Roentgenol Radium Ther Nucl Med 78:499–501
160. Wiss DA (1981) Metaphyseal cupping. A case report. Orthopedics 4(6):649–652

Disuse

2.1 Introduction

Growth of bone is determined not only by heredity and nutrition, but also by the work it has to perform. The mechanical factors which influence and are essential for normal longitudinal growth, are movement and weight bearing [2]. Disuse of an extremity from any cause results in atrophy of muscle and other soft tissues in both adults and children. Osteoporosis is a well known feature of inactivity and disuse in adults. Osteoporosis from disuse also occurs in children, but to a lesser extent. If disuse is prolonged in children, growth of bone length is also diminished. Since growth retardation occurs before growth arrest, the process may be reversed if discovered and treated early. If disuse is marked, some physes may cease growing completely. The most commonly reported sites of growth slow down and arrest from disuse are the distal femur and proximal tibia [3]. Unfortunately these physes rank first and second in the amount of longitudinal growth they provide.

The incidence of growth arrest associated with disuse is difficult to measure because the disuse is variable and because recognition of the arrest may require years of observation. Prolonged disuse secondary to bed rest, traction, cast immobilization, braces, crutches, and delayed weight bearing, have all been associated with growth slow down or arrest of one or more physes of the involved extremity. These treatment modalities, previously used in management of children with tuberculosis of the hip, poliomyelitis, lower extremity diaphyseal fracture, Perthes disease, developmental hip dislocation, osteomyelitis, and slipped capital femoral epiphysis, are today used more sparingly for a number of reasons, one of which is the occurrence of growth arrest.

The degree to which growth reduction is associated with neurologic conditions (discussed in Chap. 6) cannot be separated from the accompanying disuse. The statement "that education in the performance of exercises designed to increase the use of the limb to the greatest possible extent may lead to marked reduction of the discrepancy in growth" [1] was written in the context of neurologic conditions, but can be applied to all causes of disuse.

2.2 Tuberculosis

Prior to the mid twentieth century tuberculosis of the hip was common in children and the treatment was "rest, uninterrupted, continuous, and prolonged." [4] Bed rest, balanced traction, and casts were commonly used for months to years [5, 6, 10]. The duration of treatment was chosen arbitrarily to allow completion of destruction of the femoral head to improve probability of successful hip fusion [10]. One regimen included continuing immobilization and delaying hip fusion until the child had "reached his tenth year of age, providing the acute manifestations of the disease have disappeared." [6] These children were often more disabled from secondary complications of disuse than from their hip joint tuberculosis [10]. One patient with bilateral tuberculosis of the hip developed growth arrest of both knees [3].

Arrest of physes distal to the hip would often occur even though none of these physes or their accompanying joints were infected [7]. The longer the duration of disuse the more extensive the growth arrest about the knee (Table 2.1) [9]. The limb length discrepancy varied from minimal up to 7 in. [3, 10]. In one series [10],

Table 2.1 Incidence of knee physeal arrest with hip tuberculosis in children

Year	Author	No. cases	No. arrests	Percentage[a]
1944	Gill [7]	150	10	6.7
1947	McCarroll and Heath [10]	43	28	65.1
1948	Ross [3]	92	9	9.8
1949	Parke et al. [11]	91	29	31.0
TOTAL		376	76	20.2

[a]The lower percentage of arrests is probably due to earlier hip surgery and shorter time of immobilization [3]. Length of follow-up was not well documented in these series, which also impacts the results

of 43 hips completely immobilized for 2–8 years, 28 (65%) showed limb shortening of from 2 to 7 in. The degree of shortening was in direct proportion to the length of immobilization. The loss of limb length was estimated to be 12% from the diseased and fused hip, and 88% due to premature closure of the distal femur and proximal tibia physes.

The physes most often affected from disuse are the distal femur and proximal tibia, separately or both [3, 7–9, 11]. The fibula and distal tibia physes are never involved [11]. The central portion of the physis is affected first producing cupping (Sect. 1.3), which if left untreated progresses from mild to moderate, to marked (Fig. 1.13) [7, 12]. When the cupping is eccentric, angular deformity occurs [7, 12]. When the proximal tibia is involved, normal fibular growth proceeds to relative overgrowth.

Although observers recognized that growth arrest was associated with prolonged immobilization, the explanation for it was often speculative. It was difficult for authors to separate the accompanying and often more noticeable osteoporosis from the growth arrest [3]. Some authors [7, 8, 13] speculated that in some cases the accompanying osteoporosis predisposed the physis or the accompanying small vessels to microfractures. Others suggested that the arrest was due to a secondary factor, such as a faulty gait [3]. These early attempts to explain arrests by mechanical causes were gradually replaced by vascular insufficiency explanations, confirmed by the work of Trueta and colleagues in the 1950s (Sects. 1.2 and 1.3). The presence of soft tissue atrophy and the absence of pain support the concept of impaired vascular supply [9].

Long periods of immobilization in casts should be avoided unless it is absolutely necessary [8, 13]. Although the distal physeal arrests can be found 6–8 months following the hip disease, the clinical features of growth impairment are often not detected for 2–3 years [9]. Gill [8] advocated the surgical placement of metal markers in the femoral diaphysis, followed by a repeat scanogram every 6 months to observe the amount of growth. The ensuing relative limb discrepancy was usually treated by a shoe lift, contralateral surgical physeal arrest or bone shortening, or ipsilateral bone lengthening. On occasion severe leg length discrepancy resulted in amputation and prosthetic fitting [5, 12].

2.3 Poliomyelitis

In the aftermath of poliomyelitis, recovery of useful function in the paralyzed limb is sometimes remarkable, but growth of the limb is usually disturbed [27]. Adults who contract poliomyelitis develop no limb length discrepancy. In children, paresis caused by poliomyelitis often results in growth retardation of a lower limb by 5%; i.e. about 4 cm in the average adult. Growth of the tibia is affected to a greater extent than the femur by a ratio of 3:2, regardless of the distribution of the paralysis (Fig. 2.1) [26]. Central physeal closure with cupping (Sect. 1.5) was found in several distal femoral and proximal tibial physes [16]. The age of onset of the disease has little influence on the annual increment of shortening, but influences the final inequality due to the number of years to maturity [26].

The etiology of diminished bone growth in the paralytic limb is most likely due to secondary disuse rather than primary nerve dysfunction. The functional use of the involved extremity plays a large role in determining its longitudinal growth [18, 28]. Disuse of the extremity alters the circulation and nutrition of the extremity. Delayed weight bearing is thought to be a greater factor than paralysis. Intermittent weight bearing is a necessary stimulus for optimal growth. The

2.3 Poliomyelitis

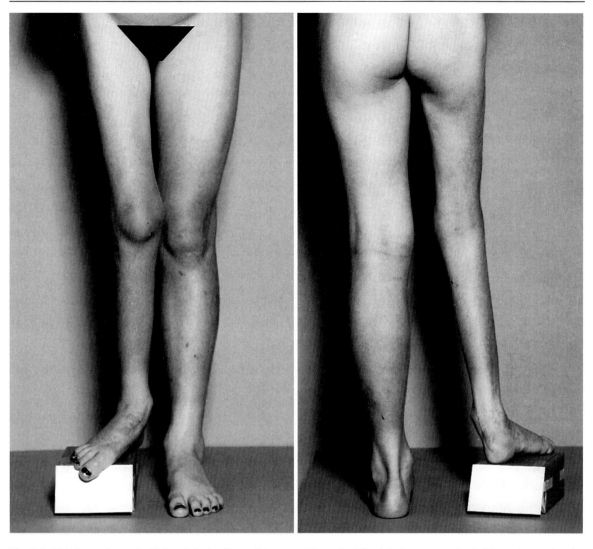

Fig. 2.1 This 8 year 7 month old female had poliomyelitis at age 20 months. The right lower extremity is 5.7 cm shorter than the left (femur 2.0 cm, tibia 3.7 cm)

relationship of motor paralysis and limb vasculature as a cause of diminished physeal growth has also been studied. Chronic vascular insufficiency with consequent hypoxia of growth cartilage cells is known to reduce growth in poliomyelitis patients. Harris and McDonald [19] in 1936 noted that the increase in blood supply which follows lumbar sympathectomy in poliomyelitis patients was capable of inducing mild acceleration of the rate of growth. The factors favorable to a good result include paralysis limited to one lower extremity, paralysis of moderate degree, operation before age 6 years, and the use of ganglionectomy rather than ramisection. Subsequent studies, however, concluded that sympathectomy does not increase the growth potential consistently or appreciably in polio limbs [15, 17, 29]. Sympathectomy performed to increase bone length in poliomyelitis patients is no longer used, most likely because the result is unpredictable, the benefit minor, the side effects permanent, and if the discrepancy is large other treatments would be needed anyway. A related experimental study in rabbits [29] concluded that "motor paralysis (with the sympathetic nerve supply intact) plays a very minor part in the retardation of growth." Another proposed concept that the circulating polio virus damages blood vessel walls directly [24], was never proven.

Barr (1948) [14] studied 371 cases in which the onset of poliomyelitis was before the age of 16 years. Forty-one percentage had ½ in. or less of shortening, 24% had between ½ and 1½ in. shortening, and 35% had 1½ in. or more of shortening. The age of onset was an important factor. Leg length inequality of moderate or marked severity was greater in boys, due to longer growing period and greater length potential. Premature cessation toward the end of growth was noted in the femur and tibia, together or separately. Although qualitative measurement of the circulatory status was not done, decreased circulation was felt to cause the growth retardation.

Stinchfield et al. (1949) [28] examined 166 adults in whom poliomyelitis developed before age 11 years and found a definite relationship between the muscle strength in the two lower extremities and the discrepancy in limb length, but no relationship between the age of onset and the amount of length discrepancy.

Gullickson et al. (1950) [18] reviewed 88 chronic poliomyelitis patients with unilateral lower extremity involvement and found a definite correlation between atrophy of the thigh or leg and shortening of the femur or tibia, between total atrophy and shortening of the involved extremity, and between total strength of the involved extremity and shortening in that extremity. The age at which acute poliomyelitis occurred affected the percentage of shortening; the younger the onset the greater the percentage of growth retardation (Table 2.2). They concluded that in poliomyelitis there is a decreased blood flow due to increased sympathetic activity or decreased function of the leg, causing an interference with soft tissue and bone metabolism and therefore growth.

Ring (1957) [27] evaluated 55 patients with residual unilateral paralysis and noted that in young children the effect of paralysis on growth increased as age advanced, and that this effect is maximal at age 10 years and then rapidly diminished. Since no mechanical cause could be found, he concluded that since the paralyzed limb is often cold and blue and has a lower resting blood flow than the contralateral leg, bone growth is diminished due to vascular insufficiency.

Ratliff (1959) [25] found leg shortening in 215 of 225 (96%) patients. Most of the shortening was in the tibia rather than in the femur. He noted that although a mild degree of paresis produced a small amount of shortening, severe paresis might produce either a little or more significant shortening.

Table 2.2 Relation between age of onset of acute poliomyelitis and retardation of bone growth expressed as percentage shortening in relation to the normal extremity [18]

Age at onset years	No. cases	Shortening of femur (%)	Shortening of tibia (%)	Shortening of lower extremity (%)
0–5	47	2.52	2.44	2.64
6–10	29	1.96	2.37	2.14
11–14	12	1.40	1.39	1.27

Makin (1965) [22], reviewed 112 patients with unilateral paralysis with leg length discrepancy of more than 2.5 cm, measured by scanography. The onset of poliomyelitis was 6 years or less in all patients. The length deficit was primarily in the tibia in 51 patients, in both the femur and tibia and 48, and in the femur in 13. Shortening of the fibula was greater than that of the tibia in 87 patients (78%). Fibula shortening resulted in valgus and instability of the ankle, and if marked predisposed to genu valgum and lateral tibial torsion.

In addition to relative shortening of the tibia and femur, the fibula and the fourth metatarsal have also been found to be affected. Shortening of the fibula, relative to the tibia, results in a wedge shaped distal tibial epiphysis and ankle valgus [30], just as in other cases of other developmental fibular deficiency (Sect. 19.3). Currarino (1966) [16], found that of 250 unselected patients with poliomyelitis, 22 (9%) had premature closure with shortening of the fourth metatarsal in the paretic limb.

The period of immobilization of poliomyelitis patients should be as short as possible [13]. The "natural history" of the polio disease in an individual case as measured by the recovery of function, is variable and unpredictable early on. Careful follow-up will help identify cases which might benefit from treatment such as physeal arrest of the longer extremity. Polio residuals of genu valgum [21] and genu recurvatum [23] may also be related to the disuse and may be treated by staple hemiepiphyseodesis and osteotomy respectively, provided there is no physeal bar. A procedure to stimulate growth in the affected leg by the surgical creation of an arteriovenous fistula was successful in many cases of poliomyelitis (Fig. 2.2) [20], but was abandoned because the amount of correction achieved was unpredictable, and subsequent repair of the AV fistula is an operation of considerable magnitude. The procedure and

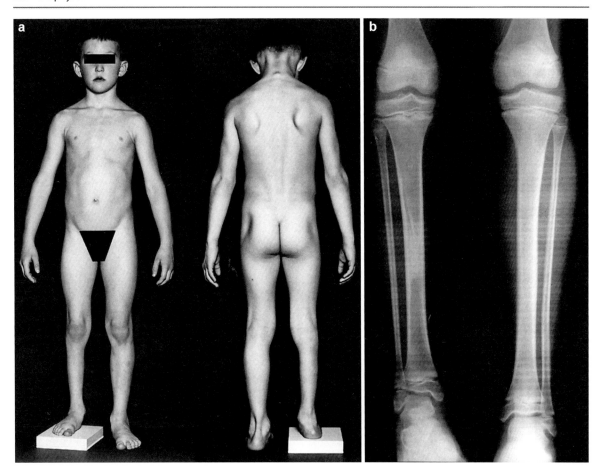

Fig. 2.2 This boy had poliomyelitis at age 6 months. (**a**) At age 7 years 4 months the right lower extremity is 3.5 cm shorter than the left, primarily in the tibia. An arteriovenous fistula was surgically created in the right mid superficial femoral vessels at age 7 years 4 months. (**b**) At age 10 years 9 months the right tibia and fibula have grown faster than the left and the discrepancy is now only 2.4 cm. The bone and physeal structure is comparable to the left

results, however, support the premise that reduction of bone growth in poliomyelitis is a vascular deficiency associated with disuse, and not a primary neurologic deficit of the physis.

2.4 Diaphyseal Fracture

Prolonged immobilization of diaphyseal fractures in children can result in considerable physeal damage, including premature and often eccentric closure, resulting in relative shortening and angular deformity [32]. The physeal arrest does not appear to be related to the severity of injury [31]. Recognition of the arrest is delayed for an average of 1 year 10 months [34]. Femoral and tibial diaphyseal fractures are the bones of concern in the literature.

Fractures of both the proximal and mid femur, when treated by prolonged immobilization, can develop premature arrest of physes distal to the fracture. The arrest may occur in only one, or in any combination of physes distal to the fracture [35, 38], but most often affects the distal femur and proximal tibia (Fig. 2.3) [8, 31, 32]. In one series [39] of 132 femoral fractures, there were 6 cases of arrest of the distal femur (4.5%), all considered to be due to prolonged immobilization in plaster associated with secondary salvage procedures. In most cases the precise cause of the arrest, whether from prolonged disuse or initial vascular insufficiency (Table 1.1), cannot be determined.

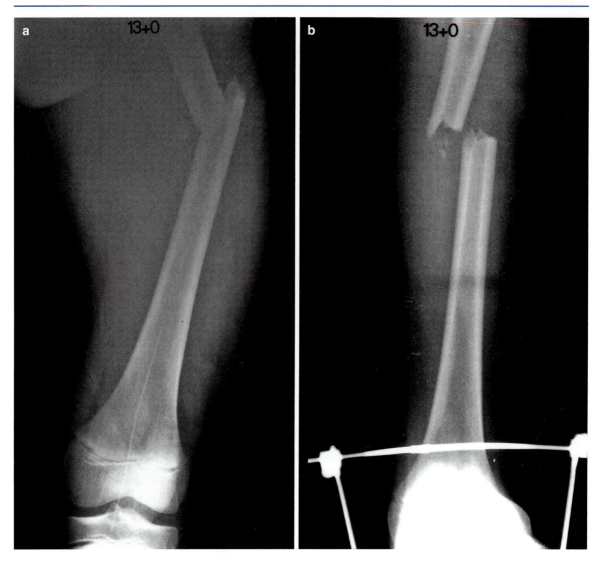

Fig. 2.3 Premature arrest of the distal femur and proximal tibial physes associated with a femoral diaphyseal fracture and prolonged disuse. This 13 year 0 month old male fell from a dirt bike injuring his left thigh. (**a**) There is a displaced femoral diaphyseal fracture. The distal femoral and proximal tibial physes are normal. (**b**) Reduction was incomplete after 7 days in 90/90, 20 lbs. skeletal traction. Traction continued 22 days at which time the traction pin was removed and a spica cast applied. The cast was worn 28 days. (**c**) Status of healing 52 days post fracture 2 days after cast removal. Note maintenance of length despite poor fracture healing. No new bone formation on the lateral side suggests that the distal fragment may have a button-hole through the periosteum (**a**). (**d**) Refracture 5 days post cast removal. The fracture was manipulated and a spica cast reapplied. The second cast was worn 44 days, followed by crutches. Delayed malunion resulted in open intramedullary nailing and bone grafting 6 weeks later. Crutches were again used and discontinued 8 months post fracture. (**e**) Scanogram 13 months post fracture, age 14 years 1 month. The left femur is 22 mm shorter and left tibia 12 mm shorter than the right. The femoral fracture was healed. (**f**) Four coronal tomograms of the uninjured right knee show open femoral and tibial physes. (**g**) Four coronal tomograms of the left knee show significant narrowing of the distal femoral and proximal tibial physes. Two months later the patient underwent rod removal and right distal femoral and proximal tibial surgical epiphysiodeses. (**h**) Age 16 years 4 months. The patient was normally active and asymptomatic and played high school hockey goalie. Scanogram showed a leg length discrepancy of 27 mm (femoral 16, tibial 11). All physes are closed. The patient wore a permanent shoe lift except for athletic shoes. The left foot is two shoe sizes smaller than the right (implying premature arrest of metatarsals and/or phalanges). The patient's height was equal to his father: 177.7 cm. Note: This fractured right femur was treated by 22 days traction, 72 days spica cast, intramedullary nailing, and crutches for 8 months. There was significant slow-down of growth of knee physes distal to the fracture as documented by relative shortening compared with the opposite extremity. The surgical physeal arrests on the normal knee prevented the discrepancy from increasing. The patient was left with a 27 mm leg length discrepancy. In this case the premature physeal closures could have been due to prolonged disuse, to initial vascular insufficiency (Sect. 1.3), or to both

2.4 Diaphyseal Fracture

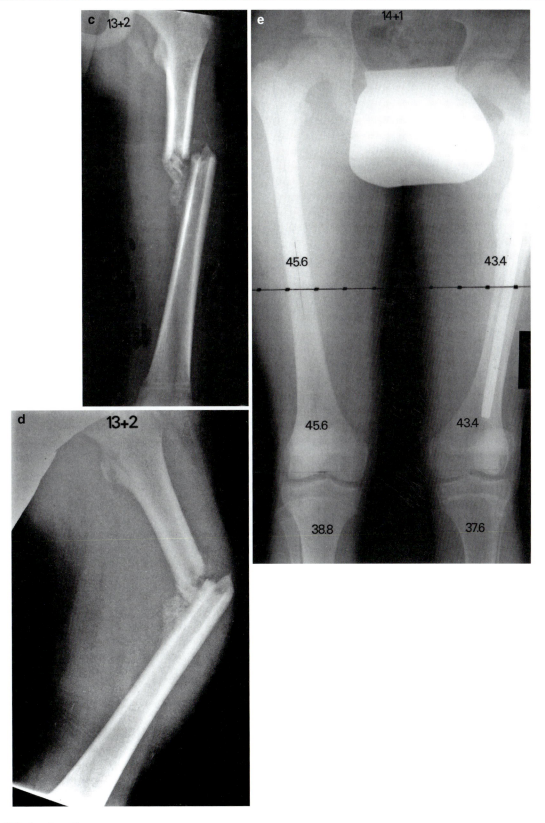

Fig. 2.3 (continued)

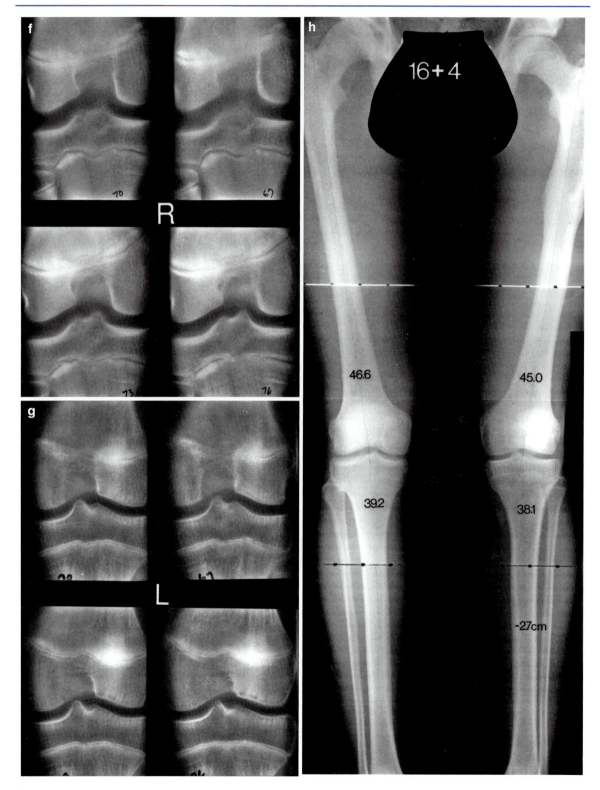

Fig. 2.3 (continued)

When the tibial diaphysis is fractured, however, the arrest may occur proximal to the tibial fracture (Fig. 1.10) [36, 37]. When this occurs vascular insufficiency due to disuse may be more plausible than vascular insufficiency due to the fracture. In one series of 354 adolescents with tibial fractures there were 7 cases (2%) of premature physeal closure [33]. All fractures resulting in arrest occurred in children between 12 and 15 years of age [33, 36, 37]. Consequently, when fracture-associated arrest occurs in this age range, the length discrepancy is often discovered too late for surgical arrest on the contralateral side. Thus, either surgical lengthening of the injured tibia or shortening of the normal femur is often required. Adolescents with tibial diaphyseal fractures should be monitored until growth is complete because of the risk of developing leg length discrepancy as a consequence of premature closure of one or more of the leg physes [37].

The physes exhibiting premature closure are always large, i.e., the distal femur, proximal and distal tibia (Table 1.1). Except for the closure of one proximal fibula [35], no other small physes, such as the metatarsals or phalanges have been recorded. This is similar to physeal arrest with vascular deficiency due to decreased quantity discussed in Sect. 1.3, but different from poliomyelitis where the fourth metatarsal is sometimes affected [16].

It is essential to treat fractures in children effectively and in the shortest possible time [32]. Early recognition of limb length discrepancy can be treated with surgical arrest of one or more physes. If the discrepancy is discovered later, physeal arrest will only prevent the discrepancy from increasing, and bone shortening or lengthening operations might be necessary.

2.5 Developmental Dislocation of the Hip

Premature closure of the distal femur and proximal tibia physes occurred on the side of the developmental hip dislocation (DDH) in three children immobilized in frog position casts for 12, 16, and 19 months [40]. The authors concluded that "relative ischemia of the involved physes is the most likely cause." Kestler [9] illustrated one case but did not specify the type or duration of treatment. Although ischemia explains the physeal arrest in the absence of trauma or toxic effect, the reason for involvement of only the ipsilateral knee (not the ipsilateral fibula or distal tibia, or the contralateral extremity) is not known. Complete immobilization should be as brief as possible [13].

When DDH is associated with avascular necrosis of the femoral head, the proximal femoral physis is at an even higher risk of arrest. If immobilization in a hip spica cast is prolonged, disuse compounds the underlying vascular deficiency of the epiphysis (Chapter 1B).

2.6 Perthes Disease

Premature closure of the distal physis has been noted to occur in the same femur as the Perthes disease [41]. Disuse, the cast, and position in the cast (similar to the discussion in Chap. 1, DDH), could all be factors. Of 147 patients with unilateral Perthes disease followed 5 years or more, the average femoral shortening was 1.38 cm, and the average tibial shortening was 0.93 cm (total 2.14 cm) [42]. The extent of the tibial discrepancy correlated well with the time of immobilization in the unilateral abduction ischial weight-bearing brace.

2.7 Osteomyelitis

Physeal arrest associated with osteomyelitis is usually thought to be due to infection in the metaphysis or epiphysis directly affecting the physis (Chap. 3). On occasion, however, the osteomyelitis is in the diaphysis, well away from the physis. If immobilization is prolonged, the arrest may be due to vascular insufficiency associated with disuse. The fact that osteomyelitis of the femoral diaphysis is associated with arrest in the proximal tibia [3, 43], as well as in the distal femur, supports this premise.

2.8 Slipped Capital Femoral Epiphysis

In the past, slipped capital femoral epiphysis (SCFE) was sometimes treated by prolonged traction or cast. One 11-year-old boy immobilized in plaster for 7½ months developed arrest of the proximal tibial physis [3].

Physeal arrest of the involved hip is more likely to occur, partly due to disuse. In one series 37 hips were treated with bed rest and traction for relief of symptoms, followed by spica cast immobilization, 8–16 weeks, until the physis reverted from increased width to normal width [44]. Fourteen of the 37 hips (38%) developed premature closure of the physis of the involved hip. Because the proximal femur has little growth remaining in these older children the resulting limb length discrepancy was no more than 2 cm (average 1.1 cm). In a second series, 10 of 17 hips (59%) treated by initial traction to allow pain and spasm to resolve, followed by a one and one-half or a bilateral spica cast (requiring bed rest) for 3–4 months, developed partial or complete physeal arrest of the proximal femur [45]. The high rate of complications, including physeal arrest, resulted in abandonment of the use of the spica cast [45].

2.9 Chemically Induced Immobilization

Induction of rigid immobilization with decamethonium bromide and flaccid immobilization with panuronium bromide in chick embryos *in ovo* for 3 days resulted in greatly reduced limb lengths and decreased width of epiphyses, most marked and more pronounced distally [46]. Could induced prolonged coma in a very young child have a similar effect?

2.10 Author's Perspective

After reading Chaps. 1 and 2 it is easy to conclude that the basic cause of most of the conditions discussed in Chap. 2 are the result of vascular deficiency due to reduced quantity discussed in Chap. 1. The conditions discussed in Chap. 2 are presented separately, because disuse is the primary event that initiates the vascular deprivation. Disuse is mentioned as an adjunct cause of physeal arrest in several other chapters, most notably Chap. 5, Metabolic Injuries, and Chap. 6, Neural Injuries. In these and other injuries it is more difficult to determine the precise role of disuse from the specific injury. Disuse of any part of the body increases risk of complications including growth arrest, and should be as short as possible.

References

Introduction

1. Gillespie JA (1954) The nature of the bone changes associated with nerve injuries and disuse. J Bone Joint Surg 36B(3):464–473
2. Golding JSR (1994) The mechanical factors which influence bone growth. Eur J Clin Nutr 48(Suppl 1):S178–S185
3. Ross D (1948) Disturbance of longitudinal growth associated with prolonged disability of the lower extremity. J Bone Joint Surg Am 30A:103–115

Tuberculosis

4. Barr JS (1947) Tuberculosis of the hip in children (discussion). J Bone Joint Surg 29:905
5. Chandler FA, Fox TA (1949) Amputation for discrepancy of limb length in tuberculosis of the hip. J Bone Joint Surg Am 31A:420–425
6. Gill AB (1947) Tuberculosis of the hip in children (discussion). J Bone Joint Surg 29:906
7. Gill GG (1944) The cause of discrepancy in the length of the limbs following tuberculosis of the hip in children. J Bone Joint Surg 26:272–281
8. Gill GG (1947) Tuberculosis of the hip in children (discussion). J Bone Joint Surg 29:905
9. Kestler OC (1947) Unclassified premature cessation of epiphyseal growth about the knee joint. J Bone Joint Surg Am 29:788–797
10. McCarroll HR, Heath RD (1947) Tuberculosis of the hip in children: certain roentgenographic manifestations, secondary changes in the extremity, and some suggestions for a program of therapy. J Bone Joint Surg Am 29:889–906
11. Parke W, Colvin OS, Almond AH (1949) Premature epiphyseal fusion at the knee in tuberculous disease of the hip. J Bone Joint Surg Br 31B:63–73
12. Sissons HA (1952) Osteoporosis and epiphyseal arrest in joint tuberculosis: an account of the histological changes in involved tissues. J Bone Joint Surg Br 34-B:275–290
13. Slee GC (1966) Premature fusion of the knee epiphyses (abstr). J Bone Joint Surg 48B:589

Poliomyelitis

14. Barr JS (1948) Growth and inequality of leg length in poliomyelitis. N Engl J Med 238:737–743
15. Barr JS, Stinchfield AJ, Reidy JA (1950) Sympathetic ganglionectomy and limb length in poliomyelitis. J Bone Joint Surg Am 32A:793–802
16. Currarino G (1966) Premature closure of epiphyses in the metatarsals and knees: a sequel of poliomyelitis. Radiology 87:424–428
17. Goetz RH, Du Toit JG, Swart BH (1955) Vascular changes in poliomyelitis and the effect of sympathectomy on bone growth. Acta Med Scand Suppl 306:56–83

18. Gullickson G, Olson M, Kottke FJ (1950) The effect of paralysis of one lower-extremity on bone growth. Arch Phys Med Rehabil 31:392–400
19. Harris RI, McDonald JL (1936) The effect of lumbar sympathectomy upon the growth of legs paralyzed by anterior poliomyelitis. J Bone Joint Surg 18:35–45
20. Janes JM, Jennings WK Jr (1961) Effect of induced arteriovenous fistula on leg length: 10-year observations. Proc Staff Meet Mayo Clin 36:1–11
21. Kai Lai S, Hahn Sheng P, Kao Wha C, Po Ling L (1994) Partial medial epiphysiodesis for genu valgum in poliomyelitis. J Surg Assoc Republic China 27(2):2261–2267
22. Makin M (1965) Tibio-fibular relationship in paralyzed limbs. J Bone Joint Surg Br 47:500–506
23. Mehta SN, Mukherjee AK (1991) Flexion osteotomy of the femur for genu recurvatum after poliomyelitis. J Bone Joint Surg Br 73(2):200–202
24. Prick JJG (1958) On morbidly changed bloodvessels as the central aspect of the pathological anatomy of poliomyelitis, also in connection with clinical observations. Folia Psychiatr Neurol Neurochir Neerl 61:593–604
25. Ratliff AHC (1959) The short leg in poliomyelitis. J Bone Joint Surg Br 41-B:56–69
26. Ring PA (1958) Prognosis of limb inequality following paralytic poliomyelitis. Lancet 2:1306–1308
27. Ring PA (1957) Shortening and paralysis in poliomyelitis. Lancet 273:980–983
28. Stinchfield AJ, Reidy JA, Barr JS (1949) Prediction of unequal growth of the lower extremities in anterior poliomyelitis. J Bone Joint Surg Am 31A:478–486, 500
29. Troup H (1961) Nervous and vascular influence on longitudinal growth of bone. An experimental study on rabbits. Acta Orthop Scand Suppl 51:1–78
30. Westin GW, Dingeman RD, Gausewitz SH (1988) The results of tenodesis of the tendo achillis to the fibula for paralytic pes calcaneus. J Bone Joint Surg Am 70(3):320–328

Diaphyseal Fracture

31. Beals RK (1990) Premature closure of the physis following diaphyseal fractures. J Pediatr Orthop 10:717–720
32. Chapchal G (1979) Late complications of fractures in children. Reconstr Surg Traumatol 17:130–138
33. Gonzalez-Lopez JL (2000) Letter to the editors. J Pediatr Orthop 20:826
34. Hresko MT, Kasser JR (1989) Physeal arrest about the knee associated with non-physeal fractures in the lower extremity. J Bone Joint Surg Am 71:698–703
35. Hunter LY, Hensinger RN (1978) Premature monomelic growth arrest following fracture of the femoral shaft. J Bone Joint Surg Am 60:850–852
36. Morton KS, Starr DE (1964) Closure of the anterior portion of the upper tibial epiphysis as a complication of tibial-shaft fracture. J Bone Joint Surg Am 46:570–574
37. Navascués JA, Gonzalez-Lopez JL, Lopez-Valverde S, Soleto J, Rodriguez-Durantez JA, Garcia-Trevijano JL (2000) Premature physeal closure after tibial diaphyseal fractures in adolescents. J Pediatr Orthop 20:193–196
38. Poznanski AK (1978) Diagnostic clues in the growing ends of bones. J Can Assoc Radiol 29:7–21
39. Ratliff AHC (1970) Complications after fracture of the femoral neck in children and their treatment (abstr). J Bone Joint Surg 52B:175

Developmental Dislocation of the Hip

40. Botting TDJ, Scrase WH (1965) Premature epiphysial fusion at the knee complicating prolonged immobilization for congenital dislocation of the hip. J Bone Joint Surg Br 47:280–282

Perthes Disease

41. Barnes JM (1980) Premature epiphyseal closure in Perthes' disease. J Bone Joint Surg 62B:432–437
42. Shapiro F (1982) Legg-Calve-Perthes disuse: a study of lower extremity length discrepancies and skeletal maturation. Acta Orthop Scand 53(3):437–444

Osteomyelitis

43. Caffey J (1970) Traumatic cupping of the metaphysis of growing bones. Am J Roentgenol Radium Ther Nucl Med 108:451–460

Slipped Capital Femoral Epiphysis

44. Betz RR, Steel HH, Emper WD, Huss GK, Clancy M (1990) Treatment of slipped capital femoral epiphysis. Spica cast immobilization. J Bone Joint Surg Am 72(4):587–600
45. Meier MC, Meyer LC, Ferguson RL (1992) Treatment of slipped capital femoral epiphysis with a spica cast. J Bone Joint Surg Am 74(10):1522–1529

Chemically Induced Immobilization

46. Osborne AC, Lamb KJ, Lewthwaite JC, Dowthwaite GP, Pitsillides AA (2002) Short-term rigid and flaccid paralyses diminish growth of embryonic chick limbs and abrogate joint cavity formation but differentially preserve pre-cavitated joints. J Musculoskelet Neuronal Interact 2(5):448–456

Infection

3.1 Introduction

This chapter presents the harmful effects of infection on the physis, according to the anatomic site of the infection. The sites of infection include both bones and joints. Osteomyelitis and septic arthritis have many similar features, frequently occur concurrently, and are often reported together [3, 4, 22, 43, 46, 47, 149, 153, 160]. The chapter gives little attention to clinical, imaging, and laboratory evaluation of bone or joint infection in general, since these subjects are well covered in other sources. The diagnosis and treatment of infection are discussed primarily as they pertain to subsequent damage of the physis. Much of the discussion on diagnosis and treatment of both the infection and the complication of physeal arrest in Sect. 3.2 is appropriate for the remaining sections in this chapter and is not repeated.

Infection in the vicinity of the physis places it at risk of injury. Several concerns significantly impact this association: (a) the infection can be due to a variety of microorganisms, each having a different virulence, (b) the age, health and resistance of the host, (c) determination of the precise site of origin of the infection is often difficult or impossible, particularly when the infection is found in both bone and the joint, or in both the metaphysis and epiphysis crossing the physis, (d) concurrent bone and joint infection increases the risk of subsequent physeal damage, and (e) the mechanism by which the infection causes growth plate damage in any specific case is usually unknown.

3.2 Metaphyseal Osteomyelitis

Approximately 70% of osteomyelitis in children originates in the metaphyseal region of long bones [53]. It is often referred to in the literature as hematogenous osteomyelitis [3, 5, 20, 25, 32, 36, 37, 39, 47, 54, 57, 59, 60, 62, 63, 65, 69], implying a vascular transference of a pathogen (bacteremia, septicemia) to bone. Compound fractures, puncture wounds, and surgery are additional sources of infection [8, 36, 46, 66–68, 71, 72]. Blunt trauma or closed fracture as a co-requisite for the development of osteomyelitis may be present in some cases [10, 25, 37, 62]. The focus of this section is the association of *acute* metaphyseal osteomyelitis to subsequent physeal injury.

3.2.1 The Organism

Any bacterium, virus, or fungus can cause osteomyelitis. Little is known, however, concerning the correlation of a specific organism to the occurrence or incidence of subsequent physeal abnormality. The most frequent pathogen causing both osteomyelitis and subsequent physeal damage is *Staphylococcus aureus*, followed by *β-hemolytic streptococcus*. Residual physeal damage may be greater following *Staph. aureus* osteomyelitis than *streptococcal* osteomyelitis [21], but statistical analysis is lacking. Other micro-organisms reported to be associated with physeal arrest are *Variola* virus (small pox) [12–14], *Mycobacterium tuberculosis* [11, 52, 73], *Escherichia coli* [5, 46], *Klebsiella* species [46], and *Salmonella* species [7]. If cultures fail to isolate a pathogenic organism, the likelihood of physeal arrest is less [36].

Luckily smallpox is no longer prevalent. When it was, children who survived sometimes developed unique bone lesions, osteomyelitis variolosa [13, 14]. This condition frequently developed detachment or destruction of the epiphysis, which seemed to be the result of "transverse metaphysitis". Epiphyses were tilted, and in some cases completely displaced. The loose bodies so formed gradually diminish in size, and eventually become absorbed, or extruded through sinuses. Antibiotics administered to patients initially or after the onset of complications had no influence on the course. Premature physeal closure and joint ankylosis were common. Bones so affected (in descending order of frequency) were the radius, ulna, humerus, metatarsals, fibula, os calcis, tibia, talus, metacarpals, and phalanges.

Physeal arrest associated with *Salmonella* osteomyelitis is usually, but not always, due to sickle cell ischemia [7], rather than abscess, and is therefore reported in Sect. 1.4, Vascular Deficiency. Cupping (Sect. 1.5) is frequent.

3.2.2 Age of the Patient

Clinical characteristics of acute hematogenous osteomyelitis varies according to the age of the patient. Osteomyelitis in the infant (0–1 year), child (1–16 years), and adult (16 years plus) constitute three separate clinical entities with few features in common [59]. Infants have greater propensity to develop osteomyelitis than children, and acquire more serious growth deformities [4–6, 16, 24, 30, 32, 33, 43, 57, 60]. Children with osteomyelitis have fewer general sequelae [30], and permanent damage to the physis is less common [59].

The differences in pathogenesis between infants and children include: (1) in most newborns the infection, especially the severe forms of osteomyelitis, is acquired in the newborn nursery [33], (2) infants have less natural immunity to infection, due to changing patterns of immune status and response [16, 43], (3) pathogens resistant to antibiotics are more common in newborns, (4) the presence of blood vessels crossing the physis in children less than 2 years of age (Sect. 3.5), (5) the bone trabeculae in the metaphysis in infants are weak compared to that of the child and are more readily broken down by the inflammatory process [44], (6) penetration from the primary focus in bone into the joint occurs more often among infants less than 1 month of age [32], (7) younger children may be more susceptible to physeal chondrocyte destruction [30], and (8) more rapid absorption of dead bone and formation of new bone in infants. These differences could affect principles of treatment, such as the urgency of surgery, and the subsequent development of growth arrest.

3.2.3 Pathogenesis

Acute septicemia invokes immediate slowing of chondroplasia in the germinal zone of the physis, with more extensive calcification in the zone of provisional calcification than is normal. As growth resumes this may leave a "growth arrest line" as a marker in the metaphysis [1].

Seeding of pathogens in the metaphysis by the septicemia, is the underlying etiology of most cases of osteomyelitis in both infants and children [24, 53]. The metaphysis has a lively blood flow which slows down in the finer capillaries of the juxtaphyseal arterioles (Fig. 1.2) and the wide venous sinusoids which follow [18, 32, 43, 59]. The earliest evidence of involvement is the accumulation of inflammatory cells and bacteria in the primary spongiosa [43]. Pathogens congregate in the sluggish circulation of the larger metaphyseal sinusoidal veins where defensive mechanisms are poor. In many cases the infection remains confined to the metaphysis and does not disturb growth [30, 43].

If the metaphyseal infection is allowed to continue and become well established, it follows the path of least resistance and may spread in one of several directions [24, 44]. The highly vascular and actively remodeling chondro-osseous skeleton is characterized by relatively larger cancellous spaces. This allows the infection to develop more rapidly and to spread latitudinally by osteolytic destruction of the primary spongiosa. Penetration into the subperiosteal space may occur through metaphyseal cortical fenestrations without necessarily causing a large cortical defect [43, 44].

Physeal arrest due to metaphyseal osteomyelitis may occur by one of several discrete mechanisms, is highly variable, and is mostly due to differences in circulatory patterns [43, 59]. The interval between infection and physeal arrest may be years. Typically, there is no residual infection at the time the arrest is discovered. Explaining the pathophysiology requires some speculation (Fig. 3.1) [43].

3.2.3.1 Transphyseal Vessels

Infants and children less than 2 years of age, whose epiphyses are mainly composed of cartilage, may have a few transphyseal vessels which could allow direct transference of infection through the physis into the epiphysis [3, 18, 29, 32, 43, 44, 46, 59]. Even though the normal blood flow into the physis is from the epiphysis (Figs. 1.1 and 1.2), osteomyelitis may spread retrogradely from the metaphyseal sinusoids along these transphyseal vessels into the epiphyseal vascular system (Fig. 3.1a). The epiphyseal arcade of vessels arborize at the top of the proliferative zone of the physis in a "rake-like" configuration into small arterioles. These arterioles divide into capillaries which extend into terminal spurs before turning back as larger veins. The infectious products effectively occludes these arborizing epiphyseal arterioles and capillaries, causing ischemia of the physis, resulting in death of the chondrocytes in the germinal and proliferating zones [43, 44, 56]. When the inflammatory process occupies both the metaphyseal and epiphyseal sides of the growth plate, rendering it ischemic, the physis becomes susceptible to direct destruction [44, 46]. As a result of this vascular connection, the infection can also spread from the metaphysis through the epiphysis into the joint in infants [29, 43]. In children over age 2 years there usually are no transphyseal vessels and the avascular cartilaginous physis is regarded as a barrier [29, 43, 59, 106] In these children the effectiveness of the physis as a barrier to the spread of infection is confirmed by the less common extension to the epiphysis, destruction of the physis, or growth disturbance [53, 106].

3.2.3.2 Direct Chondrolysis

A second pathway is the spread of a purulent abscess in the metaphysis to the physis directly by chondrolysis, rather than spread along a vessel (Fig. 3.1b). The inflammatory process fills the cell columns, destroying the transverse septa and replacing the chondrocytes [43]. Because of the excellent resistance of the physis to infection, direct infection to the germinal cell layer occurs only occasionally [56]. However, the possibility

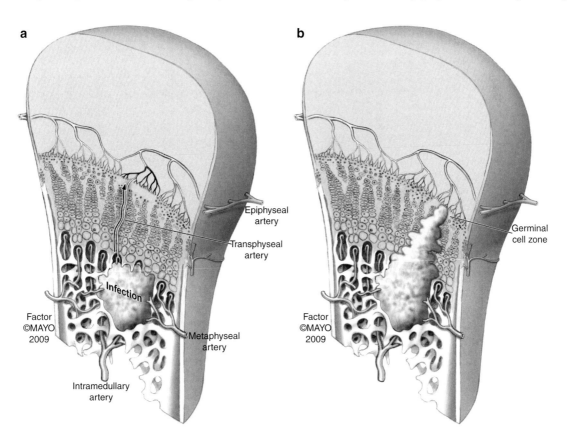

Fig. 3.1 Pathways metaphyseal osteomyelitis affects the physis. A metaphyseal abscess can affect the physis by five pathways: (**a**) Transphyseal blood vessels (present in some physes from birth to age 2 years) allow vascular extension of bacteria and inflammatory cells to cross the physis. The epiphyseal arcade of vessels becomes occluded and cause ischemia of the physis. (**b**) Direct destruction of the germinal cell zone of the physis by chondrolysis. If the vascular arcade is unaffected, the remaining physis may continue to grow relatively normally. (**c**) Lateral extension of the abscess in the primary spongiosa and or the hypertrophic zone of the physis promotes mechanical loosening (slipping) of the epiphysis. (**d**) Lateral extension through the cortex into the subperiosteal space where the metaphysis is completely extra articular (e.g., the proximal tibia). The epiphyseal vessels are externally compressed or internally infected causing thrombosis in the epiphyseal arcade and ischemia of the physis. (**e**) Lateral extension through the cortex and subperiosteal space where the metaphysis is intraarticular (e.g., the proximal femur). The infection extends into the joint. Increased joint pressure can compress the epiphyseal vessels, or the intraarticular sepsis can enter the epiphyseal vessels

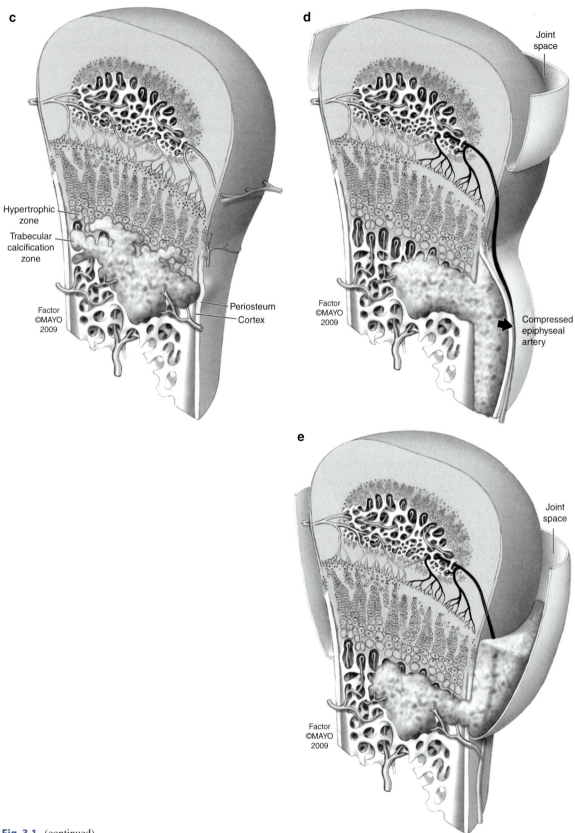

Fig. 3.1 (continued)

that the physis was preemptively rendered ischemic by transphyseal or epiphyseal vascular invasion, and thus more susceptible to chondrolysis, must be considered [43]. It is surprising how few authors implicate direct chondrolysis [30, 43, 44]. Siffert stated that direct bacterial invasion of the physis from the metaphysis is extremely rare [56]. Nothing is recorded relating this mechanism to the age of the patient.

3.2.3.3 Lateral Extension with Slipping of the Epiphysis

Lateral or centrifugal extension of a metaphyseal abscess in the zone of trabecular calcification and hypertrophic zone of the physis is associated with variable osteolysis, with or without cortical perforation and periosteal stripping (Fig. 3.1c) [43]. This promotes mechanical loosening of the epiphysis and predisposes to complete separation and slipping. This uncommon occurrence is found most often in the proximal femur, less often in the distal femur [4, 44], proximal tibia [44], and distal humerus [23]. These slipped epiphyses do not necessarily develop growth arrest because the germinal cell layer is spared.

3.2.3.4 Spread to Compress or Enter the Epiphyseal Vessels

At any age the infection most commonly spreads from its metaphyseal origin by way of the Haversian system through fenestrations in the thin peripheral cortical bone to the subperiosteal space [24, 29, 30, 43, 53, 106]. The loosely attached periosteum is dissected from the cortical bone, and the consequent subperiosteal abscess may rupture into the soft tissues without necrosis of the shaft [24, 55]. This process progresses rapidly so that gross sequestration is uncommon [24].

When the metaphysis is extra-articular (as in the proximal tibia) the tense subperiosteal infection may elevate the periosteum, stretching and compressing the epiphyseal vessels in the soft tissues thereby reducing the blood supply to the epiphysis (Fig 3.1d), or enter the epiphyseal vessels to occlude the blood supply to the physis.

3.2.3.5 Spread to the Joint

When the metaphysis is intra-articular (as in the proximal femur), the subperiosteal abscess may perforate directly into the joint space (Fig. 3.1e) [16, 29, 30, 32, 43, 44, 53, 56, 106]. The ensuing suppurative arthritis increases inarticular pressure compressing the epiphyseal vessels sufficiently to cause physeal ischemia, or alternatively may enter the epiphyseal circulation supplying the physis [30, 38, 43]. Children who present with combined osteomyelitis and septic arthritis have a greater potential for subsequent growth disturbance [57]. Neonates (age 1–28 days) are the most likely to have concomitant joint involvement: 12 of 17 (71%) in one series, and half of these had residual growth deficit [61].

Many physes (for example the proximal humerus) are both intra and extra articular. Depending on the configuration of the capsular attachment, the metaphyseal abscess may decompress into either the joint or the subperiosteal space or both [43]. In these physes, physeal arrest could occur with the mechanism prop-osed in either Fig. 3.1d or e. These last two mechanisms are by far the most commonly mentioned in the literature.

3.2.3.6 Blunt Trauma

Blunt or closed trauma, with or without fracture, may be an underlying etiologic factor with any of the five mechanisms described above [10, 25]. The association of blunt trauma to the development of osteomyelitis [37, 62, 112] is reasoned as follows. Bacteremia is frequent in infants and children and rarely causes bone or joint infection. Blunt trauma, however, causes soft tissue swelling, occasional closed fracture, decreased local blood flow, and a possible lowered resistance to infection [62]. If bacteremia is present at the same time as the trauma, bone abscess formation is more likely to develop (Fig. 3.2). In one series of 75 children of all ages with acute hematogenous osteomyelitis, there was a history of trauma in 41 cases (55%) [63]. Most reported series of osteomyelitis do not record concurrent blunt trauma or do not follow the patients long enough to document subsequent growth arrest.

3.2.3.7 Avascular Necrosis

In infants both increased density and disappearance of the femoral head may be forms of "avascular necrosis", and occur occasionally following both osteomyelitis and septic arthritis. These cases are likely an aseptic process, due to compression of blood vessels supplying the femoral capital epiphysis, rather than a spread of infection through the bone [3, 27]. Lack of histologic or autopsy material makes pathogenesis conjectural [3]. Physeal arrest with either occurrence has been recorded in a minority of cases [3, 27].

3.2.3.8 Summary of Pathogenesis

In summary, a metaphyseal septic process can damage physeal chondrocytes directly by chondrolysis, or indirectly by ischemia of the epiphyseal arcade of vessels [43, 55]. The prognosis may be better when ischemia (rather than direct lysis) is the cause of physeal damage [55]. The pathomechanics by which the metaphyseal osteomyelitis causes physeal damage is rarely determined in a given case. While it is recognized that osteomyelitis in infants varies clinically from that occurring in children, the pathomechanisms in either group have remained speculative due to a paucity of substantiating pathologic material [44]. There is a need for further investigation of the pathomechanics of infectious processes near the growth plate as they relate to subsequent growth disturbances [30].

3.2.4 Pathologic Anatomy

Children who develop long-term growth disturbance often have extensive tissue damage during active infection, but not all children with initial extensive tissue damage have growth disturbance [30]. If the physeal damage is localized to a small area, the dead portion of the physis may be reparable. Undamaged regions of the discoid growth plate may expand horizontally into the damaged area by centripetal expansion. This depends on the amount and location of damage and the state of epiphyseal maturation. New peripheral expansion may also occur, and may lead to the development of unusual physeal contours [43].

Physeal abnormalities caused by metaphyseal osteomyelitis include premature complete or partial closure, horizontal dissolution of the hypertrophic zone of the physis with or without epiphyseal displacement (Fig. 3.1c), and longitudinal transphyseal extension across all layers of the physis (Sect. 3.5, Fig. 3.1b).

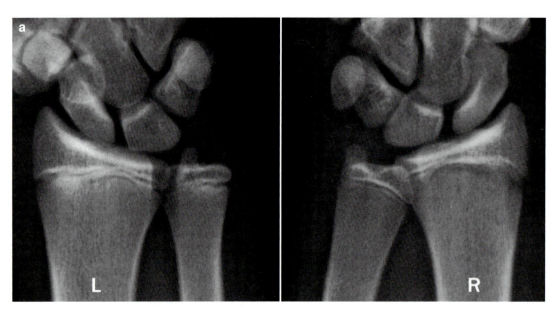

Fig. 3.2 Osteomyelitis following blunt trauma. This 13 year 9 month old boy was struck on the radial side of his right radius while playing football. Pain at the site of impact subsided promptly, but returned a few hours later and continued for the next 6 days. Roentgenograms taken at 6 days post injury were negative and the wrist was placed in a splint. The pain persisted and 3 days later a short arm cast was applied. Eleven days post injury "pain medication" was started. (**a**) Thirteen days post injury the hand began to swell, the temperature was 104°F, and the patient was given IM penicillin. The cast was removed. The distal forearm was swollen. Roentgenograms revealed demineralization of the metaphysis on the radial side of the distal right radius. The diagnosis of osteomyelitis was made and the patient given Ampicillin 500 mg q.i.d., and Vigramycin 100 mg q 12 h orally. (**b**) Fifteen days post injury the patient held the wrist in 10° flexion, extension of the fingers was painful, and there was redness and "extreme tenderness" on the radial side of the distal forearm. The WBC was 15,000 with 82% neutrophils, and the sedimentation rate was 95. There was increased lytic destruction extending to the medial side of the distal radial metaphysis. (**c**) Sixteen days post injury the patient was taken to surgery. Thick yellow pus was found within tendon sheaths, subperiosteally for several inches proximal to the physis, and within the metaphysis. An estimated 20 cc of pus was removed. The physis was visible and was cleaned with irrigation and gauze wipes. The wound was irrigated freely and packed with conforming gauze soaked in liquid furacin. The cultures returned *Staph. aureus*. Four days later the wound was clean and was closed. A forearm splint was applied. Recovery was progressive, uncomplicated, and complete. (**d**) At age 16 years 7 months, 2 years 10 months post injury the forearm and hand were clinically normal. The forearms were of equal length and there was no radial-ulnar variance. Note: The association of trauma and osteomyelitis is strong in this case and best explained by transient bacteremia present at the time of injury. At the time of injury there was an estimated 2 cm growth remaining in the distal radius [48], yet no growth impairment occurred. This case illustrates strong resilience of the physis, despite close contact to osteomyelitis

3.2 Metaphyseal Osteomyelitis

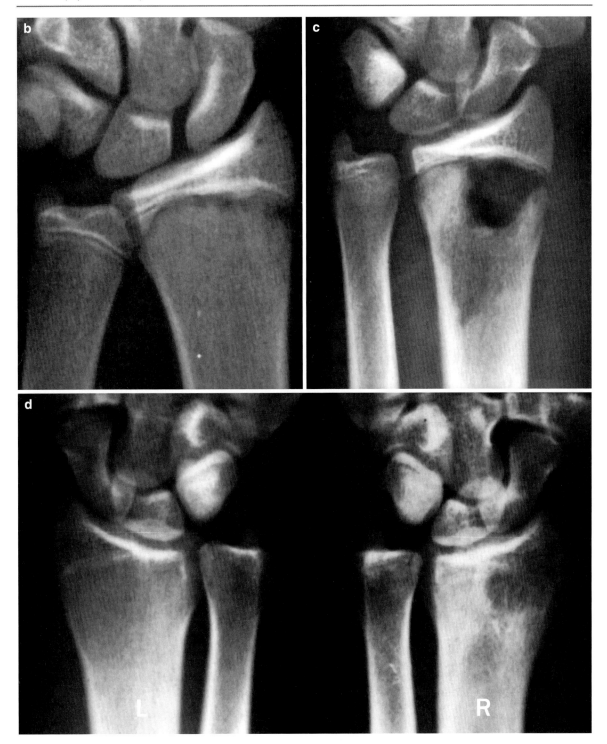

Fig. 3.2 (continued)

Premature complete physeal closure is uncommon and may take months or years to develop. The subsequent relative bone shortening is dependent on the age of closure. The bones most commonly requiring treatment are those with the most growth: the femur, tibia/fibula, or humerus.

Premature partial physeal closure (a physeal bar) may occur at any age during growth and often cannot be predicted (Fig. 3.3a–g). The size and location of the bar determine the clinical deformity [49]. Partial central physeal closure is relatively common following metaphyseal osteomyelitis. This results in diminished

Fig. 3.3 Metaphyseal osteomyelitis followed by premature partial physeal arrest. This infant girl had a cut-down on the right ankle saphenous vein on her second day of life. (**a**) On the 16th day of life there was swelling and tenderness over the right distal femur and faint roentgenographic lysis of the distal femoral metaphysis. The WBC was 19,900, the ESR 47. (**b**) Incision and drainage on the 17th day of life revealed pus confined within the center of the metaphysis. This intraoperative roentgenogram was taken to document the most distal penetration of the curette, approximately 5 mm from contact with the physis. Cultures grew *Staph. aureus*. Antibiotics were given. (**c**) At age 36 days the patient was doing well and the distal femur had subperiosteal new bone. (**d**) Scanogram at age 1 year 0 months shows the right femur 2 mm shorter than the left, but growing well. (**e**) The new sclerotic bone indicating growth in the right metaphysis is incomplete and the physis is irregular. (**f**) Scanogram at age 2 years 0 months shows both femora growing and equal in length. The metaphysis and physis are more irregular on the right than the left. The parents were advised to return in 1 year. (**g**) The patient and parents returned nearly 3 years later when leg malalignment became obvious. Photograph at age 4 years 11 months shows right genu valgum and pelvis tilt down on the right. (**h**) Scanogram at the same time as g shows right distal femoral valgus angulation and relative shortening of the femur (1.2 cm). Note the proximal femoral shaft–femoral articular condyle angle of 62°, due in part to bowing of the femur and in part to valgus angulation of the epiphysis. Both are due to impaired growth of the physis. (**i**) Tomogram of right knee confirms a mildly excentric central bar. (**j**) Age 5 years 0 months; an operative roentgenogram during removal of the central bar through a window in the cortex [48, 49]. There was no sign of infection and cultures were subsequently negative. The metal pin was used to determine medial extent of the bar excision and a rough estimate of the size of the bar, and was removed after completion of the roentgenogram. The cavity was filled with cranioplast. (**k**) Close-up of a scanogram 5 months post operatively. The physis remained open. The two metal markers inserted at the time of operation are now 28 mm apart. The proximal femoral shaft-femoral condyle angle is essentially unchanged. Note that the cranioplast lucency is very close to the proximal marker. (**l**) Scanogram almost 4 years postoperatively (age 8 years 11 months) shows the metal markers 83 mm apart. Both femora have grown 1.3 cm in the past year, and equally since operation (the discrepancy remains 1.2 cm). The femoral shaft-femoral condyle angle is unchanged (compare with (**i**)). The orientation of the metal markers to each other remains unchanged. (**m**) Close-up of the scanogram of the right knee in (**l**). The physis is open throughout. Because this is taken from a scanogram, there is no magnification of the distance between the two metal markers. Note that the cranioplast plug initially stayed with the epiphysis, as evidenced by the increased distance of the plug from the proximal metal marker (compare with (**k**)). Later, the epiphysis grew away from the plug, as evidenced by the increased distance of plug from the distal metal marker. Surgical physeal arrests were performed on the normal left distal femur and proximal tibia at age 12 years 0 months. (**n**) Photograph at age 13 years 6 months. The legs are straight and body alignment is good. The right knee and pelvis are lower than the left. (**o**) Scanogram at same time as (**n**) showed the right lower extremity 2.9 cm shorter than the left. All physes were closed. The left femur was surgically shortened 3 cm. (**p**) At age 14 years 9 months a scanogram showed the right leg was 1 mm longer and the metal markers were 11.2 cm apart. There is mild knee height discrepancy. All metal was removed 15 months after insertion. Note: Several items warrant further comment. The first is that the faint osteopenia along the metaphyseal border of the physis in (**a**), possibly due to vascular deficiency, preceded the roentgenographic lytic area representing the osteomyelitis in the center of the metaphysis (**b**). Second is that care was taken to avoid surgical damage to the physis (**b**). These two observations suggest that the subsequent bar was due to vascular deficiency rather than infection or surgical encroachment. Third is the need for close follow-up. At age 2 years the parents ignored the recommendation to return at age 3 years. When they noticed right genu valgum at age 4 years 11 months, the bar, the deformity, and the relative shortening were well established (**g, h**). Fourth, the long duration between surgery and the appearance of the physeal bar, and absence of infection at time of bar removal, also supports the supposition that the bar was secondary to vascular deficiency rather than direct infection. Fifth, the bar excision was successful despite the underlying etiology of osteomyelitis. Unfortunately, the distance between the metal markers was first roentgenographically measured 5 months post bar excision. The amount of growth in these 5 months cannot therefore be determined, but it is well known that greatest acceleration of growth after bar excision occurs in the first year [48]. Post bar excision documented growth of the distal right femoral physis was 8.4 cm (11.2–2.8), not counting the amount of undocumented growth during the first 5 months post bar excision. Sixth, the valgus angulation of the right distal femur corrected well following bar excision (compare (**g**) and (**n**), and (**h**) and (**o**)). No osteotomy was necessary. Seventh, the timing of contralateral physeal arrest is difficult. The contralateral epiphyseodesis performed at age 12 years 0 months had little effect because this patient ceased growth early, sometime before age 13 years 6 months. Earlier arrest would have equalized the extremity lengths, and negated surgical contralateral femoral shortening. Eighth, the decision for treatment of relatively mild residual leg length inequality is subjective. At the time of growth completion the discrepancy was 2.9 cm, the legs were straight, and pelvic tilt was mild. Counseling the patient and parents in this situation was difficult. The choices were doing nothing, wearing a shoe lift for life, or surgically equalizing the leg lengths. The parents chose the latter and a good result was obtained, but it required two operations (bone shortening on the normal femur and metal removal). Was this the correct decision and what weight should be given to the parents in the decision making process? (Reproduced from Peterson [49], with permission and additional follow-up)

3.2 Metaphyseal Osteomyelitis

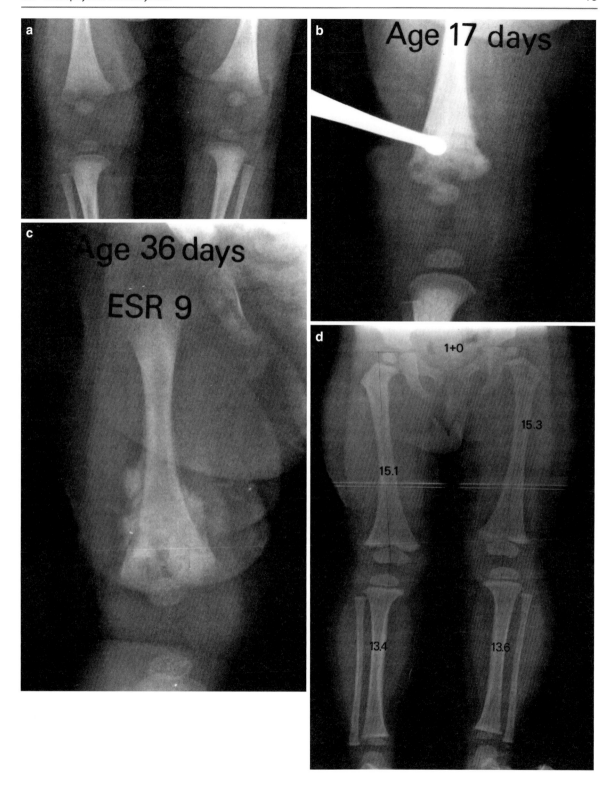

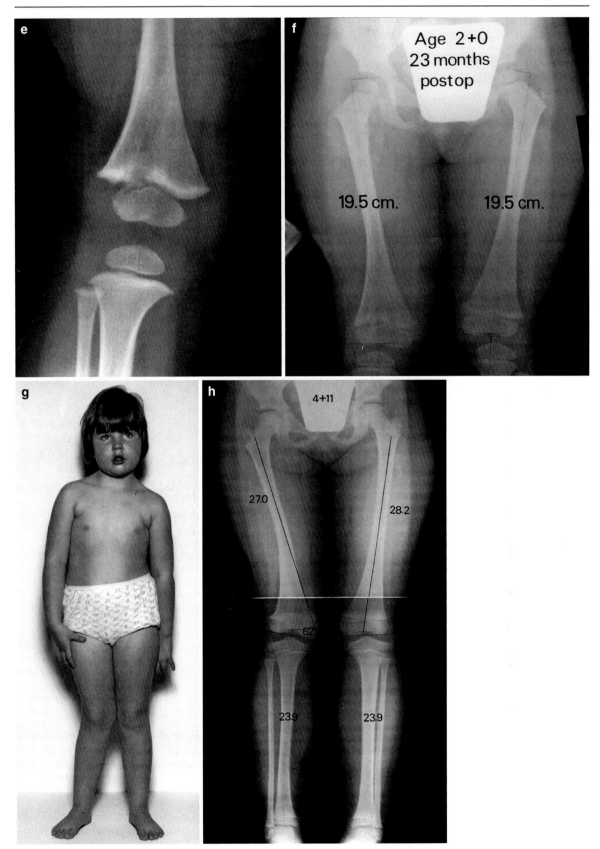

Fig. 3.3 (continued)

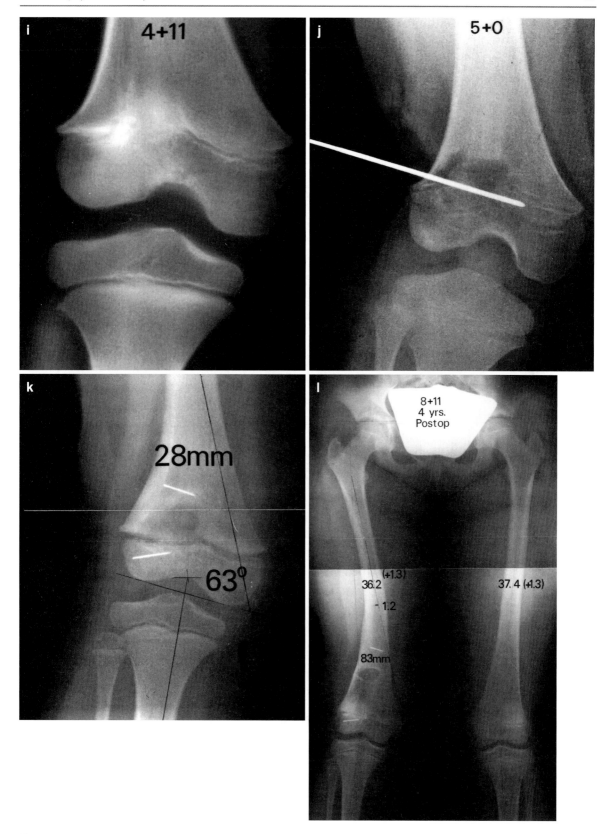

Fig. 3.3 (continued)

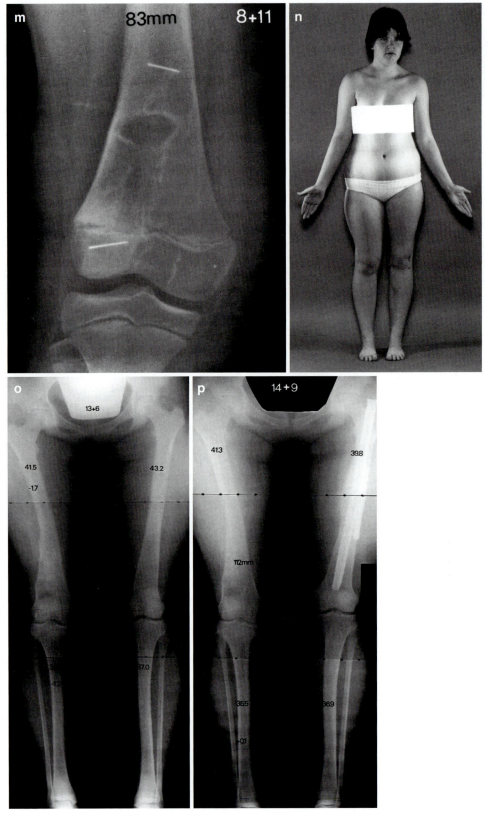

Fig. 3.3 (continued)

longitudinal growth, frequent cupping (Sect. 1.5) [9, 12], and angular deformity if the central closure is eccentric (Fig. 3.3f–h) [2, 30, 65].

Displacement or complete separation of the epiphysis from the metaphysis is an uncommon complication of metaphyseal osteomyelitis and occurs primarily in the neonatal age group [4, 14, 16, 23, 24, 43, 44, 56], and less common in older children [17]. The separation occurs on the metaphyseal side of the physis (Fig. 4.1c) and may result in significant displacement of the epiphysis. Accompanying local cortical perforation and periosteal stripping can significantly aid the slipping [44, 56]. The entire juxtaepiphyseal metaphysis and circumferential cortex may be involved. The most common sites are the proximal and distal femur [4, 44]. A sometimes difficult differential diagnosis is traumatic epiphyseal separation, especially after complicated delivery such as breech presentation and cesarean section [4].

Increased sclerosis of the femoral capital epiphysis following osteomyelitis of the femoral neck is usually referred to as "avascular necrosis". It is aseptic, due to interference with the vascular supply rather than to the spread of infection into the joint [27]. The roentgenographic changes so closely resemble those of Perthes disease that osteomyelitis has been proposed as the etiology of Perthes disease [27, 147]. The roentgenographic increased density is only recognizable 6–8 weeks after the onset of infection, supporting the vascular etiology. Healing occurs with variable femoral head deformity, and in a minority of cases, physeal arrest. The danger of avascular necrosis demands an aggressive approach to the management of femoral neck osteomyelitis. Drainage of the primary focus should be forthwith and include inspection of the joint [27].

In summary, the nature and degree of growth disturbance following metaphyseal osteomyelitis is related to damage directly to the physeal cartilage or by ischemia of the arcading arterial system of the chondroepiphysis [43]. This determines (1) the amount of physis destroyed (relative to the total area of the plate), (2) the anatomic location of the destroyed area of the physis (i.e., central vs. peripheral), and (3) the degree of concomitant destruction of the hyaline cartilage of the chondroepiphysis (Sect. 3.3).

3.2.5 The Bone Involved

The incidence of osteomyelitis in each bone closely parallels the amount of growth contribution of the physes of that bone [43]. Similarly, the incidence of physeal arrest also closely correlates with the amount of growth contributed by the physes of that bone. Thus, of all long bone physeal closures following osteomyelitis, the proximal and distal femur are involved in almost 50% of cases [6, 20, 34, 55, 101], followed in frequency by the proximal and distal tibia [31, 33, 58], the proximal humerus [23, 26, 46], distal radius [8, 20, 33, 34, 40, 45, 46, 50, 58], distal ulna [20], distal fibula [34], metacarpals and phalanges [12, 34], and metatarsals [54]. The majority of infections involve only a single bone [57]. Multifocal metaphyseal osteomyelitis occurs occasionally [5, 12–14, 27, 34, 40, 43, 44, 46, 55, 61]. In one series of 100 children of all ages, seven had more than one lesion [60]. In another series of neonates age 1–28 days, 7 of 17 (41%) had multiple bone infections [60]. Multifocal physeal arrest as a result of multiple site acute osteomyelitis is less common and less frequently documented [12–14, 34, 43, 44, 46, 55]. Multifocal physeal arrest associated with multifocal septic arthritis is more common (Sect. 3.9).

3.2.6 Diagnosis

The importance of establishing an etiologic diagnosis from material aspirated or obtained at the time of incision and drainage of the infected bone and joint cannot be overemphasized. All joint fluid specimens should be sent immediately to the laboratory for microbiologic studies and cell count. Bone and tissue specimens should be sent to the microbiology laboratory for appropriate stains, cultures, and sensitivity testing, and to the pathology laboratory for histopathology. When the patient's history, physical examination, roentgenograms, or intraoperative findings suggest an unusual infection, additional cultures and histopathological techniques for mycobacteria, fungi, and other microorganisms may be indicated. Failure to submit surgical specimens at the time of initial incision and drainage may result in unnecessary procedures to obtain additional microbiologic and histologic material, or may result in therapeutic failure despite adequate debridement [19].

3.2.7 Treatment of Infection

Early detection and treatment of bone and joint infection are the best ways to avoid or reduce the complication of growth arrest. The meaning of the word "early" is rarely, and not uniformly, defined [33, 47, 51].

The debates for and against surgical drainage occurred before and continue after the advent of antibiotics [5, 6, 21, 24, 28, 32, 36, 39–41, 43, 46, 53, 54, 56, 57, 59–62, 64, 117].

Prior to the discovery of antibiotics, infants and children with osteomyelitis were frequently very ill and the mortality rate was high [55, 57]. Early surgical drainage of the pus was often life saving and helped prevent or minimize tissue destruction. Healing without sequestration was the desired result. The urgency of surgery was often stressed [23, 42], resulting in the dictum that in pediatric orthopedics the only true surgical emergencies other than trauma, were acute hematogenous osteomyelitis and septic arthritis [15]. Growth disturbance among the survivors was correspondingly high.

With the introduction of penicillin for civilian use (circa 1944), the incidence of mortality and morbidity from acute hematogenous osteomyelitis in children fell precipitously [18, 39, 56, 57, 63]. The emphasis of treatment shifted to early diagnosis by aspiration, followed by intravenous antibiotics [18, 28, 39, 55, 64]. From 1945 to 1951, before penicillin-resistant staphylococci evolved, most cases of acute hematogenous osteomyelitis were treated by antibiotics without surgery [18, 39]. These previous surgical emergencies now became candidates for urgent chemotherapy with more specialized indications for surgical drainage [28, 32, 65]. With the emergence of strains of bacteria resistant to antibiotics there was an increase in incidence of the disease, with more failures of treatment [39, 56]. The reintroduction of early surgery combined with antibiotics became common [5, 32, 36, 60]. Even with a combined antibiotic and surgical approach, subsequent physeal arrest occurred in 20% of 100 cases collected from 1943 to 1970 [36].

Today, osseous limb infections in children remain emergencies [15]. Increased awareness, improving diagnostic techniques [15, 22, 29, 35, 53], and the development of more specific and potent antibiotics, favor treatment by antibiotics without surgery [20, 22, 54, 57]. However, the emergence of more drug resistant organisms shifts the emphasis back to early surgery.

The often unappreciated issue affecting the decision for or against surgical intervention is the stage of the infection at time of presentation. If the diagnosis can be made before roentgenographic evidence of bone destruction, antibiotic therapy without surgery may be successful [36]. In rabbits, roentgenographic lytic changes of osteomyelitis were present in traumatized tibiae 48 h after an intravenous injection of *Staphylococcus aureus* [62]. Unfortunately, human cases in which antibiotics are started early enough to prevent the appearance of detectable bone changes are rarely seen [60]. Antibiotics attack microorganisms. Once leukocyte and tissue debris (pus) have caused bone lysis sufficient to be discernable on a roentgenogram, antibiotics are less accessible to the bacteria, and the abscess cannot be sterilized by the systemic administration of antibiotics [18, 63]. In addition, aspiration is seldom successful in evacuating all of the pus [63]. The concept that the longer the infectious process persists the greater the likelihood of physeal damage, favors early surgical intervention [51]. New imaging techniques aiding early diagnosis, such as scintigraphy [29, 35, 55], CT and MRI [57] have an increasing role to play. In patients with photopenic osteomyelitis, CT and MRI may identify a coexisting abscess requiring drainage [20, 53].

So long as patients present for care with pus already formed, surgical intervention will continue to be necessary. Surgical debridement removes the osteolytic effects of pus and allows better antibiotic access to the bacteria. A wise precaution is to avoid the physis during the surgery (Fig. 3.3b). Delicate operative technique is required to avoid further damage to the physis [52]. If the physis is exposed, wiping it with gauze is less damaging than using a curette [58].

The treatment of separation or displacement of the epiphysis is decompression and debridement of the abscess, followed by reduction of the epiphysis. If reduction cannot be maintained with external immobilization, pins across the physis, despite the presence of infection, have been successful [4]. A large amount of callus can be expected to form around the metaphysis, just as in birth fractures. If discovered early, before the germinal and proliferating cell layers of the physis are affected, and treated vigorously, the prognosis is often surprisingly good due to remodeling [56]. Growth disturbance is rare and deformity is unusual [4].

In summary, if no osseous destruction has occurred and the clinical response to aspiration and antibiotics is good, surgical intervention may not be necessary [36]. The circumstances requiring surgery are when the diagnosis is in doubt, and the aggressive and established cases in which antibiotic therapy alone is insufficient [22, 54, 117]. This includes the presence of roentgenographic osseous destruction, with or without evidence of soft tissue abscess, aspirated pus, or a draining sinus tract [61, 117]. When osteomyelitis is associated with septic arthritis the prognosis is poor, with no improvement even with long term antibiotic therapy [36]. Early, effective radical aspiration, or preferably incision and drainage of the infected bone or joint, are the most conservative procedures for the preservation of blood flow in the affected bone or joint [18, 59]. No antibiotic will reach the foci of infection without the preservation of some local blood flow [59]. Surgical debridement not only facilitates antibiotic delivery, but can also shorten the duration of antibiotic therapy [57, 117]. Osteomyelitis in children should be treated aggressively with both surgical drainage and antibiotics [43, 46, 50].

Morbidity following acute hematogenous osteomyelitis is primarily due to delays in diagnosis and inadequate treatment [57, 60]. The main reason for growth arrest following infection is tardiness of surgical drainage [6, 59, 60]. The relationship of post operative delayed wound closure or continuous suction irrigation to subsequent physeal arrest has not been reported. Physeal arrest associated with prolonged immobilization of patients with osteomyelitis is documented in Sects. 2.2 and 2.7.

Arrest of the physis may occur at any time following infection [55]. Frequently however, it may not become clinically manifest for years (6–12 years in one study [101], and a mean of 9 years in another [46]). Since restitution of growth following osteomyelitis is unpredictable, all infants and children with metaphyseal osteomyelitis need to be followed at least yearly until maturity [46, 60, 101]. The most serious and unhappy long term complication of acute metaphyseal osteomyelitis in infants and children is growth disturbance [58].

3.2.8 Treatment of Physeal Arrest

Treatment of physeal arrest caused by infection is the same as for cases due to fracture. Treatment options are chosen based on the bone and physis involved, the amount of relative shortening, and the age of the patient which determines the amount of growth remaining [48, 49].

Complete physeal closure of large physes is not common following osteomyelitis. Complete closure in the femur or tibia in an older child may need only a shoe lift, or surgical arrest of the contralateral normal physis, or both. In a middle age child bone lengthening (injured side) or bone shortening (contralateral side), or both, are additional options. In a young child repeat lengthening is added to the list. Proximal humerus arrest resulting in relative shortening of 6 cm or more is best treated by surgical lengthening [26, 188]. When one of two paired bones (such as the tibia/fibula or radius/ulna) are involved the result is relative overgrowth of the companion uninfected bone [58]. This usually requires secondary length equalization surgery [8, 40, 45, 46, 50].

Partial physeal arrest (a physeal bar) is more common than complete arrest after infection (Fig. 3.3g–i). It may be peripheral or central. Peripheral partial arrest produces angular deformity which is rarely controlled or corrected by nonoperative treatment, such as bracing [55]. In an older child corrective osteotomy, combined with closure of the remaining physis and of the contralateral physis, is a reasonable solution. In a younger child, excision of the bar has the potential to reestablish growth [101], and allow the angular deformity to correct. Osteotomy, if necessary, can be done concurrently, or later. Concurrent osteotomy may negatively affect the bar excision, and may not be necessary as reestablished growth may correct the angular deformity (Fig. 3.3j–p). Repeat corrective osteotomies (3–6 in each patient in one series [101]) can be avoided if the bar excision is successful. Uncorrected angular deformity resulting in knee instability may require corrective osteotomy combined with knee arthrodesis [55]. Bone lengthening surgery is infrequently necessary [55].

Central partial closure results in relative shortening with little or no angular deformity. The object of treatment is to equalize the bone lengths and avoid cupping (Sect. 1.5) from becoming marked resulting in articular incongruity. This can be done by surgical arrest of the remaining physis of the partially arrested physis combined with arrest and/or shortening of the contralateral normal bone, or by excision of the bar. Successful bar excision may be less predictable than in cases caused by fracture [46], but no statistics exist. Following infection, the bar found at surgery is sometimes larger than anticipated from the preoperative evaluation [44, 46]. An additional fear of bar excision is failure due to recurrent infection. Nevertheless, even though bar excision may be unpredictable it has been successful following osteomyelitis using both fat [31, 46] and cranioplast [48, 49] (Fig. 3.3j) as interposition materials. Bar excision offers the only chance of reestablishing growth, and when successful and combined with arrest of the opposite limb physis, avoids or reduces the amount of bone lengthening or bone shortening (Fig. 3.3n, o). Interestingly, no pus or bacteria have been visualized histologically or cultured from tissue removed at time of bar excision. Does this bolster the theory that the original damage to the physis was vascular rather than infectious?

3.2.9 Stimulation of Growth

Temporary stimulation of growth in a long bone may occur during and shortly after osteomyelitis. This "overgrowth" is attributed to hyperemia of epiphyseal vessels as a result of local inflammation [34, 56, 59, 106]. Articles discussing this phenomenon do not usually separate diaphyseal from metaphyseal osteomyelitis, and follow-up to maturity is rare. The patient age at time of surgical drainage has no bearing on the extent of overgrowth [65]. Leaving the operative incision open to drain was associated with cavitation and sequestration in a number of limbs, with resulting overgrowth [63].

In one series of 100 patients, 32 had some increased length of the infected bone compared with its contralateral member [60]. In no case was the increase more than 2 cm. In another series, 1–3 cm increase in length occurred in 13 of 24 bones (54%) before the penicillin era, and an increase of no more than 1 cm in 82 patients treated after 1947 with penicillin [63].

When only one of two paired bones is infected (for example the tibia or fibula), the increase in length affects both bones equally [63, 65]. This confirms a more general vascular influence. Stimulation ceases when the inflammatory phase is over and osseous vascularity is restored to normal [56, 60]. A gradual correction then occurs. Permanent increase in bone length due to physeal stimulation from osteomyelitis has not been noted [39, 56].

3.2.10 Metaphyseal-Equivalent Osteomyelitis

Approximately 30% of cases of metaphyseal hematogenous osteomyelitis occur in metaphyseal-equivalent sites [53, 57, 69]. Metaphyseal-equivalent locations are those which have a cartilagenous physis adjacent to metaphyseal bone, but no epiphysis. They include flat and irregular bones such as the pelvis (Fig. 3.4a–d), calcaneus, scapula, talus, patella, sternum, vertebrae, carpal and tarsal bones, and mandible; in other words, all bones other than tubular bones. The vascular anatomy of the metaphysis and physis in these locations is comparable to that in long bones and results in sluggish

Fig. 3.4 Metaphyseal-equivalent osteomyelitis of the ischium with arrest of the triradiate cartilage. This newborn male was normal at a 2 week check-up. (a) At age 4 weeks he was noted to hold the left hip in flexion and abduction and the buttock was mildly swollen and discolored ("*black* and *blue*"). Roentgenographs were reported normal. In retrospect the left ischium is more wide than the right and has irregular lysis and sclerosis. A better quality film would have been helpful. There is periosteal new bone formation on the left pubis. (b) At age 6 weeks the left buttock was hugely swollen. The left femur was held in marked flexion and abduction, and the hip had limited motion. The groin was not swollen or tender. Roentgenographs showed the left ischium to be wider than the right with patchy sclerosis and a round lytic area (*arrow*). The patient was hospitalized and given ampicillin, oxacillin, and gentamycin intravenously. The temperature varied between 37.0°C. to 38.0°C. (c) Three days later pus began to drain from a sinus tract on the inferior aspect of the left buttock (*arrow*; the patient's body is on the *right*, the *left* leg is vertical). (d) A CT scan showed osteolysis, sclerosis, and deformity of the left ischium, and swelling of the left buttock. An incision was made over the draining osteum and the sinus tract followed to the ischium. The gluteus muscle was white and did not contract well. The lateral wall of the ischium was nonexistent. Debris and pus were removed. The hip joint, triradiate cartilage, and ileum were not directly involved. The wound was packed and a figure-of-eight soft dressing applied. Cultures revealed *Staph. aureus* and the antibiotics were changed to vancomycin. (e) The drainage site was closed secondarily at age 8 weeks. The triradiate cartilage is open and the hip is located. (f) At age 10 months he was standing, beginning to take a few steps, and had no discernable pain. He had been wearing a Craig abduction splint full time. The left triradiate cartilage is indistinct, the femoral neck is valgus and the femoral head is subluxated. At age 11 months a proximal femoral varus derotation osteotomy was done. (g) At age 1 year 3 months the ischium is sclerotic and the triradiate cartilage indistinct. With the legs abducted the femoral head is well located. The triradiate physis is beginning to close. (h) At age 3 years 2 months the left triradiate cartilage is closed and the acetabulum is shallow. A second proximal femoral varus derotation osteotomy was done. (i) At age 7 years 1 month the patient was normally active and asymptomatic, but had a bizarre gait with marked pelvic obliquity and adduction of the left leg. The left hip is lateralized and the femoral head poorly covered. (j) A Chiari osteotomy was performed at age 7 years 4 months. (k) At age 12 years 1 month he was doing remarkably well clinically. He had no pain and was a fast runner compared with his sixth grade classmates. There was 1 cm leg length discrepancy, significant pelvic obliquity, and a marked Trendelenburg gait. The ischium is underdeveloped, the acetabulum shallow, the femoral head is poorly covered, and the femoral neck is in valgus. The parents declined further surgery. (l) At age 20 years 6 months he remained pain free, had an abnormal gait and a clinical 1 cm relative shortening of the left lower extremity. The most recent scanograms showed the left femur 3 mm longer than the right and the tibiae equal in length. When weight bearing the left hip adducts, producing contact between the ischium and lesser trochanter which have hypertrophied and formed a false joint. He declined additional treatment

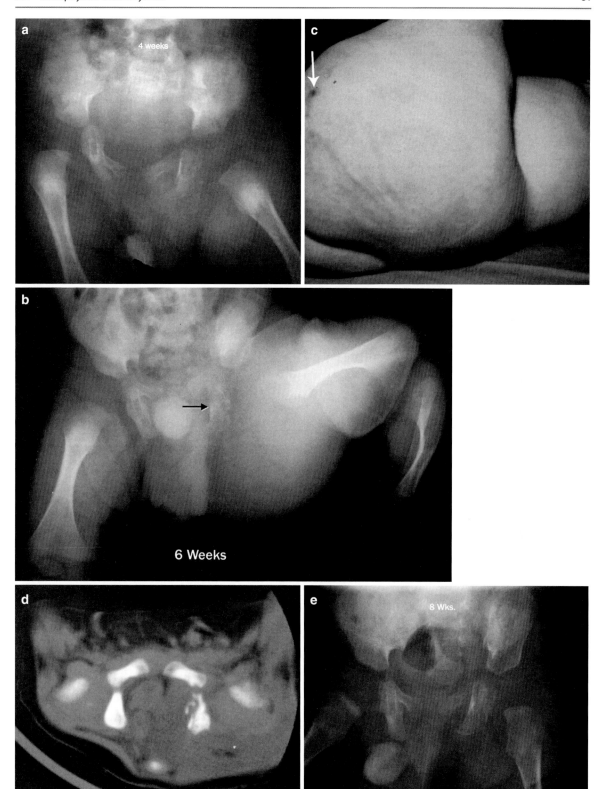

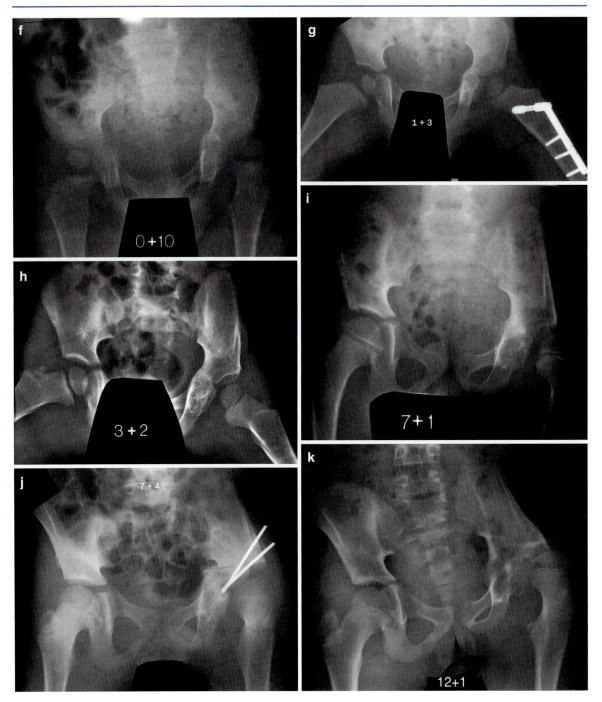

Fig. 3.4 (continued)

3.3 Epiphyseal Osteomyelitis

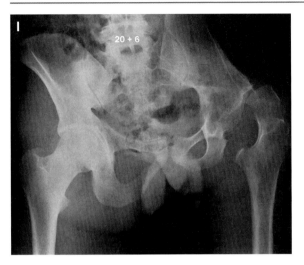

Fig. 3.4 (continued)

end-arterial blood flow [35, 53, 59]. Infection in these sites originates in subchondral metaphyseal areas [69] and is more likely to be due to a penetrating injury [66–68, 71, 72], than in long bone metaphyseal osteomyelitis. The basic clinical, laboratory, and radiographic features are similar to those of osteomyelitis in long bones [69]. Early diagnosis can be elusive because of the vagueness of symptoms, clinical findings and roentgenographic evaluation [35, 69]. Once the site of metaphyseal-equivalent infection is identified, CT can document precise anatomic changes in the cortex and adjacent soft tissues, especially when diagnostic or therapeutic intervention is being contemplated [35]. The most common organism in the adolescent is *Staph. aureus*. Before 10 years of age no identifiable organism is common [35].

Some of these infections progress to physeal closure. For example, infection in the os calcis can occur after heel puncture in the newborn and result in a small heel [66, 67]. The short heel causes shoe fitting problems. Osteomyelitis of tarsal bones occurs frequently following puncture wounds of the foot [68, 71, 72]. The ensuing osseous abnormalities are the result of collapse, loss of structure, or growth arrest. Osteomyelitis in the pelvis close to the acetabulum may result in premature closure of the triradiate cartilage and have disastrous results (Fig. 3.4e–l). In the spine it is difficult to determine if the infection process begins primarily in metaphyseal bone or in the intervertebral disk [29, 69, 70, 74]. The anterior aspects of the vertebral bodies are typically affected because the major arterial vessels enter the vertebral body anteriorly [29, 74]. The result is nearly always a predominantly kyphotic deformity due to continued growth of the uninfected posterior elements [21, 73]. Younger patients have progression of kyphosis during their growing years. The younger the child is at time of infection, the greater the deformity [73]. This implies that the final kyphotic deformity is due more to growth impairment than structural collapse [73].

The treatment of metaphyseal-equivalent osteomyelitis is similar to that of metaphyseal osteomyelitis. The treatment of growth arrest in a metaphyseal-equivalent site is much more individualized.

3.3 Epiphyseal Osteomyelitis

Osteomyelitis that begins in the epiphysis, just like metaphyseal osteomyelitis (Sect. 3.2), is also often referred to as hematogenous osteomyelitis [75–78, 92], implying a vascular transference of a pathogen (bacteremia, septicemia) to bone. The infection may be acute or chronic.

3.3.1 Acute

Acute primary osteomyelitis confined to the epiphysis has been defined as rapid onset and progression of systemic symptoms of less than 2 weeks [75, 78, 84]. It is rare [34, 52, 76–78, 85] and occurs primarily in infants and young children [16, 32, 75, 78, 79], but children up to 11 years of age have been reported [75, 77, 78]. Most cases are due to *Staphylococcus aureus*. One patient with hemolytic uremic syndrome developed fungal sepsis and epiphyseal osteomyelitis due to *Candida albicans* [79]. It occurs most often in the distal femur and proximal tibia [80]. Roentgenographs will be normal early in the course of the infection [78]. Early diagnosis by scintigraphy shows a focal area of isotope deposition [80], and favors treatment with antibiotics. When the diagnosis is delayed and a well-defined lytic lesion has developed on roentgenographs, surgical intervention should be considered [80]. Although no subsequent physeal growth abnormalities have been reported, even with up to 6 years follow-up, observing these children until skeletal maturity is recommended [78].

3.3.2 Subacute

Subacute epiphyseal osteomyelitis develops as a result of increased host resistance and/or decreased bacterial virulence. It may be a continuance of the acute form [75], but usually has a more insidious onset [78]. Osteomyelitis of the epiphysis is so often subacute that some authors use the terms *subacute osteomyelitis* and *epiphyseal osteomyelitis* synonymously.

The age range at time of onset is from infancy to 13 years, and more than half are less than 5 years [16, 81, 86, 87, 90, 94]. It usually affects the distal femur or proximal tibia [81, 82, 86, 87, 92, 129], but may occur in any epiphysis [85, 91]. It presents with moderate local symptoms, such as nonspecific pain, decreased joint mobility, limp, or refusal to walk for weeks or months without general illness [76, 81, 84, 87, 89, 94]. Local tenderness may accompany swelling and effusion of the contiguous joint [82, 85, 108]. The sedimentation rate and white cell count are of little diagnostic value, but a bone scan is positive [94].

The pathogenesis is theoretical. The epiphyseal abscess may be primary, or secondary to unrecognized septic arthritis [84]. Or pathogens may travel from the metaphysis via persistent transepiphyseal cartilage canals into the epiphyseal arteries as described in metaphyseal osteomyelitis (Fig. 3.1a) [3, 78, 84]. In the early stages bacterial proliferation, adherence of bacteria to cartilage (both physeal and articular), cartilage destruction, and subsequent spread along vascular channels is common [3]. The differential in blood flow and lower oxygen tension represent a possible explanation for osteomyelitis in the epiphysis [77]. Once the secondary center of ossification forms and begins to enlarge, the pattern of epiphyseal vessels changes. The previous end-arterial cartilage canal systems send vessels into the ossification center, thereby creating anastomoses between canal systems. Thus, the ossification center becomes a focus for more diffuse spread of infection. This is most evident in the larger epiphyses (distal femur, proximal tibia) [43, 94]. Most epiphyseal abscesses are in the subchondral areas of the epiphysis, well away from the physis, giving credence to the concept of pathogens entering directly from unrecognized septic arthritis.

The infecting organism is most often *Staph. aureus* [3, 81, 82, 85, 87, 108, 129]. Other reported pathogens are Group A *Streptococcus* [53, 81], *Streptococcus pneumoniae* [81], *M. tuberculosis* [93], *Salmonella* species without sickle cell disease [77], and one case of *Escherichia vulneris* associated with a wooden foreign body [90].

The diagnosis is often delayed due to an insidious onset, lack of general illness, and a paucity of determining symptoms [81, 83, 89]. The usual roentgenographic picture is a well demarcated radiolucent area in the epiphysis accompanied by a rim of sclerosis emulating tumor [81, 83, 84]. The differential diagnosis includes chondroblastoma, osteoid osteoma, osteoblastoma, enchondroma, chondromyxoid fibroma, eosinophilic granuloma, chondrosarcoma, epiphyseal osteosarcoma and foreign body granuloma [81–84]. Technetium-99 bone scans shows significant increased local uptake and hyperemia in the early phases, and may lead to earlier diagnosis and more effective treatment [35, 80, 82, 88]. Excisional biopsy is often required to confirm the diagnosis [84]. If biopsy is anticipated, accurate localization of the infectious process to a specific geographical area of bone is extremely important. MRI may help define the lesion, detect radiolucent foreign bodies, and aid in selection of the surgical approach [89, 90].

Epiphyseal osteomyelitis is often treated initially by parenteral antibiotics alone [75, 81, 83, 120]. If the response is suboptimal, surgical drainage is indicated [81, 108]. Open biopsy and curettage will both confirm the diagnosis and facilitate delivery of the antibiotic [85–87].

The long term prognosis is generally favorable [81, 87, 94, 97, 104]. In most cases regeneration of the destroyed epiphyseal area is good, even when the radiolucency crosses the physis into the metaphysis [16, 83, 122]. Joint damage is usually not a problem, since these lesions rarely involve the articular surface [85]. Most reported cases have not been followed long enough to determine the presence or absence of growth arrest. One 2 year old boy was followed 9 years with no evidence of growth disturbance [94].

3.3.3 Epiphyseal Disappearance and Regeneration

Roentgenographic disappearance of the epiphysis, or a portion thereof, has been recorded by multiple authors [3, 7, 9, 13, 14, 16, 34, 55, 56, 96–99, 101–105, 147, 155, 176, 179]. The epiphyseal disappearance may be due to primary epiphyseal infection, or associated with metaphyseal osteomyelitis or septic arthritis (Fig. 3.5a–g). The original site of infection may be difficult to determine [3, 101]. The cartilage canal system within the epiphysis allows a pathway for extension of the infection throughout the chondroepiphysis into the secondary center of ossification, where trabecular destruction similar to that in the metaphysis may occur [43]. The cartilaginous epiphysis, or the secondary center of ossification if present, can be partially or totally destroyed by the infection, by thrombosis or interruption of its blood supply [3, 96, 98], or by persistent decalcification rather than by loss of bone substance [105]. The remaining cartilaginous portion may collapse, resulting in a flattened deformed epiphysis [96]. Disappearance of a portion of the adjacent metaphysis is common [55, 56, 96, 99, 101, 104, 105]. The proximal and distal femur or proximal tibia are the most common sites, and varus or valgus deformity is common [55, 56, 96, 98, 99, 101–105, 155].

Prior to the advent of antibiotics these patients were treated only with surgical debridement [96, 97]. Later some were treated only with antibiotics [55, 99, 101, 102, 104, 105], and some with surgery and antibiotics [103, 104]. One case was aided by an iliac bone graft [105].

Curiously, sometimes the epiphysis regenerates after it disappeared (Fig. 3.5h–k); often years later, and sometimes with improvement or correction of deformity and bone length [55, 56, 96, 97, 99, 101, 147]. This may be more appropriately called survival and growth of remnants of the physis, rather than regeneration [100]. This reparative phenomenon has been documented to occur following infections with *Staph. aureus* [55, 56, 96, 98, 101, 104, 105] and *M. tuberculosis* [96, 103, 113]. The loss of growth, and resumption of growth, can both be unexpected [100]. Roentgenographically, there is no way to predict the extent of the physeal loss or the anticipated subsequent recovery [96]. Even if roentgenograms show extensive loss of epiphyseal bone, the appearance may be deceptive as the remaining chondroepiphysis can restore the epiphysis and proceed with normal joint development [104]. The bone is destroyed, but the physis survives, possibly because of the paucity of circulation [100]. Regeneration of the epiphysis after destruction is directly related to the amount of cartilage that survives [96]. It is possible that in the infant relatively undifferentiated hyaline cartilage cells might be capable of forming cell populations that would regenerate the growth plate, just as similar hyaline cartilage cells formed the original physis in utero [44]. The younger the patient the more regeneration may be expected. No regeneration occurred in rats and rabbits after complete surgical excision of physeal cartilage [95]. The ossification and reformation of the cartilaginous epiphysis is influenced by revascularization from adjacent epiphysis and marginal capsular vessels [98]. Remarkably, in some cases after the epiphysis regenerated, growth in the physis resumed [56, 101] aided by its well known resistance to infection [24]. The initiation of reossification may be delayed for several years after the infection. In the meantime it is prudent to treat the bony epiphyseal defect expectantly [104].

Regeneration of the epiphysis proper is difficult to influence by operative treatment [101]. Residual angular deformity has been treated by corrective osteotomy (Fig. 3.5i–k), and sometimes multiple osteotomies [101, 102, 104]. One case was aided by iliac bone graft [105]. Initiation of reossification of the defective epiphysis often occurs after osteotomy. Therefore, it may be beneficial to perform the osteotomy sooner rather than later [104].

There is some residual relative shortening in every case [55]. The final length discrepancy is usually mild, but can be significant [55]. In one case growth resumed from the physis without regeneration of the epiphysis [101]. Regeneration of lesions in the distal femur [55, 56, 96, 98, 99, 101, 102], the proximal tibia [55, 104], the proximal femur [96], a proximal metacarpal [97], and two metaphyseal-equivalent sites (the ilium and talus) [103], have been documented.

The largest series of disappearance and regeneration of the epiphysis is 15 cases [55]. The infection began in all cases in children ages 11 days to 3 months. Only one patient had documented septicemia. *Staph. aureus* was cultured in eight patients. Involvement was in the distal femur in 13 cases, and the proximal tibia in 2 cases. Knee deformity was established by age 18 months and could not be prevented or controlled by nonoperative treatment. Corrective osteotomy and repeat osteotomies were frequently used to control deformity. Roentgenographically there was no way to predict regeneration, although islands of new bone appeared within the epiphyseal defect preceding the appearance of the rest of the bony epiphysis. The patients were followed 11–32 years. Grading of epiphyseal regeneration was descriptive, and included no evidence, no significant, minimal (3), little, some (3), considerable, almost complete, and complete. Final relative shortening was from 1 to 14 cm. Most other articles report more positive regeneration and subsequent growth.

Attempts to explain regeneration of a roentgenographically absent epiphysis have been made by Siffert [56] and Ogden [43, 44]. The initial damage leads to replacement of segments of the physis, epiphysis, and metaphysis by fibrous tissue, which will not necessarily cause epiphyseodesis. The remaining hyaline cartilage is undifferentiated and eventually becomes part of the secondary center of the ossification center. It seems likely that undifferentiated hyaline cartilage cells might be capable of forming cell populations that would regenerate the physis, just as similar hyaline cartilage formed the original physis in utero. It is not untenable to suggest that hyaline cartilage may help regenerate portions of the damaged physis, especially if the damaged area is small. Also, diametric expansion of the still intact physis could slowly fill in the defect. Thus, by gradual replacement and differentiation, the defect could be filled in, so that it would seemingly regenerate.

3.4 Physeal Chondritis

Infection originating in the physis is exceedingly rare or does not occur. In all illustrated cases where the physis is involved the infection appears to have begun in the metaphysis, the epiphysis, or the joint. Only one author discusses the possibility of primary infection originating in the physis [56, 106]. Since the physis is cartilage, infection originating in the physis would be best called physeal chondritis.

No convincing cases have been reported or illustrated. On record is "a case of very slight osteomyelitis of the lateral side of the epiphyseal cartilage of the tibia at the age of three which gave rise very slowly to a genu valgum at the age of twelve." [107] A roentgenogram of both knees standing at age twelve showed mild right genu valgum with normal articular and osseous structures. Unfortunately, there were no illustrations at a younger age to document the precise locus of the initial infection.

3.5 Transphyseal Osteomyelitis

An infection which includes metaphysis, physis and epiphysis is an infrequent occurrence [109, 114]. Roentgenographically there is a lucency in the metaphysis and epiphysis crossing the physis (Fig. 3.6a, b). Sometimes the margins are well-demarcated by surrounding sclerosis [112]. The extent of involvement is best seen on MRI (Fig. 3.6c) [29, 114]. The exact locus of origin of the infection is rarely, if ever, determined. In many cases the larger involvement is in the metaphy-

Fig. 3.5 Septic arthritis of the knee with disappearance and regeneration of the epiphysis and cupping of the physis. At age 5 months this girl was given amoxicillin for an upper respiratory tract infection. Six days later she was hospitalized with swelling and erythema of the right knee and temperature 105°. Three days after admission, aspiration was followed by arthrotomy and synovectomy. The cultures grew *Staph. aureus* and gram-positive Enterococci. The patient was given nafcillin followed by Ceclor. Sixteen days later increased pain in the right knee prompted readmission. Blood cultures were negative. Unasyn, rifampin, and gentamicin were given. (**a**) A roentgenograph at age 7 months shows distal femoral physeal irregularity and mild cupping. (**b**) MR T2 imaging showed nonspecific bone edema in the epiphysis, widening of the physis, and reactive nonspecific edema in the metaphyses and surrounding soft tissues. (**c**) At age 8 months the physeal widening and cupping were increased. (**d**) Aspiration of the physeal widening revealed 2–3 cc of bloody fluid that grew nothing. She was dismissed from the hospital wearing a knee brace to combat flexion contracture. (**e**) At age 9 months the epiphysis was beginning to disappear. Note growth arrest lines of the distal femur and proximal tibia, documenting growth from time of infection 4 months earlier. (**f**) At age 11 months the epiphysis was roentgenographically absent, but the physeal cupping was less and the metaphysis more normal with evidence of continuing growth documented by the growth arrest line in the metaphysis. (**g**) MR T1 imaging shows focal marrow fat replacement of the ossified portion of the epiphysis extending across the physis into the metaphysis. Note the amount of growth of the normal distal left femur documented by the growth arrest line in the metaphysis. (**h**) At age 1 year 6 months the epiphysis was beginning to reossify, but mild cupping had increased. (**i**) At age 2 years 7 months the patient had occasional knee pain and no swelling. There was moderate genu valgum and equal bone lengths. (**j**) The epiphysis had partially regenerated and the physeal cupping was increased, but without a physeal bar. A bar later occurred and was excised at age 3 years 7 months. Growth resumed for a year before the bar recurred. Open wedge femoral osteotomy was performed at ages 7 years 3 months, and femoral lengthening at age 8 years 10 months. (**k**) At last follow-up, age 10 years 3 months the knee was functioning well, the femur and tibia were appropriately aligned and the femoral condyles have developed and ossified reasonably well. The distal femoral physis was closed. Increasing leg length discrepancy, and possibly joint obliquity, will require more treatment (This case contributed by Dr. Stig Jacobsen, Marshfield, Wisconsin, with permission)

sis, suggesting that the infection began in the metaphysis and spread to the epiphysis [114]. But this is difficult to prove. In other cases the lytic area first appears in the epiphysis and soon thereafter in the metaphysis [112].

Transphyseal osteomyelitis may present as an acute [111], subacute [108, 113, 115, 116] or chronic [109, 110, 112] infection. It is usually subacute, with few, if any, systemic signs. A lapse of time of one or more months from the beginning of symptoms to the first physician visit is not unusual [112]. The causative organism is usually *Staph. aureus*, but cases are recorded due to *M. tuberculosis* [109, 112, 113, 115, 117], *Salmonella species* [108, 115], and *Haemophilus influenza* [111]. Cultures are often negative, but histology confirms infection. The differential diagnosis includes both benign and malignant tumors [109, 112]. Recorded sites include the proximal tibia [110, 111, 113–118], distal femur [29, 108, 110, 112, 114], distal tibia [29, 109, 110, 112], proximal femur [117], and proximal humerus [109].

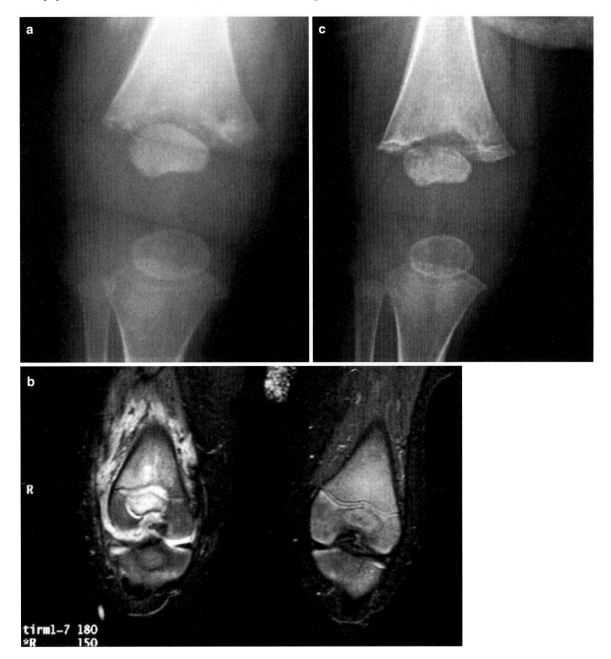

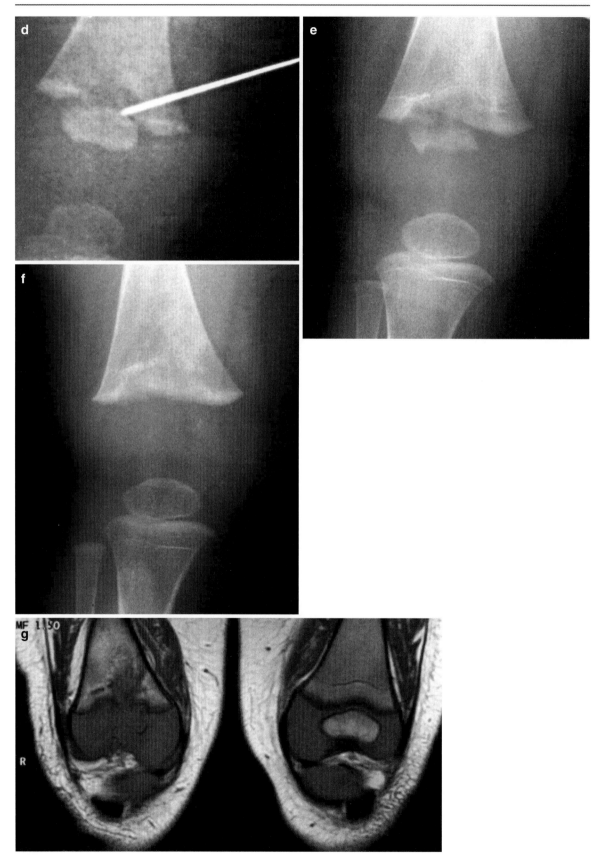

Fig. 3.5 (continued)

3.5 Transphyseal Osteomyelitis

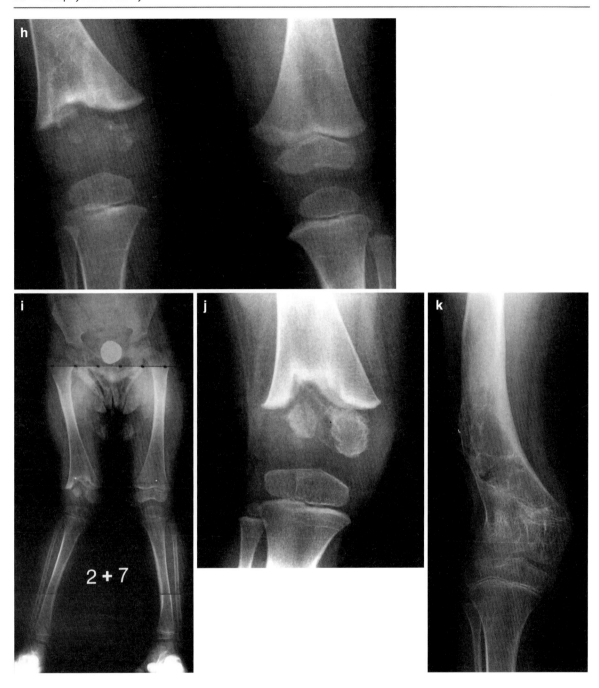

Fig. 3.5 (continued)

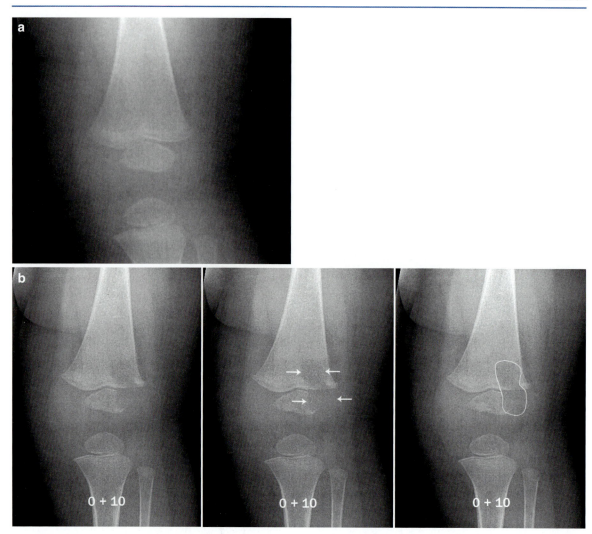

Fig. 3.6 Transphyseal osteomyelitis with pseudo-bar formation. At age 10 months this female was thought to have "a viral prodromal upper respiratory infection." She stopped crawling and standing. (**a**) A roentgenogram of the left knee was normal. Intermittent fever reached a maximum of 100.2 °F. Only "anti-inflammatory" medication was given. (**b**) At the first orthopedic examination 7 days later a roentgenogram was reported normal, but the left view shows a faint loss of bone architecture in the lateral distal metaphysis and epiphysis. The *middle* and *right* views are the same image with *arrows* and a continuous line added to delineate the lesion. The white blood count was 16.44, the sed rate 30, and the CRP 0.8. She was admitted to a hospital for observation of suspected septic arthritis of the left knee. Aspiration of knee fluid cultured methicillin sensitive staph aureus. (**c**) MRI 2 days after (**b**). *Top view* shows abnormality consistent with osteomyelitis located primarily in the lateral metaphysis. The middle view, a more posterior slice, shows involvement across the physis into the epiphysis. The *bottom view* further posterior shows greatest involvement in the epiphysis. (**d**) Curettement of the lesion through a window in the lateral metaphyseal cortex on same day as (**c**). The curette crosses the physis into the epiphysis. Cultures were negative. (**e**) At age 2 years 3 months the femur is growing, with mild genu valgum. (**f**) A persistent transphyseal defect on CT scan was of concern and was associated with mild valgus deformity. No bar is present. (**g**) A second curettement of the lesion was performed at age 2 years 4 months; only "fibrous tissue" was encountered in the defect. Fat was inserted as an interposition material. Breakoff titanium wires were inserted in the metaphysis and epiphysis. Gram stain and cultures of the fibrous tissue were negative for infection. (**h**) A scanogram at age 2 years 5 months. The physis is open. The more distal metal marker is not in the bone. (**i**) At last evaluation, age 3 years 11 months, the femur is growing well. A scanogram showed the right femur 22.98 cm, the left 22.85 cm. The distance from the proximal marker to the physis has increased. The distal metal marker became dislodged. (**j**) Lateral view shows posterior displacement of the distal marker. Note: The original knee aspiration confirmed the diagnosis of septic arthritis, but the pathomechanism of the transphyseal defect is unknown. Was the transmetaphyseal defect due to infectious material sterilized by methicillin, or was it secondary to vascular ischemia? Since there was never a definite osseous bridge from metaphysis to epiphysis, and the growth impairment (both length and angulation) was minor, this might be best called a *pseudo-bar*

3.5 Transphyseal Osteomyelitis

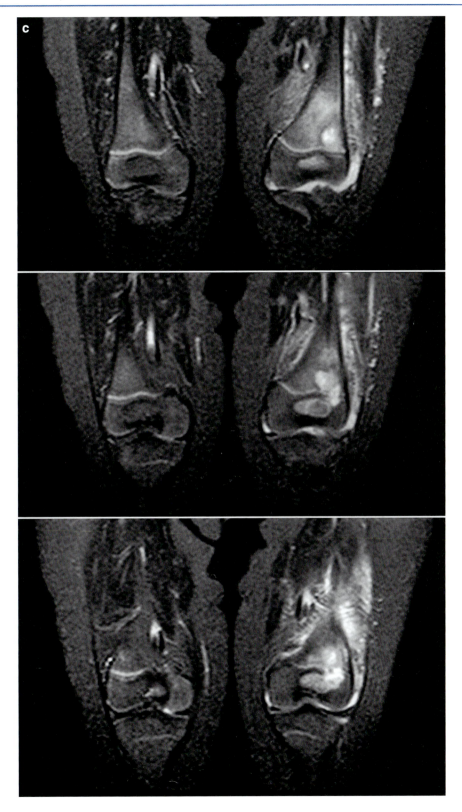

Fig. 3.6 (continued)

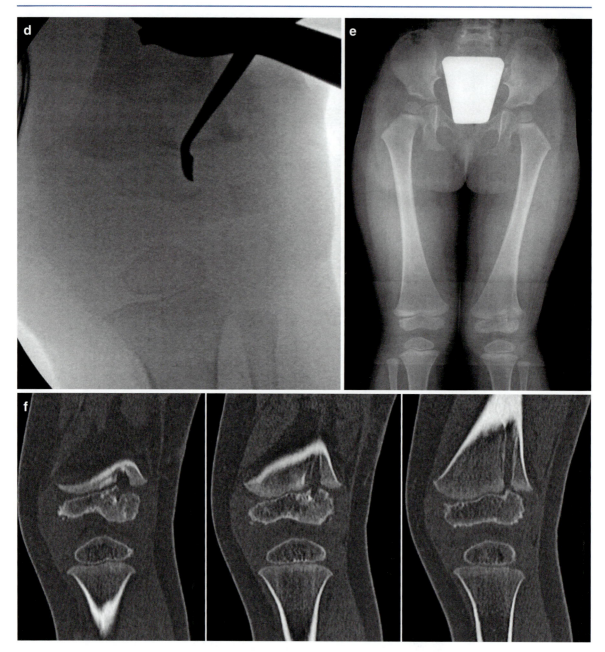

Fig. 3.6 (continued)

3.5 Transphyseal Osteomyelitis

Fig. 3.6 (continued)

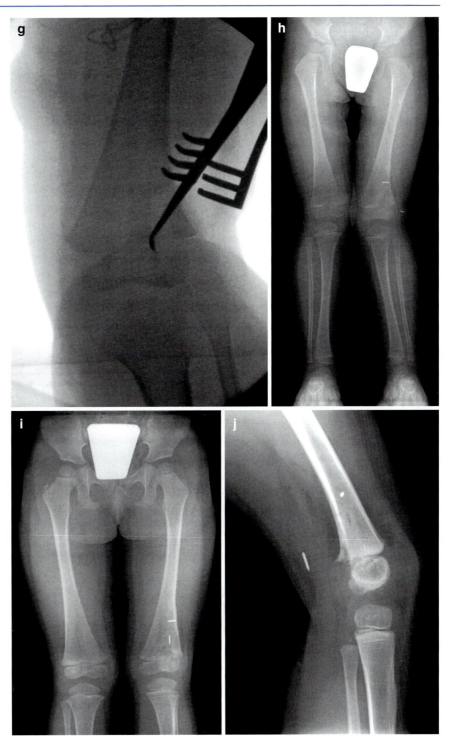

The pathogenesis is not well understood. A metaphyseal abscess may spread directly into the epiphysis via transphyseal vessels (Fig. 3.1a), or there may be direct destruction and lysis of the physis by bacterial/enzymatic activity and/or polymorphonuclear leucocytes (Fig. 3.1b) [3]. The concept that the physis is a barrier to the spread of infection is challenged by cases in which the infection crosses the physis [112, 114]. The lesion sometimes has a hourglass configuration with the narrowest point at the physis [112], suggesting a resistive component to the physis. In children less than 2 years of age metaphyseal vessels penetrate the physis into the epiphysis, and are called "transphyseal" or "communicating" vessels (Fig. 3.1c) [43, 44, 59]. By the time the secondary ossification center forms a discrete subchondral bone plate adjacent to the physis, no vessels cross the growth plate [43]. However, there are more recordings of transphyseal osteomyelitis in the literature in children over 2 years of age [109, 110, 112–116, 118], than in children below 2 years of age [108, 111, 117]. The fact that the overwhelming number of cases occur in children over age 2 years suggests that transphyseal osteomyelitis rarely occurs via transphyseal vessels, or that transphyseal vessels do occur in some children after age 2 years.

Most cases of transphyseal osteomyelitis are subacute in nature and many resolve with antibiotic therapy alone [83, 109, 110, 114]. Combining surgical debridement (Fig. 3.6d) with antimicrobial therapy is preferred in most reports [85, 106, 112, 113, 115–118]. This usually results in eradication of the infection with subsequent improvement of the normal architecture of the physis and normal growth (Fig. 3.6e–j). Surgical evacuation of the lesion is indicated: to confirm the diagnosis, for acute infection, for extension of infection into the joint, for sinus formation, and for failure of the patient to respond to antibiotics [110]. Computed tomography-guided surgery allows for precise curettage with less compromise of the contiguous normal physis [108, 112]. Curettage of the lesion including the damaged portion of the physis has no apparent harmful effect on future growth [112, 116, 117].

In almost all reports, symmetrical growth has continued despite known penetration of the physis [112, 113]. The fact that major growth abnormalities occur infrequently is probably due to the central location of the penetrating abscess, which does not form a bar, and to the growth potential of the remaining peripheral physis [43].

3.6 Subacute Osteomyelitis

Subacute osteomyelitis develops as a result of increased host resistance and/or decreased bacterial virulence, or by the use of inadequate antibiotic therapy [121]. It has milder systemic signs, which may have been present a number of weeks [36], and is less severe than acute osteomyelitis. When a membrane lines the abscess it is called a Brodie's abscess [43]. When considering both acute and subacute osteomyelitis approximately 33% are subacute. Subacute osteomyelitis occurs most often in the diaphysis, followed by the metaphysis, and the epiphysis [125]. This differs from acute osteomyelitis which is most commonly metaphyseal. Subacute osteomyelitis affecting the epiphysis is not common [83]. However, because primary infection in the epiphysis is usually subacute, the term subacute epiphysitis is sometimes used synonymously with epiphyseal osteomyelitis (see Sect. 3.3). Subacute osteomyelitis in the metaphysis can occur in any bone, but most frequently is in the distal femur or proximal tibia [124]. Subacute osteomyelitis can occur at any age, but it is relatively uncommon in infants. In a retrospective study of 18 patients with subacute osteomyelitis, the youngest child reported was 6 months of age [127].

Subacute osteomyelitis may be difficult to diagnose because of lack of characteristic signs and symptoms of infection. Fever, leukocytosis and elevated sedimentation rate may be lacking [88, 120]. Subacute metaphyseal osteomyelitis often extends across the physis into the epiphysis (see Sect. 3.5) [120, 123]. The roentgenographic features often mimic benign or malignant skeletal neoplasia and non-pyogenic infections [124, 125]. Diagnostic delay is common [83]. MR imaging reveals the extent of subperiosteal and epiphyseal involvement not seen on plain roentgenograms [125]. Cultures are frequently negative; *Staph. aureus* is the most frequently cultured organism [119, 121, 124–128]. Histologic confirmation is necessary to avoid delay in diagnosis [125, 126], and to rule out skeletal neoplasm.

Treatment consisting of biopsy, curettage, and antibiotics in varying combinations usually concludes with a good result and no growth impairment [119, 120, 123–126, 128]. The debridement facilitates antibiotic access to the offending pathogens. In general, patients with subacute osteomyelitis follow a benign course and have few or no complications. No growth arrests have been reported. This could be associated with lack of long term follow-up.

3.7 Chronic Osteomyelitis

Chronic osteomyelitis may be defined as the presence of devitalized bone with ongoing infection for longer than 1 month [29]. It is usually a consequence of acute hematogenous osteomyelitis which develops sequestra harboring bacteria. Spontaneous drainage from the affected site and low-grade fever are common. A chronic focus of osteomyelitis near a physis can cause destruction of major areas of the physis. The remaining cartilage has fibrous replacement in some areas, and in other areas clusters of cartilage in the metaphysis left behind by longitudinal growth [43]. This results in partial growth arrest and subsequent deformity [131, 132]. In one series of 26 children with chronic osteomyelitis followed an average of 23 years, 4 (15%) had irreversible physeal damage, with relative shortening and angular deformity of the affected limb, due to either the virulence of the pathogen or inadequate medical and/or surgical treatment [132].

Surgical debridement is essential for the drainage of chronic osteomyelitis abscesses [22]. However, in an effort to avoid physeal damage from surgical insult one group treated five patients solely with antibiotics [130]. Surgical biopsy was done only to rule out malignancy. All five recovered completely. Recurrence of bone infection in children or later in life, and the subsequent development of chronic osteomyelitis are unusual [16, 32].

In summary, the usual treatment of chronic osteomyelitis is surgical debridement and antibiotics. The ensuing osteopenia, joint stiffness, or the reconstructive procedures used to treat the condition, may result in disuse and growth arrest (see Sects. 2.2 and 2.7). Under these circumstances there is usually little to be done for the physis and treatment revolves around the primary condition and its residue.

3.8 Chronic Recurrent Multifocal Osteomyelitis

Chronic recurrent multifocal osteomyelitis (CRMO) is an unusual form of inflammatory bone disease characterized by multiple exacerbations and spontaneous remissions in children and young adults. The clinical symptoms and signs include the insidious onset of multiple episodes of localized pain, swelling, redness, tenderness, and low grade fever, with spontaneous regression. These signs of inflammation occur in multiple skeletal sites, most commonly involving metaphyses of the long bone, clavicles, metatarsals, phalanges, or vertebral bodies, and less commonly in the pelvis or rib cage [35, 134, 137, 140, 141, 145]. The lesions are almost always multiple and often symmetric. Most patients are female and between the ages of 8 and 14 years at presentation [35, 134, 136–141].

The etiology is unknown and the pathogenesis is unexplained. No causative agent has been isolated [143]. Histopathologic examination of lesions show changes suggestive of osteomyelitis. Staining for bacteria and fungi is negative [140]. Cultures of biopsied material typically yield no growth of microorganisms, including fungi and mycobacteria [136, 138, 140].

The diagnosis of CRMO is essentially one of exclusion. Roentgenographic areas of lysis, mixed lytic-sclerotic lesions, and reactive periosteal sclerosis are usually in the metaphysis [134, 136–138, 140, 141, 143]. Epiphyseal lesions are uncommon, usually small, and may be easily overlooked unless adjunctive imaging techniques are performed [135, 137, 139]. The lytic area may encompass the entire metaphysis immediately adjacent to the physis [138]. When present this characteristic appearance may be pathognomanic [140], but is also very similar to the metaphyseal/physeal abnormality seen in child abuse [144]. If the patient is active athletically the diagnosis maybe confused with chronic stress (Chap. 12) [142]. Extension into the epiphysis (transphyseal) is rare [137, 139, 140]. Because the lesions are close neighbors of the joint, "sympathetic arthritis" with synovitis is often seen [145]. The lesions can mimic conditions such as Ewing's sarcoma, metastatic neuroblastoma, Langerhans cell histiocytosis, and eosinophilic granuloma. Bone scintigraphy is helpful in recognizing multifocal disease and may identify clinical and roentgenographically silent lesions [29, 35, 137, 140, 143]. Whole body scintigraphy is therefore helpful in identifying all the lesions and in choosing the best one for biopsy. Without whole body scintigraphy the patient may present several times before the correct diagnosis is made [35]. MRI is a sensitive method of determining the extent of the disease and excluding soft tissue abscess [143]. With multifocal disease, the lack of specific clinical laboratory criteria for differentiation from multifocal malignancy (Ewing sarcoma or osteosarcom) or metastatic disease (leukemia, lymphoma) may force the biopsy of one or more lesions [35]. Histology reveals an abundance of plasma cells, with an abundance of polymorphonuclear cells in acute lesions, and an admixture of lymphocytes, multinucleated giant cells, and fibrosis in older lesions [35]. The correct diagnosis will avoid expensive therapies and unnecessary prolonged hospitalization [35].

Therapeutically there has been no consistent clinical or roentgenographic improvement with courses of antibiotics, corticosteroids, nonsteroidal antiinflammatory drugs, and gamma interferon [133, 137]. Recent trials with indomethacin have been encouraging [133].

The usual natural history of CRMO is slow spontaneous resolution of the osseous lesions without specific treatment. Sequelae, and particularly growth disturbance are infrequent, probably because the metaphyseal foci of inflammation damage only the adjacent hypertrophic and provisional calcification zones of the physis [136]. These regions can be replaced by growing cartilage from the germinal and proliferative zones. However, occasional subsequent premature physeal arrest with significant deformity, length discrepancy and degenerative arthrosis, [136, 137, 139, 141, 143, 144] dictates that these patients be followed until skeletal maturity.

3.9 Septic Arthritis

Septic arthritis is the result of: (a) septicemia with seeding of the highly vascular synovial membrane, (b) rupture into the joint from an adjacent osteomyelitis abscess, or (c) a penetrating injury with direct inoculation into the joint. The route of infection is of major importance. Cases of septic arthritis caused by hematogenous implantation of pathogens into the synovium do much better than when joints are infected secondarily by osteomyelitis [147]. The relationship of concurrent blunt trauma to septic arthritis is seldom discussed [194], just as it is infrequently discussed in hematogenous osteomyelitis [37, 62, 63]. The age of the patient is also important. When the underlying cause of septic arthritis is septicemia, the children are invariably less than 1 year old [160]. Infants do less well than children [147] for the same reasons discussed in Sect. 3.2.

Staphylococcus aureus is by far the most common cause of septic arthritis in all ages, although Group B *streptococcus* is also a common cause in neonates. Additional potential bacterial pathogens may include *Streptococcus pneumoniae*, Group A *streptococcus*, *Pseudomonas aeruginosa*, meningococcus, *E. coli* and others [147, 150, 155, 160]. *Haemonphilus influenza* type B was a common cause of septic arthritis in children, but has become rare in areas of high vaccine coverage since the use of conjugated vaccine in the 1990s [149]. In neonates, coliform bacteria and Neisseria gonorrhea are also prevalent [29]. *Kingella kingae* has become a frequent gram-negative organism causing septic arthritis in young children [153]. Sterile cultures are common, even when bacteria are visualized by microscopy [147]. Physeal arrest is most likely to occur with *Staph. aureus* and less likely with *Haemonphilus influenza* and *pneumococcus* [147, 150], Meningococcal septicemia causes physeal arrest by vascular deprivation without abscess formation, and is therefore presented in Sect. 1.4.

The precise mechanism leading to physeal arrest is often not discernable in a given case. The synovial fluid cushions, lubricates, and supplies nutrients to the surface of joint cartilage which is avascular. Intraarticular inflammation leads to the elaboration of cytokines and proteolytic enzymes. This results in destruction of the cartilaginous matrix. Increased intraarticular pressure from the purulent exudate exacerbates the destructive process [29, 155]. Eventually inflammatory occlusion of the epiphyseal blood supply results in vascular ischemia of the physis [43, 46]. This occlusion could be due to either increased intraarticular pressure compressing the epiphyseal vessels, or intra arterial presence of bacteria and purulent material causing thrombosis in the smaller arterioles (Fig. 3.1e). At the time of infection the degree of physeal damage and the eventual outcome are difficult to predict [46].

Traditionally the imaging evaluation begins with conventional roentgenography. Plain films may be normal or demonstrate joint space widening with adjacent soft tissue swelling and loss of normal tissue planes. In neonates dislocation of the hip may be present [29]. Ultrasound is highly sensitive for the detection of joint effusion and can be used to guide needle aspiration. MR imaging is extremely sensitive for the detection of even a tiny joint effusion [29]. Scintigraphy and CT are less sensitive for identification of joint effusion, but may detect areas of adjacent osteomyelitis [148]. Bone destruction is usually not evident until late in the course of the disease unless septic arthritis is secondary to osteomyelitis [35]. Sometimes the diagnosis of septic arthritis is made months or years later based on physical or roentgenographic findings consistent with the diagnosis [195].

Roentgenographic disappearance of an ossified epiphysis may occur during or shortly after an acute episode of septic arthritis (Fig. 3.5e–g), similar to the process discussed in osteomyelitis of the epiphysis (Sect. 3.3). This has been noted most commonly in the hip and shoulder [155, 156]. The fact that the cartilage epiphysis has the potential to reappear suggests that reparative revascularization, rather than enzymatic dissolution of bone and cartilage by the infecting organism, is responsible for the disappearance of the ossification center [156].

The management of acute joint infections is a race against time, with nature grudgingly allowing a brief period of time from the onset of symptoms when the disease may be completely cured by the prompt administration of the right antibiotic in an adequate dose. This period may be shorter than 24 h, and is probably never longer than 5 days [147]. Once this golden opportunity is missed, the incidence of disappointing results begins to rise [147]. The most beneficial influence of antibiotics has been on the septicemic phase of the disease. The mortality rate of 10–20% in 1920 was reduced to less than 1% by 1970 [147].

Septic arthritis in infants and children is a surgical emergency [35]. Every hour an acute suppurative process continues within a joint affects the prognosis [155]. Delay in diagnosis and treatment have disastrous consequences to the infected joint, primarily permanent growth deformity and degenerative arthritis, and is the most important factor in determining prognosis in children [147, 150, 151, 154, 162, 167]. Once an effusion has been detected, prompt arthrocentesis should be carried out, followed by appropriate antibiotic therapy. In addition, most authorities recommend open surgical drainage of the hip joint, whereas management of other joints is somewhat controversial between repeated aspirations or surgical drainage [29, 46, 154]. Surgical drainage should be used as soon as it is clear that aspiration is inadequate and should always be carried out without delay in the case of the hip joint [147, 150].

The prognostic factors associated with poor results of septic arthritis are premature birth, age of onset of infection, virulence of the organism, and delay in diagnosis and treatment. Physicians have some control only on the last factor. When diagnosis and treatment are prompt the long term prognosis is generally good [47, 152]. Children with sequelae tend to have been sick longer before diagnosis, and drainage of pus delayed [150]. Of cases with an unsatisfactory outcome, 75% involve the hip joint [147]. Growth abnormalities, particularly physeal bars, may not be clinically evident for months or years [150]. The need for long term follow-up of infants and children with septic arthritis cannot be overemphasized [43, 150].

3.9.1 Monoarticular Septic Arthritis

Over 90% of cases of septic arthritis following septicemia occur in a single joint. The most commonly affected sites are the hip, knee, shoulder, ankle, elbow, and wrist, approximately in that order [147, 155]. The size of the joint may be a factor in this order. Larger joints predominate in both infants and children [147]. Septic arthritis affects weight-bearing joints in three fourths of cases [150].

3.9.1.1 Hip

Septic arthritis of the hip is the most commonly encountered joint infection, and has the highest rate of unsatisfactory results [35, 147, 155, 163]. It is frequently associated with osteomyelitis of the proximal femoral metaphysis [156, 160, 163], as high as 70% in one series [147]. The pitfalls in diagnosis are many, and in neonates plain roentgenograms of the unossified epiphysis are often misleading. The differential diagnosis includes birth trauma, scurvy, and non-accidental injury. A high index of suspicion and the use of multiple imaging modalities are useful in making an early diagnosis. Ultrasound of the hip usually shows an effusion. Photopenia of the femoral head by radionuclide bone scanning is secondary to transient ischemia caused by the pressure of the intraarticular fluid [35, 38] and carries a poor prognosis [163].

The generally accepted principles of treatment are early adequate incision and drainage, and appropriate and ample antibiotics [164, 170]. Urgent surgical decompression and drainage is essential if vascularity is to be re-established before bone death has occurred [155, 163]. When septic arthritis and osteomyelitis of the femoral neck co-exist it is difficult to establish the primary source. Both the joint and the femoral neck abscess need decompression and surgical debridement to minimize irreversible damage. Cases which respond quickly to treatment usually have no coexisting osteomyelitis [147]. In some cases post operative immobilization in plaster cast or traction may contribute to physeal arrest (Sects. 2.2 and 2.7) [155].

The long term prognosis depends on survival of the epiphysis and the physis [160], and may be more dependent on the primary site of origin (intraarticular synovial arthritis or interosseous osteomyelitis), than the type of organism [157]. The final roentgenographic anatomic appearance and Harris rating system may be far worse than the clinical results, and activities may be only mildly restricted [158]. Preservation of even a slight amount of hip motion may be better than an arthrodesis [158]. In one study prior to the advent of antibiotics, only 7 of 113 cases of hip septicemia concluded treatment with a normal hip [157]. The prognosis has improved in recent years, possibly aided by a more vigorous policy of early arthrotomy [167]. No unsatisfactory results are expected if treatment is instituted less than 4 days after onset of symptoms [167]. The final residual deficits can be best minimized by early diagnosis and treatment [162].

A variety of sequelae have been described, ranging from minimal femoral head contour changes to complete destruction of the head and neck with dislocation of the hip [159, 165, 166]. This section will discuss only those sequelae pertaining to the physis, and includes premature physeal closure of the femoral capital physis, avascular necrosis of the epiphysis, separation (slipping) of the epiphysis, destruction of the epiphysis, and closure of the triradiate physis.

Arrested or delayed growth of femoral head physis is a common outcome [164]. The arrest may be complete or partial. Complete physeal closure leaves a short femoral neck and a small inadequate femoral head leading to joint incongruity and relative overgrowth of the greater trochanters [173]. A frequent outcome of partial arrest is coxa vara if the arrest is medial, and coxa valga if the arrest is lateral. Medial arrest results in gradual relative overgrowth of the greater trochanter, and relative femoral shortening (Fig. 3.7). Lateral arrest results in coxa valga, a short femoral neck, lateral tilt of the femoral physis and the femoral head, and mild relative femoral shortening [169]. Bar excision in the proximal femoral physis is very rarely done following fracture, and probably has not been done following infection. If the bar is small and peripheral, as in Fig. 3.7a, it could be excised intraarticularly. A small central the bar could be removed through the metaphysis. If this is not feasible, repeated valgus osteotomies are probably preferable to attempting physeal closure of the remaining head and greater trochanter physes, followed by arrest of the contralateral distal femoral physis at a later date or femoral lengthening at conclusion of growth, if necessary. Most of these children are infants at the time of infection and have considerable growth of the opposite normal femur.

Avascular necrosis of the femoral head is a common complication of septic arthritis of the hip in infants. It occurs when the pressure of the intraarticular pus exceeds the arterial pressure of the retinacular vessels (approximately 40 mmHg), which supply the immature femoral head [163]. It occurs in three forms: absence or delayed appearance of the epiphyseal ossification center, disappearance of an existing center, or increased bone density (sclerosis) of the center [171]. Once the femoral head is dead, modeling deformities of the femoral head inevitably occur, even if the sepsis is drained and eradicated. Joint stiffness, femoral shortening, and painful degenerative arthritis are frequent sequelae [163].

Complete separation (slipping) of the proximal femoral epiphysis is a rare complication of neonatal septic arthritis [4, 56, 158]. It results from mechanical loosening of the epiphysis rather than infective destruction of the growth plate. Since the germinal and proliferating layers of the physis are resistant to infection, physeal growth is maintained despite the slipping [4, 20]. The prognosis of an epiphyseal separation is dependent on the degree of damage to the blood supply of the epiphysis, rather than the mechanical disturbance of the physis [4]. The potential for recovery is good provided the diagnosis is made early and prompt treatment by anatomic reduction is obtained [4]. Internal fixation with a transarticular Kirschner wire through the center of the physis and femoral head has resulted in a viable, growing hip followed for 7½ years [4]. If the femoral head is not secured a non-union between the head and neck can develop [166].

Roentgenographic disappearance or failure of development of the bony nucleus of the capital femoral epiphysis is most likely to occur in children from birth through age 2 years [156, 157, 160, 164], and is almost always due to *Staphylococcus aureus* [156, 160, 164]. Reduction of the remnant femoral head or neck into

Fig. 3.7 Septic arthritis of the hip followed by premature partial physeal closure. At 1 week of age this female had septic arthritis of the right hip which was aspirated and treated with IV antibiotics. (**a**) At age 4 years 0 months she had occasional vague right hip complaints without symptoms or signs of infection. The hip had excellent range of motion with no tenderness. There is a small bar in the femoral capital physis medially (*arrow*), producing mild coxa vara and decreased femoral head-greater trochanter distance (*lines*). A scanogram showed the right femur 8 mm shorter than the left. (**b**) At age 9 years 4 months the coxa vara and greater trochanter relative overgrowth had increased. (**c**) A frog leg lateral view at the same time as (**b**) shows more marked deformity. (**d**) At age 10 years 7 months a valgus derotation osteotomy was combined with arrest of the greater trochanteric physis. The subsequent maximal leg length discrepancy was 3 cm. Physeal arrest of the distal left femur resulted in equal femoral lengths documented on scanogram at age 13 years 0 months. (**e**) At age 19 years 5 months the patient was normally active and asymptomatic. The mild femoral head deformity and femoral neck shortening need ongoing observation (Case contributed by Dr. Michael Busch, Atlanta, GA, with permission)

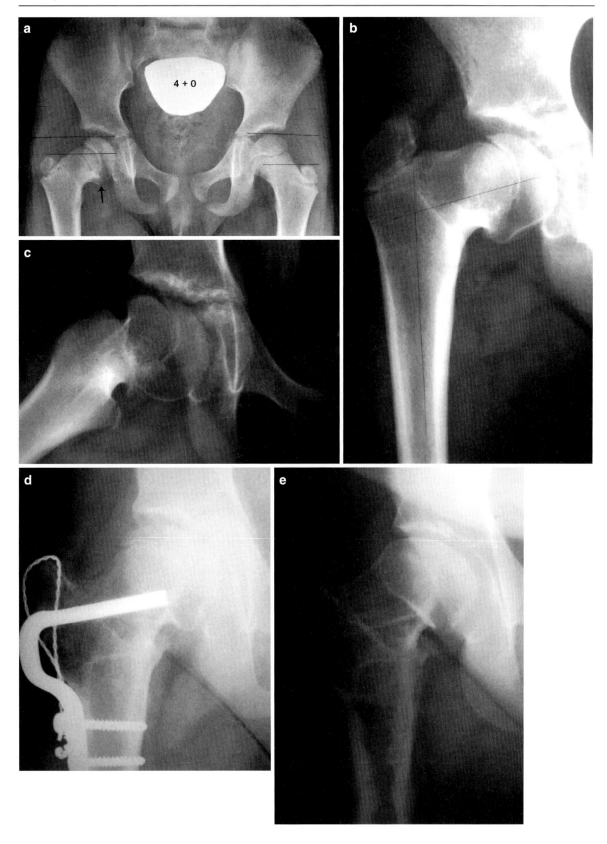

the acetabulum by holding the leg in an abduction cast, brace, or traction, has had some success in achieving well formed femoral heads [164]. Arthrography assessment of unossified remnants [156] has been replaced today by CT and MRI. Later return or partial reappearance (see Sect. 4.3) are less likely to occur in the proximal femur than at other sites [160, 164].

Premature closure of the triradiate physis is not commonly reported following septic arthritis of the hip in infants [161, 172]. If the mechanism of closure is the intraarticular release of proteolytic enzymes by pus in the synovial fluid, closure of the triradiate cartilage should be much more common [161]. When it occurs, the acetabulum is shallow with a disproportion in the size of the head (large) and the acetabulum (small). In one case of partial triradiate physeal closure bar excision failed, complicated by postoperative deep infection [161]. Bar excision of the triradiate cartilage has, however, been successful following trauma [168], and therefore could be considered in selected cases of partial closure following infection.

3.9.1.2 Knee

Septic arthritis of the knee accounts for approximately 40% of septic joints in children [176]. Most of the statements concerning clinical data and imaging techniques found in the preceding sections H, Septic Arthritis, and Hip, are applicable to the knee as well. One major difference is that in the acute stage of a septic knee repeated aspiration [150], or arthroscopic evacuation, debridement, and irrigation [178], may be sufficient in preventing joint or epiphyseal/physeal destruction.

Physeal problems due to septic arthritis of the knee are similar to those at the hip; namely premature complete and partial arrest, slipping of epiphysis, and epiphyseal destruction and regeneration, of either the distal femur or proximal tibia. Premature central physeal closure producing cupping of the physis (Sect. 1.5) is perhaps most common in the knee and may be accompanied by soft tissue flexion contracture [175]. The potential of severe deformity due to asymmetrical loss of the epiphysis or severe bone length loss is greatest at the knee [147]. In general, residual physeal abnormalities occur more often, and are more severe, in the distal femur than in the proximal tibia [179]. Sometimes focal physeal disruption occurs which slows growth, but does not stop it. The physis, though irregular remains intact (Fig. 3.8 and 3.6). This could be called a *pseudo-bar*. Physeal damage in both the distal femur and proximal tibia in the same patient is rare or non-existent. Interestingly, when septic tuberculosis of the knee joint was common, it appeared not to cause premature arrest of the femoral or tibial physis [174].

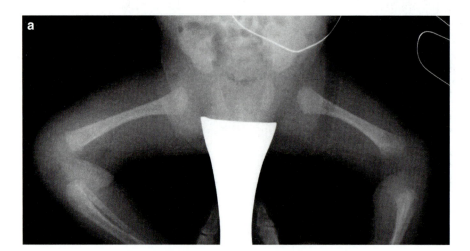

Fig. 3.8 Septic arthritis of the knee with subsequent pseudo physeal bar of the femur. Premature infant treated with an umbilical artery catheter, developed septic arthritis of the knee and a physeal pseudo-bar. This male was born prematurely weighing 1,300 g. He was transferred to a tertiary hospital, intubated, placed on a ventilator, and an umbilical artery catheter inserted. Ampicillin and cefotoxamine were given IV for 7 days. (**a**) At age 5 weeks the right knee was swollen and tender. A roentgenogram showed moderate right knee soft tissue swelling. Cultures of blood, right knee joint fluid, and distal right femoral bone aspiration each grew *Staph. aureus*. Vancomycin and oxacillin were given followed by rifampin. The knee swelling subsided and at 6 weeks of age a bone scan was negative for focal uptake. He was dismissed from the hospital at age 3 months with the diagnosis of septic arthritis of the knee.

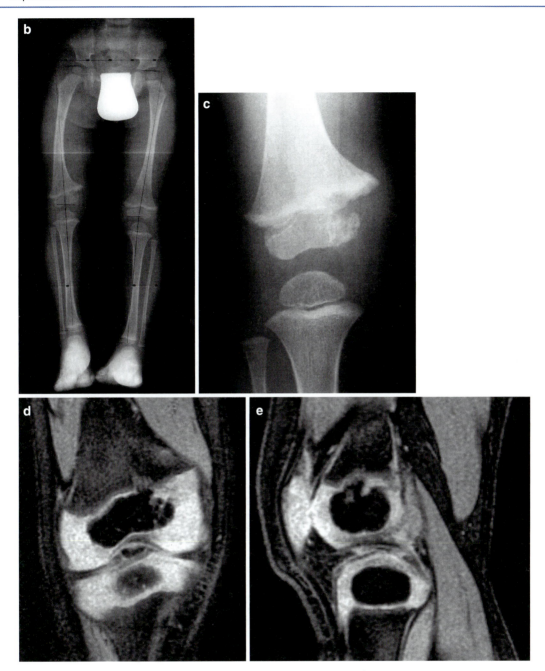

Fig. 3.8 (continued) (**b**) At age 2 years 5 months a scanogram showed the right femur 12 mm shorter than the left, with medial bowing of the mid and distal femoral shaft. (**c**) The medial metaphysis and epiphysis were irregular. No physeal cupping or bar was present. (**d**) An MRI was recorded as showing a "fairly well defined physeal bar just medial to the midline in the distal femoral growth plate". In addition, "there are small patchy ill-defined areas of lower signal within the epiphyseal cartilage adjacent to the medial physis". The radiologist also commented that "the physeal abnormality is not well defined yet because the cartilage has not yet ossified". (**e**) A lateral view confirms that the physis, though irregular, has continuity throughout and that no osseous bridge is present from metaphysis to epiphysis.

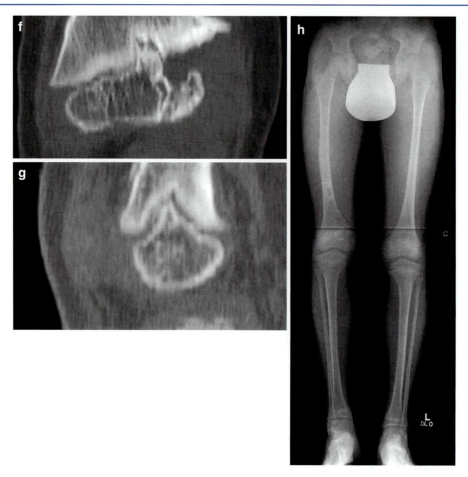

Fig. 3.8 (continued) (**f**) Two months later a CT scan shows sclerosis, irregularity and slanting of the medial aspect of the metaphysis, and fragmentation of the medial portion of the epiphysis. A portion of the mid epiphysis projects into the metaphysis, but is not joined to the metaphysis. (**g**) A lateral view at the same time confirms cupping of the physis, but no true bar. This is similar to the pseudo-bar seen in Fig. 3.6f. At age 2 years 7 months the irregular area was excised, like a bar would be excised, and the cavity filled with cranioplast. Titanium break-off wires were placed parallel in the metaphysis and epiphysis 27 mm apart. (**h**) At age 9 years 0 months, 6 years 5 months post bar excision, the right femur was growing well. On scanogram the right femur was 13 mm shorter than the left and the metal markers were 89 mm apart. Thus the right femur was growing essentially equal to the left (compare with **b**). Interestingly, his bone age at this time was 11 years 0 months, representing an advancement of two standard deviations from the mean. Note: Unknowns in this case are: (1) the mechanism by which the septic arthritis caused the distal femoral physeal abnormality, (2) the amount and pattern of growth had the "bar excision" not been done, (3) the association of rapid growth, as documented by advanced bone age, with the absence of formation of a true bar, and (4) had the area not been operated would a true bar have formed? This is another example of a pseudo-bar (see Fig. 3.6f)

The most common disabling deformity is premature closure of the distal femur or the proximal tibia. If physeal closure is peripheral, angular deformity may be present by 10 months post infection [178]. Since these physes contribute the major growth of the leg, their arrest can produce major angular and length abnormalities. All treatment options must be considered. These include bar excision, osteotomy, multiple osteotomies, closure of the contralateral physis, closure of the remaining ipsilateral physis, bone lengthening, and contralateral bone shortening [46].

Destruction and partial or complete reappearance of the distal femoral and proximal tibial epiphysis have been reported a number of times (see Sect. 4.3 and Fig. 4.1) [55, 99, 101, 102, 104, 105, 152, 176, 177, 179]. The causes and results are similar to those in the hip. If destruction occurs before ossification of the ossific nucleus, ossification may be delayed for months or years. The epiphysis does not regrow, it simply remains unossified for a greater period of time [177]. The unossified epiphyseal center continues to enlarge. The size and shape of the ossific nucleus visualized on roentgenograms do not represent the entire cartilaginous epiphysis [179]. During growth arthrograms or MRI are necessary to accurately assess epiphyseal shape and volume [177, 179]. Though a portion of the epiphysis remains unossified for years, it may ultimately prove to have normal shape. Deformity can take the form of smaller size, flattening, or uncommonly, enlargement [177]. Reappearance of the epiphysis may be accompanied with central physeal arrest with cupping, angular deformity, and bone relative shortening [177]. Bar excision and corrective osteotomy should not be delayed while waiting for further epiphyseal reossification [177].

Slipping of knee epiphyses is a rare complication of neonatal septic arthritis [4]. Epiphyseal slipping results from mechanical loosening of the epiphysis rather than from infective destruction of the physis [56]. Roentgenograms of unossified epiphyses are often misleading. A high index of suspicion and the use of imaging modalities are useful in making the diagnosis of epiphyseal slip. The differential diagnosis includes birth trauma, nonaccidental trauma, and scurvy. The potential for recovery is good, provided an early diagnosis is made and prompt anatomic reduction is achieved [4].

3.9.1.3 Shoulder

Septic arthritis of the shoulder and osteomyelitis of the proximal humeral metaphysis have similar presentations [183, 186], and often coexist. This highlights the problem of determining the original site of infection and has prompted one group to establish the diagnosis by aspiration, followed by surgical drainage of the joint and bicipital recess, and drilling of the proximal humeral metaphysis to rule out osteomyelitis or to more adequately decompress the bone [191].

The prognostic factors associated with poor results of septic arthritis of the shoulder are the same as for the hip and knees. These are premature birth, age of onset of infection, virulence of the organism, and delay in diagnosis and treatment. Physicians have some control only on the last factor. In one series [180], five shoulders in which the diagnosis was made within 1 day of the onset of symptoms had normal humeral heads and normal humeral lengths. When the diagnosis was made after 1 day, 3 of 5 humeral heads were abnormally shaped, motion (particularly humeral rotation) was restricted, and relative humeral shortening (10 cm in one patient) was present.

When physeal arrest is complete or nearly complete proximal humeral anatomy remains relatively good, but there may be significant humeral relative shortening [180]. Partial physeal arrest has predilection to occur on the medial side ultimately producing an extreme varus position of the head and significant relative humeral shortening. This is frequently called "humerus varus" (Fig. 3.9a, b). It occurs most often following infection, less commonly following trauma and tumor, and is called developmental humerus varus when the underlying etiology is unknown [186].

From a functional point of view sequelae of septic arthritis of the shoulder, despite delay in diagnosis and what might be called less than optimal treatment, are much less than following septic arthritis of the hip or knee [185]. Most need no reconstructive surgery. Despite the extreme varus angulation of the humeral head causing limited abduction, patients have reasonably good shoulder function and the usual main complaint is relative shortening of the arm (Fig. 3.9c). Corrective valgus osteotomy improves shoulder abduction [193], but is not routinely done since patients infrequently complain of limited abduction. There are no reports of bar excision in the proximal humerus done following infection. Surgical lengthening for relative humeral shortening has been uniformly successful (Fig. 3.9d–h) using a variety of devices and techniques [181, 182, 184, 187–189, 192]. It is probably indicated only when the relative shortening exceeds 6 cm [188]. Separation of the epiphysis from the metaphysis in conjunction with septic arthritis is relatively rare in the proximal humerus. In one case reduction was not attempted due to the active infection and the epiphysis was removed since it was acting as a sequestrum [190]. No follow-up was given.

3.9.1.4 Wrist

Septic arthritis of the wrist in children is infrequent. Only one paper is devoted to the subject [195]. Case reports can be found in multiple site series [46] and in series which included both children and adults [194]. In studies of multiple site septic joints, the wrist is involved in 0–4% of cases [147, 195]. Septic arthritis of the wrist is a surgical emergency requiring immediate arthrotomy [194]. Distal radial growth arrest occurs if the diagnosis is delayed. Less commonly the distal ulnar physis is also involved and may be accompanied by subsequent fusion of the proximal row of carpal bones [195].

Arrest of the distal radial physis with subsequent shortening of the radius relative to the ulna can be treated by surgical shortening and/or arrest of the distal ulna, or radial lengthening, just as with osteomyelitis of the distal radius [50].

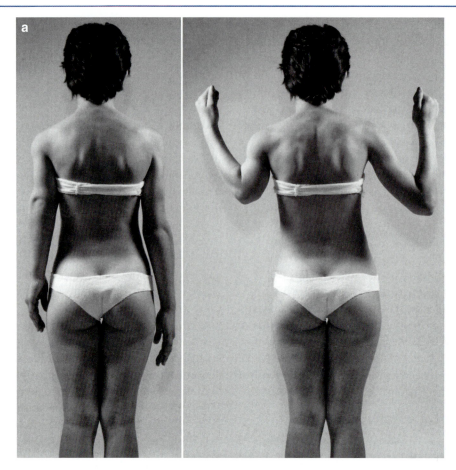

Fig. 3.9 Septic arthritis of the shoulder with subsequent humerus varus. At age 1 month, this female patient had septicemia, was treated with antibiotics, and recovered. At age 7 months, she had an acute episode in which she was unable to move her left arm. The problem appeared to be in the left shoulder. Inability to move the arm lasted several days. The patient was examined by an orthopedist, but no diagnosis was made. The same symptoms recurred a few weeks later, but this time the symptoms lasted only a few hours. No medical attention was sought. With these last two episodes, there was no history of injury or fever. When she was 4 years old, her parents noted that her left upper arm was shorter than the right. An orthopedist recommended surgical shortening of the normal right humerus. This advice was not followed. Over the next 7 years, there was occasional mild discomfort in the left shoulder. Minor limitation of motion did not disrupt activities of daily living or sports. The patient became ambidextrous, able to write with either hand. (**a**) At age 12 years 3 months the chief complaint was arm length discrepancy. There was no pain. She had difficulty with certain activities such as basketball, volley ball, and diving because of arm length inequality and inability to abduct the left shoulder completely. She could not play the flute as well as she would like because of inability to reach as far with the left arm. She preferred to wear only long-sleeved blouses. Shoulder abduction was 100° on the left and 180° on the right. The left shoulder was more full than the right in the anterior posterior projection, but there was otherwise no palpable abnormality. Clinically, the left humerus was 9 cm shorter than the right. (**b**) The left humeral head is in 90° varus relative with the shaft of the humerus. It articulated well with the glenoid. The physis was closed. (**c**) At age 13 years 1 month a scanogram showed the left humerus to be 12.3 cm shorter than the right. The left forearm was 0.8 cm shorter than the right, for a total arm length discrepancy of 13.1 cm. The right proximal humeral physis was open. Skeletal age was 11 years 0 months. Surgical lengthening of the humerus was begun. (**d**) Age 13 years 4 months, 89 days after lengthening was started. Nearly full correction of length discrepancy had occurred despite continued normal growth of right humerus. (**e**) Interoperative roentgenogram at the conclusion of lengthening after application of a plate, and before removal of the Wagner apparatus. Actual length gained after 12.5 weeks was 10.1 cm by direct measurement before application of plate. (**f**) Age 15 years 1 month, 2 years after lengthening was started. The right humerus is 4.2 cm longer than the left due to continued growth of the right proximal humerus. The plate and screws were removed. (**g**) Age 16 years 4 months. Solid bone union and return to preoperative functional status. (**h**) Residual mild humeral length discrepancy, due to continued growth of the right humerus, caused no impediment to activities of daily living. Left coat sleeves need to be shortened. No further treatment was desired or recommended (Reprinted from Peterson [188], with permission)

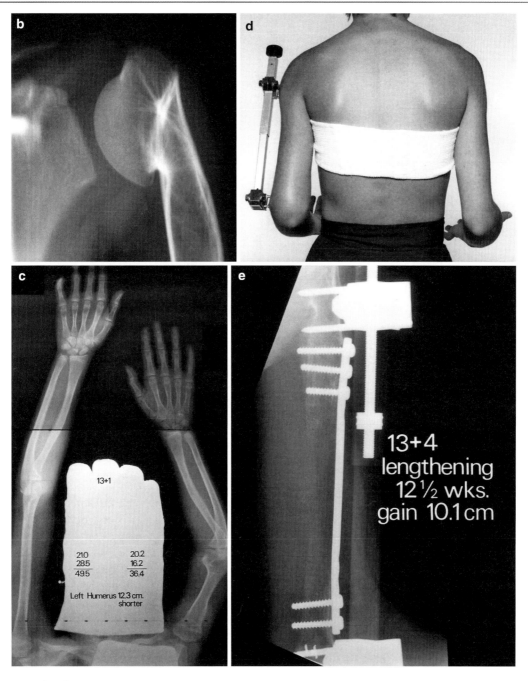

Fig. 3.9 (continued)

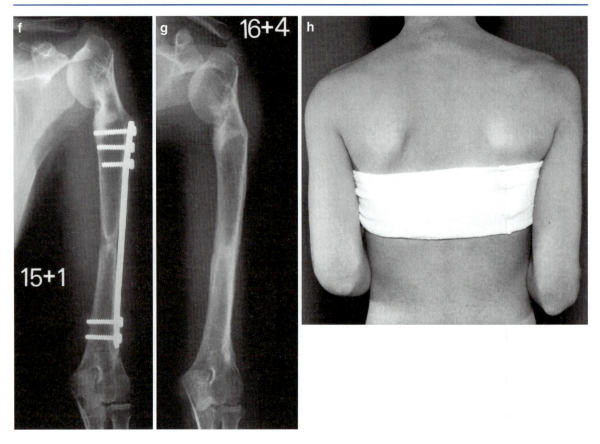

Fig. 3.9 (continued)

3.9.2 Multiarticular Septic Arthritis

Septicemia has the potential to infect multiple joints simultaneously. The mortality and morbidity associated with this crippling disease has declined substantially in the last few decades, due to better understanding of neonatal infection, availability of better imaging techniques for early diagnosis, and prompt intervention with antibiotics and surgery [4].

The most commonly reported infecting organism is *Staph. aureus*, but a variety of lesser known pathogens reported from Africa may cause multiple phalangeal and metacarpal physeal arrests [146]. At the time of acute sepsis some infected joints may be unrecognized due to the examiner's attention being focused on other septic joints [195]. Multifocal septic arthritis resulting in multifocal physeal arrest is uncommon but may be disastrous (Fig. 3.10) [4, 46, 175].

Fig. 3.10 Septicemia with multiple site involvement. This female developed septicemia at approximately 10 days of age from contaminated IV fluids. Septic arthritis in multiple joints, including both shoulders, hips, and knees, the left elbow and left hand was accompanied by osteomyelitis in some of these areas. Later corrective surgical procedures included osteotomy of the proximal femora bilaterally and staple epiphyseodesis of the right distal femur and proximal tibia, and medial side of the left distal femur. (**a**) Scanogram at age 14 years 11 months shows good limb alignment. Relative shortening of the left femur is 8.9 cm and of the left tibia 0.2 cm despite staple physeal arrests of the right distal femur and proximal tibia. The patient ambulated with a marked limp. (**b**) There is fishtail deformity of the right distal humerus. (**c**) There is marked shortening of the left third metacarpal. The normal appearance of the proximal end of the third proximal phalanx suggests this infection was primarily osteomyelitis in the metacarpal head.

3.9 Septic Arthritis

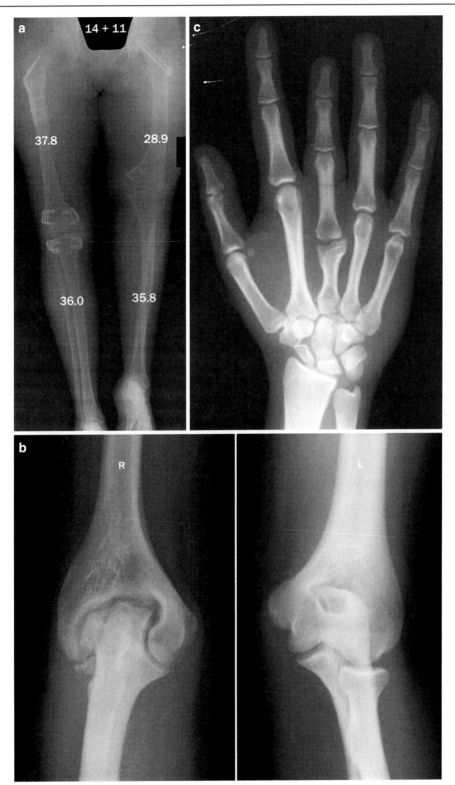

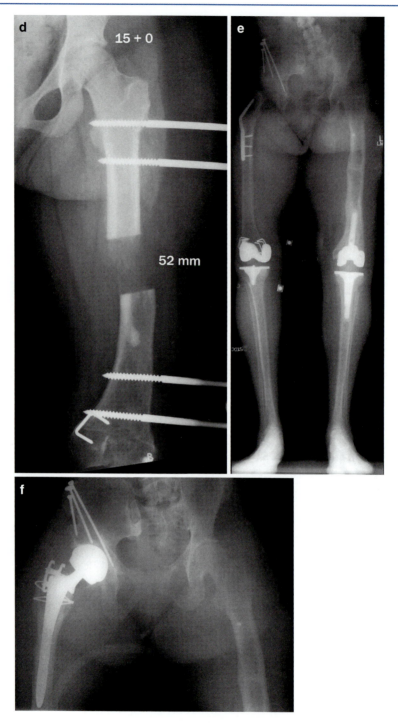

Fig. 3.10 (continued) (**d**) Left femoral lengthening at age 15 years 0 months shows 5.2 cm of lengthening with beginning ossification of the osteotomy diastasis. A second femoral lengthening of 4.8 cm was subsequently achieved and was followed later by bilateral total knee replacements and osteotomy of the right ileum. (**e**) At age 41 years 3 months the patient was ambulating well, but was having right hip pain. Standing roentgenogram of lower extremities shows reasonable alignment and length equality. Note residual lumbar scoliosis from having significant leg length discrepancy throughout the growing years. (**f**) Right hip replacement performed at age 42 years 3 months. Note: The septicemia in this patient may have resulted in both multiple site septic arthritis and multiple site osteomyelitis. The articular abnormality of both hips and right knee with normal growth is best explained by residuals of septic arthritis. The deformity and shortening of the left distal femur, right distal humerus, and left third metacarpal are explained by either septic arthritis or osteomyelitis affecting their respective physes

3.10 Author's Perspective

After review of the data in this chapter, the basic underlying cause of growth impairment associated with most cases of bone and joint infection appears to be vascular compromise of the physis, rather direct lysis of the physis. If this is true, a major objective of treatment of acute infection should be to preserve or reestablish adequate blood flow. The overall lesson to be learned is that *early* diagnosis and treatment is key to a good outcome. A high index of suspicion is helpful. A time honored dictum is that the only true pediatric orthopedic emergencies other than trauma, in which surgery should be done *now* and not wait until morning, are acute osteomyelitis and septic arthritis. Early aspiration and surgical debridement are the most expeditious means of achieving a specific diagnosis and the optimal environment for specific antibiotic efficacy. Having spent my career in a tertiary medical center seeing numerous disastrous effects of delay, I endorse this regimen. Hopefully, better means of early diagnosis and the institution of more specific and potent antibiotics may improve the course of nonoperative treatment in the future.

I also firmly subscribe to the position that bar excision should be considered in selected cases of partial arrest due to infection. The selection is similar to cases due to fracture (less than 50% of the physis involved and 2 years of growth remaining). The time interval between infection and bar excision should be long enough to ensure eradication of the infection. Bar excision requires attention to detail, but is not a difficult operation. It can be done as an outpatient or one night hospital stay, and complications are uncommon. If successful it can obviate the need for bone lengthening and shortening procedures, and if unsuccessful all other treatment operations are still available.

References

Metaphyseal Osteomyelitis

1. Acheson RM (1939) Effects of starvation, stepticemia and chronic illness on the growth cartilage plate and metaphysis of the immature rat. J Anat 93:123–130
2. Ahstrom JP (1965) Epiphyseal injuries of the lower extremity. Surg Clin North Am 1:119–134
3. Alderson M, Speers D, Emslie K, Nade S (1986) Acute hematogenous osteomyelitis and septic arthritis – a single disease. An hypothesis based upon the presence of transphyseal blood vessels. J Bone Joint Surg 68B:268–274
4. Aroojis AJ, Johari AN (2000) Epiphyseal separations after neonatal osteomyelitis and septic arthritis. J Pediatr Orthop 20:544–549
5. Bergdahl S, Ekengren K, Eriksson M (1985) Neonatal hematogenous osteomyelitis: risk factors for long-term sequelae. J Pediatr Orthop 5:564–568
6. Blanche DW (1952) Osteomyelitis in infants. J Bone Joint Surg 34A:71–85
7. Bohrer SP (1974) Growth disturbances of the distal femur following sickle cell bone infarcts and/or osteomyelitis. Clin Radiol 25:221–235
8. Burgess RC (1991) Use of the Ilizarov technique to treat radial nonunion with physeal arrest. J Hand Surg 16A:928–931
9. Caffey J (1970) Traumatic cupping of the metaphyses of growing bones. Am J Roentgenol Radium Ther Nucl Med 108:451–460
10. Canale ST, Puhl J, Watson FM, Gillespie R (1975) Acute osteomyelitis following closed fractures. Report of three cases. J Bone Joint Surg 57A(3):415–418
11. Chen SC, Huang SC, Wu CT (1998) Nonspinal tuberculous osteomyelitis in children. J Formos Med Assoc 97(1):26–31
12. Cockshott P (1963) Dactylitis and growth disorders. Br J Radiol 36:19–26
13. Cockshott P, MacGregor M (1958) Osteomyelitis variolosa. Q J Med 27:369–387
14. Cockshott P, MacGregor M (1959) The natural history of osteomyelitis variolosa. J Faculty Radiologists 10(2):57–63
15. Ducou Le Pointe H, Sirinelli D (2005) Limb emergencies in children [French]. J Radiol 86(2 II):237–249
16. Einstein RAJ, Thomas CG Jr (1946) Osteomyelitis in infants. Am J Roentgenol Radium Ther 55:299–314
17. Farrington DM, Melini de Paz F, Moral Pinteno JC (2001) Slipped capital femoral epiphysis associated with peripheral osteoarticular tuberculosis. Case report. J Pediatr Orthop B 10(2):96–100
18. Ferguson AB Jr (1973) Osteomyelitis in children. Clin Orthop 96:51–69
19. Fisher RG, Boyce TG (2005) Orthopedic syndromes. In: Fisher RG, Boyce TG (eds) Moffet's pediatric infectious diseases, 4th edn. Lippincott, Williams and Wilkins, Philadelphia, pp 527–554
20. Fitoussi F, Litzelmann E, Ilharreborde B, Morel E, Mazda K, Pennecot GF (2007) Hematogenous osteomyelitis of the wrist in children. J Pediatr Orthop 27:810–813
21. Fox L, Sprunt KS (1978) Neonatal osteomyelitis. Pediatrics 62(4):535–542
22. Gomis Gavilan M, Barberan Lopez J, Sanchez Artola B (1999) Peculiarities of osteo-articular infections in children. Baillieres Clin Rheumatol 13(1):77–94
23. Green WT (1935) Osteomyelitis in infancy. JAMA 105:1835–1839
24. Green WT, Shannon JG (1936) Osteomyelitis of infants. A disease different from osteomyelitis of older children. Arch Surg 32:462–493
25. Hardy AE, Nicol RO (1985) Closed fractures complicated by acute hematogenous osteomyelitis. Clin Orthop 21:190–195
26. Janovec M (1991) Short humerus: results of 11 prolongations in 10 children and adolescents. Arch Orthop Trauma Surg 111:13–15

27. Kemp HBS, Lloyd-Roberts GC (1974) Avascular necrosis of the capital epiphysis following osteomyelitis of the proximal femoral metaphysis. J Bone Joint Surg 56B:688–697
28. Key AJ (1952) Osteomyelitis in infants (discussion). J Bone Joint Surg 34A:85
29. Kothari NA, Pelchovitz DJ, Meyer JS (2001) Imaging of musculoskeletal infections. Radiol Clin North Am 39(1):653–671
30. Kylberg NK (1983) Descriptions of growth disturbances in children with osteomyelitis at different ages. Orthop Nurs 2(6):28–32
31. Langenskiöld A (1981) Surgical treatment of partial closure of the growth plate. J Pediatr Orthop 1(1):3–11
32. Lindblad B, Ekengren K, Aurelius G (1965) The prognosis of acute haematogenous osteomyelitis and its complications during early infancy after the advent of antibiotics. Acta Paediatr Scand 54:24–32
33. Lindell L, Parkkulainen KV (1960) Osteitis in infancy and early childhood with special reference to neonatal osteitis. Ann Paediatr Fenn 6:34–52
34. Macey HB (1939) Epiphyseal changes resulting from acute infections of bone. Thesis written to qualify for membership in the American Orthopedic Association.
35. Mandell GA (1999) Nuclear medicine in pediatric musculoskeletal imaging. Semin Musculoskelet Radiol 3(3):289–315
36. Morrey BF, Peterson HA (1975) Hematogenous pyogenic osteomyelitis in children. Orthop Clin North Am 6(4): 935–951
37. Morrissy RT, Haynes DW (1989) Acute hematogenous osteomyelitis: a model with trauma as an etiology. J Pediatr Orthop 9:447–456
38. Mortensson W, Nybonde T (1984) Ischemia of the childhood femoral and humeral head epiphyses following osteomyelitis. A hypothesis on its cause. Acta Radiol Diagn 25(4):269–272
39. Nade S (1983) Acute haematogenous osteomyelitis in infancy and childhood. J Bone Joint Surg 65B:109–119
40. Netrawichien P (1995) Radial clubhand-like deformity resulting from osteomyelitis of the distal radius. J Pediatr Orthop 15(2):157–160
41. Nicholson JT (1952) Osteomyelitis in children (discussion). J Bone Joint Surg 34A:85
42. Ober FR (1935) Osteomyelitis in infancy (discussion). JAMA 105:1839
43. Ogden JA (1979) Pediatric osteomyelitis and septic arthritis: the pathology of neonatal disease. Yale J Biol Med 52(5): 423–448
44. Ogden JA, Lister G (1975) The pathology of neonatal osteomyelitis. Pediatrics 55(4):474–478
45. Ono CM, Albertson KS, Reinker KA, Lipp EB (1995) Acquired radial clubhand deformity due to osteomyelitis. J Pediatr Orthop 15(2):161–168
46. Peters W, Irving J, Letts M (1992) Long-term effects of neonatal bone and joint infection on adjacent growth plates. J Pediatr Orthop 13:806–810
47. Petersen S, Knudsen FU, Andersen EA, Egeblad M (1980) Acute haematogenous osteomyelitis and septic arthritis in childhood. A 10-year review and follow-up. Acta Orthop Scand 51:451–457
48. Peterson HA (2007) Epiphyseal growth plate fractures. Springer, Heidelberg, p 914
49. Peterson HA (1984) Partial growth plate arrest and its treatment. J Pediatr Orthop 4(2):246–258
50. Price CT, Mills WL (1983) Radial lengthening for septic growth arrest. Case report. J Pediatr Orthop 3:88–91
51. Prokopova LV, Nikolaeva NG, Bugaeva TL, Kisilevich IM (1989) Early decompression of an osteomyelitic focus in children [Bulgarian]. Ortop Travmatol Protez 7:4–7
52. Ratliff HC (1958) Tuberculosis of the femoral neck in childhood. J Bone Joint Surg 40A:1365–1373
53. Rehm PK, Delahay J (1998) Epiphyseal photopenia associated with metaphyseal osteomyelitis and subperiosteal abscess. J Nucl Med 39(6):1084–1086
54. Robb JE (1984) Primary acute haematogenous osteomyelitis of an isolated metatarsal in children. Acta Orthop Scand 55:334–338
55. Roberts PH (1970) Disturbed epiphysial growth at the knee after osteomyelitis in infancy. J Bone Joint Surg 52B:692–703
56. Siffert RS (1957) The effect of juxta-epiphyseal pyogenic infection on epiphyseal growth. Clin Orthop 10:131–139
57. Song KM, Sloboda JF (2001) Acute hematogenous osteomyelitis in children. J Am Acad Orthop Surg 9:166–175
58. Speed K (1922) Growth problems following osteomyelitis of adolescent long bones. Surg Gynec Obst 34:469–476
59. Trueta J (1959) The three types of acute haematogenous osteomyelitis. A clinical and vascular study. J Bone Joint Surg 41B:671–680
60. Trueta J, Morgan JD (1954) Late results in the treatment of one hundred cases of acute haematogenous osteomyelitis. Br J Surg 41:449–457
61. Weissberg ED, Smith AL, Smith DH (1974) Clinical features of neonatal osteomyelitis. Pediatrics 53:505–510
62. Whalen JL, Fitzgerald RH Jr, Morrissy RT (1988) A histological study of acute hematogenous osteomyelitis following physeal injuries in rabbits. J Bone Joint Surg 70A: 1383–1392
63. White M, Dennison WM (1952) Acute haematogenous osteitis in childhood. A review of 212 cases. J Bone Joint Surg 34B:608–623
64. Wilkinson FR (1952) Osteomyelitis in children (discussion). J Bone Joint Surg 34A:84–85
65. Wilson JC, McKeever FM (1936) Bone growth disturbance following hematogenous acute osteomyelitis. JAMA 107: 1188–1193

Metaphyseal-Equivalent Osteomyelitis

66. Abril Martin JC, Aguilar Rodriguez L, Albinana Cilveti J (1999) Flatfoot and calcaneal deformity secondary to osteomyelitis after neonatal heel puncture. J Pediatr Orthop B 8:122–124
67. Borris LC, Helleland H (1986) Growth disturbance of the hind part of the foot following osteomyelitis of the calcaneus in the newborn. A report of two cases. J Bone Joint Surg 68A:302–305
68. Lang AG, Peterson HA (1976) Osteomyelitis following puncture wounds of the foot in children. J Trauma 16(12): 993–999
69. Nixon GW (1978) Hematogenous osteomyelitis of metaphyseal-equivalent locations. AJR Am J Roentgenol 130(1): 123–129

70. Peterson HA (1983) Disk-space infection in children. In: Evarts CM (ed) Instructional course lectures: American Academy of Orthopaedic Surgeons, vol 32. CV Mosby Co, St. Louis, Chapter 3 (Part VII), pp 50–60
71. Peterson HA (1977) Skin puncture… bone disease. Emerg Med: 187–188
72. Peterson HA, Tressler HA, Lang AG, Johnson EW Jr (1973) Puncture wounds of the foot. Minn Med 56:787–794
73. Rajasekaran S, Shanmugasundaram TK, Prabhakar R, Dheenadhayalan J, Shetty AP, Shetty DK (1998) Tuberculous lesions of the lumbosacral region: a 15-year follow-up of patients treated by ambulant chemotherapy. Spine 23(10): 1163–1167
74. Song KW, Ogden JA, Ganey T, Guidera KJ (1977) Contiguous discitis and osteomyelitis in children. J Pediatr Orthop 17:470–477

Epiphyseal Osteomyelitis

Acute

75. Gibson WK, Bartosh R, Timperlake R (1991) Acute hematogenous epiphyseal osteomyelitis. Orthopedics 14(6): 705–707
76. Kao FC, Lee ZL, Kao HC, Hung SS, Huang YC (2003) Acute primary hematogenous osteomyelitis of the epiphysis: report of two cases. Chang Gung Med J 26(11):851–861
77. Kramer SJ, Post J, Sussman M (1986) Acute hematogenous osteomyelitis of the epiphysis. Case report. J Pediatr Orthop 6:491–495
78. Longjohn DB, Zionts LE, Stott NS (1995) Acute hematogenous osteomyelitis of the epiphysis. Clin Orthop Relat Res 316:227–234
79. Nissen TP, Lehman CR, Otsuka NY, Cerruti DM (2001) Fungal osteomyelitis of the distal femoral epiphysis. Case report. Orthopedics 24(11):1083–1084
80. Rosenbaum D, Blumhagen D (1985) Acute epiphyseal osteomyelitis in children. Radiology 156:89

Subacute

81. Andrew TA, Porter K (1985) Primary subacute epiphyseal osteomyelitis: a report of three cases. J Pediatr Orthop 5:155–157
82. Azouz EM, Greenspan A, Marton D (1993) CT evaluation of primary epiphyseal abscesses. Skeletal Radiol 22(1):17–23
83. Ezra E, Cohen N, Segev E, Hayek S, Lokiec F, Keret D, Wientroub S (2002) Primary subacute epiphyseal osteomyelitis: role of conservative treatment. J Pediatr Orthop 22:333–337
84. Gardner DF, Azouz EM (1988) Solitary lucent epiphyseal lesions in children. Skeletal Radiol 17:497–504
85. Green NE (1988) Osteomyelitis of the epiphysis. In: Uhthoff HK, Wiley JJ (eds) Behavior of the growth plate. Raven, New York, pp 323–329
86. Green NE (1983) Primary subacute epiphyseal osteomyelitis. Instructional Court Lectures 32, pp 37–40
87. Green NE, Beauchamp RD, Griffin PP (1981) Primary subacute epiphyseal osteomyelitis. J Bone Joint Surg 63A: 107–114
88. Hall FH (1993) CT evaluation of primary epiphyseal bone abscesses. Letters to the editors. Skeletal Radiol 22(6): 439–440
89. Hempfing A, Placzek R, Göttsche T, Meiss AL (2003) Primary subacute epiphyseal and metaepiphyseal osteomyelitis in children. J Bone Joint Surg 85B(4):559–564
90. Levine WN, Goldberg MJ (1994) *Escherichia vulneris* osteomyelitis of the tibia caused by a wooden foreign body. A case report. Orthop Rev 23:262–265
91. Malfulli N, Fixsen JA (1990) Osteomyelitis of the proximal radial epiphysis. A case report. Acta Orthop Scand 61(3):269–270
92. Murray P, Youel L, Buckwalter J (1992) Hematogenous epiphyseal osteomyelitis: three case reports. SOMOS, Colorado Springs, pp 11–30
93. Rasool MN (2001) Osseous manifestations of tuberculosis in children. J Pediatr Orthop 21:749–755
94. SØrensen TS, Hedeboe J, Christensen RE (1988) Primary epiphyseal osteomyelitis in children. Report of three cases and review of the literature. J Bone Joint Surg 70B:818–820

Epiphyseal Disappearance and Regeneration

95. Banks SW, Compere EL (1941) Regeneration of epiphyseal cartilage. An experimental study. Ann Surg 114(6): 1076–1084
96. Banks SW, Krigsten W, Compere EL (1940) Regeneration of epiphysial centers of ossification following destruction by pyogenic or tuberculous infection: report of five cases. JAMA 114(1):23–27
97. Bennett CB (1931) A case of continued growth after loss of bony epiphysis. J Bone Joint Surg Am 13:158–159
98. Halbstein BM (1967) Bone regeneration in infantile osteomyelitis. Report of a case with fourteen-year follow-up. J Bone Joint Surg 49A:149–152
99. Hall RM (1954) Regeneration of the lower femoral epiphysis. Report of a case. J Bone Joint Surg 36B:116–117
100. Key JA (1940) Regeneration of epiphyseal centers of ossification (Discussion). JAMA 114(1):23–27
101. Langenskiöld A (1984) Growth disturbance after osteomyelitis of femoral condyles in infants. Acta Orthop Scand 55:1–13
102. Miller B (1969) Regeneration of the lateral femoral condyle after osteomyelitis in infancy. A case report with 20-year follow-up. Clin Orthop 65:163–166
103. Papavasiliou VA, Petropoulos AV (1981) Bone and joint tuberculosis in childhood. Acta Orthop Scand 52:1–4
104. Song KS, Kim HKW (2005) Regeneration of the proximal tibial epiphysis after infantile osteomyelitis. Report of three cases with an eight-to-22-year follow-up. J Bone Joint Surg 87B:979–983
105. Vizkelety TL (1985) Partial destruction of the distal femoral epiphysis as a consequence of osteomyelitis: regeneration after transplantation of a bone graft. Case report. J Pediatr Orthop 5:731–733

Physeal Chronditis

106. Siffert RS (1966) The growth plate and its affections. J Bone Joint Surg 48A:546–563
107. Verbrugge J, Verjans H (1958) Small lesions of the growth-plate of the knee with severe anatomic and clinical complications [French]. Acta Orthop Belg 25(6):791–794

Transphyseal Infection

108. Abdelgawad AA, Rybak LD, Sheth M, Rabinowitz SS, Jayaram N, Sala DA, van Bosse HJP (2007) Treatment of acute salmonella epiphyseal osteomyelitis using computed tomography-guided drainage in a child without sickle cell disease. J Pediatr Orthop B 16(6):415–418
109. Bagaria V, Harshvardhna NS, Desai M, Sonowane S (2005) Transphyseal spread of benign tumors and infections in pediatric patients: a series of six cases. Indian J Med Sci 59(6):259–264
110. Bogoch E, Thompson G, Salter RB (1984) Foci of chronic circumscribed osteomyelitis (Brodie's abscess) that traverse the epiphyseal plate. J Pediatr Orthop 4:162–169
111. Cramer KE, Green NE (1993) Acute transphyseal hematogenous osteomyelitis caused by haemophilus influenzae with 5-year follow up. A case report. Orthop Rev 22:1027–1032
112. González Herranz J, Farrington DM, Gutiérrez J, Rodriguez Ferrol P (1997) Peripheral osteoarticular tuberculosis in children: tumor-like bone lesions. J Pediatr Orthop B 6:274–282
113. Hayes JT (1961) Cystic tuberculosis of the proximal tibial metaphysis with associated involvement of the epiphysis and epiphyseal plate. A report of two cases. J Bone Joint Surg 43A:560–567
114. Jäger HJ, Schmitz-Stolbrink A, Götz GF, Roggenkamp K, Mathias KD (1995) Invasion of the growth plate by bone tumors and osteomyelitis in childhood [German]. Radiologe 35(6):409–413
115. Marui T, Yamamoto T, Akisue T, Nakatani T, Hitora T, Nagira K, Yoshiya S, Kurosaka M (2002) Subacute osteomyelitis of long bones. Diagnostic usefulness of the "penumbra sign" on MRI. Clin Imaging 26(5):314–318
116. Ohtera K, Kura H, Yamashita T, Ohyama N (2007) Long-term follow-up of tuberculosis of the proximal part of the tibia involving the growth plate. A case report. J Bone Joint Surg 89A:399–403
117. Shih H, Hsu RW, Lin T (1997) Tuberculosis of the long bone in children. Clin Orthop 335:246–252
118. Simmons BP, Southmayd WW, Schwartz HS, Hall JE (1975) Wood, an organic foreign body of bone. A case report. Clin Orthop 106:276–278

Subacute Osteomyelitis

119. Blyth MJG, Kincaid R, Craigen MAC, Bennet GC (2001) The changing epidemiology of acute and subacute haematogenous osteomyelitis in children. J Bone Joint Surg 83B(1):99–102
120. Gledhill RB (1973) Subacute osteomyelitis in children. Clin Orthop 96:57–69
121. González-López JL, Soleto-Martín FJ, Cubillo-Martín A, López-Valverde S, Cervera-Bravo P, Navascués del Río JA, García-Trevijano JL (2001) Subactue osteomyelitis in children. J Pediatr Orthop B 10(2):101–104
122. King DM, Mayo KM (1969) Subacute haematogenous osteomyelitis. J Bone Joint Surg 51B(3):458–463
123. Letts RM (1988) Subacute osteomyelitis and the growth plate. In: Uhthoff HK, Wiley JJ (eds) Behavior of the growth plate. Raven, New York, pp 331–338
124. Lindenbaum S, Alexander H (1984) Infections simulating bone tumors. A review of subacute osteomyelitis. Clin Orthop Relat Res 184:193–203
125. Poyhia T, Azouz EM (2000) MR imaging evaluation of subacute and chronic bone abscesses in children. Pediatr Radiol 30(11):763–768
126. Rasool MN (2001) Primary subacute haematogenous osteomyelitis in children. J Bone Joint Surg 83B(1):93–98
127. Roberts JM, Drummond DS, Breed AL, Chesney J (1982) Subacute hematogenous osteomyelitis in children: a retrospective study. J Pediatr Orthop 2:249–254
128. Robertson DE (1967) Primary acute and subacute localized osteomyelitis and osteochondritis in children. Can J Surg 10:408–413
129. Ross ERS, Cole WG (1985) Treatment of subacute osteomyelitis in childhood. J Bone Joint Surg 67B:443–448

Chronic Osteomyelitis

130. Reinehr T, Burk G, Michel E, Andler W (2000) Chronic osteomyelitis in childhood: is surgery always indicated? Infection 28(5):282–286
131. Siegling JA (1937) Lesions of the epiphyseal cartilages about the knee. Surg Clin North Am 17:373–379
132. Tudisco C, Farsetti P, Gatti S, Ippolito E (1991) Influence of chronic osteomyelitis on skeletal growth: analysis at maturity of 26 cases affected during childhood. J Pediatr Orthop 11(3):358–361

Chronic Recurrent Multifocal Osteomyelitis

133. Abril JC, Ramirez A (2007) Successful treatment of chronic recurrent multifocal osteomyelitis with indomethacin. J Pediatr Orthop 27(5):587–591
134. Brown T, Wilkinson RH (1988) Chronic recurrent multifocal osteomyelitis. Radiology 166:493–496
135. Cuende E, Gutierrez MA, Paniagua G, Feito C, Gonzalez M, Sanchez J (1995) Chronic recurrent multifocal osteomyelitis: report of a case with epiphyseal and metaphyseal involvement. Clin Exp Rheumatol 13(2):251–253
136. Kasser JR (1986) Case records of the Massachusetts General Hospital. Presentation of a case. N Engl J Med 315:178–185
137. Manson D, Wilmot DM, King S, Laxer RM (1989) Physeal involvement in chronic recurrent multifocal osteomyelitis. Pediatr Radiol 20:76–79

138. McCoy SH, Pritchard DJ, Bianco AJ Jr, Millar EA (1977) Arthritides and osseous lesions of unknown etiology: is a viral cause worth considering? Orthopedics Digest 5:15–26
139. Mortensson W (1990) Physeal and epiphyseal involvement in chronic recurrent multifocal osteomyelitis (CRMO). Letters to the editor. Pediatr Radiol 20:570
140. Mortensson W, Edeburn G, Fries M, Nilsson R (1988) Chronic recurrent multifocal osteomyelitis in children. A roentgenologic and scintigraphic investigation. Acta Radiol 29:565–570
141. Pelkonen P, Ryoppy S, Jääskeläinen J, Rapola J, Repo H, Kaitila I (1988) Chronic osteomyelitis like disease with negative bacterial cultures. Am J Dis Child 142:1167–1173
142. Peterson HA (2001) Premature epiphyseal fusion and degenerative arthritis in chronic recurrent multifocal osteomyelitis. In: Morrey BF (ed) Year book of orthopedics. Mosby, St. Louis, pp 47–48
143. Piddo C, Reed MH, Black GB (2000) Premature epiphyseal fusion and degenerative arthritis in chronic recurrent multifocal osteomyelitis. Skeletal Radiol 29:94–96
144. Prose NS, Fahrner LJ, Miller CR, Layfield L (1994) Pustular psoriasis with chronic recurrent multifocal osteomyelitis and spontaneous fractures. J Am Acad Dermatol 31(2):376–379
145. Shilling F, Kessler S (2001) Chronic recurrent multifocal osteomyelitis – 1. Review [German]. Klin Padiatr 213(5):271–276

Septic Arthritis

General Considerations

146. Cockshott WP (1963) Dactylitis and growth disorders. Br J Radiol 36:19–26
147. Gillespie R (1973) Septic arthritis of childhood. Clin Orthop 96:152–159
148. Herndon WA, Alexieva BT, Schwindt ML, Scott KN, Shaffer WO (1985) Nuclear imaging for musculoskeletal infections in children. J Pediatr Orthop 5(3):343–347
149. Howard A, Viskontas D, Sabbagh C (1999) Reduction in osteomyelitis and septic arthritis related to *Haemophilus influenzae* type B vaccination. J Pediatr Orthop 19(6):705–715
150. Howard JB, Highgenboten CL, Nelson JD (1976) Residual effects of septic arthritis in infancy and childhood. JAMA 236(8):932–935
151. Kabak S, Halici M, Akcakus M, Cetin N, Narin N (2002) Septic arthritis in patients followed-up in neonatal intensive care unit. Pediatr Int 44(6):652–657
152. Lloyd-Roberts GC (1960) Suppurative arthritis of infancy. Some observations upon prognosis and management. J Bone Joint Surg 42B:706–720
153. Lundy D, Kehl D (1998) Increasing prevalence of *Kingella kingae* in osteoarticular infections in young children. J Pediatr Orthop 18(2):262–267
154. Nade S (1983) Acute septic arthritis in infancy and childhood. J Bone Joint Surg 65B:234–241
155. Paterson DC (1970) Acute suppurative arthritis in infancy and childhood. J Bone Joint Surg 52B:474–482
156. Wood BP (1980) The vanishing epiphyseal ossification center: a sequel to septic arthritis of childhood. Radiology 134:387–389

Hip

157. Badgley CE, Yglesias L, Perham WS, Snyder CH (1936) Study of the end results in 113 cases of septic hips. J Bone Joint Surg Br 18:1047–1061
158. Betz RR, Cooperman DR, Wopperer JM, Sutherland RD, White JJ, Schaaf HW, Aschliman MR, Choi IH, Bowen RJ, Gillespie R (1990) Late sequelae of septic arthritis of the hip in infancy and childhood. J Pediatr Orthop 10:365–372
159. Choi H, Pizzutillo PD, Bown JR, Dragann R, Mathis T (1990) Sequelae and reconstruction after septic arthritis of the hip in infants. J Bone Joint Surg 72A(8):1150–1165
160. Eyre-Brook AL (1960) Septic arthritis of the hip and osteomyelitis of the upper end of the femur in infants. J Bone Joint Surg 42B:11–20
161. Dias L, Tachdjian MO, Schroeder KE (1980) Premature closure of the triradiate cartilage. Report of a case. J Bone Joint Surg 62B:46–48
162. Fabry G, Meire E (1983) Septic arthritis of the hip in children: poor results after late and inadequate treatment. J Pediatr Orthop 3:461–466
163. Gash A, Walker CR, Carty H (1994) Cast report: complete photopenia of the femoral head on radionuclide bone scanning in septic arthritis of the hip. Br J Radiol 67:816–818
164. Hallel T, Salvati EA (1978) Septic arthritis of the hip in infancy: end result study. Clin Orthop 132:115–128
165. Hunka L, Said SE, MacKenzie DA, Rogala EG, Cruess RL (1982) Classification and surgical management of the severe sequelae of septic hips in children. Clin Orthop 171:30–36
166. Kaye JJ, Winchester PH, Freiberger RH (1975) Neonatal septic "dislocation" of the hip: true dislocation or pathological epiphyseal separation? Radiology 114:671–674
167. Morrey BF, Bianco AJ, Rhodes KH (1976) Suppurative arthritis of the hip in children. J Bone Joint Surg 58A:388–392
168. Peterson HA, Robertson RC (1997) Premature partial closure of the triradiate cartilage treated with excision of a physeal osseous bar. J Bone Joint Surg 79A(5):767–770
169. Song HR, Oh CW, Guille JT, Song KS, Kyung HS, Kim SY, Park BC (2006) Lateral growth disturbance of the proximal femur in premature infants who had neonatal sepsis. J Pediatr Orthop B 15(3):178–182
170. Umer M, Hashmi P, Ahmad T, Ahmed M, Umar M (2003) Septic arthritis of the hip in children – Aga Khan University Hospital experience in Pakistan. J Pak Med Assoc 53(10):472–478
171. Vidigal EC Jr, Vidigal EC, Fernandes JL (1997) Avascular necrosis as a complication of septic arthritis of the hip in children. Int Orthop 21:389–392
172. Wientroub S, Lloyd-Roberts BD, Fraser M (1981) The prognostic significance of the triradiate cartilage in suppurative arthritis of the hip in infancy and early childhood. J Bone Joint Surg 63B:190–193

173. Wopperer JM, White JJ, Gillespie R, Obletz BE (1988) Long-term follow-up of infantile hip sepsis. J Pediatr Orthop 8:322–325

Knee

174. Girdlestone BR (1931) The pathology and treatment of tuberculosis of the knee-joint. Br J Surg 19:488–507
175. Kumar SJ, Forlin E, Guille JT (1992) Epiphyseometaphyseal cupping of the distal femur with knee-flexion contracture. Orthop Rev 21(1):67–70
176. Lejman T, Strong M (1998) Septic arthritis. In: de Pablos J (ed) The immature knee. biblio stm, Barcelona, Chapter 14, pp 113–126
177. Lejman T, Strong M, Michno P (1995) Septic arthritis in newborns and infants – the value of arthrography in diagnosis of post-inflammatory knee defects [Polish]. Chir Narzadow Ruchu Ortop Pol 60(3):199–204
178. Stanitski CL, Harvell JC, Fu FH (1989) Arthroscopy in acute septic knees. Management in pediatric patients. Clin Orthop Relat Res 241:209–212
179. Strong M, Lejman T, Michno P, Hayman M (1994) Sequelae from septic arthritis of the knee during the first two years of life. J Pediatr Orthop 14(6):745–751

Shoulder

180. Bos CFA, Mol LJCD, Obermann WR, Tjin a Ton ER (1998) Late sequelae of neonatal septic arthritis of the shoulder. J Bone Joint Surg 80B:645–650
181. Cattaneo R, Villa A, Catagni MA, Bell D (1990) Lengthening of the humerus using the Ilizarov technique. Clin Orthop Relat Res 250:117–124
182. Dick HM, Tietjen R (1978) Humeral lengthening for septic neonatal growth arrest: case report. J Bone Joint Surg 60A:1138–1139
183. Ellefsen BK, Frierson MA, Raney EM, Ogden JA (1994) Humerus varus: a complication of neonatal, infantile, and childhood injury and infection. J Pediatr Orthop 14:479–486
184. Janovec M (1990) Prolongation of the humerus in children and adolescents. In: DePablos J, Cãnadell J (eds) Bone lengthening: current trends and controversies. Servico de Publicationes de la Universidad de Navarra, S.A, Pamplona, pp 463–465
185. Lejman T, Strong M, Michno P, Hayman M (1995) Septic arthritis of the shoulder during the first 18 months of life. J Pediatr Orthop 15:172–175
186. Ogden JA, Weil UH, Hempton RF (1976) Developmental humerus varus. Clin Orthop 116:158–166
187. Olerud S, Henriksson T, Engkvist O (1983) A free vascularized fibular graft in lengthening of the humerus with the Wagner apparatus. J Bone Joint Surg 65A:111–114
188. Peterson HA (1989) Surgical lengthening of the humerus: case report and review. J Pediatr Orthop 9(5):596–601
189. Poul J (2001) Svebis: results of 20 lengthening of the humerus. Acta Chir Orthop Traumatol Cech 68(5):289–293
190. Rankin KC, Rycken JM (1993) Bilateral dislocation of the proximal humeral epiphyses in septic arthritis: a case report. J Bone Joint Surg 75B:329–330
191. Schmidt D, Mubarak S, Gelberman R (1981) Septic shoulders in children. J Pediatr Orthop 1:67–72
192. Timperlake RW, Degnan GG (1992) Transient radial nerve palsy during humeral lengthening in a child. Contemp Orthop 25(5):499–503
193. Ugwonali OFC, Bae DS, Waters PM (2007) Corrective osteotomy for humerus varus. J Pediatr Orthop 27(5):529–532

Wrist

194. Rashkoff ES, Burkhalter WE, Mann RJ (1983) Septic arthritis of the wrist. J Bone Joint Surg 65A:824–828
195. Strong M, Lejman T, Michno P (1995) Septic arthritis of the wrist in infancy. J Pediatr Orthop 15:152–156

Tumor

4.1 Introduction

The focus of this chapter is the effect of tumors on physeal growth, and not on the details of patient demographics, imaging, histology or treatment of the tumor. Tumor and tumor-like conditions that injure the physis may be benign or malignant and occur primarily in the metaphysis. Some cross the physis into the epiphysis (transphyseal). Tumors, benign or malignant, located exclusively in the epiphysis which cause injury to the physis, are a rare occurrence [4]. For the purpose of this chapter a tumor or tumor-like condition is defined as a space occupying lesion of normal or abnormal tissue for that location, rather than some expression of neoplasia.

Radionuclide bone scanning will readily identify areas where vascularity or osteogenesis is disturbed [3]. Bone scans are therefore valuable in evaluating the physis and identifying osteoblastic reaction and metastatic disease. Tumors near the growth plate are well demonstrated by modified coronal computerized tomography (CT) [2]. Fast contrast-enhanced MR imaging assists differentiation between aggressive and nonaggressive lesions [1].

4.2 Benign Bone Tumors

Benign bone tumors occur most commonly in the metaphysis and less commonly in the epiphysis [5, 6]. They often have clinical and roentgenographic features similar to subacute osteomyelitis [5, 8]. Benign tumors often abut against the physis, which has only a partial or temporary inhibitory effect preventing penetration of the tumor into the epiphysis. The physis may close prematurely when the tumor is untreated or following treatment, particularly curettage and bone grafting procedures. Examples are solitary bone cyst, aneurysmal bone cyst, osteochondroma, enchondroma, chondroblastoma, giant cell tumor of bone, histiocytosis X, osteoid osteoma, focal fibrocartilaginous dysplasia, and fibrous dysplasia of bone. Most of these cause little or no pain and remain undetected for considerable periods of time [5–7].

Transition of a primary benign bone tumor to a malignant tumor is rare, and when it occurs it is often in connection with radiation treatment [7]. Other effects of radiation treatment [9], such as physeal arrest producing limb length discrepancy, angular deformity, exostoses, scoliosis, short stature, and slipped capital epiphysis are discussed in Chap. 13.

4.2.1 Solitary Bone Cyst

A bone cyst is a resorbtive lesion of bone. The cavity is characterized by a thin lining of connective tissue, occasionally containing giant cells, and a variable amount of clear or yellow fluid which is not under increased pressure [14, 25, 36]. Trabeculae frequently traverse the cavity. The cortices are often thin and expanded. Spontaneous new bone formation does not occur, except near a fracture [14]. These cysts appear as a radiolucent defect on roentgenogram. They have been called solitary [5, 11, 12, 21, 23, 30, 38, 43], simple [13, 14, 25, 31, 32, 39, 47], unicameral [14–17, 19, 21, 24, 28, 33–37, 41, 45], essential [10], and benign [18]. The term solitary is used here because they usually are single (two cysts occurring in the same patient is exceedingly rare [14]), and on occasion can be anything but "simple" [25]. Using the term simple also conveys a misleading message to parents. The terms unicameral (one chamber) or uniloculated exclude those cysts that are multicameral or multiloculated.

Metaphyseal "cysts" occur in a small number of patients with Perthes' disease [26, 27, 29, 44]. Their etiology is unknown. Although they have some similarity to solitary bone cysts, and on occasion are accompanied with "physeal irregularity", their histology is that of fibrous connective tissue, or cartilage [29, 44]. Reports of growth arrest are lacking and therefore they are not discussed further.

The etiology of solitary bone cysts remains elusive. Proposed theories include vascular events such as interosseous hemorrhage [36] and venous obstruction [19, 30]. The rapidity with which bone is deposited and absorbed also suggests a vascular mechanism [17]. The cysts have been found in patients as young as 2 years [11, 14], and as old as 60 years [15], but are usually discovered during the first two decades of life, particularly between the ages of 9 and 15 years [14, 15]. Males predominate 3:1 [11, 14, 15]. Bone cysts are nearly always located in the metaphysis of tubular long bones, most frequently in the proximal humerus, followed by the proximal femur [11, 14–16, 19, 37]. They occur less commonly in metaphyseal equivalent sites, most often in the ilium and calcaneus [14, 15, 37]. They have been called "active" if near the physis, and "latent" or inactive if in the diaphysis [19]. This may just reflect the time of discovery since the epiphysis may grow away from an active cyst allowing it to reside in the diaphysis (a latent cyst) [23, 24].

Clinically the only presenting symptoms may be a mild ache in the affected area. Pain and swelling secondary to pathologic fracture through the cyst associated with minor trauma is the most frequent presentation [11, 14, 19, 35, 41]. The fracture heals rapidly, apparently not influenced by the pathologic process. Muscle atrophy and palpable prominence may be present following multiple fractures through a cyst treated symptomatically [25]. Many cysts disappear after fracture or when the patient reaches maturity (Fig. 4.1). Some persist into adulthood (Fig. 4.2) or are first discovered in adulthood.

Treatment of the cyst includes observation, immobilization of the fracture if present, needle aspiration, two needle aspiration-irrigation, instillation of sclerosing agents, steroids or prepared bone substances, open evacuation and excisional curettement, and sauceriza-tion with bone grafting using autogenous bone or prepared bone substances. When curetting a cyst the exposed physis can be wiped with a sponge rather than excoriated with a curette in an attempt to lessen damage to the physis [34]. The effect of treatment on the physis is case dependent and often speculative. Nonoperative treatment of an active cyst is an attractive temporary measure, allowing the epiphysis to grow away from the cyst to lessen the chance of injury

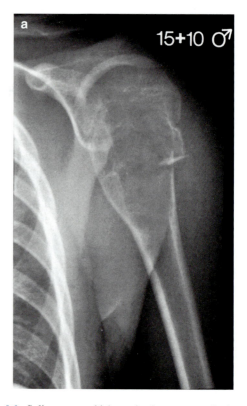

Fig. 4.1 Solitary cyst which resolved spontaneously, but with growth impairment. This 15 year 10 month old boy felt pain in the left shoulder while turning the handle bar on the bicycle he was riding. He did not fall. (**a**) There is expansion, thinning, and fractures of the cortex of the proximal humeral metaphysis. This has all the characteristics of a solitary cyst. The physis is not well visualized. A shoulder immobilizing splint was applied and worn 6 weeks. The lesion was not aspirated, injected, or operated. (**b**) At age 16 years 9 months the patient is normally active and asymptomatic. His only complaint is that his shirt sleeve hangs lower at his left wrist. (**c**) Scanogram shows the healing of the lesion. The left humerus is 2.9 cm shorter than the right. All physes are essentially closed. Note: This fracture was confined to the metaphysis and occurred during an atraumatic minor event. Humeral lengths at the time of fracture were not recorded. Since there was no treatment other than a shoulder immobilizer for 6 weeks it can be concluded that the premature physeal closure was due to direct involvement of the cyst

4.2 Benign Bone Tumors

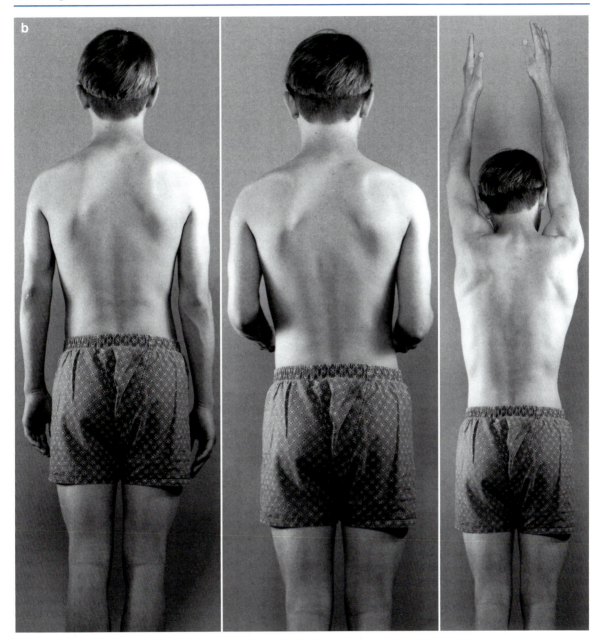

Fig. 4.1 (continued)

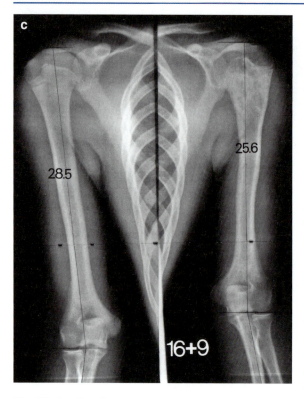

Fig. 4.1 (continued)

to the physis during surgery [14, 41]. Growth arrest can occur with or without surgical intervention [18, 34]. Neer [37] reported growth arrest in 9.9% of cysts treated nonoperatively, and 3.1% of cysts treated by curettage and bone grafting (Table 4.1). Therefore the risk of growth arrest need not be a contradiction to surgical intervention [18, 34].

Physeal arrest probably occurs in less than 10% of cases (Table 4.1). The etiology of the arrest remains controversial [45, 47]. Large cysts located close to the physis are most prone to be associated with growth arrest. Theories that might explain physeal arrest include local erosion of the physis by the cyst, increased cyst pressure, fracture through the cyst, or treatment of the cyst [18, 19, 23, 32, 34, 39, 47]. Fracture or multiple fractures through the cyst are an unlikely source of growth arrest because they are usually the result of minor trauma, are through the middle portion of the cyst, have minimal displacement, and involvement of the physis is not usually apparent [35, 45]. In addition, the cyst sometimes disappears after fracture. Treatment may certainly damage a physis, but in some instances physeal arrest is noted prior to treatment [34, 45], or without treatment (Figs. 4.1 and 4.2). A vascular etiology for physeal closure has also been proposed [23, 39], based on work of previous authors who suggested hyperemia, increased pulsatile pressure [33], or alterations in venous drainage leading to increased venous pressure within the metaphysis [45] as causes of erosion of the physis. When physeal arrest occurs it is complete in almost all cases. Relative shortening of the involved bone is common and may be present without any prior treatment [10, 25]. This suggests that in these cases the physis is affected directly by the tumor, or by the vascular mechanisms mentioned above. Separation of the epiphysis (slipped epiphysis) through the physis [13] is uncommon in the absence of transphyseal extension of the cyst into the epiphysis.

Extension of a bone cyst from the metaphysis transphyseally into the epiphysis is uncommon [12, 14, 23, 24, 28, 31, 33, 38, 39, 43, 44]. Most reports are of single cases. In one series of 607 unicameral cysts, 12 (2%) exhibited combined metaphyseal-epiphyseal or

Fig. 4.2 Solitary cyst which did not resolve spontaneously, with growth impairment. While throwing a ball this 12 year 3 month old boy was struck on the right arm by another boy attempting to knock the ball out of his hand. (**a**) There is a fracture through the distal portion of a solitary bone cyst in the proximal right humeral metaphysis abutting the physis. A sling was applied. (**b**) Five weeks later the fracture was healed and the physis was open. (**c**) Seven months post injury the right shoulder had normal motion and no tenderness, but the right humerus was clinically one inch shorter than the left. The proximal humeral physes were open, but more narrow on the right. (**d**) At age 14 years 8 months, 2 years 5 months post fracture the physis had grown away from the cyst (compare with **c**). At age 18 years he fell while climbing a hill dislocating his right shoulder which required anesthesia for reduction. There was no fracture. He was denied enlistment into the Air Force because of the persistent cyst in the humerus. (**e**) At age 18 years 11 months scanograms showed the right humerus 4.5 cm shorter and the right forearm .4 cm longer than the left, for an overall arm length discrepancy of 4.1 cm. The right proximal humerus has normal contours, but enlargement of the cyst now appears to involve a portion of the epiphysis. The cyst was grafted with homogenous cancellous bone chips. Clear yellow fluid and soft tissue lining of the cyst containing giant cells confirmed the diagnosis. He became normally active and asymptomatic. He did not join the Air Force as planned. When last seen at age 20 years 2 months he was employed operating a fork lift. He was normally active and asymptomatic with full shoulder motion. He noted mild inconvenience from asymmetric sleeve lengths of shirts and coats. Note: The clinical 1 in. relative shortening noted only 7 months post fracture (**c**) suggests immediate cessation of growth. However this was followed by some growth as noted in (**d**) by new metaphyseal bone adjacent to the physis (compare with **c**)

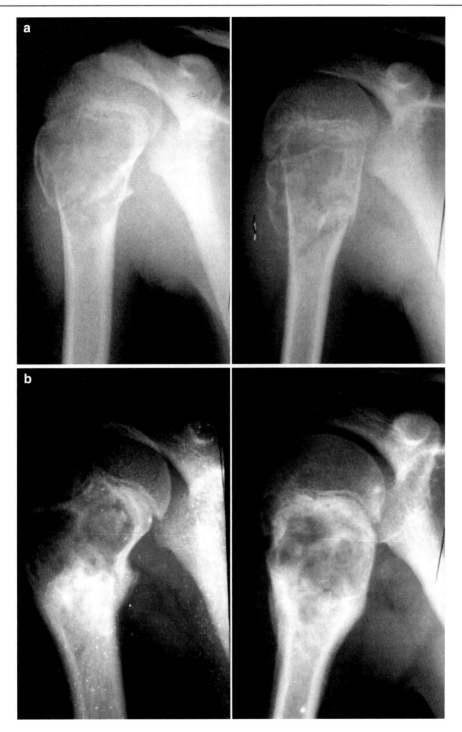

Fig. 4.2 (continued)

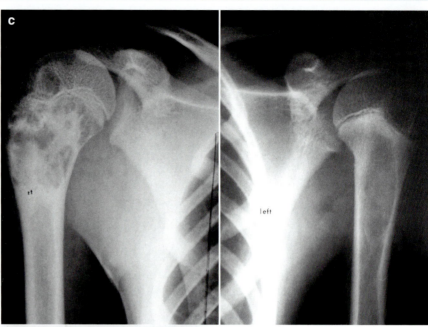

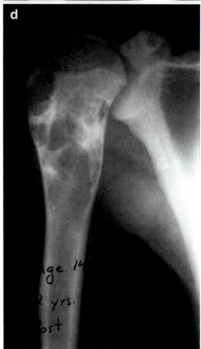

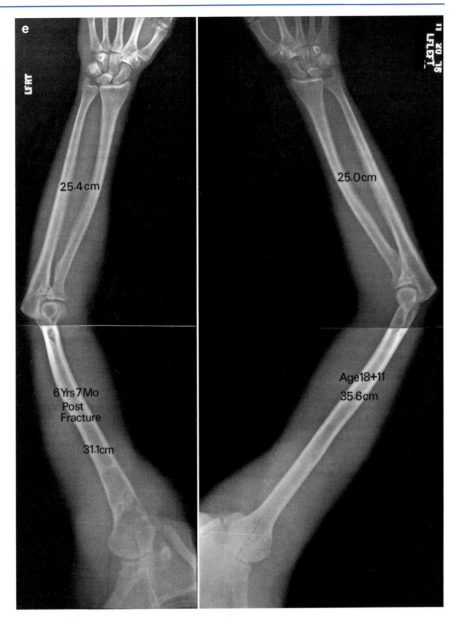

Fig. 4.2 (continued)

Table 4.1 Solitary bone cysts: incidence of growth arrest

Year	Author[a]	No.	No. arrests	Percent
1952	Graham [22]	31	2	6.5
1966	Neer [37]	41[b]	4	9.9
1966	Neer [37]	129[c]	4	3.1
1968	Boseker [14]	145	3	2.1
1977	McKay [34]	16	5	31.3
1986	Campanacci [15]	416	28	6.7
1998	Stanton [45]	51	5	9.8

[a]Most articles have multiple authors. See references
[b]Proximal humeral cysts treated nonoperatively out of a total of 175 patients
[c]Proximal humeral cysts treated by curettage and bone grafting out of a total of 175 patients. It is inappropriate to total these columns to determine a combined percentage of arrest because of differences in the proportion of active to latent cases, number of patients treated and not treated, the treatment used, and length of follow-up

apophyseal involvement through an open physis [16]. This suggests that the resistance of physeal cartilage to tumor invasion is at best only partial and should not be depended upon in any patient [16]. Transphyseal cysts are well exhibited by the injection of contrast fluid [16] or by MRI [11, 20, 23, 24, 31, 39]. The presumed etiology is erosion of the physis by the cyst in the metaphysis [20, 23]. A pulsatile, elevated pressure measurement in two cases, suggest a vascular etiology [33, 38]. The penetration is typically in the center of the physis [16, 39]. Growth of the normal peripheral physis can produce cupping (Sect. 1.5). The remaining physis surrounding the central protrusion may appear wider than normal [16, 39]. Expansion of the epiphysis [24] as well as slipping of the epiphysis [24, 39] are also reported. Accompanying growth arrest is more common (Table 4.2) than in cysts without extension into the epiphysis (compare with Table 4.1) [11, 21, 23, 24, 31, 33, 37, 38], but does not always occur [28], and is not well explained. In patients below the age of 10 years not only is the chance of cyst recurrence greater, but so also is the probability that a growth disturbance will follow after the cyst has extended into the epiphysis [16]. Relative bone shortening of 2–11 cm has been recorded [39].

The treatment of the physeal arrest is dependent upon the amount of discrepancy anticipated at maturity. Partial arrest with progressive angular deformity is rare [35] and only one bar excision is reported [25]. No follow-up was given. The treatment options for complete arrest include surgical lengthening of the involved bone, or physeal arrest or bone shortening on the contralateral side. In the case of the humerus and forearm, contralateral surgical physeal arrest and bone shortening need never be considered. Children with humeral discrepancy of 5 cm or less usually have no functional impairment or cosmetic concerns, and therefore no treatment is necessary. Relative humeral shortening of 6 cm or greater can cause interference with activities of daily living particularly sports, as well as clothes fitting problems and body image concerns. Progressive distraction lengthening of the humerus is highly successful using monolateral external fixation devices [10, 40, 42]. Ideally the lengthening should be delayed until near maturity to avoid guessing at the amount to be lengthened, and to avoid recurrence of the discrepancy due to unexpected additional growth of the normal humerus (Fig. 3.9). The

Table 4.2 Transphyseal solitary bone cysts: incidence of growth arrest

Year	Author[a]	No.	No. arrests	Percent
1986	Capanna [16]	12[b]	4	33.3
2003	Ovadia [39]	8[c]	7	87.5

[a]Both articles have multiple authors. See references
[b]All 12 cysts were treated: 8 with steroid injections, 3 with curettage and bone grafting, and 1 with curettage and bone grafting followed by steroid injection
[c]Treatment consisted of biopsy, aspiration, and injection of methylprednisolone acetate in four and autologous bone marrow in seven. Neither curettage nor bone grafting was used

osteotomy for lengthening may be through the cyst [10], or through normal bone adjacent to the cyst. The amount to be lengthened in the humerus is typically between 6 and 12 cm. Limited shoulder abduction and elbow flexion that occurs late during the lengthening usually resolves spontaneously [10]. Persistent limited shoulder abduction due to premature medial arrest causing proximal humerus varus can be treated by corrective valgus osteotomy, if necessary [46, 47].

4.2.2 Aneurysmal Bone Cyst

Aneurysmal bone cyst (ABC) is an expansive osteolytic lesion (Fig. 4.3a,b) consisting of blood-filled spaces and channels separated by connective tissue septa containing fibroblasts, osteoclast-like giant cells, and reactive woven bone. Changes resembling aneurysmal bone cyst are frequently encountered in, or co-existing with, other benign tumors, but ABC is an entity of its own [15, 50]. Only the primary lesions are discussed here.

One of the previous concepts of pathogenesis was that it is a secondary hyperplastic reactive lesion of bone occurring from a hemodynamic disturbance resulting in increased venous pressure and development of a dilated vascular bed within the involved bone. It was felt to be hyperplastic rather than neoplastic [51], and has been likened to aneurysmal fistulae of bone [49]. Trauma has been implicated as a factor, but most authors agree that the injury merely draws attention to a pre-existing lesion. Recently, chromosomal aberrations have shown ABC to indeed be neoplastic [63–65].

Angiography shows an intense, diffuse, and persistent accumulation of contrast media [15]. Intratumoral

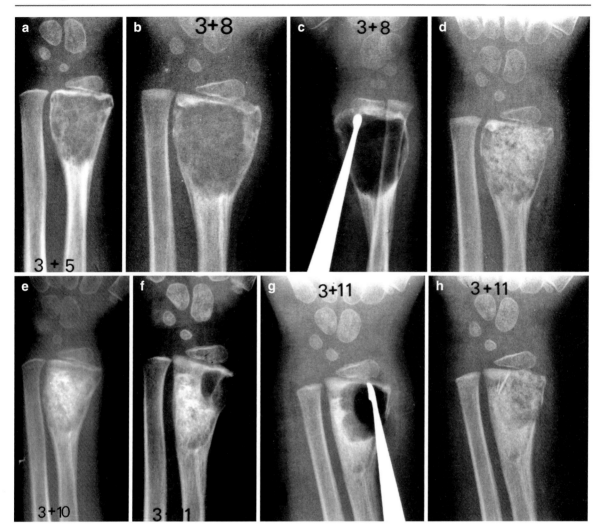

Fig. 4.3 Aneurysmal bone cyst. The presenting symptom in this 3 year 5 month old boy was swelling of the wrist, first noted by the mother. (**a**) A lytic lesion of the distal radial metaphysis has expansion and thinning of the cortex, and extends to within 3 mm of the distal radial physis. A cortisone injection was accompanied by significant bleeding. (**b**) Three months later, age 3 years 8 months, the cortical expansion was increased. Slight positive ulnar variance has increased in this 3 month interval. (**c**) Surgical exposure was obtained by removing a window of the thin cortical bone with a scalpel. Hemorrhagic grayish-white soft tissue was confirmed to be ABC. Bleeding stopped once the soft tissue was removed. The inside of the thin cortical bone was excoriated with a motorized burr. The bone adjacent to the physis was gently curetted, but not subjected to the burr. This roentgenogram was taken to document the position of the curette relative to the physis. (**d**) The cavity was filled with homogenous femoral head bone chips from the bone bank. A long arm compression bandage was changed to a long arm cast 4 days later. (**e**) Six weeks post surgery, age 3 years 10 months, there is new bone growth of the metaphysis, between the physis and the operated area. (**f**) Nine weeks post operative, age 3 years 11 months the cyst had partially recurred. (**g**) A second re-excision, re-grafting procedure was similarly performed. The curette is closer to the physis, but the physis was not visualized. (**h**) The cavity was again packed with homogenous femoral head bone chips from the bone bank. (**i**) At age 9 years 5 months, 5½ years post second surgery, the patient was normally active and asymptomatic. The radius was growing normally and the radio-ulnar variance was zero. The nature of the residual lytic defect in the diaphysis (*arrow*) is unknown, but could be the entry point of the curet from (**h**) or residual tumor which has become excentrically located in the cortex due to metaphyseal remodeling. The increasing distance between the lytic defect and the physis documents excellent growth of the physis (compare with (**g**, **h**)). The patient needs follow-up until growth is complete. Note: This juxtaphyseal ABC was successfully eradicated by two curettements without disturbing growth

Fig. 4.3 (continued)

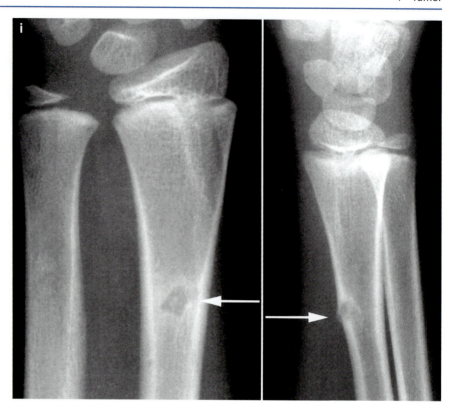

monometric vascular pressures may be as high as arteriolar levels [49]. Arteriography demonstrates no significant afferent or efferent vascular branches. Therefore ABC behaves like a sponge, absorbing blood relatively slowly from the bone capillaries and periosteal vascular network [15]. Bone scans usually shows minimal increased uptake, sometimes with a central cold area [15, 54]. The natural history of ABC is that of a progressive, expansile, osteolytic, and aggressive lesion leading eventually to a pathologic fracture [67].

ABC accounts for 1–6% of all primary bone tumors and occurs at all ages, primarily in the first and second decades of life, but less common before age 5 years [67]. These cysts occur in metaphyses of all parts of the skeleton, most often in long bones, as well as in metaphyseal equivalent sites, most often in the spine and pelvis. The cyst frequently abuts the physis (juxtaphyseal). Contrary to most tumors there is modest female gender predominance [15, 49–51, 55]. Pain, swelling, and fracture are the main reasons for seeking medical attention [50, 59, 67]. Pathologic fractures are less frequent than in patients with solitary bone cysts [15, 67].

The ABC is treated in multiple ways, usually including surgery [15, 53, 67]. Although high-energy, low-dose radiation therapy has achieved successful eradication of ABC without growth retardation [59], it is generally agreed that radiation therapy should not be used for ABC in children to avoid jeopardizing the physis [55, 59], and because of concern of a post-radiation sarcoma. The commonest operation is curettage and bone grafting using autogenous bone, homologous bank bone, or bone substitutes (Fig. 4.3c–i). When the ABC is in contact with the physis (juxtaphyseal), curettage must be done carefully to avoid disturbing growth [68]. Blunt curettage (rather than sharp curettage or a high speed burr) against the physis is preferred in an effort to preserve growth potential [50, 57, 58, 67]. Embolization of vessels supplying a distal femur tumor a few days prior to curettement and bone grafting, was accompanied by subsequent partial physeal arrest and cannot be excluded as a possible contributory factor, as embolization of any vessels supplying a physis may cause growth arrest [56]. Juxtaphyseal lesions have also been successfully treated by total subperiosteal resection of the tumor with insertion of autogenous or allogenic bone grafts including cortical struts, without invoking growth arrest [51, 57, 66]. This may require Ilizarov apparatus fixation [52]. If the resection or the bone graft transgresses the physis, arrest will of course ensue [62].

Table 4.3 Aneurysmal bone cysts: incidence of growth arrest

Year	Author[a]	No.	No. arrests	Percent
1985	Capanna [51]	30[b]	2	6.7
1990	Farsetti [55]	12	5[c]	41.7
1995	Marcove [60]	8	3	37.5
1998	Bollini [50]	27	2	7.4
2002	Rodriguiz [67]	29	3	10.3

[a]All articles have more than one author. See references
[b]All cysts were in long bones adjacent to an open physis (juxtaphyseal)
[c]Radiation therapy was used in two patients of these five
It is inappropriate to total these columns to determine a combined percentage of arrest because of differences in the number of patients treated and not treated, the treatment used, and length of follow-up

Table 4.4 Transphyseal aneurysmal bone cysts: incidence of growth arrests

Year	Author[a]	No.	No. arrests	Percent
1985	Capanna [51]	9	5	55.6
1995	Margrove [60]	3	3	100.0

[a]Both articles have more than one author. See references

The major complication of juxtaphyseal ABC is growth arrest and preservation of the physis remains a high priority [58, 67]. Since few ABC's are treated nonoperatively, it is difficult to determine whether an arrest is a result of the tumor or of its treatment [53]. The incidence is difficult to determine because of differences in reporting, particularly the location of the cyst relative to the physis, the treatment, and the length and focus of the follow-up (Table 4.3). Any overly aggressive approach that involves the physis or articular cartilage is not warranted. Reluctance by the surgeon to perform a sufficiently extensive curettage could result in local recurrence. The curettage is either aggressive, risking a physeal arrest, or is limited risking tumor recurrence. A blunt dissector near the physis may lessen the chance of damage to the physis. Incomplete tumor removal with subsequent recurrence is usually easier to treat than a physeal bar and its consequences [50, 53]. In one series of 30 juxtaphyseal ABC's treated by curettage, only 2 developed growth disturbance after curettage (Table 4.3) [51].

Extension of a metaphyseal ABC through an open physis (transphyseal) into the epiphysis occurs in 6–23% of cases [15, 49, 51, 69]. The extension is best visualized on MRI [54, 67] and is usually in the center of the physis [61]. The edge of the physis adjacent to transphyseal deficit may consist of intact growing physis or an epiphyseal-metaphyseal osseous bridge [61]. As the ABC expands within the epiphysis the physis becomes progressively ischemic in the more central portions [61]. Latitudinal physeal growth continues since the zone of Ranvier, which has a peripheral extraosseous blood supply (Fig. 1.2), is not affected by the expanding intraosseous cyst [61]. Patients near completion of growth are more likely to have invasion of the plate [51]. Presumably proliferating tissue of the ABC expands, or replaces some of the small vessels that cross the physis [54]. Thus the physis is a relative, but not complete barrier to tumor extension [51]. A physis invaded by an ABC should not be expected to grow normally. In a review of 39 ABC's adjacent to the physis, 9 (23%) extended into the epiphysis. Among the nine patients with transphyseal invasion treated by curettage, five had growth disturbance (Table 4.4). Thus, this study suggests that the transphyseal extension of the tumor was a greater factor in developing growth disturbance than the curettage. In rare cases with extension into the epiphysis, collapse of the epiphysis may cause joint deformity and limitation of joint function [15]. As expected, cysts with transphyseal involvement have a higher risk of premature growth arrest (Table 4.4, compare with Table 4.3). One ABC of the distal ulnar metaphysis with premature arrest of its physis, caused enough ulnar shortening to produce developmental dislocation of the proximal radius [48].

Close surveillance is essential in all cases to follow both the tumor and the physis. Premature partial physeal closure following treated or untreated ABC can be treated by bar excision [50], but no cases have been recorded. Complete physeal closure with resulting significant limb length discrepancy is treated by contralateral physeal arrest or bone shortening, or ipsilateral bone lengthening.

4.2.3 Osteochondroma

An osteochondroma is a projection of bone capped by cartilage. Heterotopic proliferation of peripheral physeal chondroblasts results in defective metaphyseal remodeling and retardation of enchondromal bone growth. It is the most common benign bone forming tumor [106] and is usually reported in the literature under the title osteochondroma, osteochondromata, exostosis, cartilaginous exostosis, diaphyseal aclasia, metaphyseal aclasia, or dyschondroplasia. The lesions may be solitary or multiple, the two forms having the same essential anatomic structure [106]. Multiple osteochondromas may be hereditary or due to a new mutation [115, 120]. The lesions most commonly reside on the surface of metaphysis directly adjacent to the physis, appear in a variety of shapes and sizes, and may be either sessile or pedunculated. Because it is a mass of new space occupying tissue which persists and grows independently of its surroundings, it qualifies as a tumor. The literature is voluminous; the major portion concerned with growth impairment is recorded here.

Osteochondromas may be found on all tubular long bones, occasionally on the pelvis, scapula, ribs and spine, and less commonly on the patella, sternum, and tarsal and carpal bones [86, 110, 115, 117, 120]. The lesions are rarely noticed before age 1 year, and often not until age 2 or 3 years. The majority of exostoses are clinically evident in the first decade of life [72, 74, 115]. The size and number of the exostoses vary considerably, some patients having hundreds of individual lesions. The natural history of these lesions is gradual increase in size, undesirable cosmetic appearance, retardation of growth, and function impairment. Osteochondromas enlarge while the physis is open, and stop growing with physeal closure [117, 120]. No new exostoses arise after cessation of growth [115]. Enlargement of a lesion after cessation of growth is most likely a malignant transformation. Relative bone shortening is a function of retarded physeal growth rather than premature physeal closure [86]. Sessile lesions have been associated with more shortening and deformity than pedunculated lesions [117]. No deformity, once identified, improves with growth [110]. Short stature is present in most, but not all, affected individuals [83, 110, 117], and becomes more evident at the end of the growing period [114]. The supposition that short stature is due to precocious skeletal maturation or early physeal closure lacks documentation [114]. Male prevalence is approximately 1.5 to 1 female [76, 106, 114, 115, 120].

Little is known concerning the pathogenesis of osteochondromas. Basically there is aberrant growth of a peripheral segment of the growth plate which increases in size by enchondral ossification with extension primarily toward the metaphysis, but it also impairs growth of adjacent areas of the physis [76, 89, 100]. The skeletal growth disturbance can be interpreted as a local effect of benign neoplastic behavior. In effect the osteochondroma saps growth from the remaining normal physis causing the overall length of the bone to be shorter than it would otherwise be. Growth of the osteochondroma overwhelms and retards growth of any closely associated physis, resulting in a tethering effect on paired structures [105, 117]. The faster-growing end of a long bone has the greater likelihood of involvement [115]. There is an inverse correlation between osteochondroma size and relative bone length [105, 117]. As the physis continues to grow the osteochondroma may be left behind in the metaphysis or even the diaphysis [115]. An alternative etiology for diaphyseal osteochondromas is the proliferation of persistent chondrogenic cells in the periosteum [91]. Even though the lesion may be in the diaphysis, far from the physis, longitudinal growth slow-down continues [73]. Although limb angular deformity is also common, it is usually due to growth differential between the tibia and fibula, or ulna and radius, rather than to a physeal bar. No specific treatable physeal bar has been reported as a result of osteochondroma.

The treatment of osteochondromas is basically observation or surgery. Radiation therapy has no positive affect on this tumor [115]. Observation can result in significant functional impairment in some cases (Figs. 4.4, 4.5 and 4.12). In general, surgical excision of osteochondromas is usually performed to alleviate symptoms due to the mass, for cosmetic reasons, or for disproportionate bone growth. In addition, elective removal of selected osteochondromas may prevent some growth problems from occurring [96, 101–103, 113, 117]. Ablation of rapidly enlarging lesions close to important physes reduces the rate of subsequent growth retardation [105]. The entire bony base and cartilage cap should be completely removed, or recurrence is possible. No partial growth arrests have been reported from overly aggressive removal of lesions.

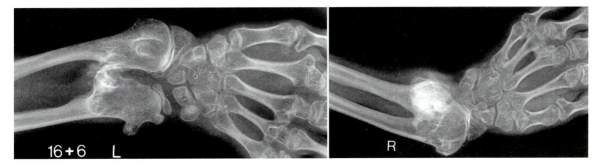

Fig. 4.4 Untreated osteochondromas of the distal forearms with loss of function. The parents of this 16 year 6 month old boy consistently declined excision of lesions because of perceived absence of functional impairment. However, there is now complete loss of forearm rotation bilaterally and the right wrist is fixed in ulnar deviation and flexion. The use of a computer is severely limited. Note osteochondromas on the metacarpals and phalanges (Reprinted from Peterson [101], with permission)

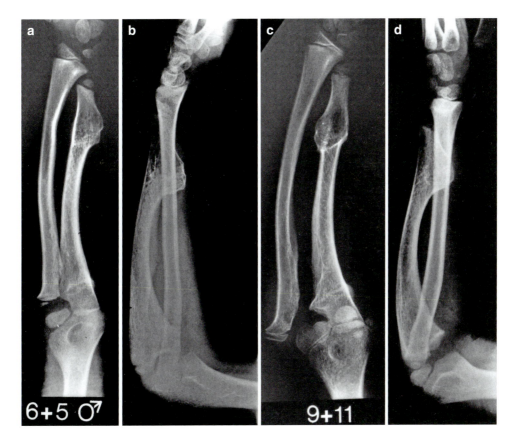

Fig. 4.5 Untreated solitary sessile osteochondroma of the distal ulnar metaphysis associated with gradual dislocation of the proximal radius. (**a**) At age 6 years 5 months the radial head is located. (**b**) A lateral view at the same time shows the true size of the osteochondroma and bowing of the ulna. A recommendation to excise the osteochondroma was declined by the parents because the patient had no symptoms or functional impairment. (**c**) At age 9 years 11 months the patient returned with elbow pain and loss of forearm and elbow motion. The radial head is dislocated. Note the mild adaptive lateral angulation of the proximal radius. The distal radial articular angle and carpal slip have improved (compare with (**a**)), probably due to loss of the tethering effect of the ulna secondary to developmental dislocation of the radial head. The distal ulnar physis has grown away from the lesion. (**d**) Lateral view at the same time as (**c**) Note: excision of the osteochondroma at age 6 years 5 months (**a**, **b**) would likely have prevented the dislocation (Reprinted from Peterson [101], with permission)

The most frequent serious clinical problem is when two paired bones, the radius and ulna or tibia and fibula, are involved to different degrees resulting in less growth in one or the other [110]. The wrist, elbow, ankle, and knee are particularly vulnerable to deformity [110]. Bones with the relatively smallest cross-sectional physis (such as the distal ulna and fibula) are the most severely shortened [114]. The articular surfaces of the distal ends of the radius and tibia are tilted toward the shorter bone (the ulna and fibula) and the shape of the epiphysis is secondarily altered [110].

The forearm is involved in approximately 60% of patients with multiple exostoses [80, 110, 114]. Forearm deformities are the most frequent cause of functional impairment [101, 102], are usually not symmetrical [80, 103], and are "always" accompanied by a length discrepancy between the radius and ulna [80, 81, 110, 120]. Although both the radius and ulna are characteristically involved, growth of the ulna is invariably more affected (Fig. 4.6) [110]. This may be because (1) the distal ulnar physis contributes more forearm length than the distal radial physis, and (2) the cross sectional area of the distal ulnar physis is less than a quarter of the area of the distal radial physis [73, 80, 95, 107, 114]. Equivalent involvement by osteochondromas of both bones would therefore mean greater proportionate involvement of the ulnar physis [73, 114, 115]. Relative ulnar shortening is accompanied by increased distal radial articular angulation, ulnar deviation of the carpus and hand, displacement of the carpus ulnarward, bowing of the radius (Fig. 4.7), and decreased wrist and forearm motion [101, 102]. If left unattended long enough, these act as a tether causing radial head dislocation (Fig. 4.5) [74]. Radial head dislocation limits elbow and forearm motion and may be painful [80, 101, 102, 107, 117].

Distal ulnar osteochondromas should be treated early and aggressively if progression of functional and cosmetic impairment is to be prevented [80, 85, 95, 101, 102, 120]. Lesions never excised have the potential to cause serious functional impairment (Fig. 4.4). The three most common operations are, (1) excision of the osteochondromas, (2) excision of the osteochondromas combined with ulnar lengthening, and (3) excision of the osteochondromas with ulnar lengthening and distal radial stapling, depending on the severity of deformity [80, 101, 102].

Excision of osteochondromas is the principle procedure in all cases [95]. The surgical excision is accomplished much easier when the lesions are small. Excision of an osteochondroma must include removal of the active cartilage cap, avoiding violation of the physis [101, 102]. Adjacent palpable cartilage bumps should also be removed. Although the physis may not have normal growth potential there is some recovery of growth potential after excision of an osteochondroma [100]. If the lesions are detected with little relative ulnar shortening

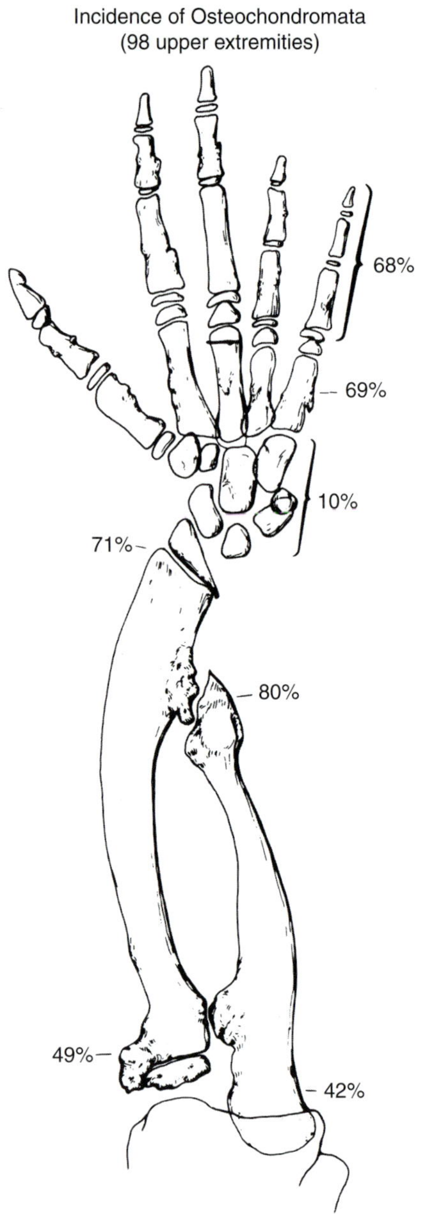

Fig. 4.6 Incidence of osteochondromas in 98 forearms according to location (Reprinted from Fogel et al. [80], with permission)

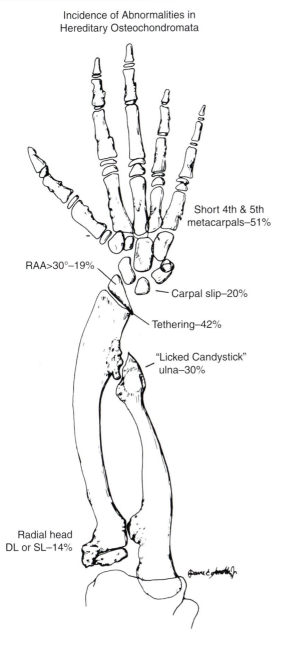

Fig. 4.7 Incidence of deformities in 98 forearms. *RAA* radial articular angle, *DL* dislocation, *SL* subluxation (Reprinted from Fogel et al. [80] with permission)

(1 cm or less), surgical excision of the ulnar osteochondroma will allow more normal ulnar growth and may obviate radial head dislocation [71, 95]. If the negative ulnar variance is 1 cm or greater, excision of the ulnar osteochondroma should be performed promptly [85, 120]. If the osteochondroma is circumferential, or nearly circumferential, it may be necessary to remove half at one surgery, followed by the other half 3–4 months later through a different incision, to allow enough cortical bone to form to prevent collapse of the metaphysis. Excision of the entire distal ulna should be considered only if a one bone forearm is the best result expected from any treatment (Fig. 4.8) [101, 102, 104].

Indications for lengthening the ulna are symptomatic loss of movement of the wrist, elbow or forearm, radial head instability, and ulnar shortening of two centimeters or more [75]. The lengthening can accompany osteochondroma excision provided there is enough cortical bone remaining in the distal ulna to prevent collapse at the site of osteochondroma removal. The ulna can be lengthened by one stage oblique or step-cut osteotomy (Fig. 19.7), by transverse osteotomy with bone graft if the distance to be lengthened is minor [80, 81, 101, 107, 118, 120], or by callus distraction if the distance is major (Fig. 4.9). Both monolateral [70, 71, 75, 79, 80, 85, 92, 94, 95, 101, 102, 107, 118] and circular [78, 84, 108] external fixator-distractors work well. Division of the cordlike portion of the interosseous membrane facilitates advancement of the distal ulna [93]. Partial recurrence of relative ulnar shortening occurs in young patients due to persistent limited growth of the ulna with continued growth of the radius [107, 118]. Over lengthening the ulna in anticipation of recurrent relative shortening, is recommended for young patients [75, 85, 107]. Bone grafting after distraction by an external fixator is usually not necessary [107]. Fracture following removal of the fixator-lengthening device [94] can be prevented by the insertion of an intramedullary rod in the ulna at time of osteotomy of the ulna (Fig. 4.9d). The intramedullary rod also corrects ulnar bowing and significantly shortens the duration the lengthener needs to be in place. If the entire forearm is excessively short, both the radius and ulna can be lengthened at the same time [94]. In this case two monolateral distracters are used to achieve disparate lengthening.

The accompanying increased radial articular angle can be treated, if necessary, by inserting staples on the radial side of the distal radial physis [80, 81, 101, 102, 112, 120]. This retards the radial side of the physis and allows the ulnar side to grow (Fig. 19.7). The staples are removed once the correction (or slight over-correction) has been achieved [80, 101, 102]. If the patient has little distal radial growth remaining, closing wedge radial osteotomy [87, 94, 95, 118, 120] is an alternative to staples. Ulnarward carpal slip may be enhanced by

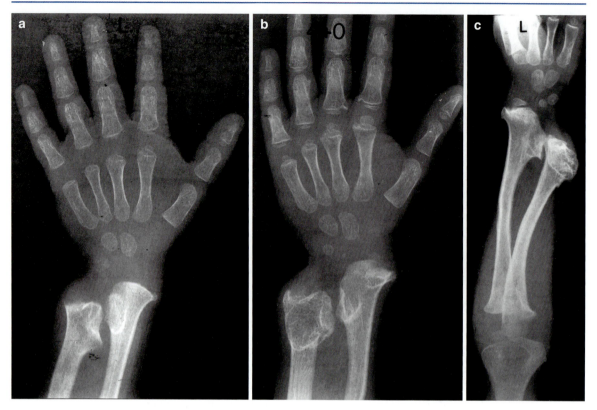

Fig. 4.8 Osteochondromas with rapid growth, developmental dislocation of the proximal ulna, and creation of the one bone forearm. (**a**) At age 2 years there are osteochondromas of the left distal radius and ulna. Forearm pronation. (**b**) At age 4 years the lesions have enlarged. Forearm pronation. (**c**) At age 5 years 4 months there is marked increase in lesion size, along with carpal slip and loss of forearm rotation. Forearm supination. (**d**) Lateral view at same time as c shows true size of the distal ulnar lesion. (**e**) At age 5 years 5 months the distal ulna was excised with immediate resumption of full forearm rotation. The distal radial osteochondroma was excised after the roentgenogram was taken. The radial head is located in (**a**–**e**). (**f**) Within 6 months (age 5 years 11 months) the radial head is completely dislocated. Subsequent surgical relocation of the radial head resulted in prompt redislocation. (**g**) At age 9 years 2 months there is elbow deformity associated with pain and decreased forearm rotation. (**h**) The radial head remains dislocated anteriorly and has become painful, with reduced forearm rotation. The increased radial articular angle persists and the carpus is subluxated ulnarward (carpal slip), both associated with distal ulnar deficiency and reduced development of the lateral distal radial epiphysis. The radial head was excised, and the proximal radius joined to the proximal ulna to make a one-bone forearm, the ulnius [104]. (**i**) Four and a half years later, age 13 years 8 months, there is no pain or instability, full elbow motion, normal wrist position and function, and no forearm rotation. The proximal radius and ulna are fused. (**j**) Age 17 years 3 months. Excision of the osteochondromas from both distal radii, combined with the left proximal radio-ulnar synostosis, has allowed normal development and growth of both distal radii. The left increased RAA, carpal slip and radial epiphyseal wedge deformity have recovered spontaneously. (**k**) At age 25 years 4 months there was full wrist and elbow motion (double exposure photo) and stability, and no forearm rotation. (**l**) The forearm was fused in neutral rotation (the left image shows an anterior-posterior view of the elbow and a lateral view of the wrist: the right image shows a lateral view of the elbow and an anterior-posterior view of the wrist). Note: It is easy to speculate that early excision of the lesions (**a** or **b**), could have avoided the subsequent surgeries. The additional lesson to be learned is that the distal ulna of a child should never be excised, unless a one bone forearm is the best final solution. Performing the surgical synostosis at the same time as distal ulnar excision (**e**) would have saved this patient from the failed surgical radial head relocation (Reprinted from Peterson [101, 104], with permission and additional follow-up)

4.2 Benign Bone Tumors

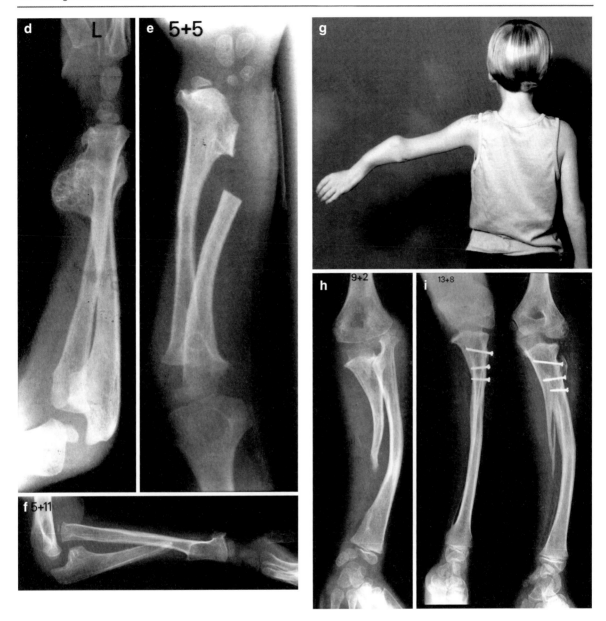

Fig. 4.8 (continued)

Fig. 4.8 (continued)

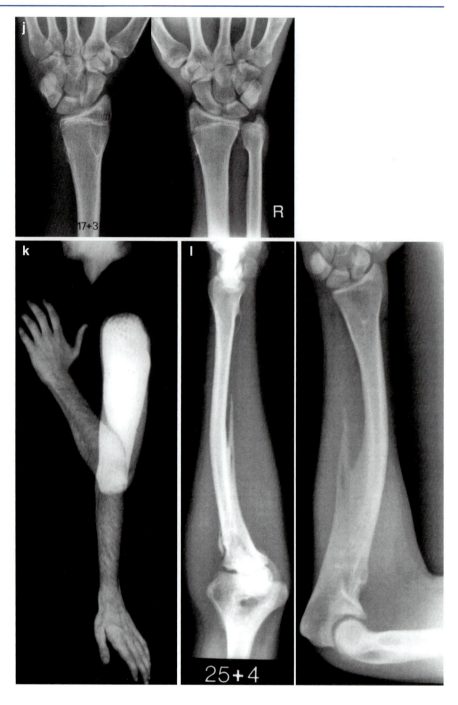

the tethering effect of the fibrous ligamentous ulnar collateral ligament at the wrist, and its release or excision has been recommended [120]. The timely application of these procedures should obviate the use of the Kapandji procedure [87, 111, 119], which is arthrodesis of the distal radial and ulnar metaphyses combined with creation of a distal ulnar shaft pseudarthrosis.

Accompanying significant radial bowing can be corrected by osteotomy [85]. Although surgical arrest of the distal radial physis or radial shortening [88] can normalize radio-ulnar relative length, each has the disadvantage of shortening the shorter forearm even more. This might be functionally insignificant, but cosmetically undesirable to the patient [75, 85].

4.2 Benign Bone Tumors

Proximal radial head dislocation is common and was recorded in 22% of untreated forearms in one series [110]. It is usually associated with a loss of forearm pronation [116]. Dislocation occurs gradually and is usually accompanied by relative shortening of the ulna, and bowing of the radius and ulna (Figs. 4.5 and 4.10). Relative ulnar shortening of more than 8% is significantly associated with radial head dislocation [74]. In rare cases osteochondroma of the proximal ulna or radius can cause dislocation by displacing the ulna laterally producing proximal radius-ulna diastasis [94, 95, 101, 102, 120]. Gradual dislocation causes deformity of the radial head, loss of radial head articular cartilage concavity, and is sometimes accompanied by an outward adaptive bow of the proximal radius (Fig. 4.5c). Thus, contrary to sudden radial head dislocations seen with trauma, once the radial head has gradually dislocated, surgical reduction and reconstruction of the annular ligament is rarely, if ever, successful in terms of either maintaining reduction or improving normal forearm or elbow motion (Fig. 4.10) [118, 120]. If pain is significant, excision of the radial head or surgical construction of a one bone forearm, the ulnius, are possible solutions. Excision of the radial head is an alternative best left until completion

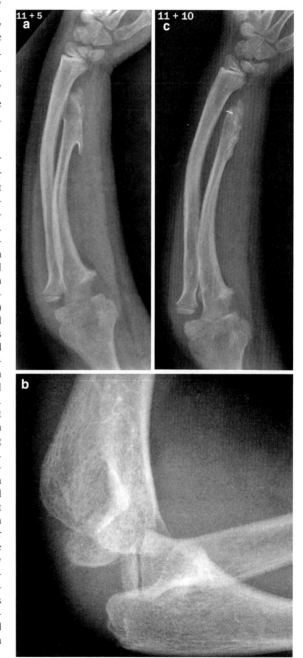

Fig. 4.9 Ulnar lengthening by callous distraction. This 11 year 5 month old boy noted limited left forearm supination (sufficient to be unable to catch a baseball in a glove), decreased left forearm strength, aching pain in the wrist, ulnar deviation and weakness of the hand, and prominence of the posterolateral left elbow. Two previous orthopedic evaluations recommended only observation. (**a**) Distal ulnar osteochondromas are accompanied with relative ulnar shortening of greater than 2 cm, ulnar and radial bowing and radial head subluxation. (**b**) Radial head subluxation is more obvious on this lateral view. The distal ulnar osteochondromas were removed in preparation for ulnar lengthening. (**c**) At age 11 years 10 months the distal ulna was sufficiently healed to proceed with lengthening. (**d**) A Rush intramedullary rod was inserted retrograde into the proximal ulna. The rod was advanced until it became impinged in the curve of the ulna. A one cm incision was made over the ulna at the level of the point of the Rush rod (as measured with a second rod of the same length external to the forearm) and the ulna divided with a small oscillating saw. This process was repeated twice more resulting in a straight ulna. An Orthofix lengthener was attached to two screws in each of the proximal and distal ulnar fragments and lengthening begun. (**e**) Three weeks later 14 mm of length had been achieved. The lengthening was continued another week, and the lengthener removed at 8 weeks. (**f**) At age 12 years 5 months the ulna was straight and of reasonable length. (**g**) The radial head remained subluxated posteriorly. The Rush rod was removed at this time. Hand strength and function and forearm supination were improved; elbow prominence was not. A second similar lengthening was performed at age 14 years 10 months. At age 16 years 6 months he had no complaints, there was full elbow motion despite posterior prominence of the radial head, the forearm supination was mildly limited, and hand function was normal despite radial deviation only to neutral. This case illustrates radial head subluxation secondary to a distal ulnar osteochondroma, and the improbability of achieving a stable reduced proximal radius in the face of gradual dislocation and loss of a convex articular surface of the radial head

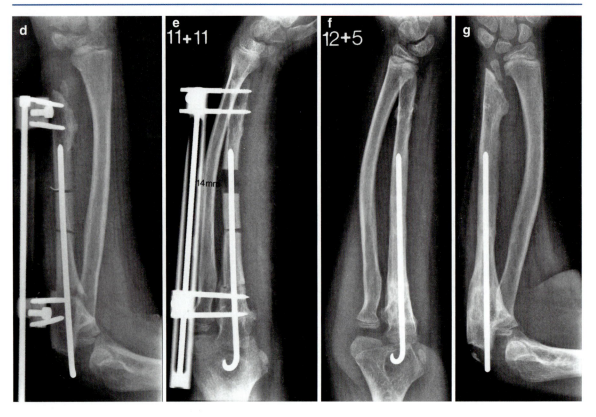

Fig. 4.9 (continued)

of growth or avoided altogether [110, 120]. The one bone forearm (Fig. 4.8h–l) maintains wrist and elbow stability and motion, and allows for more normal growth of the distal radius (Fig. 4.8j) [104, 109, 110, 118]. The only negative aspect is absence of forearm rotation, which is often significantly diminished preoperatively. The best way to prevent proximal radial head dislocation is by early excision of osteochondromas from both the distal and proximal ulna (and proximal radius if present), followed by straightening and lengthening the

Fig. 4.10 Unsuccessful radial head reduction. This is a continuation of the case shown in Fig. 4.5. (**a**) At age 10 years 1 month the osteochondroma was removed from the distal ulna, and a metal marker inserted to monitor future growth. The paucity of remaining cortical bone precluded concomitant ulnar lengthening. (**b**) By age 10 years 5 months the new cortical bone of the distal ulna was sufficiently strong to proceed with lengthening. Note persistent outward angulation of the proximal ulna and more normal growth of distal ulna by comparing metal marker and epiphysis with (**a**). At age 10 years 8 months ulnar lengthening was accomplished using two osteotomies, a Rush intramedullary rod, and a unilateral lengthener (by the method described in Fig. 4.9d). (**c**) After 7 weeks of lengthening, age 10 years 10 months, the radial head was sufficiently distracted. (**d**) The outward angulation of the proximal radius and convexity of the radial head articular surface both persist. Radial head reduction was achieved by recontouring the radial head articular surface into concavity and by a partial osteotomy to straighten the proximal radius. A second Rush pin was inserted to maintain the radial head reduction and the proximal radial osteotomy straightening. The ulna lengthener was removed. (**e**) Four weeks later, age 10 years 11 months, the radius remains reduced. The Rush pins were removed and a long arm cast applied. (**f**) Four weeks later, age 11 years 0 months the cast was removed. There was mild anterior and lateral subluxation of the radial head. (**g**) At age 11 years 4 months the wrist was functionally normal, but the radial head articular surface is convex and subluxated posterolaterally. The prognosis includes progressive pain and motion limitation of the radial-capitellar joint. Should the radial head dislocate completely, wrist positive ulnar variance could also become a problem. Note: The lesson to be learned from this case is to prevent radial head dislocation, which could likely have been be accomplished by early removal of the osteochondromas (Fig. 4.5a, b)

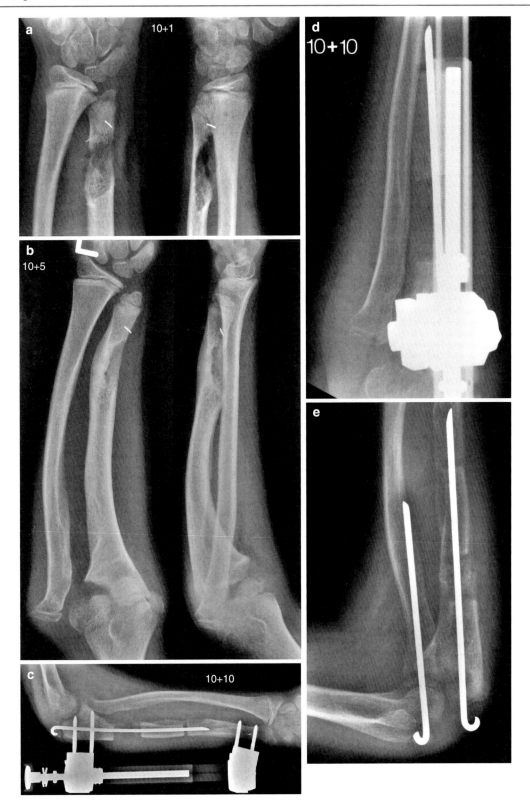

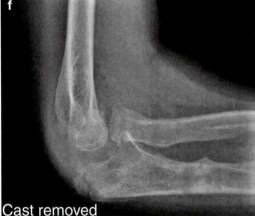
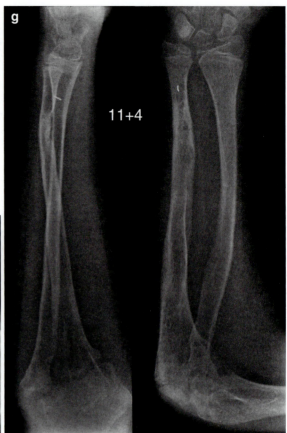

Fig. 4.10 (continued)

ulna (Fig. 19.7), and if necessary straightening the radius [101, 118]. Repeat lengthenings are sometimes appropriate and beneficial (Fig. 19.7) [118].

Distal radial osteochondromas causing significant growth problems are decidedly less common [74, 75, 81, 85]. Relative shortening of the radius is usually minor (Fig. 4.11) [101, 102, 120]. These are relatively easy to treat by excision of the radial osteochondromas. Distal ulna surgical physeal arrest or shortening of the ulna is rarely necessary, and should not be allowed to progress to negative ulnar variance.

In the lower leg the problem is similar, but less troublesome because neither proximal fibular head dislocation nor distal tibia-fibula synostosis cause functional impairment. Nevertheless, prolonged observation can result in significant functional impairment in some cases (Fig. 4.12). Osteochondromas on the distal fibular metaphysis are associated with relative fibular shortening which cause developmental ankle valgus (Fig. 19.2). Commonly, a large osteochondroma present on the lateral side of the distal tibial metaphysis causes plastic deformation of the fibula which is thereby shortened, accompanied by increased distal tibial valgus angulation [76, 82]. Valgus obliquity of the distal tibial joint surface is found in approximately 50% of the ankles assessed [86, 110, 114]. The valgus deformity is almost entirely a deformity of the tibial epiphysis, which is wedge-shaped in all cases [86, 114],

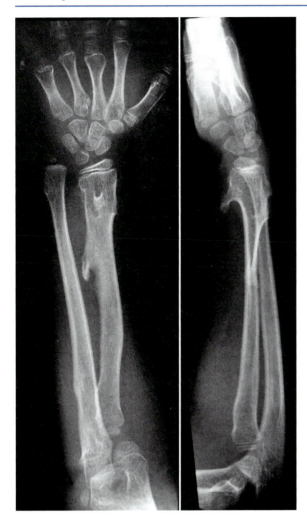

Fig. 4.11 Major involvement in the distal radius with minor involvement of the ulna in a 7 year 9 month old girl. Note relative radial shortening and medial subluxation of the proximal radius, both of which occur rarely (Reprinted from Peterson [101], with permission)

accompanied by a relatively short fibula. Residual ankle valgus of only a few degrees persisting into adulthood is a strong precursor for arthritic changes and diminished ankle motion [97]. Distal tibia-fibula synostosis is frequently present in long standing cases (Fig. 4.12b), is usually asymptomatic, and ankle motion is unimpaired [86, 113, 114].

Nonoperative treatment of symptomatic ankle lesions is rarely successful [76]. Early removal of lesions often obviates the need for further treatment. Once ankle valgus is present it is best corrected by distal tibial medial physeal stapling (Fig. 19.4) [113] or transphyseal screw [117], or supra malleolar osteotomy (closing medially, or opening laterally if more length is desired), accompanied by lengthening of the fibula [110, 113]. A one stage step-cut sliding osteotomy is often sufficient to lengthen the fibula. Complex multiplanar, multifocal deformities in the lower extremities have been successfully corrected with osteotomy combined with Ilizarov apparatus fixation [99].

At the knee genu valgum of 5° or greater was noted in 33% of cases assessed in a Growth Study Unit in one study [110]. The valgus deformity is usually within the tibia and 20% of the patients were treated with proximal tibial osteotomy. The risk of vascular compromise known to occur with high tibial osteotomy for any reason is further increased by exostoses which compromise the space available for neurovascular structures [110]. The effect of the invariably present short fibula on this deformity has not been adequately investigated. However, if the valgus deformity is identified early, it can be nicely

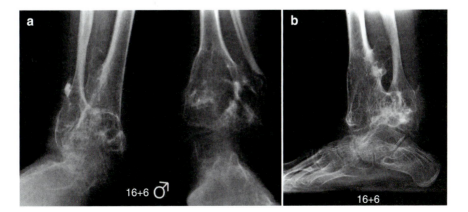

Fig. 4.12 Untreated osteochondromas of the distal lower legs with loss of function. The parents of this 16 year 6 month old boy consistently declined excision of lesions due to perceived lack of functional impairment. He now has shoe fitting problems on the right and ambulation is limited to two blocks. (**a**) The standing AP roentgenogram shows the right superior talar articular surface tilted to 80° valgus. (**b**) The lateral view shows probable distal tibio-fibular synostosis

corrected by the insertion of staples over the medial proximal tibial or distal femoral physis (Fig. 4.13), rather than by osteotomy [113].

Limb length discrepancies are common. Lower limb inequality of greater than 2 cm has been reported in 10–50% of patients with multiple osteochondromas [117]. Shortening may be in the femur and/or the tibia. In one study the discrepancy was sufficient to warrant surgical physeal arrest in the long leg in 50% of the patients referred to a Growth Study Unit [110]. Any significant residual leg length discrepancy after completion of growth could be treated with bone shortening on the long side or lengthening on the short side.

Short metatarsals and metacarpals are the most common small bone abnormalities associated with osteochondromas. Fortunately, they produce few symptoms and are therefore not commonly treated [117]. However, even relatively small exostoses of metacarpals, metatarsals and phalanges may require early surgical removal if impaired growth is causing deviation or functional limitations [86, 120]. In the hand good restoration of motion and function can be achieved by excision of lesions combined with collateral ligament reconstruction [90, 96], if necessary. However, if the shortening is more significant and symptomatic, either the metatarsal or metacarpal can be lengthened with good overall results. Operations include osteotomy and one stage distraction with or without bone grafting, and osteotomy with gradual distraction with or without bone grafting [77].

The proximal humeri and femora frequently have osteochondromas. Contrary to elbows, knees, wrists, and ankles, these lesions are more symmetrical and cause less length discrepancy and angular deformity. Lesions in the hips and shoulders cause fewer symptoms and less functional impairment. Also, surgical exposure is more difficult. Therefore, surgery around the shoulder and hip is less frequent.

The risk of complications from the surgical management of osteochondromas is low and comparable to the risk of other related elective procedures [119]. However, osteochondromas should not be routinely excised unless indications exist for their removal. Enlargement of an osteochondroma in a skeletally immature patient seldom indicates malignancy [76]. Malignant transformation during childhood is exceedingly rare [110, 115, 120]. The chance of malignant transformation even in adulthood is so low (approximately 1% [89]), that it is not feasible to excise all lesions in each patient in an effort to prevent such transformation [103].

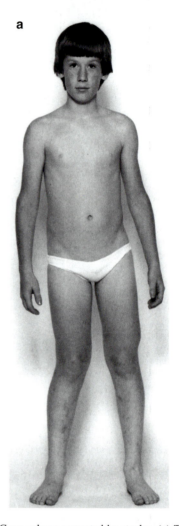

Fig. 4.13 Genu valgum corrected by staples. (a) This 12 year 6 month old boy was noted to have mild asymptomatic right knee genu valgum. Note pelvic tilt down on the right. (b) A scanogram showed genu valgum 13° on the right, a normal 4° on the left. The right femur was 2.8 cm shorter and the right tibia 0.2 cm longer than the left, for a total discrepancy of 2.6 cm. The right distal femoral physis is more tilted than the left, whereas the tibial physes are perpendicular to the tibial shafts. Osteochondromas were removed and staples inserted over the medial distal right femur. (c) Six months post operative, age 13 years 0 months, the genu valgum was 8°. (d) At age 13 years 6 months the increased genu valgum was fully corrected. (e) The right femur was now 3.6 shorter that the left. The staples were removed and the distal left femoral physis was surgically arrested. (f) At age 17 years 5 months he was asymptomatic and normally active including competitive tennis. The left lower extremity was 3 mm longer that the right. All physes were closed

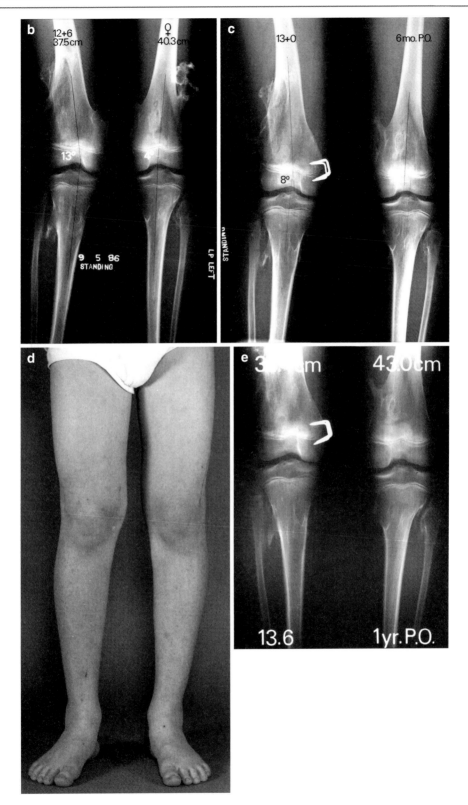

Fig. 4.13 (continued)

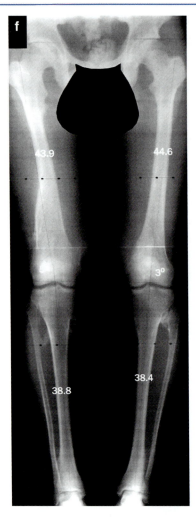

Fig. 4.13 (continued)

In summary, most authors advise early excision of symptomatic or growth troublesome osteochondromas. Surgical treatment should be considered as soon as it is clear that the growth pattern of bones is being significantly altered. The younger the patient, the greater the potential for remodeling and the better the surgical result [95]. Excision of osteochondromas before ulnar shortening and radial bowing have become severe, may avoid both ulnar lengthening and radial osteotomy [95]. Prevention of progression of deformity and functional impairment, particularly radial head dislocation, are paramount goals [101]. Three articles advocate a less aggressive approach, citing a paucity of documented functional impairment, or improvement with "aggressive" surgical treatment [72, 116, 119]. Two additional recent articles are the beginning studies of comparing the functional status of osteochondroma patients with and without surgery [97, 98].

4.2.4 Enchondroma

Enchondromas are nonhereditary benign rests of ectopic hyaline cartilage that most likely arise from normal physeal cartilage cells [127, 130], and have the incapacity to mature [132]. Histologically the cellularity of the lesions exceed that of resting articular cartilage, with small nuclei, uniform nucleoli, and abundant cytoplasm [130, 133]. There is very little mitotic activity, although a limited number of binucleate lacunae are occasionally seen [130]. The abnormal accumulation of this tissue may be the result of abnormal proliferation of chondroblasts or failure of maturation and resorption of chondroblasts of the physis [121, 129]. The lesions typically affect the metaphyseal regions of tubular bone, usually in close proximity to the physis [91]. On occasions lesions occur in the epiphysis [127, 130] and on rare occasions in both the metaphysis and epiphysis (transphyseal) [124, 130]. A patient may have a solitary or multiple lesions. Patients who have predominantly unilateral lesions are referred to as having Ollier's disease. Patients who have enchondromas in association with hemangiomas are referred to as having Maffucci syndrome. Additional synonyms are chondrodysplasia [91, 122] and dyschondroplasia [133]. There are variable expressions of the disorder, and many borderline cases [129]. They are frequently misdiagnosed as chondroblastoma. There is an equal distribution between genders and between the right and left sides [131].

The important clinical problems are progressive relative bone shortening, angular deformity, and pathologic fracture. Affected long bones grow normally in width, but poorly in length [133]. The extent of relative bone shortening parallels the roentgenographic involvement [131] and may be many centimeters [122, 125]. Length discrepancy increases progressively throughout the growth period [131]. Retardation of growth is caused by the presence of enchondromas that do not degenerate, and thus interrupt orderly enchondral ossification sufficiently to reduce growth [121]. The mechanism of how an occasional physeal bone bridge occurs has not been determined [121].

Angular deformities, particularly knee varus, are common with enchondromatosis [121, 131]. Angular deformity occurs when the metaphyseal involvement is not uniform. The concavity of the angular deformity is always on the side of the more extensive enchondromatous involvement [131]. There is no correlation between the degree of angulation and the extent of shortening [131]. Lesions of the proximal femur may result in coxa valga, but the deformity is usually mild and non-progressive, and rarely results in subluxation or dysplasia of the hip [131]. An occasional fracture through a lesion heals uneventfully and without additional physeal growth impairment.

Historically, management of the relative shortening and angular deformity has required multiple operations [124, 131]. Traditional methods of surgery, such as curettage, bone grafting and repeated osteotomies, are inefficient for the most part due to difficulties in internal stabilization and because the length discrepancy is usually large [126, 132]. One patient with lesions in both the distal femur and proximal tibia had 14 operations, 10 of which were osteotomies with single stage lengthening, producing a total of 23 cm [133]. Hemiepiphyseal stapling or surgical partial physeal arrest of the normally growing portion of the physis in an effort to correct angular deformity is ineffective [131], because the involved portion of the physis does not grow well, and the overall result is further shortening of the already short extremity.

Today treatment includes open-wedge angular-correction osteotomy, and bone lengthening on the involved side, and physeal arrest or bone shortening on the less involved or normal side. Frequent short stature reduces the potential use of physeal arrest and bone shortening on the less involved side. Bone lengthening using monolateral straight [71, 131], monolateral multiaxial [132], bilateral straight [131], and circular [108, 123, 125, 126, 128] lengthening devices have all be used with success. Callus distraction through the abnormal bone using circular, or multiaxial multiple-wire or pin fixation-distraction devices allows concurrent correction of angular deformities and elongation of bone, and seems to stimulate the conversion of the abnormal cartilage into normal bone, without curettage of the lesion [125, 126, 128, 132]. The rare lesions confined to the epiphysis can be managed by intralesional curettage and bone grafting [130].

The choice of management depends on the severity of limb inequality, the degree of angulation and the maturity of the child. If the patient is young and the deformity gross, repeated lengthening combined with overcorrection of angular deformity is appropriate. With increasing age and lesser deformity, a single lengthening combined with correction of deformity, at the site of the lengthening if possible, and contralateral physeal arrest, would be appropriate. If the patient is close to maturity and has mild deformity, surgical partial arrest of the ipsilateral physis (which stops angular deformity from increasing), and complete arrest of the contralateral physis might be sufficient [121].

4.2.5 Chondroblastoma

Chondroblastoma is a benign bone tumor of cartilage origin located preferentially in the epiphysis or apophysis of long bones, and are "always" contiguous with the physis [134, 135]. Almost half display extension into the metaphysis [134, 138]. Most authorities agree that the cell of origin arises from the physis or some remnant of it [138]. Since they have their origin in physeal cartilage, they do not arise after growth has ceased and the physeal cartilage has disappeared [140]. Despite this strong implication of physeal involvement very few growth problems have been recorded. This is most likely due to the age of development and discovery of the lesions. Epiphyseal chondroblastomas originate during the adolescent years, or just after epiphyseal closure has been completed [140]. Most cases are discovered in the second decade of life with only an occasional pre-teenage patient noted (Table 4.5) [136, 140]. The distal femur is the most common site.

The presenting symptom is usually pain, and the treatment is curettage and filling the defect with bone

Table 4.5 Chondroblastoma: age at time of discovery

Year	Author[a]	No.	Mean age (years)	Average age (years)	Range (years)
1985	Edel [135]	52	19.2	–	–
1992	Bloem [134]	104	16	–	–
1996	Pösl [137]	56	20.4	–	–
2000	Ramappa [138]	47	–	22±9.9	11–56

[a]All articles have more than one author. See references

grafts or polymethlmethacrylate [134, 138, 140]. The status of the growth plate has no significant effect on tumor recurrence rate following treatment [138]. Because the tumor is usually located near a physis, growth disturbances could be expected. It is surprising that this rarely happens. In the only article that is focused on the growth problem, only 6 of 81 patients (7%) in the growing age group (17 years or younger) developed growth changes [139]. All six of these patients were 14 years or younger with open physes. There were two cases in the proximal femur with 2 cm shortening, two cases in the proximal humerus with 2–4 cm shortening, one in the distal femur with 1 cm shortening, and one in the distal femur causing minimal varus of the knee. None of these required corrective surgery. In another article [138] one of 47 (2%) patients (all ages) had a limb-length discrepancy and angular deformity post operatively. Neither of these two articles speculated on whether these changes were due to the tumor or the treatment.

4.2.6 Giant Cell Tumor

Giant cell tumor of bone (GCT) is one of the more common tumors encountered by an orthopedic surgeon. In children, GCT is usually located in the metaphysis, in contrast to the predominantly epiphyseal or epiphyseal-metaphyseal location in adults [141, 143–145, 147, 151, 152]. Extension of the tumor from the metaphysis into the epiphysis (transphyseal) occurs commonly after closure of the physis, but only occasionally in children with open physes [145–147, 150, 153, 154]. GCT confined within the epiphysis of a child with an open physis is rare [144, 146, 150]. The metaphyseal localization of GCT in children is a decisive clue to the diagnosis [145].

GCT generally occurs in skeletally mature individuals, with its peak incidence in the third decade of life. The incidence in patients 20 years or less is 14% (143 of 1,019 patients accumulated from 17 articles [149]).

A more meaningful age separation is 15 years, the approximate average time of physeal closure considering both boys and girls, The incidence in patients 15 years or less is 2% (20 of 982 patients accumulated from 8 articles prior to 1983 [150]). The two youngest reported patients were 8 years old [145, 148]. There is a marked female preponderance in these patients with an open physis [142, 150, 151, 153]. The most common location in children is the proximal tibia [145, 147, 150]. Pain is the predominant presenting complaint.

The treatment is usually intralesional curettage with or without adjuvants such as cryotherapy, phenol or hydrogen peroxide, followed by defect reconstruction using autograft, banked allograft, methylmethacrylate, or a combination thereof. Internal fixation is sometimes used if the structural stability of the bone is significantly compromised [151]. More extensive resection is required in some cases [145, 156]. One 14 year old girl with a recurrent GCT in the distal radial metaphysis with an open physis was treated by resection of the distal radius and bone graft from the ileum, fusing the wrist [149]. Two 14 year old patients with rare multifocal GCT of the lower extremity were both treated with above knee amputation [156].

Growth related problems and angular deformities might be expected in these patients with lesions near an open physis, and where there has been surgical intervention in and around the physis. However, this hardly ever occurs. A probable explanation is that most patients are nearing skeletal maturity, and the potential for additional growth is limited. Additionally, both the disease and the resulting surgical intervention usually involve a large area of the physis, thus limiting angular deformity [151]. One case with slight clinical genu varus "which is inconspicuous" was noted in follow-up of a 12 year old boy with a GCT in the medial distal femoral epiphysis [155]. However, the tumor had been treated with both surgery and irradiation (3,850 rad over a period of several months). In another 15 year old boy with GCT of the distal radius treated with curettage and bone graft using the distal ulna developed increased radial articular angle [154]. The ulnar deviation of the hand in this case appeared to be a result of surgical removal of the distal ulna rather than from the tumor.

4.2.7 Langerhan's Cell Histiocytosis

Langerhan's cell histiocytosis (LCH) is a non-neoplastic lesion of unknown etiology characterized by a proliferation of reticulo-histocytic structures, polynuclear eosinophils, neutrophils, lymphocytes, plasma cells, and multinucleate giant cells [157]. LCH was previously categorized as histiocytosis X, eosinophilic granuloma, Letterer-Siwe disease and Hand-Schüller-Christian syndrome. These entities are only different clinical manifestations of a single pathologic disorder. LCH can involve virtually any organ and site of the body and can occur as a widespread systemic disease.

Bone can be involved either as a part of a generalized disease or as a specific entity [159]. The lesions may be solitary or multiple [157]. The most common locations for a bone lesion are the skull, spine, pelvis, and diaphysis of long bones [159]. On occasion, however, lesions appear in the epiphysis [163, 164], or are transphyseal [157, 165]. One article documents ten cases occurring in epiphyses [162]. All of these children were less than 8 years old. In five of the ten cases the lesions extended into the adjacent metaphysis (transphyseal). Only one of these developed growth arrest. The occurrence of lesions in the growing epiphysis is so rare that biopsy is imperative to confirm the diagnosis [157, 162]. The surgical approach required to obtain tissue for diagnosis must avoid endangering the physis, the articular surface, or both.

The treatment most commonly used is curettage alone or with bone grafting [158, 160, 161, 163, 165]. Chemotherapy [157], cryosurgery [163], radiation therapy [157, 159, 163], and cortisone injection [158, 159] have been used in conjunction with surgery and separately.

The prognosis is good for both solitary and multiple lesions regardless of type of treatment [157, 160]. Post operative complete regression of the lesion and "speedy growth" are significant features of this disease [161]. However, when the tumor has already crossed the physis, development of a bony bridge and growth arrest or angular deformity is a concern and requires careful management and follow-up [162]. Only patients with transphyseal involvement have developed growth arrest [162, 165], and only one required surgical bone lengthening [165].

4.2.8 Osteoid Osteoma and Osteoblastoma

Osteoid osteoma is a tumor-like lesion of bone. Its hallmark is well localized pain at night relieved, or partially relieved, by salicylates. Soft tissue atrophy in the area of the lesion is common. Roentgenographically there is a small calcified nidus surrounded by decreased bone density, which in turn may be surrounded by a zone of reactive sclerosis. The lesion may occur in any location in any bone.

The traditional treatment has been surgical biopsy with en bloc removal or curettage of the lesion. Radiofrequency ablation has been increasingly used in the past decade and is now the most common form of treatment. When the lesion abuts against the physis the decision for either treatment depends upon its potential damage to the physis.

When an osteoid osteoma is located in the metaphysis near a physis, premature physeal closure has been observed prior to treatment, possibly due to local damage to the physis directly [180], or to the secondary effects of increased vascularity and regional osteoporosis [169]. Three cases of osteoid osteoma associated with premature physeal arrest all occurred in distal phalanges of the little finger or the great toe prior to biopsy. The physis of a little finger distal phalanx in an 11 year old boy closed prematurely at age 12 years [180]. The metaphyseal lesion appeared to abut against the physis causing the closure. A 14 year old boy had a lesion in the distal phalanx of a big toe [169]. A 15 year old girl with enlargement of the terminal phalanx of a little finger over the preceding 2½ years was found to have complete closure of the distal phalanx and all other hand physes open and normal [182]. In all three cases the bone was already of sufficient size that no noticeable relative shortening or morbidity was recorded.

Two unusual cases of long standing osteoid osteoma in the proximal femoral shaft (near the intertrochanteric area) resulted in severe growth disturbance of the hip [172]. The physis did not close prematurely and the relative femoral shortening was believed to be due to "intense hyperemia and muscle contracture existing for a long period during growth." Disuse could have been a feature (see Chap. 2).

An osteoid osteoma residing within or on the surface of an epiphysis with an open physis has been reported many times, usually in single case reports [166–168, 170, 171, 173–179, 181, 185, 186]. Most have been treated with complete resection without injuring the physis or articular surface. Interestingly, no growth disturbance has been recorded with lesions confined within the epiphysis.

Most articles that describe "intraarticular" osteoid osteoma are describing lesions within an epiphysis which happens to be intra articular (the epiphysis lies within the confines of the synovial space). However, an unusual extra osseous, intra articular osteoid osteoma in the coronoid space of the distal humerus noted in two children caused enlargement, sclerosis, advanced maturation, and premature closure of the distal humeral physis [183, 184], and of the proximal radial physis in one [184]. The mechanism that leads to such profound changes due to a near-by intraarticular osteoid osteoma is unknown [184].

Osteoblastoma is a name given to a large osteoid osteoma, and is often called "giant osteoid osteoma" [179]. By definition it is larger than 2 cm. Histologically the two are virtually identical. Osteoblastoma may arise in any bone, but has a predilection for the spine. Localization of osteoid osteoma in long bones is most often in the diaphysis, where as osteoblastoma tends to occur more often in the metaphysis. Both can occur in the epiphysis [179]. No cases of growth arrest from osteoblastoma are recorded.

4.2.9 Focal Fibrocartilaginous Dysplasia

The condition known as focal fibrocartilaginous dysplasia (FFCD) consists of abnormal development of fibrocartilage at the site of tendon insertions [189]. It typically occurs unilaterally at the metaphyseal-diaphyseal junction in young children. No patient with bilateral involvement has been described. It is manifest by angular deformity and mild relative shortening of the involved bone.

Roentgenographically the cortex is deficient with thickening and sclerosis extending toward the epiphysis. The physis is not directly involved and in contrast to Blount's disease no roentgenographic abnormality of the physis has been noted [195]. The plain films are usually diagnostic, rendering CT and MRI unnecessary. However, MRI may be indicated as a problem-solving examination in the presence of an atypical clinical presentation [200]. CT and MRI clearly define the abnormal tissue as fibrocartilage and tendon-like tissue, obviating the need for biopsy [192]. Histologically there is dense hypocellular tissue resembling fibrocartilage in some areas and tendon in others. The differential diagnosis includes infection and trauma (see humerus varus, Fig. 3.9).

The etiology is unknown. One report described four femoral lesions with thick fibrous cords in the metaphysis, two of which attached to the periphery of the physis [188]. This robust tether was suspected of causing the deformity. Two patients who were described as having a "periosteal tether" displayed features strikingly similar to FFCD [194].

Sites of involvement include the proximal tibia [187, 189–191, 195–197, 200, 201, 203], distal femur [187, 188, 191, 199], proximal humerus [193, 198], distal ulna [191, 198, 202], distal radius [202], and finger phalanges [202]. The major abnormality at all sites is angular deformity. Relative shortening varies according to site. When the lesion is in the proximal tibia the relative shortening is usually mild (1–2 cm). However, in the proximal humerus relative shortening can exceed 8 cm (enough to consider surgical lengthening), and the varus angulation of the humeral physis can exceed 90° [193]. Relative shortening associated with distal ulnar lesions can be sufficient to cause radial head dislocation [202].

The response of tibial lesions to nonoperative treatment is frequently good [192, 195, 196]. Approximately 45% of proximal tibial FFCD demonstrate progressive, spontaneous resolution [190, 191], in contrast to femoral and humeral FFCD where deformity and shortening typically persist or increase. In addition, surgical excision of the abnormal tissue and periosteal release usually results in gradual spontaneous correction of the angular deformity and relative shortening [187, 189, 203]. Corrective osteotomy was frequently done previously, but is unnecessary in many cases. Serial roentgenograms are necessary to determine progression or resolution of the deformity [197, 201]. When the deformity increases or persists in spite of a reasonable period of observation or bracing, or when the deformity is severe enough to jeopardize adjacent joint mechanics and alignment, surgical excision of the abnormal tissue, and corrective osteotomy or bone lengthening if necessary, is indicated [191]. At sites other than the proximal tibia similar recommendations for observation have not been made.

4.2.10 Fibrous Dysplasia of Bone

Fibrous dysplasia of bone is characterized by an arrest of bone maturation at the woven bone stage. The lesion consists of a delicate fibrous stroma in which the fibers are closely but randomly distributed. Within this stroma spicules and trabeculae of immature bone are formed by metaplasia [205]. The abnormal dysplastic tissue may expand and completely erode the cortex, thereby directly abutting upon the deep surface of the periosteum. Fracture is often the presenting complaint (Fig. 4.14a, b).

The lesions may be monostotic or polystotic. A third form of the disease is the McCune-Albright syndrome in which multiple lesions tend to be unilateral, accompanied by café-au-lait spots on the same side of the body in which the bone lesions occur [206]. Although the lesions are most often unicameral, roentgenographically they may appear multiloculated due to uneven erosion of the endosteal surface (Fig. 4.14a, c) [206].

Lesions may occur in any location in any bone. Bone bending and fracture are common and are the usual cause of deformity and relative bone shortening rather than physeal abnormality. Leg length discrepancy accounts for 70% of physical deformities [204]. Physeal arrest due to the lesion is uncommon (Fig. 4.14d–j).

4.2.11 Miscellaneous

Multiple additional benign bone tumors in children, which may be located near a physis, are extensively reported in the literature. These include vascular, fibrous and cartilaginous tissue tumors, lymphomas, and conditions such as dysplasia epiphysealis hemimelica.

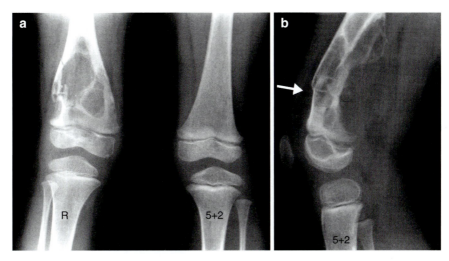

Fig. 4.14 Fibrous dysplasia of bone. This 5 year 2 month old girl noted pain above the right knee following a minor fall. (**a**) There is a multi-locutated radiolucent defect with cortical expansion in the distal femoral metaphysis with fractures of cortex laterally. The most distal extension of the tumor appears to be 5–10 mm from the physis. (**b**) A lateral view confirms a fracture (*arrow*), with mild posterior angulation of the distal fragment. The posterior cortex is absent. A long leg cast was applied. (**c**) Six weeks post injury the fracture was healing. The lytic defect was unchanged. (**d**) Ten weeks post fracture, age 5 years 5 months, the lesion was curetted and grafted with allograft from the father. (**e**) Eleven months post operative, age 6 years 3 months, the physis has grown several mm away from the grafted defect, but is narrowed and indistinct in the center. (**f**) Three years 6 months post operative, age 8 years 11 months. A scanogram shows the right femur 3 cm, and the right tibia 1 mm shorter than the left. (**g**) An AP tomogram shows a central posterior physeal bar and the remainder of the physis to be very narrow (*left*). There are two new small lytic defects in the metaphysis distal to a more proximal residual lytic defect from the original tumor. The lateral tomogram confirmed the bar to be central and posterior (*right*). Note the growth arrest line in the epiphysis confirming postoperative growth of the epiphysis. A bar excision was performed through a posterior incision at age 8 years 11 months. Cranioplast was used as the interposition material. (**h**) One month post bar excision; the metal objects are vascular clips not imbedded in bone. (**i**) Six months post bar excision the right femur has grown 16 mm, the left 14 mm, for total femoral discrepancy of 2.8 cm. (**j**) By 2 years 11 months post bar excision, age 11 years 11 months, the femoral discrepancy had increased to 3.9 cm. Surgical physeal arrest of the left distal femur and proximal tibia were performed. (**k**) At age 13 years 1 month, 4 years post bar excision, the total leg length discrepancy was 3.1 cm. All physes are closed. The patient lived normally for two decades. No shoe lift was used. (**l**) At age 35 years the patient noted right knee pain and episodes of locking, usually with the knee extended. Knee motion was from 5° to 140° flexion and she walked without limp. There was mild tenderness along the medial joint line. Standing roentgenogram shows mild right genu valgum. An MRI at the same time showed a small oblique tear of the posterior horn of the medial meniscus. Physical therapy was instituted. Over the next few months the pain posterior medial remained and was worse with standing and climbing stairs. Knee extension did not improve. Note: The cause of this growth arrest could be due to the tumor or the original surgery. The bar excision was typical in that there was good growth initially, but the physis was too narrow for growth to continue. Are her present knee problems related to the residual 3 cm femoral length discrepancy and mild genu valgum? If so, what steps should have been taken to prevent or treat them? The case needs further follow-up

Fig. 4.14 (continued)

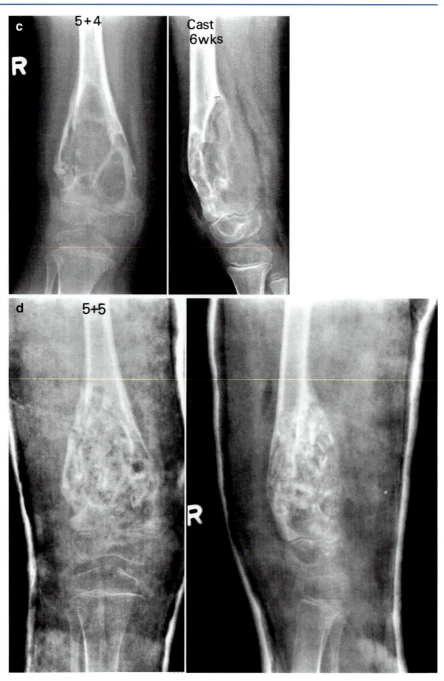

4.2 Benign Bone Tumors

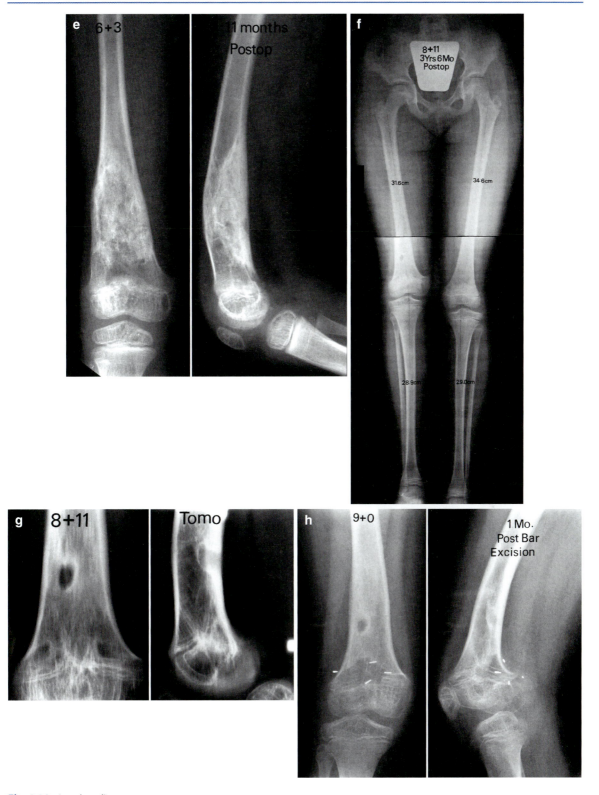

Fig. 4.14 (continued)

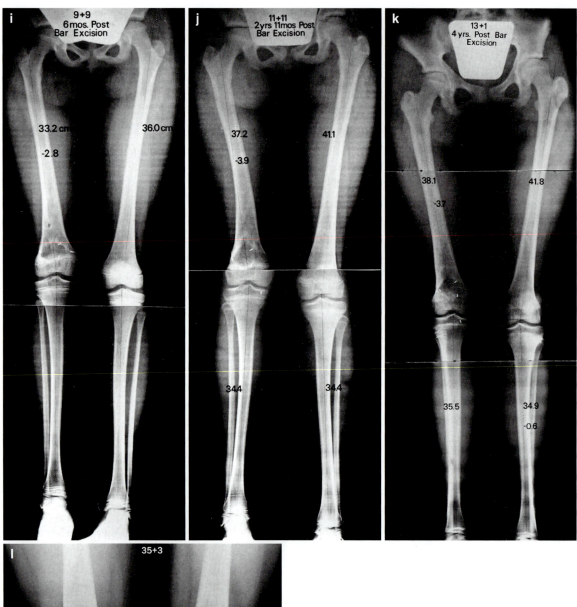
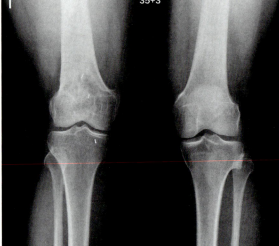

Fig. 4.14 (continued)

4.2 Benign Bone Tumors

A perusal of some of this literature uncovered no growth related problems. In addition, in reviewing the list of references by title from these articles none imply a growth problem. As an example, a benign fibrous histiocytoma in the proximal tibial epiphysis of a 12 year old girl did not cause growth abnormality [207]. However, an interosseous hemangioma of the distal femur metaphysis in our files resulted in growth arrest (Fig. 4.15). Thus, although a growth problem may occur in an occasional patient with any benign tumor, it appears to be uncommon (other than with osteochondroma).

4.2.12 Author's Perspective

Most articles concerning benign tumors emphasize the diagnosis, histology, and treatment. Follow-up is often limited, and the issue of subsequent growth arrest receives scant attention. It is remarkable that so many benign tumors which reside within the epiphysis cause no growth disturbance. These tumors apparently have little adverse effect on the blood supply to the physis which is primarily epiphyseal (Sect. 1.2). Hopefully, future literature will more frequently record the relationship between benign bone tumors and physeal growth.

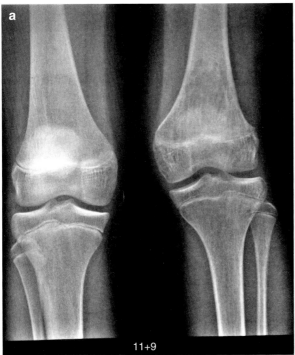
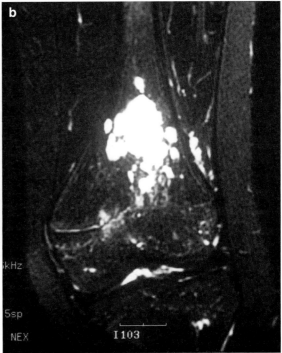

Fig. 4.15 Interosseous hemangioma. This 11 year old girl noted her own leg length discrepancy in gym class. There were no symptoms. (**a**) At age 11 years 9 months AP roentgenogram of both knees show mottled lucency in the distal left femoral metaphysis with closure of its physis. All other knee physes are open. (**b**) T2 coronal MR image of left knee at age 12 years 0 months shows irregular mottling in the metaphysis consistent with an interosseous hemangioma. Some distal femoral physis is present medially. The proximal left tibial physis is indistinct. (**c**) Scanogram at age 12 years 2 months shows bowing of the left femur. The left femur is 29 mm shorter, and the left tibia 8 mm shorter than the right, for a total discrepancy of 37 mm. (**d**) Multiple attempts to obtain tissue through a Craig needle were unsuccessful. Dye injected into the lesion suggested hemangioma. Open biopsy through a 6 cm incision revealed bits of vascular tissue and no solid tissue, confirming the diagnosis of hemangioma. Cultures were subsequently negative. The cavity was curetted and filled with cancellous bank bone. (**e**) The right distal femoral and proximal tibial physes were surgically arrested. The epiphysiodeses prevented the discrepancy from increasing. Femoral osteotomy to correct angular deformity, and lengthening with an EBI external fixator, were undertaken at age 14 years 9 months. When last seen at age 15 years 8 months the patient was asymptomatic and normally active, including participation on the school dance line. A scanogram showed a residual limb length discrepancy of 16 mm, short on the left

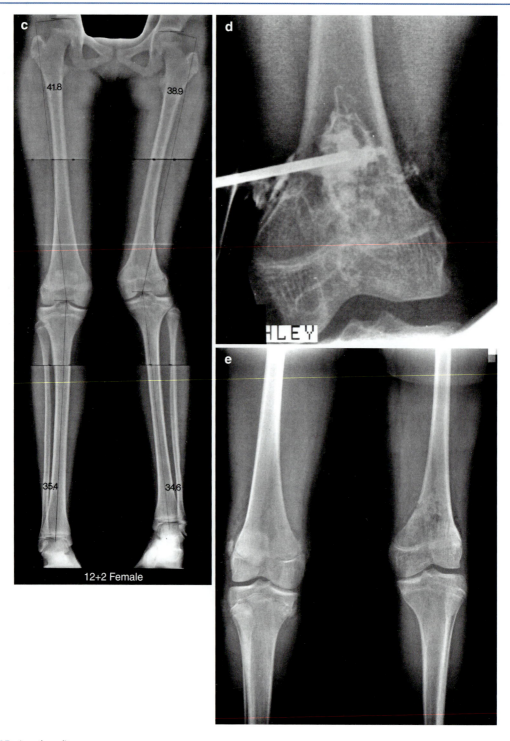

Fig. 4.15 (continued)

4.3 Malignant Bone Tumors

Malignant bone tumors occur mainly in children and 75% of cases are located near an open physis [214, 229]. The physis has only a partial inhibitory effect preventing penetration of a tumor in the metaphysis from entering the epiphysis. Preservation of limb length equality in pediatric oncology patients with reconstructed limbs is challenging because of the ongoing growth of the contralateral limb. Functional impairment secondary to residual limb length discrepancy is one of the greatest complications among survivors [230]. Most cases of residual limb length discrepancy are due to surgical removal of one or more physes, combined with difficulty estimating future growth of remaining physes due to the effects of chemotherapy. Almost two-thirds of malignant bone tumors in children are osteogenic sarcoma, and most of the rest are Ewing's sarcoma [248].

4.3.1 Osteosarcoma

Osteosarcoma is the most common malignant bone tumor and is diagnosed most frequently in the second decade of life, coinciding with maximum growth. It is most frequently found in the metaphyses of appendicular long tubular bones. Osteosarcoma confined within the epiphysis is rare [213, 251, 256, 259, 274]. In older literature the physis was regarded as a barrier to tumor spread into the epiphysis. The physeal cartilage tissue was thought to inhibit growth and invasion of the tumor by releasing anti-angiogenic or anti-proliferative factors [210, 243]. More recent literature documents that tumors in the metaphysis which abut against the physis extend into the epiphysis in more than half the cases [217, 227, 231, 234, 236, 241–243, 257, 263, 267, 269, 270, 275]. Perhaps it is an issue of better imaging or time of discovery. Invasion of the epiphysis by the tumor seems to be a matter of time [236]. Initially tumor tissue perforates the center of the physis through vascular channels (similar to the way infection perforates the physis as depicted in Fig. 3.1a, b) [227, 231, 269]. Some tumors have a sizable extra-osseous component that extends around the physis beneath the perichondral ring through epiphyseal vascular channels into the epiphysis (similar to the way infection reaches the epiphysis depicted in Fig. 3.1d, e) [227, 269].

Conventional roentgenograms are important in establishing the diagnosis [247, 263], but may not predictably determine the extent of epiphyseal involvement by the tumor [243, 269]. Scintigraphy has high sensitivity and detects multiple bone involvement, but its specificity is low; most lesions and the physis show increased uptake. [263] CT scan is complementary to roentgenography, and can be an excellent guide for needle biopsies, but does not offer multiplanar images [263, 267]. MRI most accurately detects epiphyseal extension [234, 245, 254, 255, 257, 263, 270, 281], but cannot completely rule out microinfiltration into the physis [210, 270]. Nevertheless these imaging advances have permitted radical surgery with the preservation of the limb without decreasing the survival rate or increasing local recurrences [232].

Osteosarcoma is one of the more aggressive and lethal bone neoplasms. Up through the 1970s amputation was the common treatment [219]. All physes distal to the tumor were sacrificed and substituted with an external prosthesis of increasing length as the child grew. Today "limb salvage" is an acceptable alternative to amputation due to advances in diagnostic imaging, neoadjuvant multidrug chemotherapy, biomedical engineering, and operative technique, all of which have greatly reduced morbidity and improved the functional outcome and the prognosis.

Lower limb length discrepancy is a major concern with any treatment. Attempts to maintain growth by preserving the physis are unpredictable. Growth arrest lines are commonly seen after cytotoxic chemotherapy and are valuable in assessing growth. However, plotting the growth of both the treated and untreated limbs on a Green or Mosely chart is of limited value [209]. Growth often slows after the operative procedure and during the period of chemotherapy, but may continue past the predicted time of maturity [209]. Because of these factors younger children who have more growth remaining have larger final discrepancies [209]. Once free of the disease, up to 67% of children will need some sort of limb length discrepancy compensation [232].

Limb length discrepancies may be treated with a shoe lift, physeal arrest or bone shortening on the contralateral disease-free side, or bone lengthening on the ipsilateral side [232]. To avoid complications in irradiated regions, lengthenings should be in adjacent segments [232]. Matching the length of the extremity on the tumor side with that of the normal growing limb is still difficult. Amputation and rotationplasty

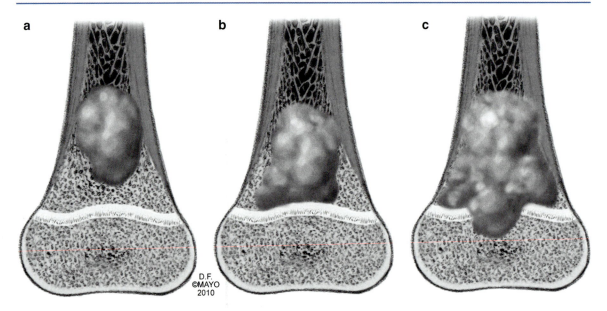

Fig. 4.16 Malignant Tumor Relationship to the Physis (**a**) Tumor in the metaphysis at least 1 cm from the physis. (**b**) Tumor in the metaphysis abuts against, but does not cross the physis. (**c**) Tumor in the metaphysis invades the epiphysis (transphyseal)

are therefore still used to some extent [218, 232, 259]. Limb salvage procedures are numerous and often ingenious. They can be classified as biologic (i.e. autograft, allograft), non-biologic (i.e. megaprosthesis, expandable prosthesis), or combined (i.e. allograft-prosthetic composite) [248]. The growth plate should be saved whenever possible. Biologic reconstruction with allografts or autografts or a combination of both is used to reconstruct large osteoarticular defects in children [245]. Metallic spacers and internal prostheses, though suitable for adults, have fixation and longevity problems when used in children [245].

The distal femur, proximal tibia, and proximal humerus are the most common sites of osteosarcoma [106]. Accurate assessment and classifying the location of the osteosarcoma with reference to the physis helps determine the optimal skeletal resection in limb salvage procedures [245, 263, 271–273]. Three possibilities exist (Fig. 4.16): (1) the tumor is not in contact with the physis, (2) the tumor is in contact with part or all of the physis, and (3) the tumor crosses the physis into the epiphysis [212, 263, 265].

1. <u>The Knee.</u> Distal femur or proximal tibia sarcomas confined to the metaphysis, but not abutting against the physis (Fig. 4.16a), can be treated in the following ways:
   (a) Intercalary Allograft [209, 230, 248, 249, 282]. Excision of a tumor in the metaphysis which does not abut against the physis and replacement with intercalary allograft or autograft is appropriate, if there is at least 1 cm of uninvolved metaphysis adjacent to the physis remaining after tumor removal. Normal growth of the physis is expected [249].
   (b) Physeal distraction [214–216, 263]. Distraction of the physis prior to tumor removal increases the safe margin of metaphysis and preserves the adjacent joint. Creating a 2 cm margin between the tumor and the physis is the goal [215]. The bone defect is reconstructed with intercalary allograft or autograft as in a. For children near the end of growth, it may be appropriate to insert an allograft longer than the resected piece [215]. This method should not be used if the tumor abuts against the physis. Local recurrences are uncommon, and the retained physis can continue growing [264].
   (c) Distraction Osteogenesis [232, 268, 271–273]. Marginal excision of the tumor preserving the physis and epiphysis can be accompanied by osseous distraction (callotasis) using bone transport of a portion of diaphysis [271–273]. Or if the tumor has been successfully removed and the bone healed, residual angular deformity and relative shortening can be corrected later by a standard osseous distraction [232, 268]. To

avoid complications, the osseous lengthening should be in a non-irradiated segment of the bone. A third option consists of removing the tumor and shortening the bone by bringing the remaining physeal-epiphyseal segment to the diaphysis. Once healed, distraction osteogenesis is applied to regain the length [271, 273].

Distal femur or proximal tibia metaphyseal sarcomas which abut against the physis (Figs. 4.16b and 4.17) can be treated by:

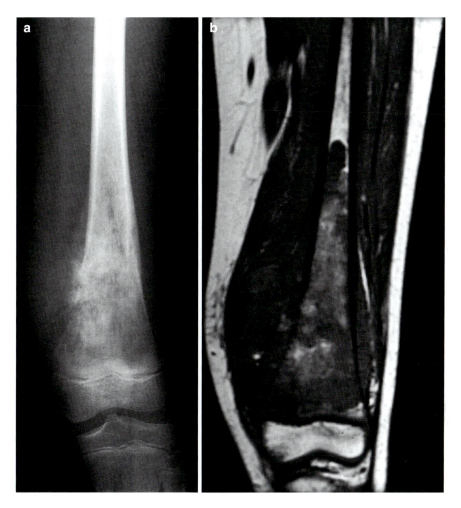

Fig. 4.17 Sarcoma adjacent to, but not crossing the physis, treated with an extendable endoprothesis. This 8 year 3 month old girl had a mass with pain in the distal left thigh. (**a**) A roentgenograph showed a permeative process involving the distal diaphysis and metaphysis and an associated soft tissue mass, but no involvement of the epiphysis. (**b**) MRI confirmed an aggressive malignant-appearing mass confined to the shaft and metaphysis of the distal femur. Chemotherapy (cisplatin and adriamycin, methotrexate) was given. (**c**) En bloc excision of the distal femur was done at age 9 years 0 months. The tumor did not cross the physis on any slab of the gross specimen, and the histologic diagnosis confirmed osteogenic sarcoma. (**d**) An extendable prosthesis was inserted. (**e**) The proximal portion of the tibial epiphysis was removed to accommodate the tibial component. The patellar tracking was excellent. (**f**) The proximal tibial physis was spared, but was crossed by the stem of the implant. Multiple lengthening procedures followed by turning the screw device proximally, allowing the spring to expand distally. (**g**) At age 9 years 9 months the proximal tibial physis was growing as noted by the growth arrest line in the metaphysis (*arrows*). (**h**) At age 11 years 2 months the lengthening was proceeding well (note elongation of the spring). The proximal tibial physis continued to grow as noted by the growth arrest line (*arrows*). Surgical physeal arrests of the right distal femur and proximal tibia were performed at age 13 years 3 months. (**i**) At age 13 years 8 months the patient was tumor free, normally active, and enjoying activities of daily living. All physes were closed and the growth arrest line had disappeared. The left lower extremity was 2 cm shorter that the right

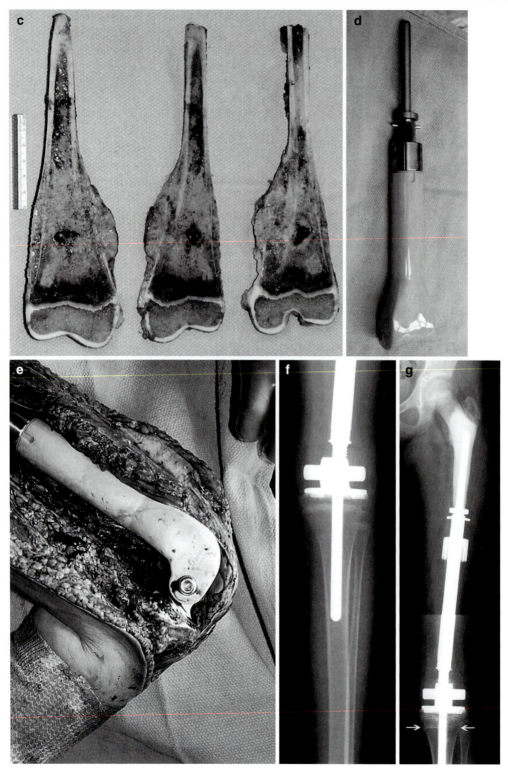

Fig. 4.17 (continued)

Fig. 4.17 (continued)

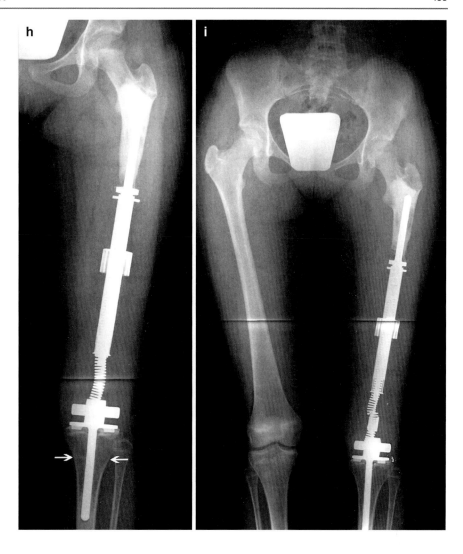

(a) Allograft reconstruction. Excision of the tumor in the metaphysis and a portion of the epiphysis containing the physis, saving the articular end of the epiphysis and replacement with bone or metal. This saves the cruciate and collateral ligaments and the menisci, enhancing joint motion. The retained articular portion of the epiphysis maintains its potential to grow spherically and subsequent degenerative joint changes are minimized [246, 258]. The cavity at the conclusion of tumor excision is reconstructed with intercalary allografts [221, 235, 246, 249, 250], autoclaved autogenous bone [210], or endo-prosthesis [233]. This epidiaphyseal reconstruction may be considered if at least 1 cm of tumor-free juxtaarticular epiphyseal bone can be preserved [221]. Most of these patients will develop leg length discrepancy as a result of loss of the physis [258]. In some patients the allograft replacement can be slightly longer than the resected part to minimize anticipated future limb length discrepancy [258]. The extent of the inequality depends on the patient age at time of resection. The adjacent normal distal femoral or proximal tibial physis will continue to grow normally [258].

(b) All of the methods mentioned in the following section where the tumor crosses the physis.

Distal femur or proximal tibial metaphyseal sarcomas which cross the physis into the epiphysis (transphyseal) (Figs. 4.16c and 4.18), or which are confined within the epiphysis, can be treated in a variety of ways:

(a) Intercalary allograft reconstruction [243]. If the physis is breached in a small area and penetrates

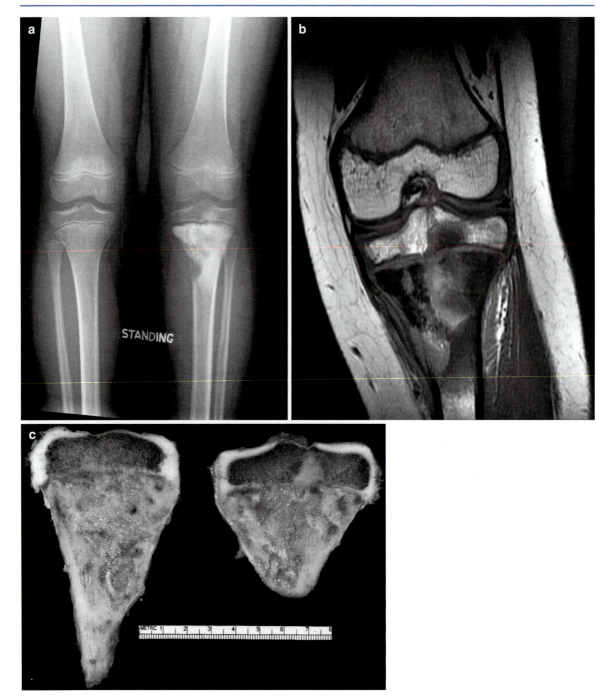

Fig. 4.18 Transphyseal osteosarcoma. This 10 year 10 month old boy noted pain in the proximal left tibia. (**a**) A roentgenogram of the knees standing shows sclerosis in the proximal left tibia with destruction of the medial metaphyseal cortex, an open physis, and faint sclerosis in the central area of the epiphysis. (**b**) Coronal T3-MRI suggests transphyseal tumor involvement in the epiphysis. (**c**) Enbloc resection of the proximal tibia confirms transphyseal extension of the tumor. The pathologic diagnosis was osteosarcoma. The patient was treated with a Van Ness rotationplasty (Fig. 4.20h–k)

into the epiphysis only a few millimeters, the metaphysis, physis and a small amount of epiphysis are removed and replaced by an allograft leaving the articular portion of the epiphysis.

(b) Osteoarticular allograft reconstruction [248, 249, 251, 258]. Excision of the entire distal femoral or proximal tibial epiphyseal-metaphyseal complex is replaced with a osteoarticular allograft. Osteoarticular allografts do less well than intercalary allografts, generally due to degeneration of the allograft articular surface secondary to chondrocyte cell death and subchondral bone resorption and collapse [248].

(c) Frozen autograft reconstruction [272]. Following preoperative chemotherapy the entire epiphyseal-metaphyseal tumor containing complex is removed en bloc. The resected specimen is treated with liquid nitrogen in a cycle of 45 min: immersion in liquid nitrogen 20 min, leaving the bone in room temperature air for 15 min, followed by immersion in distilled water for 10 min. The bone is then reimplanted and fixed with an internal fixator. The three most common complications include infection, non-union, and fracture, likely related to the avascular status of allograft bone [248].

(d) Endoprosthetic replacement [230, 237, 248, 277]. The entire end of the distal femur is removed along with the articular half of the adjacent tibial epiphysis, leaving its physis in situ. A femoral endoprosthesis with a constrained artificial knee is inserted. The stem of the tibial portion of the prosthesis crosses the physis. The stem is small in diameter, centrally located, smooth and press-fit, [252] and can be fitted with a polyethylene sleeve [225]. The ability of the tibial stem to slide within a sleeve allows the proximal tibial physis to grow somewhat normally. In some cases a cemented stem or a cemented sleeve has advanced with the growing physis [261]. This demonstrates that the physis is a formidable biologic structure, capable of overcoming partial ablation and considerable tethering forces in order to continue to grow. Endoprosthetic replacement is particularly appropriate if the prognosis is poor as in cases with lung metastases [272]. The distal tibial physis does not compensate (overgrow) for the loss of proximal tibial physeal growth.

(e) Extendable endoprosthesis replacement [218, 222–225, 228, 230, 248, 252, 253, 261, 266, 277]. After removal of the distal femur, ongoing length can be achieved by the insertion of a extendable femoral endoprosthesis, most of which have a constrained artificial knee as in d (Fig. 4.17d). Several extendable prostheses are available and can be lengthened by a variety of techniques. Most require an open surgical procedure each time the prosthesis is lengthened. Others have been developed that can be lengthened by mechanisms activated by a variety of techniques including active knee motion, passive manipulation of the knee, arthroscopic manipulation, or by an external electromagnetic field. At conclusion of growth the extendable portion is replaced with an adult type endoprosthesis. The use of these devices is most appropriate for expected growth deficit of 3 cm or more. The extension mechanism failure is high [225]. The infection risk and scarring associated with multiple surgical procedures to lengthen the expandable prosthesis is also high [222, 224]. Reoperations are frequent due to complications of restricted motion due to scar formation around the prosthesis, infection, aseptic loosening, and skin necrosis [223]. Some patients with endoprosthesis in the femur have also undergone distraction osteogenesis in the tibia [230].

(f) Distraction osteogenesis (callotasis) [271–273]. Osseous distraction with bone transport (by means of an external fixator/lengthener), to fill the area of en bloc tumor excision containing the physis has been successfully used, providing there is 1 cm of subarticular bone retained after excision of the tumor. The articular portion of the epiphysis, the transported bone, and the remaining diaphysis, are stabilized with an intramedullary nail to shorten the external fixation time. A mean gain in length of 9.7 cm was obtained in 11 patients [272].

(g) Resection arthrodesis [209, 211, 226, 230]. The entire distal femur or proximal tibia along with the articular portion of the remaining normal femoral or tibial epiphysis, are removed and replaced with massive allografts secured by an intramedullary rod [209, 226], a bridge plate [211], or external fixation [226]. Knee motion is sacrificed, but the physis of the uninvolved femur or tibia is preserved. When an intramedullary rod is used for fixation the rod crosses the remaining physis which may continue to grow. Plates and external fixation devices preclude any growth of the remaining physis. The intercalary allograft may exceed the length of the resected bone in anticipation of future progressive shortening. Nevertheless limb relative shortening of up to 7 cm is possible, despite surgical physeal arrest on the contralateral uninvolved extremity [209]. Procedures that result in knee arthrodesis are designed to conclude with 1–2 cm extremity shortening to facilitate clearing the limb during swing phase of walking [226]. The use of arthrodesis decreased after the introduction of the endoprosthesis (see below). However, arthrodesis is still considered in patients with large tumors requiring involving the joint requiring extra-articular resection, when there is a lack of replacement bone source, or when the patient prognosis is poor [230].

(h) The Van Nes rotationplasty [228, 244, 248, 276, 278, 279]. The distal femur and proximal tibia/fibula are removed. The distal tibia/fibula segment and foot are rotated 180° and fixed to the femur. The ankle joint functions like a knee (Fig. 4.20h–k). Limb relative shortening is managed by the prosthesis and no surgery on the contralateral uninvolved extremity is necessary.

2. The Shoulder. Proximal humeral osteosarcoma that does not cross the physis may be treated by the same methods as mentioned for the knee, except for intra-epiphyseal osteotomy due to irregular contour of the physis [262]. If the tumor is in contact with, or crosses the physis, the following methods have been used:
   (a) Osteoarticular allograft reconstruction [209, 264]
   (b) Ipsilateral clavicle rotation [280]. Following excision of the proximal humerus, the lateral half of the clavicle is rotated 90°, preserving the coracoacromial ligament, and fixed to distal humeral diaphysis with a metal plate. The lateral clavicular physis has the potential to grow.
   (c) Vascularized transfer of the entire proximal fibula [208, 238]. The biceps femoris tendon is used to stabilize the shoulder joint. When the anterior tibial artery is the retained blood supply, longitudinal growth of the transferred proximal fibular physis has occurred, but not at the rate of the removed proximal humerus [238].
   (d) Extendable humeral endoprosthesis [224, 225].

3. The Distal Radius. Vascularized proximal fibular transfer. Reconstruction after excision of the distal radius may be accomplished with transfer of the proximal fibula using the anterior tibial artery for vascular anastomosis [238]. When the ulna is spared, growth of the distal fibula is consistent and predictable, matching that of the host bone, with only mild final ulnar variance [238–240].

4. The Distal Tibia. Resection of the distal tibia was treated in one 9 year old boy by fusing the distal end of the fibular epiphysis to the talus, saving the distal fibular physis [260]. Follow-up at 9 months showed distal fibular growth. Physeal distraction followed by insertion of intercalary graft has also been followed by distal tibial growth [262].

5. The Distal Fibula. Resection of the distal fibula with its physis can lead to ankle instability and valgus deformity. Ligamentoplasty using peroneal tendons preserves ankle motion, but cannot avoid valgus deformity. Reconstruction with a pedicled vascularized proximal fibula with its physis is another option [220].

4.3.2 Ewing Sarcoma

Ewing sarcoma (ES) occurs most frequently during the second decade of life, and is the second most frequent malignant bone tumor found in children and adolescents. Many of the case studies of osteosarcoma include one or more ES patients [209, 214, 218, 221, 226, 230, 232, 238, 239, 246, 249, 251, 257, 258, 261–266, 273, 279, 280]. ES occurs most often in the diaphysis of long tubular bones. Lesions may be found in the metaphysis, particularly in patients over 16 years of age. Only rarely is ES located in the epiphysis. The ability of MRI to accurately define extension of ES through the physis [283] permits limb salvage, similar to that in osteogenic sarcoma. ES is one of the more aggressive tumors with a tendency toward recurrence and metastasis.

Ewing sarcoma is usually treated with multiple cycles of multidrug chemotherapies for local and metastatic disease and radiation therapy for limb salvage. The metaphyseal and epiphyseal lesions are surgically treated in the same manner as osteosarcoma. One ES in the proximal femur of a 4 year old girl was treated by an autotransplant of the ipsilateral proximal fibula with its vascular supply, inserted inside a massive bone allograft, and fixed to the residual femur by a plate [284]. Four years later the patient was weight bearing, had reasonably good hip motion, and imaging showed an open physis, with progressive tridimensional growth of the fibular epiphysis taking the shape of a femoral head.

4.3.3 Chondrosarcoma

Chondrosarcoma is rare in children [285–289]. In one series of 288 cases, only 2 patients were in the first decade of life and 8 in the second [288]. The youngest patient was 8 years old. The largest series limited to children is 12 patients [285]. In this series the average age at time of diagnosis was 14 years (range 6–20 years). Most tumors were located in the thoracic vertebrae and pelvis, and only two in the proximal femur and two in the proximal tibia. When found in a long bone, the tumor is most frequently located in the epiphysis. Some may arise in solitary or multiple osteochondromatosis or following radiation treatment, for example for Wilms tumor. [289] None of the references documented here discuss growth plate involvement or growth problems.

Prior to 1980 the usual treatment was curettage, local excision, en bloc resection, or amputation. However, it seems reasonable that the same strategies documented in the section on osteosarcoma could be used here. If staging studies show that an adequate margin can be achieved by local resection, limb-sparing techniques may be successful [289].

4.3.4 Lymphoma of Bone

Primary lymphoma of bone is a rare subset of non-Hodgkin's lymphoma in children. Only a few small series with long term follow-up are reported, and only one has appeared in the orthopedic literature [291].

The lesions may be monostatic or polystatic and occur most commonly in long bones, followed by the pelvis, skull, and vertebrae [291, 292]. In long bones the lesions may be in epiphysis, metaphysis, or diaphysis, most commonly in all three. One illustrated untreated lesion originated in the epiphysis and eventually crossed the physis into the metaphysis [290]. Plain roentgenograms often demonstrate osteolysis or osteosclerosis (Fig. 4.19a), but may fail to demonstrate a lesion at all. Computed tomography studies are more sensitive than plain roentgenograms (Fig. 4.19b). MRI consistently demonstrates low signal intensity on T1-weighted images and a hyperintense appearance on T2-weighted images (Fig. 4.19c).

Treatment consists of chemotherapy sometimes combined with radiation therapy [291, 292]. There are no reports of physeal growth arrest among survivors (Fig. 4.19d, e).

4.3.5 Author's Perspective

Every malignant tumor which resides near a physis of a growing child should include early evaluation by a pediatric orthopedist. Growth impairment among survivors can be significant and achieving limb length equality a challenge. Anticipation and early discovery of growth arrest allows the best chance of avoiding functional impairment due to limb length discrepancy.

4.4 Soft Tissue Tumors

Most soft tissue tumors do not affect the physis directly. However, treatment of the tumor may affect the physis. The growth plate should be saved

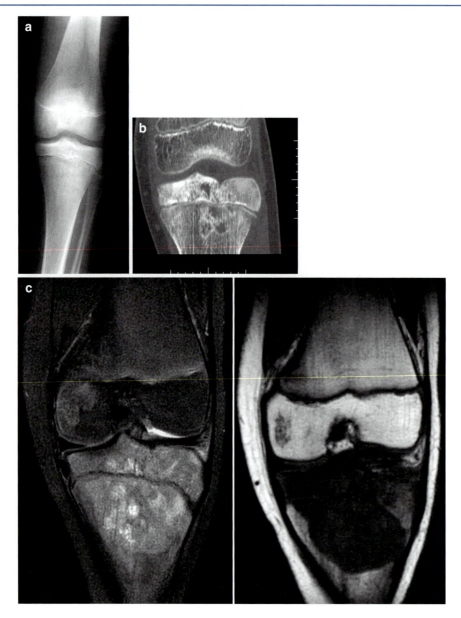

Fig. 4.19 Lymphoma of bone. This 13 year old boy noted intermittent pain in the left knee with activity for 1 year. (**a**) At age 13 years 8 months there was faint mottled lucency and sclerosis of both the metaphysis and epiphysis of the proximal tibia, and of the lateral femoral epiphysis. (**b**) CT revealed multiple small mottled lucencies within the tibial metaphysis and both epiphyses. There was no periosteal reaction or soft tissue mass. (**c**) MRI showed diffuse infiltrative process with fairly sharply defined margins in both the tibial metaphysis and epiphysis and femoral epiphysis. A biopsy of a small portion of tissue from the metaphysis through a small cortical window lateral to the tibial tubercle and adjacent to the physis revealed B cell lymphoma. Chemotherapy consisting of methotrexate, intrathecal ara-C and hyrocortisone, and leucovorin rescue were given. (**d**) At age 15 years 5 months MRI shows absence of tumor, and physes normal for that age. The round lytic defect in the left proximal tibial metaphysis is the biopsy site which was originally adjacent to the physis. (**e**) At age 16 years 6 months the patient was normally active and asymptomatic. All four major knee physes have grown equally as noted by the growth arrest lines (*arrows*). Note: the tumor involvement intimately adjacent to the physis on the metaphyseal side of the tibia was extensive (**c**), yet caused no growth impairment

Fig. 4.19 (continued)

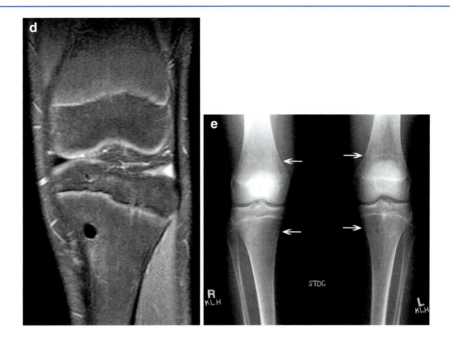

whenever possible. For example, when limb salvage procedures are not appropriate, amputation should be performed through a joint whenever possible. This avoids the problem of protrusion of the overgrowth at the stump end, which frequently requires repeated surgical revision, and the normal epiphysis provides a better weight-bearing surface. On occasion this might require surgical shortening of the bone proximal to the amputation [293]. When applied to the distal femur, it seems reasonable to expect the distal femoral physis to continue growing following the femoral shortening, but no record of this exists.

4.5 Tumor Induced Rickets

Widening of multiple physes appearing similar to rickets has been found in children at the time of discovery of a variety of tumors (Fig. 4.20a, b) [295]. Or the tumor may be present for years before the appearance of the ricketic physeal abnormality. The tumors may range from small to large, and benign to malignant. In the past tumors most often associated with this condition were benign, and included giant cell granuloma, non-ossifying fibroma, ossifying mesenchymal tumor, fibroangioma of the skin, and epidermal nevi. Today they are recognized as an extremely rare histologically distinctive tumor of a mixed connective tissue variant, recently called phosphaturic mesenchymal tumor (mixed connective tissue variant) (PMTMCT) [296]. Physeal changes and osteomalacia occur through the elaboration of a phosphaturic hormone, fibroblastic growth factor-23 (FGF-23) [294]. The physis typically returns to normal after removal of the tumor. However, premature closure of the ricketic-like physes may also occur (Fig. 4.20d, f and g).

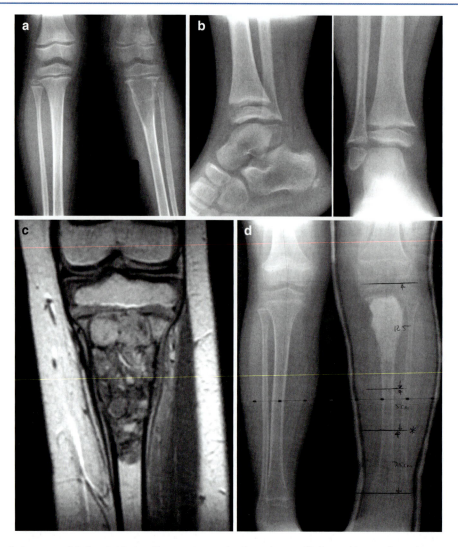

Fig. 4.20 Tumor (osteosarcoma) induced rickets with premature physeal closure. (**a**) This 7 year 5 month old female was found to have a lytic lesion in the proximal left tibia extending to the physis centrally, but not through the peripheral cortex. All physes in both knees were abnormally wide. (**b**) The distal tibial physes were also abnormally wide. Since most tumor induced rickets are secondary to benign tumor and are often present for long periods of time prior to physeal widening, the differential diagnosis of the lesion included aneurysmal bone cyst, simple bone cyst, and Brown's tumor. (**c**) MRI shows tumor involvement of the physis and metaphyseal periosteal elevation. Surgical biopsy through a small incision resulted in an initial frozen section diagnosis of aneurysmal bone cyst. The incision was enlarged to facilitate complete tumor removal by curettement. At this point Pathology changed the diagnosis to a high grade sarcoma. The cavity was filled with methacrylate as a precaution against fracture. Chemotherapy was given. (**d**) Four months later, age 7 years 9 months, the uninvolved right lower extremity physes had narrowed and appeared to be closing. An MRI showed possible tumor recurrent adjacent to the distal portion of the methacrylate. A Van Ness rotationplasty was performed at age 7 years 9 months. (**e**) Histologic analysis of the distal femoral physis at the time of rotationplasty showed marked narrowing of the proliferating, columnar, and hypertrophic zones, presumably due to the chemotherapy. (**f**) At age 11 years 8 months premature closure of the right distal femoral and proximal tibial physes was present, with persistent growth of the proximal fibular physis. (**g**) The distal right fibular physis was also open resulting in developmental relative overgrowth and ankle varus. (**h**) These unexpected premature closures resulted in the right femur and tibia being shorter than anticipated as calculated at the time of the rotationplasty. Surgical physeal arrests of both ends of the right fibula were combined with fibular shortening of 13 mm. (**i**) The left heel, which functions as a knee is lower than the right knee because of unanticipated premature closure of the right physes. (**j**) The prosthesis was constructed to equalize the leg lengths. (**k**) At age 14 years 2 months the patient was a good prosthesis wearer. At last follow-up, age 24 years, she was tumor free and physically active. Note: Removal of the tumor and chemotherapy reversed the rickets resulting in premature closure of the large physes, but not those of the fibula. Why this occurs is unknown. In this case, the unexpected closure of the distal right femoral physis resulted in the femur being shorter than anticipated, resulting in knee height discrepancy. This is not a functional problem, but when sitting the left "knee" protrudes forward more than the right. Closer observation might have resulted in earlier surgical physeal arrests of the fibula, avoiding the need for fibular shortening, but would not have prevented the knee height discrepancy

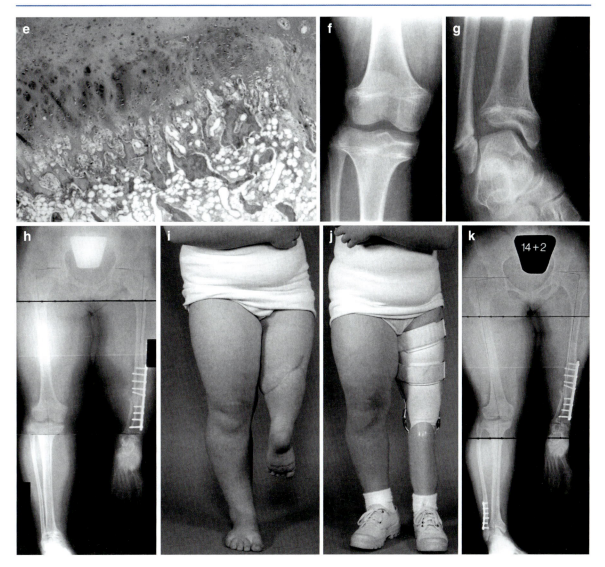

Fig. 4.20 (continued)

References

Introduction

1. Geirnaerdt MJA, Hogendoorn PCW, Bloem JL, Taminiau AHM, Van Der Woude HJ (2000) Cartilaginous tumors: fast contrast-enhanced MR imaging. Radiology 214(2):539–546
2. Murray K, Nixon GW (1988) Epiphyseal growth plate: evaluation with modified coronal CT. Radiology 166(11): 263–265
3. Murray IP (1980) Bone scanning in the child and young adult. Part I. Skeletal Radiol 5(1):1–14
4. Raymond AK, Raymond PG, Edeiken J (1989) Case report 531: epiphyseal osteoblastoma distal end of femur. Skeletal Radiol 18(2):143–146

Benign Tumors

5. Gardner DJ, Azouz EM (1988) Solitary lucent epiphyseal lesions in children. Skeletal Radiol 17(7):497–504
6. Hovy L (1996) Tumors of the epiphysis [*German*]. Z Orthop Ihre Grenzgeb 134(5):413–417
7. Jundt G (1995) Pathologic – anatomic characteristics of benign bone tumors [*German*]. Orthopade 24(1):2–14
8. Lindenbaum S, Alexander H (1984) Infections simulating bone tumors. A review of subacute osteomyelitis. Clin Orthop 184:193–203
9. Scarborough M, Zlotecki R (1999) Late effects of radiation after the treatment of musculoskeletal tumors. Curr Opin Orthop 10(6):481–484

Solitary Bone Cyst

10. Amillo S, Silberberg J, Arriagada C (2001) Lengthening of the humerus in a patient with an essential bone cyst. Orthopedics 24(3):278–280
11. Bensahel H, Jehanno P, Desgrippes Y, Pennecot GF (1998) Solitary bone cyst: controversies and treatment. J Pediatr Orthop B 7(4):257–261
12. Bernhang AM, Dua NK (1979) Solitary bone cyst with epiphyseal involvement. Orthop Rev 8:81–83
13. Bosch B, Bialik G, Bialik V (2002) Spontaneous epiphyseal injury as a complication of s simple bone cyst of the femoral neck? Case report and review of the literature [*German*]. Orthopade 31(9):930–933
14. Boseker EH, Bickel WN, Dahlin DC (1968) A clinicopathologic study of simple unicameral bone cysts. Surg Gynecol Obstet 127(3):550–560
15. Campanacci M, Capanna R, Picci P (1986) Unicameral and aneurysmal bone cysts. Orthop Clin North Am 204(3):25–36
16. Capanna R, Van Horn J, Ruggieri P, Biagini R (1986) Epiphyseal involvement in unicameral bone cysts. Skeletal Radiol 15(6):428–432
17. Clark L (1962) The influence of trauma on unicameral bone cysts. Clin Orthop 22:209–214
18. Clayer M, Boatright C, Conrad E (1997) Growth disturbances associated with untreated benign bone cysts. Aust N Z J Surg 67(12):872–873
19. Cohen J (1977) Unicameral bone cysts. A current synthesis of reported cases. Orthop Clin North Am 8(4):715–736
20. Crawford AH (1998) Growth arrest from transphyseal bone cysts (Letters to the Editors). J Pediatr Orthop 18:824–825
21. Fahey JJ, O'Brien ET (1973) Subtotal resection and grafting in selected cases of solitary unicameral bone cyst. J Bone Joint Surg Am 55A:59–68
22. Graham JJ (1952) Solitary Unicameral bone cyst. A follow-up study of thirty-one cases with prove pathological diagnosis. Bull Hosp Joint Dis 13(1):106–130
23. Gupta AK, Crawford AH (1996) Solitary bone cyst with epiphyseal involvement: confirmation with magnetic resonance imaging. A case report and review of the literature. J Bone Joint Surg Am 78(6):911–915
24. Haims AH, Desai P, Present D, Beltran J (1997) Epiphyseal extension of a unicameral bone cyst. Skeletal Radiol 26(1):51–54
25. Herring JA, Peterson HA (1987) Simple bone cyst with growth arrest. Instructional case. Guest discussant. J Pediatr Orthop 7(2):231–235
26. Hoffinger SA, Henderson RC, Renner JB, Dales MC, Rab GT (1993) Magnetic resonance evaluation of 'metaphyseal' changes in Legg-Calve-Perthes disease. J Pediatr Orthop 13(5):602–606
27. Hoffinger SA, Rab GT, Salamon PB (1991) "Metaphyseal" cysts in legg-calve-perthes' disease. J Pediatr Orthop 11(3):301–307
28. Hutter CG (1950) Unicameral bone cyst. Report of an unusual case. J Bone Joint Surg Am 32A:430–432
29. Johnson C, May DA, McCabe KM, Guse R, Resnick D (1997) Non-cartilaginous metaphyseal cysts in Legg-Calve-Perthes disease: report of a case. Pediatr Radiol 27(10):824–826
30. Komiya S, Inoue A (2000) Development of a solitary bone cyst – a report of a case suggesting its pathogenesis. Arch Orthop Trauma Surg 120(7–8):455–457
31. Lokiec F, Wientroub S (1998) Simple bone cyst: etiology, classification, pathology, and treatment modalities. J Pediatr Orthop B 7:262–273
32. Madhavan P, Dip NB, Ogilvie C (1998) Premature closure of upper humeral physis after fracture through simple bone cyst. Case report. J Pediatr Orthop B 7:83–85
33. Malawer MM, Markle B (1982) Unicameral bone cyst with epiphyseal involvement: clinicoanatomic analysis. J Pediatr Orthop 2:71–79
34. McKay DW, Nason SS (1977) Treatment of unicameral bone cysts by subtotal resection without grafts. J Bone Joint Surg Am 59A(4):515–519
35. Moed BR, LaMont RL (1982) Unicameral bone cyst complicated by growth retardation. Report of three cases. J Bone Joint Surg Am 64(9):1379–1381
36. Morton KS (1964) The pathogenesis of unicameral bone cyst. Can J Surg 7:140–150
37. Neer CS II, Francis KC, Marcove RC, Terz J, Carbonara PN (1966) Treatment of unicameral bone cyst. A follow-up of one hundred seventy-five cases. J Bone Joint Surg Am 48(4):731–745
38. Nelson JP, Foster RJ (1976) Solitary bone cyst with epiphyseal involvement. A case report. Clin Orthop Relat Res 118:147–150
39. Ovadia D, Ezra E, Segev E, Hayek S, Keret D, Wientroub S, Lokiec F (2003) Epiphyseal involvement of simple bone cysts. J Pediatr Orthop 23:222–229
40. Poul J (2001) Svebis: results of 20 lengthening of the humerus. Acta Chir Orthop Traumatol Cech 68(5):289–293
41. Robins PR, Peterson HA (1972) Management of pathologic fractures through unicameral bone cysts. JAMA 222(1):80–81
42. Schopler SA, Lawrence JF, Johnson MK (1986) Lengthening of the humerus for upper extremity limb length discrepancy. J Pediatr Orthop 6:477–480
43. Shen Q, Jia L, Li Y (1998) Solitary bone cyst in the odontoid process and body of the axis. J Bone Joint Surg Br 80(1):30–32
44. Song HR, Dhar S, Na JB, Cho SH, Ahn BW, Ko SM, Suh SW, Koo KH (2000) Classification of metaphyseal change with magnetic resonance imaging in Legg-Calve-Perthes disease. J Pediatr Orthop 20(5):557–561
45. Stanton RP (1998) Abdel-Mota'al MM: growth arrest resulting from unicameral bone cyst. J Pediatr Orthop 18(2):198–201
46. Ugwonali OFC, Bae DS, Waters PM (2007) Corrective osteotomy for humerus varus. J Pediatr Orthop 27(5):529–532
47. Violas P, Salmeron F, Chapuis M, Sales de Gauzy J, Bracq H, Cahuzac JP (2004) Simple bone cysts of the proximal humerus complicated with growth arrest. Case report. Acta Orthop Belg 70(2):166–170

Aneurysmal Bone Cyst

48. Barfod G (1987) Disturbances of growth in the forearm after a lesion of the distal epiphysis of the ulna [*Danish*]. Ugeskr Laeger 149(33):2212–2213
49. Biesecker JL, Marcove RC, Huvos AG, Miké V (1970) Aneurysmal bone cysts. A clinicopathologic study of 66 cases. Cancer 26:615–625

50. Bollini G, Jouve JL, Cottalorda J, Petit P, Panuel M, Jacquemier M (1998) Aneurysmal bone cyst in children: analysis of twenty-seven patients. J Pediatr Orthop B 7:274–285
51. Capanna R, Springfield DS, Biagini R, Ruggieri P, Giunti A (1985) Juxtaepiphyseal aneurysmal bone cyst. Skeletal Radiol 13(1):21–25
52. Carroll NC (1991) Half-pin skeletal fixation in children. Bull Hosp Jt Dis Orthop Inst 51(1):88–92
53. Cottalorda J, Bourelle S (2006) Current treatments of primary aneurysmal bone cysts. J Pediatr Orthop B 15(3):155–167
54. Dyer R, Stelling CB, Fechner RE (1981) Epiphyseal extension of an aneurismal bone cyst. AJR Am J Roentgenol 137:172–173
55. Farsetti P, Tudisco C, Rosa M, Pentimalli G, Ippolito E (1990) Aneurysmal bone cyst. Long-term follow-up of 20 cases. Arch Orthop Trauma Surg 109:221–223
56. Green JA, Bellemore MC, Marsden FW (1997) Embolization in the treatment of aneurysmal bone cysts. J Pediatr Orthop 17:440–443
57. Lampasi M, Magnani M, Donzelli O (2007) Aneurysmal bone cysts of the distal fibula in children. Long-term results of curettage and resection in nine patients. J Bone Joint Surg Br 89(10):1356–1362
58. Lin PP, Brown C, Raymond AK, Deavers MT, Yasko AW (2008) Aneurysmal bone cysts recur at juxtaphyseal locations in skeletally immature patients. Clin Orthop Relat Res 466:722–728
59. Maeda M, Tateishi H, Takaiwa H, Kinoshita G, Hatano N, Nakano K (1989) High-energy, low-dose radiation therapy for aneurysmal bone cyst. Report of a case. Clin Orthop Relat Res 243:200–203
60. Marcove RC, Sheth DS, Takemoto S, Healey JH (1995) The treatment of aneurismal bone cyst. Clin Orthop 311:157–163
61. McCarthy SM, Ogden JA (1982) Epiphyseal extension of an aneurismal bone cyst. Case report. J Pediatr Orthop 2:171–175
62. Mortensen NHM, Kuur E (1990) Aneurysmal bone cyst of the proximal phalanx. J Hand Surg Br 15(4):482–483
63. Oliveira AM, Hsi BL, Weremowicz S et al (2004) USP6 (Tre2) fusion oncogenes in aneurysmal bone cyst. Cancer Res 64:1920–1923
64. Oliveira AM, Perez-Atayde AR, Dal CP et al (2005) Aneurysmal bone cyst variant translocations upregulate USP6 transcription by promoter swapping with the ZNF9, COL1A1, TRAP150, and OMD genes. Oncogene 24:3419–3426
65. Oliveira AM, Perez-Atayde AR, Inwards CY et al (2004) USP6 and CDH11 oncogenes identify the neoplastic cell in primary aneurysmal bone cysts and are absent in so-called secondary aneurysmal bone cysts. Am J Pathol 165:1773–1780
66. Rizzo M, Dellaero DT, Harrelson JM, Scully SP (1999) Juxtaphyseal aneurysmal bone cysts. Clin Orthop Relat Res 364:205–212
67. Rodriguez Ramirez A, Stanton RP (2002) Aneurysmal bone cyst in 29 children. J Pediatr Orthop 27:533–539
68. Sakka SA, Lock M (1997) Aneurysmal bone cyst of the terminal phalanx of the thumb in a child. Arch Orthop Trauma Surg 116:119–120
69. Tillman BP, Dahlin DC, Lipscomb PR, Stewart JR (1968) Aneurysmal bone cyst: an analysis of ninety-five cases. Mayo Clin Proc 43(7):478–495

Osteochondroma

70. Abe M (1985) Lengthening of the ulna for the forearm deformity [*Japanese*]. J Jpn Soc Surg Hand 2:249–254
71. Abe M, Shirai H, Okamoto M, Onomura T (1996) Lengthening of the forearm by callus distraction. J Hand Surg Br 21(2):151–163
72. Arms DM, Strecker WB, Manske PR, Schoenecker PL (1997) Management of forearm deformity in multiple hereditary osteochondromatosis. J Pediatr Orthop 17:450–454
73. Bock GW, Reed MH (1991) Forearm deformities in multiple cartilaginous exostoses. Skeletal Radiol 20:483–486
74. Burgess RC, Cates H (1993) Deformities of the forearm in patients who have multiple cartilaginous exostosis. J Bone Joint Surg Am 75(1):13–18
75. Cheng JCY (1991) Distraction lengthening of the forearm. J Hand Surg Br 16(4):441–445
76. Chin KR, Kharrazi FD, Miller BS, Mankin HJ, Gebhardt MC (2000) Osteochondromas of the distal aspect of the tibia or fibula. J Bone Joint Surg Am 82:1269–1278
77. Choudhury SN, Kitaoka HB, Peterson HA (1997) Metatarsal lengthening: case report and review of the literature. Foot Ankle Int 18(11):739–745
78. Dahl MT (1993) The gradual correction of forearm deformities in multiple hereditary exostoses. Hand Clin 9(4):707–718
79. Dal Monte A, Andrisano A, Capanna R (1980) Lengthening of the radius or ulna in asymmetrical hypoplasia of the forearm. Ital J Orthop Traumatol 6:329–342
80. Fogel GR, McElfresh EC, Peterson HA, Wicklund PT (1984) Management of deformities of the forearm in multiple hereditary osteochodromas. J Bone Joint Surg Am 66(5):670–680
81. Fogel GR, Peterson HA (1984) Forearm deformity in multiple hereditary osteochondromata. Orthop Consult 5(7):7–12
82. Gupte CM, DasGupta R, Beverly MC (2003) The transfibular approach for distal tibial osteochondroma: an alternative technique for excision. J Foot Ankle Surg 42(2):95–98
83. Haga N, Nakamura K, Takikawa K, Manabe N, Ikegawa S, Kimizuka M (1998) Stature and severity in multiple epiphyseal dysplasia. J Pediatr Orthop 18:394–397
84. Huang SC, Kuo KN (1998) Differential lengthening of the radius and ulna using the Ilizarov method. J Pediatr Orthop 18:370–373
85. Irani RN, Petrucelli RC (1993) Ulnar lengthening for negative ulnar variance in hereditary multiple osteochondromas. J Pediatr Orthop B 1:143–147
86. Jahss MH, Olives R (1980) The foot and ankle in multiple hereditary exostoses. Foot Ankle 1(3):128–142
87. Johnson MK, Lawrence JF, Dionysian E (1995) The Kapandji procedure for the treatment of distal radioulnar joint derangement in young patients. Contemp Orthop 31(5):291–298
88. Kameshita K, Itoh S, Wada J, Yoshino M (1985) Ulnar lengthening combined with radial shortening for the forearm deformity in multiple osteochondroma [*Japanese*]. J Jpn Orthop Assoc 59:501–502
89. Karbowski A, Eckardt A, Rompe JD (1995) Multiple cartilagenous exostoses. Orthopade 24(1):37–43
90. LaFlamme GY, Stanciu C (1998) Ostéchondromes intra-articulaires isolés des phalanges chez les enfants [*French*]. Ann Chir 52(8):791–794

91. Langenskiöld A (1947) Normal and pathological bone growth in light of the development of cartilaginous foci in chondrodysplasia. Acta Chir Scand 95:367–385
92. Mader K, Gausepohl T, Pennig D (2003) Shortening and deformity of radius and ulna in children: correction of axis and length by callus distraction. J Pediatr Orthop B 12:183–191
93. Mansoor A, Beals RK (2007) Multiple exostosis: a short study of abnormalities near the growth plate. J Pediatr Orthop B 16:363–365
94. Masada K, Kojimoto H, Yasui N, Ono K (1993) Progressive lengthening of forearm bones in multiple osteochondromas. J Pediatr Orthop B 2:66–69
95. Masada K, Tsuyuguchi Y, Kawai H, Kawabata H, Noguchi K, Ono K (1989) Operations for forearm deformity caused by multiple osteochondromas. J Bone Joint Surg Br 71(1):24–29
96. Moore JR, Curtis RM, Shaw Wilgis EF (1983) Osteocartilaginous lesions of the digits in children: an experience with 10 cases. J Hand Surg Am 8(3):309–315
97. Noonan KJ, Feinberg JR, Levenda A, Snead J, Wurtz LD (2002) Natural history of multiple hereditary osteochondromatosis of the lower extremity and ankle. J Pediatr Orthop 22:120–124
98. Noonan KJ, Levenda A, Snead J, Feinberg JR, Mih A (2002) Evaluation of the forearm in untreated adult subjects with multiple hereditary osteochondromatosis. J Bone Joint Surg Am 84-A(3):397–403
99. Ofiram E, Eylon S, Porat S (2008) Correction of knee and ankle valgus in hereditary multiple exostoses using the Ilizarov apparatus. J Orthop Traumatol 9(1):11–15
100. Ogden JA (1976) Multiple hereditary osteochondromata. Report of an early case. Clin Orthop Relat Res 116:48–60
101. Peterson HA (1994) Deformities and problems of the forearm in children with multiple hereditary osteochondromata. J Pediatr Orthop 14(1):92–100
102. Peterson HA (1997) Deformities and problems of the wrist in children with multiple hereditary osteochondromata. In: Cooney WP, Linscheid RL, Dobyns JH (eds) The wrist, diagnosis and operative treatment, 2nd edn. Mosby, St. Louis, pp 991–1001, Chapter 43
103. Peterson HA (1989) Multiple hereditary osteochondromata. Clin Orthop Relat Res 239:222–230
104. Peterson HA (2008) The ulnius: a one-bone forearm in children. J Pediatr Orthop B 17:95–101
105. Porter DE, Emerton ME, Villanueva-Lopez F, Simpson AHRW (2000) Clinical and radiographic analysis of osteochondromas and growth disturbance in hereditary multiple exostoses. J Pediatr Orthop 20:246–250
106. Price CHG (1958) Primary bone-forming tumors and their relationship to skeletal growth. J Bone Joint Surg Br 40-B:574–593
107. Pritchett JW (1986) Lengthening the ulna in patients with hereditary multiple exostoses. J Bone Joint Surg Br 68:561–565
108. Raimondo RA, Skaggs DL, Rosenwasser MP, Dick HM (1999) Lengthening of pediatric forearm deformities using the Ilizarov technique: functional and cosmetic results. J Hand Surg Am 24(2):331–338
109. Rodgers WB, Hall JE (1993) One-bone forearm as a salvage procedure for recalcitrant forearm deformity in hereditary multiple exostoses. J Pediatr Orthop 13:587–591
110. Shapiro F, Simon S, Glimcher MJ (1979) Hereditary multiple exostoses. J Bone Joint Surg Am 61(6A):815–824
111. Shin EK, Jones NF, Lawrence JF (2006) Treatment of multiple hereditary osteochondromas of the forearm in children. A study of surgical procedures. J Bone Joint Surg Br 88(2):255–260
112. Siffert RS, Levy RN (1965) Correction of wrist deformity in diaphyseal aclasis by stapling. Report of a case. J Bone Joint Surg Am 47(7):1378–1380
113. Snearly WN, Peterson HA (1989) Management of ankle deformities in multiple hereditary osteochondromata. J Pediatr Orthop 9:427–432
114. Solomon L (1961) Bone growth in diaphyseal aclasis. J Bone Joint Surg Br 43-B(4):700–716
115. Solomon L (1963) Hereditary multiple exostosis. J Bone Jt Surg 45B(2):292–304
116. Stanton RP, Hansen MO (1996) Function of the upper extremities in hereditary multiple exostoses. J Bone Joint Surg Am 78(4):568–573
117. Stieber JR, Dormans JP (2005) Manifestations of hereditary multiple exostoses. J Am Acad Orthop Surg 13(2):110–120
118. Waters PM, Van Heest AE, Emans J (1997) Acute forearm lengthenings. J Pediatr Orthop 17:444–449
119. Wirganowicz PZ, Watts HG (1997) Surgical risk for elective excision of benign exostoses. J Pediatr Orthop 17:455–459
120. Wood VE, Sauser D, Mudge D (1985) The treatment of hereditary multiple exostosis of the upper extremity. J Hand Surg Am 10(4):505–513

Enchondroma

121. Chew DK, Menelaus MB, Richardson MD (1998) Ollier's disease: varus angulation at the lower femur and its management. J Pediatr Orthop 18:202–208
122. Cleveland M, Fielding JW (1959) Chondrodysplasia (Ollier's disease). Report of a case with a thirty-eight-year follow-up. J Bone Joint Surg 41-A(7):1341–1344
123. D'Angelo G, Petas N, Donzelli O (1996) Lengthening of the lower limbs in Ollier's disease: problems related to surgery. Chir Organi Mov 81:279–285
124. Gabos PG, Bowen JR (1998) Epiphyseal-metaphyseal enchondromatosis. A new clinical entity. J Bone Joint Surg Am 86:782–792
125. Jesus-Garcia R, Bongiovanni JC, Korukian M, Boatto H, Seixas MT, Laredo J (2001) Use of the Ilizarov external fixator in the treatment of patients with Ollier's disease. Clin Orthop Relat Res 382:82–86
126. Kolodziej L, Kolban M, Zacha S, Chmielnicki M (2005) The use of Ilizarov technique in the treatment of upper limb deformity in patients with Ollier's disease. J Pediatr Orthop 25(2):202–205
127. Ojeda-Thies C, Bonsfills N, Albiñana J (2008) Solitary epiphyseal enchondroma of the proximal femur in a 23-month-old girl. J Pediatr Orthop 28(5):565–568
128. Pandey R, White SH, Kenwright J (1995) Callus distraction in Ollier's disease. A case report. Acta Orthop Scand 66(5):479–480
129. Paterson DC, Morris LL, Binns GF, Kozlowski K (1989) Generalized enchondromatosis. A case report. J Bone Joint Surg Am 71(1):133–140

130. Potter BK, Freedman BA, Lehman RA Jr, Shawen SB, Kuklo TR, Murphey MD (2005) Solitary epiphyseal enchondromas. J Bone Joint Surg Am 87(7):1551–1560
131. Shapiro F (1982) Ollier's disease. An assessment of angular deformity, shortening, and pathological fracture in twenty-one patients. J Bone Joint Surg Am 64(1):95–103
132. Tellisi N, Ilizarov S, Fragomen AT, Rozbruch SR (2008) Humeral lengthening and deformity correction in Ollier's disease: distraction osteogenesis with a multiaxial correction frame. Case report. J Pediatr Orthop B 17(3): 152–157
133. Urist MR (1989) A 37-year follow-up evaluation of multiple-stage femur and tibia lengthening in dyschondroplasia (enchondromatosis) with a net gain of 23.3 centimeters. Clin Orthop Relat Res 242:137–157

Chondroblastoma

134. Bloem JL, Mulder JD (1985) Chondroblastoma: a clinical and radiological study of 104 cases. Skeletal Radiol 14:1–9
135. Edel G, Ueda Y, Nakanishi J, Brinker KH, Roessner A, Blasius S, Vestring T, Muller-Miny H, Erlemann R, Wuisman P (1992) Chondroblastoma of bone. A clinical, radiological, light and immunohistochemical study. Virchows Arch A Pathol Anat Histopathol 421(4): 355–366
136. Huvos AG, Marcove RC (1973) Chondroblastoma of bone. A critical review. Clin Orthop Relat Res 95:300–312
137. Pösl M, Amling M, Ritzel H, Werner M, Stenzel I, Delling G (1996) Morphological characteristics of chondroblastoma. A retrospective investigation of 56 cases from the Hamburg Bone Tumor Registry [German]. Pathologe 17:26–34
138. Ramappa AJ, Lee FYI, Tang P, Carlson JR, Gebhardt MC, Mankin HJ (2000) Chondroblastoma of bone. J Bone Joint Surg Am 82(8):1140–1145
139. Schuppers HA, van der Eijken JW (1998) Chondroblastoma during the growing age. J Pediatr Orthop B 7(4):293–297
140. Valls J, Ottolenghi CE, Schajowicz F (1951) Epiphyseal chondroblastoma of bone. J Bone Joint Surg Am 33-A:997–1009

Giant Cell Tumor of Bone

141. Campanacci M, Baldini N, Boriani S, Sudanese A (1987) Giant-cell tumor of bone. J Bone Joint Surg Am 69(1): 106–114
142. Dahlin DC (1970) Giant-cell tumor: a study of 195 cases. Cancer 25:1061–1070
143. Fain JS, Unni KK, Beabout JW, Rock MG (1993) Nonepiphyseal giant cell tumor of the long bones: clinical, radiologic, and pathologic study. Cancer 71(11):3514–3519
144. Gandhe A, Sandhe A, Aeron G, Joshi A (2008) Epiphyseal giant cell tumour in an immature skeleton. Case report. Br J Radiol 81:e75–e78
145. Hoeffel JC, Galloy MA, Grignon Y, Chastagner P, Floquet J, Mainard L, Kadiri R (1996) Giant cell tumor of bone in children and adolescents. Rev Rhum Engl Ed 63(9): 618–623
146. Kaufman RA, Wakely PE, Greenfield DJ (1983) Case Report 224: Giant cell tumor of the ossification center of the distal end of the fibula, growing into the metaphysis. Skeletal Radiol 9(3):218–222
147. Kransdorf MJ, Sweet DE, Buetow PC, Giudici MAI, Moser RP (1992) Giant cell tumor in skeletally immature patients. Radiology 184(1):233–237
148. Pericles Ribeiro Baptista P, Donato De Prospero J, Volpe Neto F, Yumi Saito R, Montezuma Cesar De Assumpcao R, Sanmartin Fernandez M (1996) Giant-cell tumor of the sacrum [Portuguese]. Rev Bras Ortopedia 31(11):947–951
149. Peison B, Feigenbaum J (1976) Metaphyseal giant-cell tumor in a girl of 14. Radiology 118(1):145–146
150. Picci P, Manfrini M, Zucchi V, Gherlinzoni F, Rock M, Bertoni F, Neff JR (1983) Giant-cell tumor of bone in skeletally immature patients. J Bone Joint Surg Am 65(4): 486–490
151. Puri A, Agarwal MG, Shah M, Jambhekar NA, Anchan C, Behle S (2007) Giant cell tumor of bone in children and adolescents. J Pediatr Orthop 27(6):635–639
152. Rietveld LA, Mulder JD, BruteldelaRiviere G, van Rijssel TG (1981) Giant cell tumour: metaphyseal or epiphyseal origin? Diagn Imaging 50(6):289–293
153. Schutte HE, Taconis WK (1993) Giant cell tumor in children and adolescents. Skeletal Radiol 22(3):173–176
154. Sherman M, Fabricius R (1961) Giant-cell tumor in the metaphysis in a child. Report of an unusual case. J Bone Joint Surg Am 43-A(8):1225–1229
155. Siegling JA (1937) Lesions of the epiphyseal cartilages about the knee. Surg Clin N Am 17:373–379
156. Sim FH, Dahlin DC, Beabout JW (1977) Multicentric giant-cell tumor of bone. J Bone Joint Surg Am 59(8): 1052–1060

Langerhan's Cell Histiocytosis

157. Bolinni G, Jouve JL, Gentet JC, Jacquemier M, Bouyala JM (1991) Bone lesions in histiocytosis X. J Pediatr Orthop 11(4):469–477
158. Capanna R, Springfield DS, Ruggieri P, Biagini R, Picci P, Bacci G, Giunti A, Lorenzi EG, Campanacci M (1985) Direct cortisone injection in eosinophilic granuloma of bone: a preliminary report on 11 patients. J Pediatr Orthop 5(3):339–342
159. Egeler RM, Thompson RC Jr, Voute PA, Nesbit ME Jr (1992) Intralesional infiltration of corticosteroids in localized Langerhans' cell histiocytosis. J Pediatr Orthop 12(6): 811–814
160. Greis PE, Hankin FM (1990) Eosinophilic granuloma. The management of solitary lesions of bone. Clin Orthop Relat Res 257:204–211
161. Immenkamp M (1985) Eosinophilic granuloma of the spine [German]. Z Orthop Ihre Grenzgeb 123(2):227–234
162. Leeson MC, Smith A, Carter JR, Makley JT (1985) Eosinophilic granuloma of bone in growing epiphysis. J Pediatr Orthop 5(2):147–150
163. Schreuder HWB, Pruszczynski M, Lemmens JAM, Veth RPH (1998) Eosinophilic granuloma of bone: results of treatment with curettage, cryosurgery, and bone grafting. J Pediatr Orthop B 7(4):253–256
164. Stern MB, Cassidy R, Mirra J (1976) Eosinophilic granuloma of the proximal tibial epiphysis. Clin Orthop Relat Res 118:153–156

165. Usui M, Matsuno T, Kobayashi M, Yagi T, Saska T, Ishii S (1983) Eosinophilic granuloma of the growing epiphysis. A case report and review of the literature. Clin Orthop Relat Res 176:201–205

Osteoid Osteoma and Osteoblastoma

166. Baghdadi T, Mortazavi SMJ (2005) Intraepiphyseal osteoid osteoma of proximal tibial epiphysis: a case report. Acta Med Iran 43(1):75–78
167. Beerman PJ, Crowe JE, Sumner TE, Roberts JE (1981) Case report 164, osteoid osteoma of ossification center of tibia. Skeletal Radiol 7(1):71–74
168. Blair WF, Kuge WJ (1977) Osteoid osteoma in a distal radial epiphysis. Case report. Clin Orthop Relat Res 126:160–161
169. Bordelon RL, Cracco A, Book MK (1975) Osteoid-osteoma producing premature fusion of the epiphysis of the distal phalanx of the big toe. J Bone Joint Surg Am 57:120–121
170. Brody JM, Brower AC, Shannon FB (1992) An unusual epiphyseal osteoid osteoma. AJR Am J Roentgenol 158(3):609–611
171. Destian S, Hernanz-Schulman M, Raskin K, Genieser N, Becker M, Crider R, Alba Greco M (1988) Case report 468. Skeletal Radiol 17(2):141–143
172. Giustra PE, Freiberger RH (1970) Severe growth disturbance with osteoid osteoma. A report of two cases involving the femoral neck. Radiology 96(2):285–288
173. Iceton J, Rang M (1986) An osteoid osteoma in an open distal femoral epiphysis. A case report. Clin Orthop Relat Res 206:162–165
174. Kruger GD, Rock MG (1987) Osteoid osteoma of the distal femoral epiphysis. A case report. Clin Orthop Relat Res 222:203–209
175. Micheli LJ, Jupiter J (1978) Osteoid osteoma as a cause of knee pain in the young athlete. A case study. Am J Sports Med 6(4):199–203
176. Murray IPC, Rossleigh MA, Van Der Wall H (1989) The use of SPECT in the diagnosis of epiphyseal osteoid osteoma. Clin Nucl Med 14(11):811–813
177. Odaka T, Koshino T, Saito T (1987) Intraarticular epiphyseal osteoid osteoma of the distal femur. Case report. J Pediatr Orthop 7(3):331–333
178. Olley LM, Chapman-Sheath PJ, Theologis TN (2004) Dual pathology: distal tibial epiphyseal osteoid osteoma associated with ipsilateral talar dome osteochondritis dissecans in a child. J Foot Ankle Surg 10(4):217–219
179. Raymond AK, Raymond PG, Edeiken J (1989) Case report 531: epiphyseal osteoblastoma distal end of femur. Skeletal Radiol 18(2):143–146
180. Rosborough D (1966) Osteoid osteoma. Report of a lesion in the terminal phalanx of a finger. J Bone Joint Surg Br 48:485–487
181. Seitz WH Jr, Dick HM (1983) Intraepiphyseal osteoid osteoma of the distal femur in an 8-year-old girl. Case report. J Pediatr Orthop 3:505–507
182. Sevitt S, Horn JS (1954) A painless and calcified osteoid osteoma of the little finger. J Pathol Bacteriol 67:571–574
183. Sherman MS (1947) Osteoid osteoma associated with changes in adjacent joint. J Bone Joint Surg Am 29(2):483–490
184. Shifrin LZ, Reynolds WA (1971) Intra-articular osteoid osteoma of the elbow. Clin Orthop Relat Res 81:126–129
185. Simon WH, Beller ML (1975) Intracapsular epiphyseal osteoid osteoma of the ankle joint. A case report. Clin Orthop Relat Res 108:200–203
186. van Horn JR, Karthaus RP (1989) Epiphyseal osteoid osteoma. Two case reports. Acta Orthop Scand 60(5):625–627

Focal Fibrocartilaginous Dysplasia

187. Albiñana J, Cuervo M, Certucha JA, Gonzalez-Mediero I, Abril JC (1997) Five additional cases of local fibrocartilaginous dysplasia. J Pediatr Orthop B 6:52–55
188. Beaty JH, Barrett IR (1989) Unilateral angular deformity of the distal end of the femur secondary to a focal fibrous tether. A report of four cases. J Bone Joint Surg Am 71(3):440–445
189. Bell SN, Campbell PE, Cole WG, Menelaus MB (1985) Tibia vara caused by focal fibrocartilaginous dysplasia. Three case reports. J Bone Joint Surg Br 67(5):780–784
190. Bradish CF, Davies SJM, Malone M (1988) Tibia vara due to focal fibrocartilaginous dysplasia. J Bone Joint Surg Br 70(1):106–108
191. Choi IH, Kim CH, Cho TJ, Chung CY, Song KW, Hwang JK, Sohn YJ (2000) Focal fibrocartilaginous dysplasia of long bones: report of eight additional cases and literature review. J Pediatr Orthop 20:421–427
192. Cockshott WP, Martin R, Friedman L, Yuen M (1994) Focal fibrocartilaginous dysplasia and tibia vara: a case report. Skeletal Radiol 23(5):333–335
193. Eren A, Cakar M, Erol B, Ozkurt A, Guven M (2008) Focal fibrocartilaginous dysplasia in the humerus. Case report. J Pediatr Orthop B 17(3):148–151
194. Haasbeek JF, Rang MC, Blackburn N (1995) Periosteal tether causing angular growth deformity: report of two clinical cases and an experimental model. J Pediatr Orthop 15(5):677–681
195. Herman TE, Siegel MJ, McAlister WH (1990) Focal fibrocartilaginous dysplasia associated with tibia vara. Radiology 177(3):767–768
196. Husien AMA, Kale VR (1989) Case report: tibia vara caused by focal fibrocartilaginous dysplasia. Clin Radiol 40(1):104–105
197. Kariya Y, Taniguchi K, Yagisawa H, Ooi Y (1991) Focal fibrocartilaginous dysplasia: consideration of healing process. Case report. J Pediatr Orthop 11(4):545–547
198. Lincoln TL, Birch JG (1997) Focal fibrocartilaginous dysplasia in the upper extremity. J Pediatr Orthop 17(4):528–532
199. Macnicol MF (1999) Focal fibrocartilaginous dysplasia of the femur. J Pediatr Orthop B 8(1):61–63
200. Meyer JS, Davidson RS, Hubbard AM, Conard KA (1995) MRI of focal fibrocartilaginous dysplasia. J Pediatr Orthop 15(3):304–306
201. Olney BW, Cole WG, Menelaus MB (1990) Three additional cases of focal fibrocartilaginous dysplasia causing tibia vara. Case report. J Pediatr Orthop 10(3):405–407
202. Smith NC, Carter PR, Ezaki M (2004) Focal fibrocartilaginous dysplasia in the upper limb. Seven additional cases. J Pediatr Orthop 24(6):700–705

203. Zayer M (1992) Tibia vara in focal fibrocartilaginous dysplasia. A report of 2 cases. Acta Orthop Scand 63(3): 353–355

Fibrous Dysplasia of Bone

204. Harris WH, Dudley HR Jr, Barry RJ (1962) The natural history of fibrous dysplasia. J Bone Joint Surg Am 44-A(2):207–233
205. Reed RJ (1963) Fibrous dysplasia of bone. A review of 25 cases. Arch Pathol 75:480–495
206. Stanton RP, Montgomery BE (1996) Fibrous dysplasia. Review. Orthopedics 19(8):679–685

Miscellaneous

207. Azouz EM (1995) Benign fibrous histiocytoma of the proximal tibial epiphysis in a 12-year-old girl. Skeletal Radiol 24(5):375–378

Malignant Bone TumorsOsteosarcoma

208. Ad-El DD, Paizer A, Pidhortz C (2001) Bipedicled vascularized fibula flap for proximal humerus defect in a child. Plast Reconstr Surg 107(1):155–157
209. Alman BA, de Bari A, Krajbich JI (1995) Massive allografts in the treatment of osteosarcoma and Ewing sarcoma in children and adolescents. J Bone Joint Surg Am 77(1):54–64
210. Amitani A, Yamazaki T, Sonoda J, Tanaka M, Hirata H, Katoh K, Uchida A (1998) Preservation of the knee joint in limb salvage of osteosarcoma in the proximal tibia. Int Orthop 22(5):330–334
211. Amr SM, El-Mofty AO, Amin SN, Morsy AM, El-Malt OM, Abdel-Aal HA (2000) Reconstruction after resection of tumors around the knee: role of the free vascularized fibular graft. Microsurgery 20(5):233–251
212. Aquerreta JD, San-Julian M, Benito A, Cañadell J (2009) Growth plate involvement in malignant bone tumours: relationship between imaging methods and histological findings. In: Cañadell J, San-Julian M (eds) Pediatric bone sarcomas: epiphysiolysis before excision. Springer, Heidelberg, pp 79–87, Chapter 6
213. Bonar SF, McCarthy S, Stalley P, Schatz J, Soper J, Scolyer R, Barrett I (2004) Epiphyseal osteoblastoma-like osteosarcoma. Skeletal Radiol 33(1):46–50
214. Cañadell J, Forriol F, Cara JA (1994) Removal of metaphyseal bone tumours with preservation of the epiphysis. Physeal distraction before excision. J Bone Joint Surg Br 76(1):127–132
215. Cañadell J, San-Julian M, Cara JA, Forriol F (2009) Conservation of the epiphysis while removing metaphyseal bone tumours: epiphysiolysis before excision. In: Cañadell J, San-Julian M (eds) Pediatric bone sarcomas: epiphysiolysis before excision. Springer, Heidelberg, pp 101–108, Chapter 8
216. Cañadell J, San-Julian M, Fiorriol F, Cara JA (1998) Physeal distraction in the conservative treatment of malignant bone tumours in children. In: de Pablos J (ed) Surgery of the growth plate. Ediciones Ergon S.A, Madrid, pp 321–327, Chapter 40
217. Chen ML (1981) Observation on the penetration of osteosarcoma of long bone through epiphyseal plate and joint cartilage [Chinese]. Zhonghua Wai Ke Za Zhi 19(11): 696–697
218. Cool WP, Carter SR, Grimer RJ, Tillman RM, Walker PS (1997) Growth after extendible endoprosthetic replacement of the distal femur. J Bone Joint Surg Br 79(6):938–942
219. Copeland MM, Sutow WW (1979) Osteogenic sarcoma: the past, present, and future. Int Adv Surg Oncol 2: 177–200
220. de Gauzy JS, Kany J, Cahuzac JP (2002) Distal fibular reconstruction with pedicled vascularized fibular head graft: a case report. J Pediatr Orthop B 11(2):176–180
221. Deijkers RLM, Bloem RM, Kroon HM, Van Lent JB, Brand R, Taminiau AHM (2005) Epidiaphyseal versus other intercalary allografts for tumors of the lower limb. Clin Orthop Relat Res 439:151–160
222. Delepine N, Delepine G, Desbois JC (1993) Update on use of expandable prostheses in limb salvage surgery for children's bone sarcomas of lower limb. Radiol Oncol 31(2):142
223. Dominkus M, Krepler P, Schwameis E, Windhager R, Kotz R (2001) Growth prediction in extendable tumor prostheses in children. Clin Orthop Relat Res 390: 212–220
224. Eckardt JJ, Kabo JM, Kelley CM, Ward WG Sr, Asavamongkolkul A, Wirganowicz PZ et al (2000) Expandable endoprosthesis reconstruction in skeletally immature patients with tumors. Clin Orthop Relat Res 373:51–61
225. Eckardt JJ, Safran MR, Eilber FR, Rosen G, Kabo JM (1993) Expandable endoprosthetic reconstruction of the skeletally immature after malignant bone tumor resection. Clin Orthop Relat Res 297:188–202
226. El-Gammal TA, El-Sayed A, Kotb MM (2003) Reconstruction of lower limb bone defects after sarcoma resection in children and adolescents using free vascularized fibular transfer. J Pediatr Orthop B 12(4):233–243
227. EnnekingWF KIIA (1978) Transepiphyseal extension of osteosarcoma: incidence, mechanism, and implications. Cancer 41(4):1526–1537
228. Finn HA, Simon MA (1991) Limb-salvage surgery in the treatment of osteosarcoma in skeletally immature individuals. Clin Orthop Relat Res 262:108–118
229. Forriol F, San-Julian M, Cañadell J (2009) Location of sarcomas within bone: the growth plate. In: Cañadell J, San-Julian M (eds) Pediatric bone sarcomas: epiphysiolysis before excision. Springer, Heidelberg
230. Futani H, Minamizaki T, Nishimoto Y, Abe S, Yabe H, Ueda T (2006) Long-term follow-up after limb salvage in skeletally immature children with a primary malignant tumor of the distal end of the femur. J Bone Joint Surg Am 88(3):595–603
231. Ghandur-Mnaymneh L, Mnaymneh WA, Puls S (1983) The incidence and mechanism of transphyseal spread of osteosarcoma of long bones. Clin Orthop Relat Res 177:210–215
232. González-Herranz P, Burgos-Flores J, Ocete-Guzmán JG, López-Mondejar JA, Amaya S (1995) The management of limb-length discrepancies in children after treatment of osteosarcoma and Ewing's sarcoma. J Pediatr Orthop 15(5):561–565

233. Gupta A, Pollock R, Cannon SR, Briggs TWR, Skinner J, Blunn G (2006) A knee-sparing distal femoral endoprosthesis using hydroxyapatite-coated extracortical plates. J Bone Joint Surg Br 88(10):1367–1372
234. Hoffer FA, Nikanorov AY, Reddick WE, Bodner SM, Xiong X, Jones-Wallace D et al (2000) Accuracy of MR imaging for detecting epiphyseal extension of osteosarcoma. Pediatr Radiol 30(5):289–298
235. Honoki K, Kobata Y, Miyauchi Y, Yajima H, Fujii H, Kido A et al (2008) Epiphyseal preservation and an intercalary vascularized fibular graft with hydroxyapatite composites. Reconstruction in metaphyseal osteosarcoma of the proximal tibia: a case report. Arch Orthop Trauma Surg 128(2):189–193
236. Idoate MA, de Alva E, de Pablos J, Lozano MD, Vazquez J, Cañadell J (2009) Pediatric bone sarcomas: epiphysiolysis before excision. In: Cañadell J, San-Julian M (eds) A histological study of the barrier effect of the physis against metaphyseal osteosarcoma. Springer, Heidelberg, pp 71–78, Chapter 5
237. Inglis AE Jr, Walker PS, Sneath RS, Grimer R, Scales JT (1992) Uncemented intramedullary fixation of implants using polyethylene sleeves. Clin Orthop Relat Res 284:208–214
238. Innocenti M, Ceroso M, Manfrini M, Angeloni R, Lauri G, Capanna R et al (1998) Free vascularized growth-plate transfer after bone tumor resection in children. J Reconstr Microsurg 14(2):137–142
239. Innocenti M, Delcroix L, Manfrini M, Ceruso M, Capanna R (2004) Vascularized proximal fibular epiphyseal transfer for distal radial reconstruction. J Bone Joint Surg Am 86-A(7):1504–1511
240. Inocenti M, Delcroix L, Manfrini M, Ceruso M, Capanna R (2005) Vascularized proximal fibular epiphyseal transfer for distal radial reconstruction. J Bone Joint Surg Am 87(9 II Suppl 1):237–246
241. Jäger HJ, Götz GF, Schmitz-Stolbrink A, Roggenkamp K, Mathias KD (1995) Crossing of the physis by bone tumors and osteomyelitis in childhood [German]. Radiologe 35:405–413
242. Jesus-Garcia R, De Seixas MT, Da Costa SR, Petrilli AS (1997) Osteosarcoma invastion of the epiphyseal plate. Is plaque a barrier to tumor growth? [Portuguese]. Rev Brasil Ortopedia 32(11):870–874
243. Jesus-Garcia R, Seixas MT, Dosta SR, Petrilli AS, Filho JL (2000) Epiphyseal plate involvement in osteosarcoma. Clin Orthop Relat Res 373:32–38
244. Krajbich JI, Carroll NC (1990) Van Nes rotationplasty with segmental limb resection. Clin Orthop Relat Res 256:7–13
245. Kumta SM, Chow TC, Griffith J, Li CK, Kew J, Leung PC (1999) Classifying the location of osteosarcoma with reference to the epiphyseal plate helps determine the optimal skeletal resection in limb salvage procedures. Arch Orthop Trauma Surg 119(5–6):327–331
246. Manfrini M, Gasbarrini A, Malaguti C, Ceruso M, Innocenti M, Bini S et al (1999) Intraepiphyseal resection of the proximal tibia and its impact on lower limb growth. Clin Orthop Relat Res 358:111–119
247. Meyer S, Reinhard H, Graf N, Puschel W, Ziegler K, Schneider G (2002) The importance of conventional radiographs in the diagnosis of osteosarcoma [German]. Klin Padiatr 214(2):58–61
248. Most MJ, Sim F (2009) Surgical options for limb salvage in immature patients with extremity sarcoma. In: Cañadell J, San-Julian M (eds) Pediatric bone sarcomas: epiphysiolysis before excision. Springer, Heidelberg, pp 33–56, Chapter 3
249. Muscolo DL, Ayerza MA, Aponte-Tinao LA, Farfalli G (2008) Allograft reconstruction after sarcoma resection in children younger than 10 years old. Clin Orthop Relat Res 466(8):1856–1862
250. Muscolo DL, Ayerza MA, Aponte-Tinao LA, Ranalletta M (2004) Partial epiphyseal preservation and intercalary allograft reconstruction in high-grade metaphyseal osteosarcoma of the knee. J Bone Joint Surg Am 86-A(12):2686–2693
251. Muscolo DL, Campaner G, Aponte-Tinao LA, Ayerza MA, Santini-Araujo E (2003) Epiphyseal primary location for osteosarcoma and Ewing's sarcoma in patients with open physis. J Pediatr Orthop 23:542–545
252. Neel MD, Heck R, Britton L, Daw N, Rao BH (2004) Use of a smooth press-fit stem preserves physeal growth after tumor resection. Clin Orthop Relat Res 426:125–128
253. Neel MD, Letson GD (2001) Modular endoprosthesis for children with malignant bone tumors. Cancer Control 8(4):344–348
254. Norton KI, Hermann G, Abdelwahab IF, Klein JM, Granowetter LF, Rabinowitz JG (1991) Epiphyseal involvement in osteosarcoma. Radiology 180(3):813–816
255. Onikul E, Fletcher BD, Parham DM, Chen G (1996) Accuracy of MR imaging for estimating intraosseous extent of osteosarcoma. AJR Am J Roentgenol 167(5):1211–1215
256. Paltiel HJ, Wilkinson RH, Kozakewich PW (1988) Case report 507. Osteosarcoma of the distal femoral epiphysis. Skeletal Radiol 17(7):527–530
257. Panuel M, Gentet JC, Scheiner C, Jouve JL, Bollini G, Petit P et al (1993) Physeal and epiphyseal extent of primary malignant bone tumors in childhood. Pediatr Radiol 23(6):421–424
258. Ramseier LE, Malinin TI, Temple HT, Mnaymneh WA, Exner GU (2006) Allograft reconstruction for bone sarcoma of the tibia in the growing child. J Bone Joint Surg Br 88(1):95–99
259. Raymond AK, Dahlin DC, Campanacci M, Picci P, Spjut H, Unni KK et al (1987) Epiphyseal osteosarcoma. Lab Invest 56:63
260. Ribeiro Baptista PP, Guedes A, Reggiani R, Fontes Lavieri R, Sa Lopes JA (1998) Distal fibula transplantation for tibia preserving the epiphyseal plate: preliminary report [Portuguese]. Rev Brasil Ortopedia 33(11):841–846
261. Safran MR, Eckardt JJ, Kabo JM, Oppenheim WL (1992) Continued growth of the proximal part of the tibia after prosthetic reconstruction of the skeletally immature knee. Estimation of the minimum growth force in vivo in humans. J Bone Joint Surg Am 74(8):1172–1179
262. San-Julian M (2009) Other techniques for epiphyseal preservation. In: Cañadell J, San-Julian M (eds) Pediatric bone sarcomas: epiphysiolysis before excision. Springer, Heidelberg, pp 137–144, Chapter 10

References

263. San-Julian M, Aquerreta JD, Benito A, Cañadell J (1999) Indications for epiphyseal preservation in metaphyseal malignant bone tumors of children: relationship between image methods and histological findings. J Pediatr Orthop 19(4):543–548
264. San-Julian M, Cañadell J (2009) Clinical results. In: Cañadell J, San-Julian M (eds) Pediatric bone sarcomas: epiphysiolysis before excision. Springer, Heidelberg, pp 109–135, Chapter 9
265. San-Julian M, Cañadell J (2009) Imaging-based indications for resection with epiphyseal preservation. In: Cañadell J, San-Julian M (eds) Pediatric bone sarcomas: epiphysiolysis before excision. Springer, Heidelberg, pp 89–100, Chapter 7
266. Schiller C, Windhager R, Fellinger EJ, Salzer-Kuntschik M, Kaider R, Kotz R (1995) Extendable tumour endoprosthesis for the leg in children. J Bone Joint Surg Br 77(4):608–614
267. Schurawitzki H, Schratter M, Pongracz N, Braun O (1989) Determination of intramedullary extension of osteosarcomas using CT with special reference to the epiphyseal groove [*German*]. Z Orthop Ihre Grenzgeb 127(3):362–366
268. Shira T, Tsuchiya H, Yamamota N, Sakurakichi K, Karita M, Tomita K (2004) Successful management of complications from distraction osteogenesis after osteosarcoma resection: a case report. J Orthop Sci 9(6):638–642
269. Simon MA, Bos GD (1980) Epiphyseal extension of metaphyseal osteosarcoma in skeletally immature individuals. J Bone Joint Surg Am 62:195–204
270. Spina V, Torricelli P, Montanari N, Manfrini M, Picci P, Sangiorgi L et al (1994) The epiphyseal involvement of metaphyseal bone sarcomas in patients with fertile growth plates. A magnetic resonance assessment. Radiol Med 88(3):190–197
271. Tsuchiya H, Abdel-Wanis ME, Sakurakichi K, Yamashiro T, Tomita K (2002) Osteosarcoma around the knee. Intraepiphyseal excision and biological reconstruction with distraction osteogenesis. J Bone Joint Surg Br 84(8):1162–1166
272. Tsuchiya H, Abdel-Wanis ME, Tomita K (2006) Biological reconstruction after excision of juxta-articular osteosarcoma around the knee: a new classification system. Anticancer Res 26(1B):447–454
273. Tsuchiya H, Tomita K, Minematsu K, Mori Y, Asada N, Kitano S (1997) Limb salvage using distraction osteogenesis. A classification of the technique. J Bone Joint Surg Br 79(3):403–411
274. Tsuneyoshi M, Dorfman HD (1987) Epiphyseal osteosarcoma: distinguishing features from clear cell chondrosarcoma, chondroblastoma, and epiphyseal enchondroma [*Japanese*]. Hum Pathol 18(6):644–651
275. Usui M, Sasaki T, Minami A, Yagi T, Kobayashi M, Matsuno T et al (1985) A histological study on osteosarcoma. Part II: the mode of local extension of osteosarcoma [*Japanese*]. Nippon Seikeigeka Gakkai Zasshi 59(1):45–53
276. van der Eijken JW (1988) Surgical treatment of bone tumours in children [*Dutch*]. Tijdschr Kindergeneeskd 56(6):267–275
277. Ward WG, Yang R, Eckardt JJ (1996) Endoprosthetic bone reconstruction following malignant tumor resection in skeletally immature patients. Orthop Clin North Am 27(3):493–502
278. Winkelmann WW (1996) Rotationplasty. Orthop Clin North Am 27(3):503–523
279. Winkelmann WW (2000) Type-B-IIIa hip rotationplasty: an alternative operation for the treatment of malignant tumors of the femur in early childhood. J Bone Joint Surg Am 82(6):814–828
280. Woźniak W, Izbicki T, Rychlowska M, Niedzielski P (1996) Malignant humeral bone tumors in children: excision and reconstruction with the use of rotated clavicle. J Surg Oncol 62(3):183–185
281. Wu HTH, Chang CY, Lin J, Chen TH, Chein WM, Wang SF (2001) Preoperative MR imaging assessment of osteosarcoma: a radiological-surgical correlation. Chin J Radiol 26(1):9–16
282. Yu XC, Liu XP, Zhou Y, Fu ZH, Song RX, Sun HN et al (2007) Epiphyseal preservation and reconstruction with inactivated bone in distal femur for metaphyseal osteosarcoma in children. J Clin Rehabil Tissue Eng Res 11(4):758–762

Ewing Sarcoma

283. Frouge C, Vanel D, Coffre C, Couanet D, Contesso G, Sarrazin D (1988) The role of magnetic resonance imaging in the evaluation of Ewing sarcoma. A report of 27 cases. Skeletal Radiol 17(6):387–392
284. Manfrini M, Innocenti M, Ceruso M, Mercuri M (2003) Original biological reconstruction of the hip in a 4-year-old girl. Lancet 361:140–142

Chondrosarcoma

285. Aprin H, Riseborough EJ, Hall JE (1982) Chondrosarcoma in children and adolescents. Clin Orthop Relat Res 166:226–232
286. Bjornsson J, Beabout JW, Unni KK, Sim FH, Dahlin DC (1984) Clear cell chondrosarcoma of bone. Observations in 47 cases. Am J Surg Pathol 8(3):223–230
287. Gitelis S, Bertoni F, Picci P, Campanacci M (1981) Chondrosarcoma of bone. The experience at the Istituto Ortopedico Rizzoli. J Bone Joint Surg Am 63(8):1248–1257
288. Henderson ED, Dahlin DC (1963) Chondrosarcoma of bone – a study of two hundred and eighty-eight cases. J Bone Joint Surg Am 45(7):1450–1457
289. Young CL, Sim FH, Unni KK, McLeod RA (1989) Case report 559. Chondrosarcoma of the proximal humerus. Skeletal Radiol 18(5):403–405

Lymphoma of Bone

290. Giudici MAI, Eggli KD, Moser RP, Roloff JS, Frauenhoffer EE, Kransdorf MJ (1992) Case report 730. Malignant large cell lymphoma of proximal tibial epiphysis. Skeletal Radiol 21(4):260–265
291. Glotzbecker MP, Kersun LS, Choi JK, Wills BP, Schaffer AA, Dormans JP (2006) Primary non-Hodgkin's lymphoma of bone in children. J Bone Joint Surg Am 88(3):583–594
292. Wollner N, Lane JM, Marcove RC, Winchester P, Brill P, Mandell L et al (1992) Primary skeletal non-Hodgkin's lymphoma in the pediatric age group. Med Pediatr Oncol 20(6):506–513

Soft Tissue Tumors

293. Angel D, Kligman M, Roffman M (1997) The technique for growth plate sparing in soft-tissue sarcoma around the knee. J Pediatr Orthop 17:437–439

Tumor Induced Rickets

294. Bahrami A, Weiss SW, Montgomery E, Horvai AE, Jin L, Inwards CY et al (2009) RT-PCR analysis for FGF23 using paraffin sections in the diagnosis of phosphaturic mesenchymal tumors with and without known tumor induced osteomalacia. Am J Surg Pathol 33(9): 1348–1354
295. Dezner MK (1990) Tumor – associated rickets and osteomalacia. In: Favus MJ (ed) Primer on the metabolic bone diseases and disorders of mineral metabolism. William Byrd Press, Richmond
296. Folpe AL, Fanburg-Smith JC, Billings SD, Bisceglia M, Bertoni F, Cho JY et al (2004) Most osteomalacia-associated mesenchymal tumors are a single histophathologic entity. An analysis of 32 cases and a comprehensive review of the literature. Am J Surg Pathol 28(1):1–30

Metabolic

5.1 Introduction

Metabolism is the sum of all physical and chemical processes by which living organized substance is produced and maintained. Control over the metabolism of the skeleton is a process of major clinical importance. The physis, like other organ systems during growth, is sensitive to general body changes, the lack of nutrients, hormonal alterations, medications, chemotherapy, etc. The cells of the physis are the ultimate regulators of bone growth. Longitudinal growth is retarded as a result of diminished cellular activity and matrix production in the germinal cell layer (Fig. 1.1). This chapter discusses some of the conditions where the metabolism of the physis has gone awry.

The atlas of Greulich and Pyle for skeletal maturity and physeal closure is used world wide to assess skeletal age and to plan bone length-correcting orthopedic surgery. In most of the conditions outlined in this chapter the skeletal age of the children varies considerably from this atlas. Care must be exercised when using the atlas to predict years of remaining growth in children with metabolic abnormalities.

Most metabolic abnormalities that affect physes involve all of the physes in the body. Thus, the pediatric orthopedist is rarely the primary physician for children with these abnormalities. The material in this chapter is basic and is presented so that the pediatric orthopedist has a general knowledge of these conditions, and of how the presence of the condition in a child might affect the treatment of a specific problem, such as an accompanying physeal fracture with growth arrest. The molecular mechanisms which regulate and modulate the rate of progression and final outcome of longitudinal bone growth continue to be elucidated incrementally. The metabolic processes described in this chapter include basic aspects of nutrition, hormones, medications, and chemotherapy as they affect skeletal growth in both humans and animals. Not included is a host of recent human and animal research concerning genetic, molecular, and biochemical factors which affect skeletal growth. Grouping of substances mentioned in this chapter into a category of nutrition, hormones, medications, and chemotherapy is sometimes arbitrary.

5.2 Nutrition

Growth involves two factors, the capacity for growth and the nutritive material necessary for the exercise of this capacity. In children, growth of the physis is a direct reflection of the effects of nutrition. Improved nutrition following World War II is generally regarded as the major cause for the increase of average individual stature in many nations.

5.2.1 General Nutritional Deprivation

Starvation, malnutrition, acute or chronic illness or disease, or a traumatic episode can all deprive the physis of adequate essential substances necessary for rapid growth [6]. For example, low roentgenographic skeletal age found in some Malawi children was felt to be due to poor nutrition associated with chronic diseases such as malaria and diarrhea [5]. Insufficient nutrient intake has been implicated as a possible cause of short stature among adolescent elite female gymnasts [2]. Pediatric patients with small bowel disease, such as

Crohn disease, are likely to have chronic malnutrition and growth retardation at the time of diagnosis [3]. Therefore, corrective bowel surgery prior to physeal closure optimizes growth [3].

Normal bone development requires appropriate amounts of a variety of dietary substances including calories, proteins, minerals, and vitamins [7]. When nutritional deprivation occurs there is an immediate slowing of chondroplasia, with more extensive calcification of the cartilage than is normal, followed by a reduction of osteoblastic activity. Longitudinal growth is more susceptible to interference from nutritional deprivation than is skeletal maturation [1]. But even in the most unfavorable conditions, physeal cartilage growth does not come to a complete stop [1, 7]. The physis may narrow, but maintains its basic anatomy and functional integrity [6]. Reversal of the insult allows resumption of normal growth, often with a residual growth arrest line. In general, the physeal cartilage has considerable tolerance to nutritional deprivation [4].

Vitamins are essential substances in body metabolism. The effects of vitamin deficiencies on the physis include decreased chondrogenesis, disorderly palisading, alterations in remodeling, metaphyseal osteoclasis, and diminished osteogenesis. However, whether these changes are direct effects on the physis, or secondary non-specific manifestations of nutritional deficiency or excess, have not been clarified [6]. There are three vitamins that affect bone growth directly. Vitamins A and D involve physeal cell activities, and C affects bone in common with all collagenous structures [8].

5.2.2 Vitamin A Deficiency

Vitamin A is essential for the activities of physeal cartilage cells, particularly the sequence of maturation and degeneration essential for bone growth [8]. In vitamin A deficiency, all physeal functions cease. Cells cease to divide, and cells which have almost matured undergo no further change. The long bones are shorter and thicker than normal.

5.2.3 Vitamin A Excess

Vitamin A toxicity in the infant, which today rarely occurs from dietary over dosage, was recognized in the 1940s as painful periostitis with occasional progression to premature closure of lower limb physes [13]. Decades later, most cases of vitamin A-induced physeal growth retardation occur in pediatric dermatologic patients given vitamin A analogues [13]. Almost without exception vitamin A intoxication has been observed in children ages 1–5 years [12]. Children differ as to the rate at which they metabolize vitamin A, and the amount of vitamin required to cause intoxication varies considerably [11]. In addition, the metabolism of vitamin A may not be a constant factor in any given child [11]. The commonly prescribed dose of 200,000 units of vitamin A given daily to children without vitamin deficiency may be too much for some children [11]. Daily intakes of 1,500 IU/kg body weight lead to toxicity. Daily intakes of greater than 25,000 IU for more than 6 years, or greater than 100,000 IU for more than 6 months, are considered toxic [15].

Hypervitaminosis A causes accelerated maturation and degeneration of physeal cells with concurrent replacement by bone [8, 15]. The longer vitamin A is administered, the greater the retardation of growth [8]. Histologically, a lag in matrix production is associated with compression of the cartilage cells adjacent to the metaphysis, resulting in mild widening and cupping of the physis of long bones (Fig. 1.17). Mild cupping is easily reversed by withdrawal of vitamin A [12]. When hypervitaminosis A is present for longer periods physeal closure begins centrally resulting in moderate cupping [9–11, 13–15]. When the cupping is marked, there may be accompanying knee-flexion contractures. The flexion contractures have been treated with skin traction, physical therapy, splinting, and in some instances two-pin tibial traction. Bilateral hamstring lengthening or femoral and/or tibial osteotomy may be appropriate for severe cases [10].

5.2.4 Vitamin C Deficiency (Scurvy)

Vitamin C is essential for the integrity of the intercellular substance, specifically for collagen formation and matrix elaboration in both cartilage and bone. Chronic deficiency of vitamin C results in failure of formation of the osteoid matrix and osteoblasts. Normal proliferation of chondroblasts continues, causing the physis to widen [16]. The physeal widening is accompanied by significant reduction in longitudinal growth [17].

Because no collagen is formed the structural strength of the physis is weakened, and stress of weight bearing or muscular tension may produce physeal disruption with epiphyseal displacement [20, 25].

The clinical manifestations of scurvy have been well chronicled in the literature since 1757, when James Lind recommended the inclusion of lemon juice in diets of naval personnel. Scurvy develops following 6–12 months of vitamin C deficiency. Infants fed only cows' milk without any supplements are at risk. Rapid recovery occurs following daily oral or parenteral administration of ascorbic acid (vitamin C) at a dose of 100–200 mg/day.

Roentgenographic changes typical of scurvy are best visualized at the knees, wrists, and costochondral junctions, all sites of rapid bone growth. The initial picture includes generalized osteoporosis, decrease in cortical thickness, subperiosteal hemorrhage, and increase in width and opacity of the zone of provisional calcification in both the primary physis (Fig. 1.1) and around the margins of the epiphyseal secondary centers of ossification (the secondary physis, Fig. 1.2).

Spontaneous physeal disruption may occur in scurvy [16, 19–21, 23, 25]. Epiphyseal separations occur in descending order of frequency in the lower femur, upper humerus, costochondral junction, and distal tibia [21]. Separation of the epiphysis is best treated nonoperatively by splinting, rest, and observation. In young children no reduction is necessary and excellent remodeling usually occurs [16, 18–22]. Providing the underlying vitamin deficiency is corrected, complete recovery is the rule and residual deformity or disturbance in longitudinal growth is uncommon [16, 19]. In one unusual case unilateral slipped distal femoral epiphysis was found in a 6 month old infant boy [23]. The displaced epiphysis was not reduced and subsequently developed marked cupping of the physis (Fig. 1.17), which resulted in only minor loss of length and articular abnormality [24]. A mild knee flexion contracture was successfully treated with a wedging cast.

Untreated scurvy cases develop growth deficit in the center of the physes (Cupping, Sect. 1.5), particularly at the knees where it may be accompanied by knee flexion contracture [18, 24, 25]. If the cupping is mild (Fig. 1.17), it should improve with vitamin C therapy. If a bar has already formed (moderate cupping) it will not improve with vitamin therapy. Bar excision would be appropriate, but probably would not produce correction of the more severe deformities. No bar excisions associated with scurvy have been reported, probably because the incidence of scurvy has been markedly reduced in the past four decades when bar excision became available. Although scurvy universally affects the knees bilaterally, premature growth arrest may occur unilaterally [18], sufficient to require surgical leg length correction. The knee flexion contractures are rarely corrected by non-operative treatment (splints, braces, traction, or physical therapy) and usually require femoral supracondylar extension osteotomy or osteotomies [18].

5.2.5 Vitamin D Deficiency (Rickets)

The inadequate intake of vitamin D and diseases that alter vitamin D metabolism are characterized by inadequate mineralization of growing bones. The causes are multiple [27]. Nutritional deficiency, inadequate exposure to the sun, renal disease (Sect. 5.6), liver disease, and genetic enzyme defects can all lead to the development of rickets. Seasonal variation of slipped capital femoral epiphysis between northern and southern United States children, and between black and white children, has suggested a possible link to impaired vitamin D synthesis [26]. Endocrine abnormalities such as hyperparathyroidism without primary renal disease or acidosis can also result in clinical and radiologic findings identical with rickets [29].

The primary metabolic abnormality in rickets occurs at the zone of provisional calcification. Diminished calcification of cartilage cell columns, continued osteoid production by osteoblasts, and diminished resorption of osteoid result in a widened and irregularly calcified physis. The physis becomes broadened and cupped [27]. One explanation is that the withdrawal of vitamin D retards the metaphyseal vessels from growing into their proper position [28]. This prevents removal of cells in the zone of hypertrophy, allowing the physis to widen.

Roentgenograms of long bones reveal widening and irregularity of all physes, and fraying and broadening of the metaphysis. Femoral and tibial bowing are common. The bowing usually corrects with proper medical treatment, but corrective osteotomy would be appropriate for residual deformity. The physis itself rarely requires orthopedic treatment.

5.3 Endocrine

Endocrine glands secrete discrete chemical substances which have specific effects on the activities of other organs, including the physis. It is often said that normal physeal closure is mediated by interplay between growth hormones and sex hormones. But if cessation of physeal activity is under control of hormones with body wide distribution, why do the various growth plates in the body close at different times? Do different physeal sites have different receptors with different sensibilities to hormones? These questions remain unanswered. At present, all that can be said is that normal cessation of growth is controlled by heritable factors. It is known that a lowered rate of germinal cell division and early fusion of the physis can be brought about by raising the estrogen levels in girls and the testosterone levels in boys. This knowledge is of value in the management of tall stature, and possibly in the curtailment of progression of scoliosis in a tall child [30, 31].

There are many examples of growth alteration due to endocrine abnormality. As mentioned in the Introduction, all physes are invariably affected and orthopedic evaluation or intervention is seldom sought. However, of special interest to the pediatric orthopedist are endocrine abnormalities as they relate to clinical conditions, such as slipped capital femoral epiphysis.

5.3.1 Slipped Capital Femoral Epiphysis (SCFE)

There are multiple causes of SCFE, but in the majority of cases the cause is unknown. It may be associated with endocrine diseases. Any hormonal condition or therapy which aims to keep the physis open to promote growth, predisposes the proximal femoral physis to slipping (Table 5.1) [57].

As a generalization, children with SCFE accompanied by an endocrine abnormality tend to be younger or older than the usual age of 10–16 years, taller or shorter than the norm for their age, and more obese or thin than usual. There is usually delayed skeletal maturity, an absence of trauma, and the slips are more likely to be bilateral.

As an example of endocrinopathy and growth problems, consider the growth hormone (GH). SCFE has been detected in GH-deficient patients before, during, and after GH therapy [64]. However, growth hormone deficiency (GHD) in itself does not appear to be a great

Table 5.1 Examples of endocrine disorders with slipping of one or both femoral capital epiphyses

Hypothyroidism [37, 40, 42, 46–48, 52, 53, 56, 66, 68]
Hypopituitarism [41, 45, 51, 53, 56, 66]
Hyperparathyroidism [32, 35, 62, 67, 124]
Growth hormone treatment [36, 38, 41, 59, 60]
Growth hormone deficiency [54, 57]
Growth hormone excess [44]
Hypotestosteronism [55, 66]
Hypoestrogenism [51]

factor in developing SCFE [46]. In the International Cooperative Growth Study database there were 6,343 patients with GHD. Only four patients had SCFE, and two of these were obese and two had received radiation treatment [54]. However, patients with GHD given GH are at significantly greater risk of developing SCFE than are normal children [36, 43, 57]. GH is usually given to increase the longitudinal growth rate in patients with GHD. These GH treated children have been found to have a progressive increase in proximal femoral capital physis width and inclination (Southwick's angle) producing an increased risk of slipping. The effect is similar to an increase risk of SCFE during the adolescent growth spurt [59, 60]. Close observation is necessary. If SCFE occurs during GH treatment, it can be considered iatrogenic [59].

The fact that SCFE occurs most often during the rapid growth spurt of puberty led to the suggestion that an endocrine abnormality *always* plays a role in the etiology of the condition [52, 63]. Early animal research suggested that an imbalance of growth-hormone and sex-hormone was the cause of structural weakness in the physis making it more susceptible to shearing stress [44]. However attractive this hypothesis may seem, there is no evidence it operates in man [45, 58, 63]. Although some literature supports the hypothesis that every patient with SCFE has an underlying endocrine abnormality [33, 50], some contradict it [33, 52, 58].

In most patients with SCFE, rapid growth and mechanical factors which increase the stress on the physis, such as obesity, are the only predisposing causes [33, 38]. Almost half of SCFE patients are over the 90th weight percentile. This suggests that mechanical factors such as obesity are more important etiologically than endocrine abnormalities [33]. Alternatively, the obesity may be another manifestation of an undetected endocrine abnormality.

Age is another factor. If the age of SCFE presentation is outside the usual age span of 14–16 years in boys and 11–13 in girls, the possibility of endocrine abnormality is greatly increased. For example, patients who have SCFE before age 10 have a higher incidence of endocrinopathy than children over age 10 [34, 66]. Why? Also, in the third decade of life an open proximal femoral physis due to endocrine abnormalities such as hypopituitarism and hypoestrogenism is likely to slip. Is the risk of slipping increased by time, due to remaining open so long, or due to the underlying endocrine abnormality? [45, 51] If due to the endocrine abnormality, why the long delay before the slip?

None of these questions have been adequately answered. They do, however, cause conflict when considering orthopedic treatment. Any patient with a SCFE *may* have an endocrinopathy. Despite the recommendation that every child who develops SCFE should have an endocrinology evaluation [39, 42, 47, 66], no overt endocrine abnormality is found in most cases [33]. Endocrinopathy has been found in only 8% of patients [34]. Screening for the possibility of endocrinopathy in all patients with SCFE has proved to be expensive and not cost effective [34]. Some authorities believe that surgery should be delayed until an endocrine evaluation is conducted and treatment begun [35, 46, 48, 52]. This may take several weeks during which time the patient may be immobilized in bed, traction or cast [48]. During this time progressive slipping may occur [56]. Since most of these investigations are negative and some require weeks or months to conclude, such delay would likely result in less desirable outcomes.

Experts have recommended that very young patients be kept in bed or cast for months to avoid operative physeal closure with its attendant loss of length [52]. If a specific problem, such as a parathyroid adenoma is found, its removal may result in prompt correction of the physeal widening and abatement of the slipping [32]. Pinning has also been withheld in some patients because of concomitant anemia, hypertension, bleeding tendencies, and electrolyte abnormalities, making surgery too dangerous [62]. Progressive epiphyseal displacement or disability did not occur in these patients.

Today the treatment of SCFE in patients with or without known endocrine abnormality is internal fixation, usually performed with one threaded cannulated pin. The goals of pinning are stabilization, and in children of adequate height closure of the physis (Sect. 20.2). Pinning a hip provides only temporary stabilization. It may be desirable to fuse the physis as rapidly as possible by using hormonal therapy [45]. There are several examples of the physis remaining open after fixation with one or more threaded pins [35, 53, 68]. Surgical stabilization may need to be augmented by concomitant autologous bone grafting to ensure physeal closure [41, 53]. However, in a very young, short child with significant growth remaining, closure of the physis would be undesirable (Fig. 5.1a–d). Instead, a smooth pin in the center of the physis may be used, if the goals are stabilization and continued growth (Fig. 5.1e–h).

Reduction of the femoral head is usually not done for mild slipping prior to pinning. Moderate slips are often pinned in situ after placing the leg in abduction and internal rotation, without forceful manipulation. Marked slips are usually reduced, closed or open, followed by reduction and pinning [52]. Proximal femoral corrective osteotomy initially or later may also be appropriate if deformity is severe [41, 52].

Bilateral slips at the time of discovery are both pinned. Since the incidence of bilateral SCFE is quite high (60–100% [49, 66]), some authors advocate "strong consideration" for prophylactic pinning of the contralateral normal hip in a child with a known endocrine disorder presenting with a unilateral slip [45, 49, 56, 60, 66]. However, if the endocrine disorder is known and treatment has begun at the time of single slip discovery, it could also be argued that the contralateral normal hip is less likely to slip because of the treatment, and therefore is best managed by careful observation. In addition, pinning the normal contralateral hip has resulted in complication rates from 14 to 40% [66].

In summary, SCFE occurs in fast-growing adolescents who are often overweight, and who occasionally have endocrine disturbances which delays closure of the physis. It is a disorder with a multifactorial basis, sometimes caused by an imbalance of hormones coupled with biomechanical events [53, 65]. Treatment of SCFE in patients with suspected, but not established endocrine disease, should be treated by pinning of the involved hip, or hips. The endocrine investigation should begin immediately, and the uninvolved hip observed closely. If endocrine disease is found and treated, the uninvolved normal hip could be observed for the same reasons given in the preceding paragraph (Fig. 5.1i, l).

Interestingly, there are few reports of slipping of other physes associated with endocrinopathy [61], despite widening of all physes in some of the conditions.

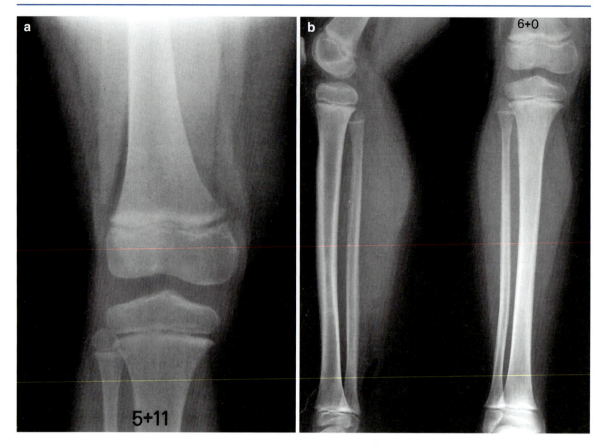

Fig. 5.1 Slipped capital femoral epiphysis in a young child with suspected endocrine abnormality. This girl was noted to limp and favor the right leg at age 5 years 11 months. (**a**) AP roentgenogram of the right knee was read normal, but there is sclerosis in the metaphyses adjacent to the physes which are mildly wide. (**b**) Nine days later, age 6 years 0 months, AP and lateral views of the right tibia were also read normal. (**c**) AP & Lat views of the right hip showed posterior inferior slip of the capital epiphysis. (**d**) The patient was referred at age 6 years 1 month. The left proximal femoral physis is widened. The evaluation noted that the patient first walked at age 13 months, but physical and mental skills were at the 3 year level, and she had been obese for the past 2 years. Endocrine work-up was begun. (**e**) The patient was placed on a fracture table with the leg in abduction and internal rotation, and the right hip pinned with a single smooth Kirschner (K) wire to allow growth. Other than leg position placement, no reduction was done. (**f**) At age 6 years 5 months no endocrine diagnosis had been made and the diagnoses of Prader-Willi syndrome* and Albright hereditary osteodystrophy (pseudohyperparathyroidism) were entertained. (**g**) At age 8 years 4 months the patient was ambulating normally without pain. Both femoral capital physes were slightly widened. The right femoral physis had grown away from the metaphysis and off the K wire. At age 8 years 5 months the diagnoses of precocious puberty with gonadotrapin independent pseudo-pseudohyproparathyroidism was made. The patient was treated with testolactone 20 mg/kg/day, qid, increasing to 40 mg/kg/day over 3–4 weeks. At age 8 years 7 months the patient was experiencing increasing right hip pain. (**h**) At age 8 years 8 months the K-wire was replaced with a longer smooth K wire, and the greater trochanteric physis was surgically arrested. (**i**) By age 10 years 7 months the patient was again having right hip pain. Scanogram showed the right femur was 1.8 cm shorter than the left. The right greater trochanteric physis was closed, but the greater trochanter-femoral head height was reversed. (**j**) The K wire was replaced with a titanium cannulated screw in an attempt to produce physeal closure. (**k**) Photograph at age 10 years 10 months. The patient walked with a right antalgic limp. (**l**) At age 13 years 4 months all physes were closed. There was mild/moderate right coxa vara. A scanogram showed the right femur 1.7 cm shorter than the left. The patient continued to have a Trendelenburg gait and sign, but did not have pain. Her I.Q. and speech capabilities never progressed past age 5 years. Her family was unable to care for her and she became a resident in a state facility. She began using a walker at age 19. She continues to be seen in other clinic departments 2–3 times a year and at last follow-up was 31 years old. No further hip roentgenograms have been deemed necessary. *Note*: This case supports the supposition that SCFE in a young child is likely to be associated with endocrine disease. The long delay in identifying the precise endocrine abnormality supports the decision to not delay surgical treatment during endocrine assessment. The smooth pin across the physis allowed continued longitudinal growth of the femoral neck. Earlier arrest of the greater trochanteric physis may have prevented the coxa vara and the antalgic limp. Should the normal left hip have been pinned? Once the endocrine abnormality was identified and under treatment was it necessary to repin the right hip (**h**, **j**)? * Prader-Willi syndrome is diagnosed on a clinical basis from a complex evolving during childhood that features hypotonia, mental retardation, gross obesity, and sexual immaturity

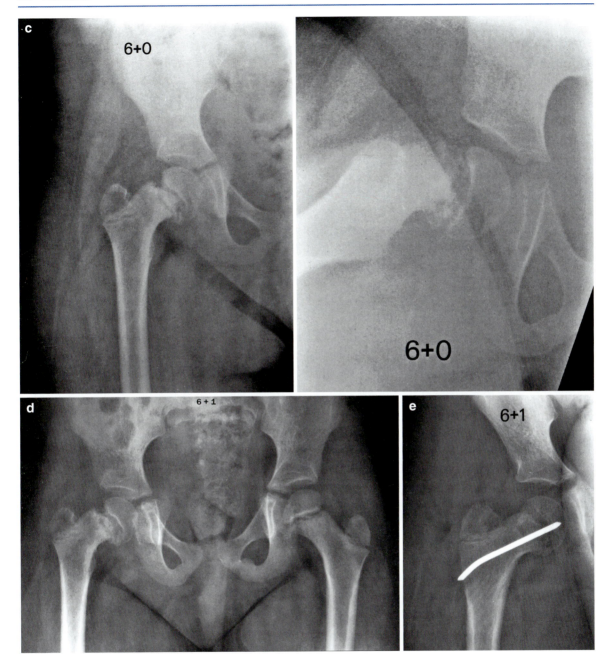

Fig. 5.1 (continued)

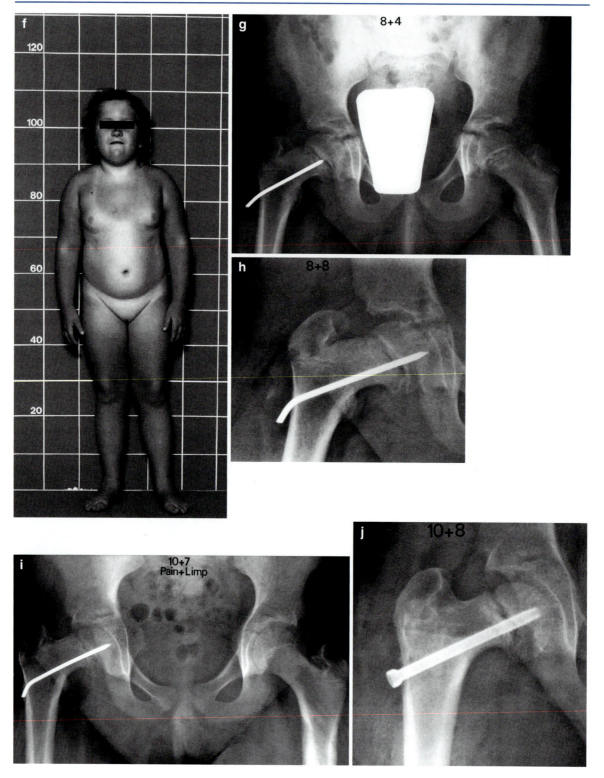

Fig. 5.1 (continued)

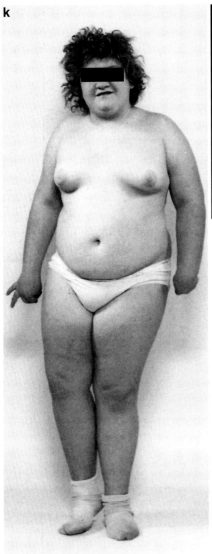
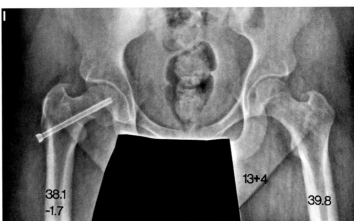

Fig. 5.1 (continued)

5.4 Medications

This section includes the administration of any chemical compound or drug that affects the integrity or growth of the physis. The examples given here are probably only a small part of the number and type of substances which have an adverse effect on the physis. In most of the examples all physes of the body are affected to some degree. The benefits of administering these drugs in children must be weighed against their adverse effects.

5.4.1 Aminonucleoside

The aminonucleoside of puromycin is a chemical homologue of yeast adenylic acid. The primary effect of the drug aminonucleoside administered to immature rats was the proliferation of chondroblasts [77]. The physis widened. This period of cellular hyperactivity was followed by one of decreasing proliferation of cartilage, growth retardation, and eventually premature physeal closure.

5.4.2 Bisphosphonates

Bisphosphonates are the mainstay of treatment in many adult forms of bone disease. In pediatric bone disease, bisphosphonates are increasingly used to treat osteogenesis imperfecta, idiopathic juvenile osteoporosis, and fibrous dysplasia, and occasionally juvenile chronic arthritis, osteonecrosis, and tibial pseudarthrosis. Bisphosphonates in children have an adverse effect on metaphyseal modeling leading to "drug induced osteopetrosis", widening of the physes, and multiple physeal arrest lines [89].

5.4.3 2-Butoxyethanol

An ethylene glycol ether, 2-butoxyethanol (BE) is a major environmental chemical used in the manufacture of industrial products – in sun coatings, as a chemical intermediate, and as a general solvent in various products, including house aerosols and cleaning agents. In immature rats, BE administration produced metaphyseal vascular thrombosis, growth plate infarction, and partial or complete premature physeal growth arrest [81]. The growth plate changes are due to thrombosis of the blood supply, similar to changes seen in sickle cell disease, thalassemia, osteotomy and mechanical injury (Chap. 1).

5.4.4 Calcitriol

Calcitriol activated Vitamin D used in the management of hypocalcemia in patients on chronic renal dialysis and in patients with hypocalcemia associated with hypoparathyroidism. High doses of calcitriol therapy adversely affects linear growth by directly inhibiting chondrocyte activity within the physis [78].

Fig. 5.2 Steroid induced premature closure of random physes. This boy was 11 months old when diagnosed with idiopathic autoimmune hemolytic anemia (IAHA). From the first year of life he received 4 mg/kg/day of prednisone gradually increasing to 80 mg/kg/day in an attempt to control hemolysis. He was on and off prednisone for the first 8 years of his life. He was also on cyclosporine and had long term iron overload due to transfusion hemosiderosis. (**a**) At age 4 years 7 months there was undermineralization of bone and marked irregularity of both distal femoral and proximal tibial physes and epiphyses. (**b**) At age 11 years 7 months his marked short stature was well below two standard deviations, and the femora and tibiae had not grown appreciably (compare with **a**). The physes of the distal femora, proximal tibiae and distal left tibia show central physeal closure with moderate to marked cupping (Fig. 1.17). The right distal tibial physis, all fibular physes, and both proximal femoral capital physes, and are open and growing, perhaps not normally. Bilateral fibular relative overgrowth is greater on the left. (**c**) Coronal MRI of the left knee shows marked cupping of the distal femoral physis and massive closure of the proximal tibial physis. Bar mapping by MRI Analyze software showed the distal femoral physis was approximately 40% closed. Identical changes were present in the right knee. (**d**) Bilateral distal femoral bar excisions were performed at age 11 years 7 months. An interoperative roentgenograph of the right knee (*left*) shows a transverse Kirschner wire used to measure the extent of bar excision. The faint stainless steel vascular clips used as markers in the metaphysis and epiphysis were placed 25 mm apart. The markers in the left knee (*right*) were 29 mm apart. Cranioplast was inserted as the interposition material. (**e**) Photograph at age 12 years 5 months show standing height 113 cm, bilateral cataracts, mild obesity, hypogonadism, and relative shortening of the left humerus and left lower extremity. The abdominal scar was from cholecystectomy (performed at age 7 years 0 months for choletishiasis, gallstone pancreatitis, and common bile duct stenosis). The following day surgical physeal arrests were performed on the right distal tibia and both distal fibulae to prevent further leg length discrepancy, and the left proximal fibular head was excised in an attempt to improve mild knee flexion contracture. (**f**) Roentgenographs at age 17 years 4 months show the residuals of marked cupping of both distal femora and proximal tibiae. All physes are closed and there is relative overgrowth of the right fibula. (**g**) A roentgenograph taken standing with a 4 in. block beneath the left foot at age 22 years 11 months shows the right tibia 4.4 cm longer, and the right femur 6.6 cm longer than the left. The distance between the metal markers in the distal femora is 57 m on right, 31 mm on the left. The right distal femur has grown 32 mm, the left 2 mm. There is relative overgrowth of both fibulae, greater on the right. There is moderate coxa valga bilaterally. *Note*: Final diagnoses included IAHA compensated on prednisone, developmental mental and growth retardation, random physeal premature closure, severe diffuse CNS deficit secondary to hypoxic ischemic encephalopathy, speech and language deficit, bilateral cataracts, myoclonic seizures, liver dysfunction secondary to transfusion hemosiderosis, cholelithiasis, and gallstone pancreatitis. This case shows premature partial arrest of random physes most likely due to prolonged overdose of prednisone. The case also shows the peril of attempting simultaneous excision of bilateral similar bars. Had the bar excision been successful on the distal left femur and not the right, the difference due to tibial length discrepancy would have been partially corrected. Instead, renewed growth from the right distal femur and none on the left increased the femoral length discrepancy. The patient walks reasonably well with a 3 in. shoe lift. He is a poor candidate for femoral lengthening due to uncontrollable hyperactivity, myoclonic seizures, mental retardation and inability to understand or follow directions

5.4 Medications

5.4.5 Corticosteroids

In mice, rats, and rabbits corticosteroids have been shown to cause narrowing of the physis and growth slow down. The dose and duration of the corticosteroid determines whether the physis recovers or proceeds to premature physeal closure [70, 85, 87]. In children cortisone tends to slow the rate of statural growth and skeletal maturation within a few weeks of onset of therapy. When the doses are sufficient to cause a reduction in the growth rate to subnormal levels, it also produces facial changes and obesity of the type seen in patients with Cushing syndrome [69]. Continuous high dose corticosteroid therapy in children causes random physeal closure and stunted growth (Fig. 5.2) [84]. However, if monitored closely, cortisone can be administered over considerable periods to growing children without necessarily altering the child's ultimate stature [69]. Continuous corticosteroid administration should be relaxed from time to time to allow for growth to resume before closure of the physis [84]. The role of hormones producing widening of the physis predisposing to slipped epiphysis is discussed in Section B of this chapter.

5.4.6 Deferoxamine

Deferoxamine is a heavy metal chelating agent, used for acute iron intoxication and chronic iron overload secondary to multiple transfusions. When used in children with thalassemia, marked abnormalities of the physis and significant decline in mean height percentile are observed [82].

5.4.7 Etretinate

Etretinate, thought to be a Vitamin A analogue, is a dermatologic medication used in the treatment of recalci-

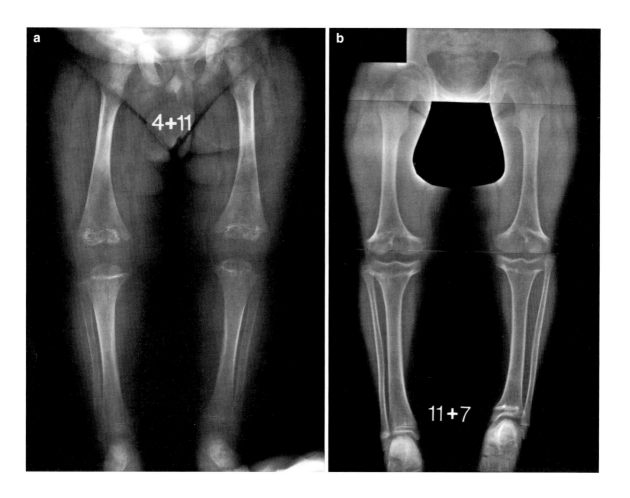

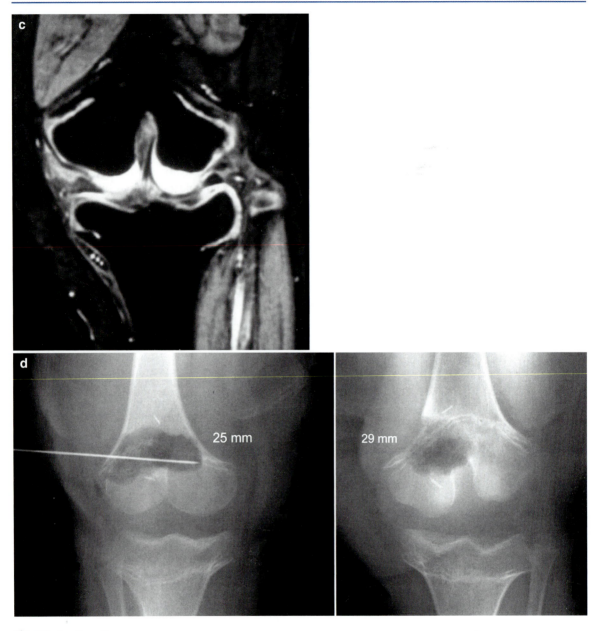

Fig. 5.2 (continued)

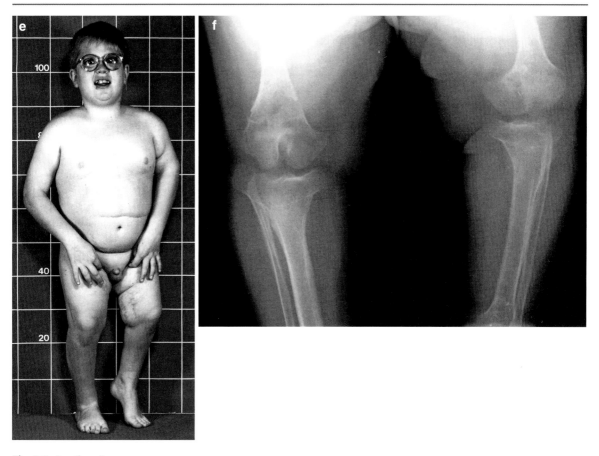

Fig. 5.2 (continued)

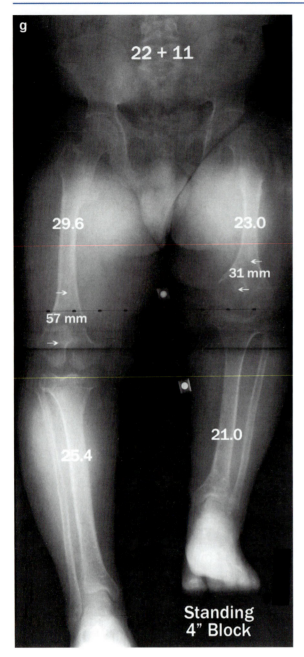

Fig. 5.2 (continued)

trant psoriasis. Shortness of stature and premature closures of random physes have been noted with the use of this drug [83]. Baseline roentgenographic skeletal surveys or whole body bone scans repeated at yearly intervals for the duration of treatment have been recommended [73].

5.4.8 Isotretinon (13-cis-Retinoic Acid)

Isotretinon, an oral synthetic vitamin A derivative, is effective in controlling a wide variety of dermatoses. In children it is used to treat hyperkeratosis and severe acne unresponsive to conventional therapy. Side effects of prolonged isotretinon therapy include premature fusion of random physes and modeling abnormalities of long bones [72]. Retinoic acid was implicated as the cause of premature closure of physes of the lower extremities resulting in short stature in a 4 year old girl with sacral ganglioneuroblastoma, who was also treated with chemotherapy and irradiation [88]. One 6 year old boy with epidermolytic hyperkeratosis treated with retinoic acid had only unilateral partial proximal tibial physeal closure at age 10 years [80].

5.4.9 Papain

Papain is a proteolytic enzyme obtained from the latex of the papaya tree, which catalyzes the hydrolysis of proteins, proteases, and peptones to polysaccharides and amino acids. It is used in dyspepsia, and as an application to warts, false membranes, etc. Papain injected repeatedly into immature animals intraperitoneally caused permanent disorganization of chondrocytes, premature physeal closure, and shortened long bones and vertebral bodies [74–76, 79]. Changes occurring after single doses of papain are reversible [74, 75].

5.4.10 ^{153}Sm-Ethylenediaminetetramethylene Phosphonate (^{153}Sm-EDTMP)

The radiopharmaceutical ^{153}Sm-EDTMP is an effective component of multimodality therapy for the treatment of primary bone tumors. When given to rabbits the physes were disrupted and chaotic in appearance [71]. The derangement of the growing physes was regarded as clinically significant.

5.4.11 Tetracycline

In the short term tetracycline slows enchondral ossification and linear growth. These effects are reversible.

Protracted tetracycline treatment at high doses more severely impairs longitudinal bone growth [86].

5.5 Chemotherapy

Chemotherapy could be thought of as a medication or drug, but is presented separately here because of its complexity, and because it is used in so many types of cancer in conjunction with other therapies such as surgery and radiation. Disturbed growth in the childhood cancer survivor is multifactorial. The definitive contribution of the tumor, each drug, radiation therapy, or endocrine imbalance often remains unclear.

Malignancy affects 1 in 1,000 children before their 15th birthday. Leukemia, lymphoma, and tumors of the central nervous system comprise the majority of childhood cancer [95]. Improvements in outcomes due to chemotherapy are being made yearly. One in every 900 young adults is a survivor of childhood cancer (2003) [91, 97]. Short stature is a well recorded long term sequela among adult survivors [90, 93, 94]. It is therefore important for pediatric orthopedists to have an understanding of the possible late effects of chemotherapy on growth.

Combining chemotherapy with mega-voltage irradiation has lowered the dose requirements for curative irradiation. However, the effects of some chemotherapy agents, such as actinomycin D, glucosteroids, adriamycin, cyclophosphamide, and methotrexate may sensitize the physis to irradiation, causing enhanced bone retardation (Chap. 13). Chemotherapy may be the most important modality of treatment for any histology, stage, or location of cancer [98]. The possibility of growth inhibition from chemotherapy alone has not been systematically studied [95]. The age at which the chemotherapy is applied may affect the onset of puberty and the final height [93]. This section attempts to document the adverse effects of chemotherapy on physeal growth.

Chemotherapy is usually accompanied by some degree of skeletal growth reduction [90, 93, 94]. The route of delivery makes a difference. Intravenous (i.v.) therapy usually affects all physes of the body. However, local intra-arterial (i.a.) therapy usually affects only physes of the involved limb. Differences between the i.v. and i.a. groups were found to be slight in one study [90]. The pattern of growth after completion of therapy can be either persistent growth deficit or catch up growth [90]. This difference may be a function of dose or of age, or both.

Most childhood normal growth takes place before the age of four years and during puberty. In these periods of rapid growth the incidence of childhood cancer is highest. Correspondingly, the effect of chemotherapy on longitudinal growth is most pronounced during these periods. The peak incidence of neuroblastoma is 2 years, acute lymphatic leukemia 3–4 years, and 50% of children with rhabdomyosarcoma and 80% of children with Wilm's tumors are less than 5 years old at diagnosis. Ewing's sarcoma is usually diagnosed between ages of 10 and 20, acute myeloid leukemia shows a peak incidence in adolescence, and the mean age of osteosarcoma is 16 years in girls and 18 years in boys [97].

Anticancer drugs have different mechanisms of action. The most commonly used chemotherapeutic agents in childhood cancer include alkylating agents, antimetabolites, antibiotics, and plant alkaloids [97]. The common multiagent adjuvant chemotherapy agents are methotrexate, vincristine, bleomycin, actinomycin D, cyclophosphamide, cisplatin, doxorubicin, cystosine arabinoside, daunomycin, ifosphamide, and dacarbazine. They are given in various combinations. The duration, interval, dose and combination of the drugs are so variable that no one drug has been implicated as the one causing growth reduction. It is difficult to distinguish the effect of one single drug on the growing skeleton from clinical studies. Some individual chemotherapeutic drug effects on the physis have been done on rats [94, 96]. Doxorubicin, actinomycin D, and cisplatin have a direct effect on physeal chondrocytes of animals resulting in decreased growth and final height [97]. Doxorubicin inhibits proliferation of immature chondrocytes leading to growth plate thinning and longitudinal growth retardation. Cisplatin decreases the height of the proliferating cell layer, but has little effect on the width of the physis. Methotrexate has an inhibitive effect on the trabecular zone, but cell proliferation is not inhibited [96].

Histologic specimens of physes of patients with osteosarcoma treated with chemotherapy have shown decrease in the number of cells in the proliferative and maturing zones, increase in the number of hypertrophic cells, minimal disruption of the columnar arrangement of the cells, and preservation of the grow thickness of the physis was preserved [90]. The gross thickness of the plate was preserved. Growth arrest lines were present in the metaphysis. Absence of complete growth arrest and evidence of a resumption of growth are relevant in planning limb salvage procedures in patients receiving pre- and postoperative chemotherapy in skeletal malignancy [90]. These findings clearly localize the effect on the physis to the proliferating zone. These findings are consistent with the clinical observation of growth slowdown followed by growth recovery [92]. A final difference in body height is usually small [92].

In summary, linear growth will continue after cessation of chemotherapy and may not be markedly affected by chemotherapy regimens. The direction and extent of possible change in final height of an individual is likely to be small and difficult to predict [92]. Long-term follow-up of pediatric cancer survivors is essential to get more insight into the long-term effect of chemotherapeutic treatment on skeletal growth and maturation [97].

5.6 Chronic Renal Failure

Children with chronic renal failure (CRF) are typically short in stature [105]. Growth retardation and delayed closure of physes are characteristic findings in juvenile CRF [106, 114]. The causes of CRF are multiple and include both congenital and acquired conditions [100, 107, 115, 118]. A wide variety of terminology for the condition includes renal osteodystrophy, azotemic osteodystrophy, chronic metabolic acidosis, end-stage renal failure, and renal rickets. The kidney problems occur in several types of combined glomerular and tubular disease resulting in disturbance of calcium and phosphorous metabolism which cause physeal disturbance [105]. The short stature may be a tissue resistance to growth hormone associated with uremia [120]. Like any severe disease, uremia causes cessation of longitudinal growth [112].

Histologic studies of physes in immature rats with induced CRF reveal disturbances in the normal pattern of chondrocyte differentiation [99, 104]. CRF is associated with variation in the rates and degree of substitution of hypertrophic cartilage with bone, resulting in accumulation of cartilage at the hypertrophic zone. The physeal widening is perceived to result from the inhibitory effect of CRF on cartilage cell progression and a lack of bone formation in the metaphysis.

Histologic studies in humans [112, 113, 115] also found a disturbance of vascularization of hypertrophic cartilage. The chondro-osseous continuity is lost by resorptive destruction at the border between the physis and the metaphysis where there is an accumulation of woven bone and/or fibrous tissue. There were notable differences between growth plates in different localizations: physes subjected to shearing forces (upper femur) are seen to slip sideways; physes subjected to axial compression (distal femur, tibia) show signs of growth arrest (reduction of the hypertrophic cartilage, and the formation of a bone bar). These histologic studies failed to show a traumatic separation as might be perceived from roentgenographs. On the contrary, epiphyseal slipping was the result of lateral movement of epiphysis due to destruction and reparative processes at the physis – metaphysis juncture. Uremic epiphyseolysis is distinguished from idiopathic epiphyseolysis by the intensive fibroosteoclastic lesions in the primary spongiosa.

The histologic studies are supported by roentgenographic studies which, in addition to showing widening of the physis, typically show disorganized structure in the metaphyseal-physeal junction with large irregular defects [109, 115]. Such findings are almost diagnostic [103]. In addition to physes in the femur and tibia, physes in the distal fibula, proximal humerus, distal radius and ulna, and metacarpals can also be involved [101, 109, 113, 115, 121]. A higher incidence of physeal abnormality occurs in CRF patients diagnosed earlier (younger than 3 years) than those diagnosed later [100, 101].

Advances in the treatment of CRF, particularly the success of renal dialysis and renal transplantation have improved survival of these children. This may increase the need for orthopedic care among survivors, although better medical care can also reduce the need for orthopedic care. For example, regression of lower extremity angular deformity in two patients was noted with improved metabolic control [107]. Subtotal parathyroidectomy has also been successful in reversing the physeal changes of renal rickets [124]. In addition, one report of five patients given 1α-hydroxyvitamin D showed remarkable physeal healing sufficient to preclude surgery in four of the patients [102]. Advances in treatment such as these must be followed closely by pediatric orthopedists so that all options can be considered before undertaking surgery.

Orthopedic treatment for children with CRF was often avoided up through the 1960s because of the short life expectancy and grave surgical risks involved, particularly of surgery which might precipitate uremia [121]. By the 1970s life expectancy had improved appreciably. The current goals of orthopedic management in these patients are to control the crippling deformities and to enhance functional capacity as much as possible. The surgical candidate should have deformities which are amenable to one or two definitive procedures and life expectancy sufficient to warrant the procedure.

Epiphyseolysis occurs where rapid growth and shear potential exist, and occurs in approximately 10% of children with CRF [99, 100, 113, 115]. Slipped capital femoral epiphyses (SCFE) is the most common condition requiring surgery and is almost always bilateral. It may be the first sign of chronic renal insufficiency [108]. Therefore renal failure should be included in the differential diagnosis of SCFE [108]. Urine albumin of all patients should be examined on several occasions [103]. Conversely, SCFE may first appear long after CRF has been diagnosed [108]. In one population of 124 children with renal failure, 16 were treated for skeletal problems, including SCFE, genu valgum, and ankle valgus [101]. Six patients had SCFE, all bilateral. Of the six with SCFE, all had concomitant genu valgum and three had ankle valgus. In another study of 112 children with CRF, SCFE was found in 10 of 30 (33%) of non-dialysized children and only 1 of 82 (< 1%) of dialysized children [115]. Regular screening of CRF patients for signs of SCFE has been advised [116].

Treatment of SCFE in CRF patients is usually surgical. One 13 year old girl with minimal slips was treated successfully in Buck's traction for one month, non-weight bearing for a second month and Vitamin D throughout this period [122]. Severe slips in two boys, ages 14 and 18 years, were stabilized following subtotal parathyroidectomies [108, 124]. Nevertheless, the standard treatment remains the use of multiple Knowles pins or a single cannulated screw fixation. Medical control of the renal disease is crucial to the success of either surgical or nonsurgical treatment [103]. Further slipping and pin protrusion are frequently noted in patients with poorly controlled metabolic disease [101]. Successful early closure of the femoral capital physis in a young child may result in greater trochanteric overgrowth and coxa vara, which in turn might require surgical arrest of the greater trochanteric physis or valgus osteotomy [101]. Therefore, in a very young child a smooth pin across the physis will allow growth of the proximal femur (Fig. 5.1) and can be successful in CRF if accompanied by proper medical treatment [110]. In unilateral cases, prophylactic pinning of the contralateral hip always needs consideration [101]. With complete displacement of the femoral head, bilateral subtrochanteric valgus osteotomies [124] and total hip replacements [109] have been done.

Angular deformities such as genu valgum, and ankle valgum also attract orthopedic attention [100, 101, 105, 106, 109]. The pattern of deformity in any specific patient is dependent on age, ambulatory status, severity of renal failure, lower extremity alignment, and iatrogenic factors [100].

Genu valgum is a common skeletal problem associated with CRF [100, 107, 117–119]. It is typically bilateral and is accompanied by a waddling gait. The pathogenesis is likely a combination of the natural valgus state of knees, which causes increased lateral knee pressure, together with metabolic abnormality and increased weight [107, 117]. Children less than 3 years of age typically have physiologic varus alignment of the lower extremities. If renal failure begins before 3 years, these children tend to have accentuation of the genu varus, instead of genu valgum [107]. Roentgenographically there is a lateral metaphyseal depression accompanied by cyst like changes along the metaphysis, similar to changes noted in the medial proximal tibia in Blount's disease [117]. Although the major roentgenographic abnormality is usually in the proximal tibial physis, the major deformity may be in the distal femur or the proximal tibia. Established genu valgum in CRF has not been improved by medical treatment [101]. The decision whether to correct the femur, the tibia, or both is made by using full length, weight bearing AP films [107, 118]. In general, if deformity is mild or moderate and sufficient growth remains, medial hemiphyseal stapling is done; if the deformity is severe, particularly in an older child, osteotomy may be necessary [101, 107, 117, 118]. Osteotomies of both the distal femur and proximal tibia have been secured with staples in younger children and with crossed wires, plates, or blade plates in older children [101, 107, 117, 118]. Although one article stated that bone healing time is normal in patients with CRF [105], others have found slow healing time, emphasizing the need for good medical management and adequate internal fixation and external immobilization [107, 111, 118].

Ankle valgus in CRF is usually associated with genu valgum. The earliest sign of impending deformity is a characteristic widening and lucency on the lateral aspect of the distal tibial physis [101, 117]. Ankle valgus is usually mild, and once genu valgum is corrected the ankle valgus is usually not a clinical problem [101]. However, three cases of slippage of both the distal tibial and fibular epiphysis bilaterally had severe valgus, enough to require varus osteotomies in two of the cases [123].

References

Nutrition
General Nutritional Deprivation

1. Acheson RM (1939) Effects of starvation, septicaemia and chronic illness on the growth plate and metaphysis of the immature rat. J Anat 93:123–130
2. Caine D, Lewis R, O'Connor P, Howe W, Bass S (2001) Does gymnastics training inhibit growth of females? Clin J Sport Med 11(4):260–270
3. Konno M, Kobayashi A, Tomomasa T, Kaneko H, Toyoda S, Nakazato Y et al (2006) Guidelines for the treatment of Crohn's disease in children. Pediatr Int 48:349–352
4. Kuhlman RE, Miller JA (1967) The biochemical changes preceding tissue death in rats. J Bone Joint Surg Am 49:90–100
5. Lewis CP, Lavy CBD, Harrison WJ (2002) Delay in skeletal maturity in Malawian children. J Bone Joint Surg Br 84(5): 732–734
6. Siffert RS (1966) The growth plate and its affections. J Bone Joint Surg Am 48:546–563
7. Winters JC, Smith AH, Mendel LB (1927) The effects of dietary deficiencies on the growth of certain body systems and organs. Am J Physiol 80:576–593

Vitamin A Deficiency

8. Wolbach SB (1947) Vitamin-A deficiency and excess in relation to skeletal growth. J Bone Joint Surg Am 29(1): 171–192

Vitamin A Excess

9. Caffey J (1970) Traumatic cupping of the metaphyses of growing bones. Am J Roentgenol Radium Ther Nucl Med 108:451–460

10. Kumar SJ, Forlin E, Guille JT (1992) Epiphyseometaphyseal cupping of the distal femur with knee-flexion contracture. Orthop Rev 21(1):67–70
11. Pease C (1962) Focal retardation and arrestment of growth of bones due to vitamin A intoxication. JAMA 182:980–985
12. Persson B, Tunnel R, Ekengren K (1965) Chronic vitamin A intoxication during the first half year of life: description of 5 cases. Acta Paediatr Scand 54:49–60
13. Rothenberg AB, Berdon WE, Woodword JC, Cowles RA (2007) Hypervitaminosis A-induced premature closure of epiphyses (physeal obliteration) in humans and calves (hyena disease): a historical review of the human and veterinary literature. Pediatr Radiol 37(12):1264–1267
14. Ruby LK, Mital MA (1974) Skeletal deformities following chronic hypervitaminosis A. J Bone Joint Surg Am 56(6): 1283–1287
15. Saltzman MD, King EC (2007) Central physeal arrests as a manifestation of hypervitaminosis A. J Pediatr Orthop 27(3): 351–353

Vitamin C Deficiency (Scurvy)

16. Aroojis A, D'Souza H, Yagnik MG (1990) Separation of the proximal humeral epiphysis. Postgrad Med J 74:752–755
17. Banks SW (1943) Bone changes in acute and chronic scurvy: an experimental study. J Bone Joint Surg 25(3):553–565
18. Hallel T, Malkin C, Orth MC, Garti R (1980) Epiphyseometaphyseal cupping of the distal femoral epiphysis following scurvy in infancy. Clin Orthop Relat Res 153: 166–169
19. Hosalkar HS, Johnston DR, Pill S, Flynn JM (2005) Multiple Epiphyseal Separations in a child with scurvy and cerebral palsy: a case report and literature review. Am J Orthop 34(6): 295–298
20. Nerubay J, Pilderwasser D (1984) Spontaneous bilateral distal femoral physiolysis due to scurvy. Acta Orthop Scand 55:18–20
21. Quiles M, Sanz TA (1988) Epiphyseal separation in scurvy. Case report. J Pediatr Orthop 8(2):221–225
22. Scott W (1941) Epiphyseal dislocations in scurvy. J Bone Joint Surg Am 41:314–322
23. Silverman FN (1953) An unusual osseous sequel to infantile scurvy. J Bone Joint Surg Am 35-A(1):215–220
24. Silverman FN (1970) Recovery from epiphyseal invagination: sequel to an unusual complication of scurvy. Follow-up notes on articles previously published in the journal. J Bone Joint Surg Am 52:384–390
25. Sprague PL (1976) Epiphyseo-metaphyseal cupping following infantile scurvy. Pediatr Radiol 4:122–123

Vitamin D Deficiency (Rickets)

26. Brown D (2004) Seasonal variation of slipped capital femoral epiphysis in the United States. J Pediatr Orthop 24(2): 139–143
27. States LJ (2001) Imaging of metabolic bone disease and marrow disorders in children. Radiol Clin North Am 39(4): 749–772

References

28. Trueta J, Buhr AJ (1963) The vascular contribution to osteogenesis. J Bone Joint Surg Br 45-B:572–581
29. Wood BSB, George WH, Robinson AW (1958) Parathyroid adenoma in a child presenting as rickets. Arch Dis Child 33:46–48

Endocrine

30. Drop SLS, De Waal WJ, De Muinck Keizer-Schrama SMPF (1998) Sex steroid treatment of constitutionally tall stature. Endocr Rev 19(5):540–558
31. Menelaus M (1981) Opening and closing the growth plate. The Anstey Giles lecture. Aust N Z J Surg 51(6):518–527

Slipped Capital Femoral Epiphysis (SCFE)

32. Bone LB, Roach JW, Ward WT, Worthen HG (1985) Slipped capital femoral epiphysis associated with hyperparathyroidism. Case report. J Pediatr Orthop 5(5):589–592
33. Brenkel IJ, Dias JJ, Davies TG, Iqbal SJ, Gregg PJ (1989) Hormone status in patients with slipped capital femoral epiphysis. J Bone Joint Surg Br 71(1):33–38
34. Burrow SR, Alman B, Wright JG (2001) Short stature as a screening test for endocrinopathy in slipped capital femoral epiphysis. J Bone Joint Surg Br 83:263–268
35. Chiroff RT, Sears KA, Slaughter WH III (1974) Slipped capital femoral epiphyses and parathyroid adenoma. Case report. J Bone Joint Surg Am 56(5):1063–1067
36. Coelho de Andrade A, Longui CA, Damasceno FLV, Santili C (2009) Southwick's angle determination during growth hormone treatment and its usefulness to evaluate risk of epiphysiolysis. J Pediatr Orthop 18(1):11–15
37. Crawford AH, MacEwen GD, Fonte D (1977) Slipped capital femoral epiphysis co-existent with hypothyrodism. Clin Orthop Relat Res 122:135–140
38. Docquier PL, Mousny M, Jouret M, Bastin C, Rombouts JJ (2004) Orthopaedic concerns in children with growth hormone therapy. Acta Orthop Belq 70:299–305
39. Ehrlich RM, Simone AM, Wedge JH, Weitzman S (1996) Slipped capital femoral epiphysis and endocrine disorders. Endocrinologist 6(4):340–342
40. Epps CH Jr, Martin ED (1963) Slipped capital femoral epiphysis in a sexually mature myxedematous female. JAMA 183(4):287–289
41. Fidler MW, Brook CGD (1974) Slipped upper femoral epiphysis following treatment with human growth hormone. J Bone Joint Surg Am 56(1):1719–1722
42. Fisher M, Frogel M, Raifman MA, Nussbaum M (1980) Hypothyroidism and slipped capital femoral epiphysis. J Pediatr 96(3):517–518
43. Frisch H (1997) Pharmacovigilance: the use of KIGS (Pharmacia & Upjohn International Growth Database) to monitor the safety of growth hormone treatment in children. J Clin Endocrinol Metab 4(Suppl B):83–86
44. Harris WR (1950) The endocrine basis for slipping of the upper femoral epiphysis. An experimental study. J Bone Joint Surg 32B(1):5–11
45. Heatley FW, Greenwood RH, Boase DL (1976) Slipping of the upper femoral epiphyses in patients with intracranial tumours causing hypopituitarism and chiasmal compression. J Bone Joint Surg Br 58(2):169–175
46. Hennessy MJ, Jones KL (1982) Slipped capital femoral epiphysis in a hypothyroid adult male. Clin Orthop Relat Res 165:204–208
47. Hirano T, Stamelos S, Harris V, Dumbovic N (1978) Association of primary hypothyroidism and slipped capital femoral epiphysis. J Pediatr 93:262–264
48. Jayakumar S (1980) Slipped capital femoral epiphysis with hypothyroidism treated by nonoperative method. Clin Orthop Relat Res 151:179–182
49. Loder RT, Wittenberg B, DeSilva G (1995) Slipped capital femoral epiphysis associated with endocrine disorders. J Pediatr Orthop 15:349–356
50. Löfgren L (1953) Slipping of the upper femoral epiphysis, signs of endocrine disturbance, size of sella turcica and two illustrative cases of simultaneous slipping of the upper femoral epiphysis and tumour of the hypophysis. Acta Chir Scand 106(2–3):153–165
51. McAfee PC, Cady RB (1983) Endocrinologic and metabolic factors in atypical presentations of slipped capital femoral epiphysis Report of four cases and review of literature. Clin Orthop Relat Res 180:188–197
52. Moorefield WG Jr, Urbaniak JR, Ogden WS, Frank JL (1976) Acquired hypothyroidism and slipped capital femoral epiphysis. Report of three cases. J Bone Joint Surg Am 58(5):705–708
53. Ogden JA, Southwick WO (1977) Endocrine dysfunction and slipped capital femoral epiphysis. Yale J Biol Med 50:1–16
54. Nishi Y, Tanaka T, Fujieda K, Hanew K, Hirano T, Igarashi Y (1998) Slipped capital femoral epiphysis, Perthes' disease and scoliosis in children with growth hormone deficiency. Endocr J 45(Suppl):S167–S169
55. Primiano GA, Hughston JC (1971) Slipped capital femoral epiphysis in a true hypogonadal male (Klinefelter's mosaic XY/XXY). A case report. J Bone Joint Surg Am 53(2):597–601
56. Puri R, Smith CS, Malhotra D, Williams AJ, Owen R, Harris F (1985) Slipped upper femoral epiphysis and primary juvenile hypothyroidism. J Bone Joint Surg Br 67(1):14–20
57. Rappaport EB, Fife D (1985) Slipped capital femoral epiphysis in growth hormone-deficient patients. Am J Dis Child 139:396–399
58. Razzano CD, Nelson C, Eversman J (1972) Growth hormone levels in slipped capital femoral epiphysis. J Bone Joint Surg Am 54(6):1224–1226
59. Rennie W, Mitchell N (1974) Slipped femoral capital epiphysis occurring during growth hormone therapy. Report of a case. J Bone Joint Surg Br 56-B(4):703–705
60. Reynaud P, Kohler R (1996) Role of growth hormone in slipped capital epiphysis genesis [*French*]. Rev Chir Orthop Reparatrice Appar Mot 82(1):76–79
61. Robin GC, Kedar SS (1962) Separation of the upper humeral epiphysis in pituitary gigantism. J Bone Joint Surg Am 44-A:189–192
62. Shea D, Mankin HJ (1966) Slipped capital femoral epiphysis in renal rickets. Report of three cases. J Bone Joint Surg Am 48(2):349–355
63. Sørensen KH (1968) Slipped upper femoral epiphysis. Clinical study on aetiology. Acta Orthop Scand 39:499–517

64. Watkins SL (1996) Bone disease in patients receiving growth hormone. Kidney Int Suppl 53:S126–S127
65. Weiner D (1996) Pathogenesis of slipped capital femoral epiphysis: current concepts. J Pediatr Orthop B 5(2):67–73
66. Wells D, King JD, Roe TF, Kaufman FR (1993) Review of slipped capital femoral epiphysis associated with endocrine disease. J Pediatr Orthop 13(5):610–614
67. Yang WE, Shih CH, Wang KC, Jeng LB (1997) Slipped capital femoral epiphyses in a patient with primary hyperparathyroidism. J Formos Med Assoc 96(7):549–552
68. Zubrow AB, Lane JM, Parks JS (1978) Slipped capital femoral epiphysis occurring during treatment for hypothyroidism. J Bone Joint Surg Am 60(2):256–258

Medications

69. Blodgett FM, Burgin L, Iezzoni D, Gribetz D, Talbot NB (1956) Effects of prolonged cortisone therapy on the statural growth, skeletal maturation and metabolic status of children. N Engl J Med 254(14):636–641
70. Bright RW, Elmore SM (1967) Some effects of immunosuppressive drugs on the epiphyseal plate of rats. Surg Forum 18:485–487
71. Essman SC, Lattimer J, Cook JL, Turnquist S, Kuroki K (2003) Effects of 153Sm-ethylenediaminetetramethylene phosphonate on physeal and articular cartilage in juvenile rabbits. J Nucl Med 44(9):1510–1515
72. Franco A, Hampton WR, Greenspan BD, Holm AL, O'Mara RE (1993) Gastric uptake of Tc99m MDP in a child treated with isotretinoin. Clin Nucl Med 18(6):510–511
73. Glover MT, Atherton DJ (1987) Etretinate and premature epiphyseal closure in children. J Am Acad Dermatol 17(5):853–854
74. Hulth A (1958) Experimental retardation of endochondral growth by papain. Acta Orthop Scand 28(1):1–21
75. Hulth A (1958) The growth inhibiting effect by papain on young rabbits. Acta Orthop Scand 27(3):167–172
76. Hulth A, Westerborn O (1959) The effect of crude papain on the epiphysial cartilage on laboratory animals. J Bone Joint Surg Br 41-B(4):836–847
77. Johnston AD, Follis RH (1961) Bone destruction associated with aminonucleoside administration. J Bone Joint Surg 43A:865–875
78. Kuizon BD, Goodman WG, Jüppner H, Boechat I, Nelson P, Gales B, Salusky IB (1998) Diminished linear growth during intermittent calcitriol therapy in children undergoing CCPD. Kidney Int 53:205–211
79. Merkow L, Lalich JJ (1961) Skeletal changes in suckling rats induced by prolonged papain administration. J Bone Joint Surg 43A:679–686
80. Milstone LM, McGuire J, Ablow RC (1982) Premature epiphyseal closure in a child receiving oral 13-*cis*retinoic acid. J Am Acad Dermatol 7(5):663–666
81. Nyska M, Shabat S, Long PH, Howard C, Ezov N, Levin-Harrus T et al (2005) Disseminated thrombosis-induced growth plate necrosis in rat: a unique model for growth plate arrest. J Pediatr Orthop 25(3):346–350
82. Olivieri NF, Koren G, Harris J, Khattak S, Freedman MH, Templeton DM et al (1992) Growth failure and bony changes induced by deferoxamine. Am J Pediatr Hematol Oncol 14(1):48–56
83. Prendiville J, Bingham EA, Burrows D (1986) Premature epiphyseal closure – a complication of etretinate therapy in children. J Am Acad Dermatol 15:1259–1262
84. Shaw NE, Lacey E (1975) The influence of corticosteroids on the normal and papain-treated epiphysial growth plate in the rabbit. J Bone Joint Surg Br 57:228–233
85. Silbermann M, Levitan S, Kleinhaus U, Finkelbrand S (1979) Long bone growth during prolonged intermittent corticosteroid treatment and subsequent rehabilitation. Cell Tissue Res 201:51–62
86. Simmons DJ, Chang SL, Russell JE, Grazman B, Webster D, Oloff C (1983) The effect of protracted tetracycline treatment on bone growth and maturation. Clin Orthop Relat Res 180:253–259
87. Sissons HA, Hadfield GJ (1955) The influence of cortisone on the structure and growth of bone. J Anat 89:69–79
88. Vassilopoulou-Sellin R, Eftekhari F, Ater JL (1998) Accelerated lower extremity epiphyseal maturation in a prepubertal, growth hormone-deficient girl after treatment for sacral ganglioneuroblastoma. Internat J Pediatr Hematology/Oncology 5(1):35–39
89. Ward K, Cowell CT, Little DG (2005) Quantification of metaphyseal modeling in children treated with bisphosphonates. Bone 36:999–1002

Chemotherapy

90. Bar-On E, Beckwith JB, Odom LF, Eilert RE (1993) Effect of chemotherapy on human growth plate. J Pediatr Orthop 13(2):220–224
91. Bottomly SJ, Kassner E (2003) Late effects of childhood cancer therapy. J Pediatr Nurs 18(2):126–133
92. Glasser DB, Duane K, Lane JM, Healey JH, Caparros-Sison B (1991) The effect of chemotherapy on growth in the skeletally immature individual. Clin Orthop Relat Res 262:93–100
93. Mohnike K, Dörffel W, Timme J, Kluba U, Aumann V, Vorwerk P, Mittler U (1997) Final height and puberty in 40 patients after antileukaemic treatment during childhood. Eur J Pediatr 156:272–276
94. Robson H, Anderson E, Eden OB, Isaksson O, Shalet S (1998) Chemotherapeutic agents used in the treatment of childhood malignancies have direct effects on growth plate chondrocyte proliferation. J Endocrinol 157:225–235
95. Spoudeas HA (2002) Growth following malignancy. Best Practice & Research Clin Endocrinol and Metabolism 16(3):561–590
96. van Leeuwen BL, Hartel RM, Jansen HWB, Kamps WA, Hoekstra HJ (2003) The effect of chemotherapy on the morphology of the growth plate and metaphysis of the growing skeleton. Eur J Surg Oncol 29:49–58
97. van Leeuwen BL, Kamps WA, Jansen HWB, Hoekstra HJ (2000) The effect of chemotherapy on the growing skeleton. Cancer Treat Rev 26:363–376
98. Wollner N, Lane JM, Marcove RC, Winchester P, Brill P, Mandell L et al (1992) Primary skeletal non-Hodgkin's lymphoma in the pediatric age group. Med Pediatr Oncol 20(6):506–513

Chronic Renal Failure

99. Álvarez J, Balbín M, Fernández M, López JM (2001) Collagen metabolism is markedly altered in the hypertrophic cartilage of growth plates from rats with growth impairment secondary to chronic renal failure. J Bone Miner Res 16(3):511–524
100. Apel DM, Millar EA, Moel DI (1989) Skeletal disorders in a pediatric renal transplant population. J Pediatr Orthop 9(5):505–511
101. Barrett IR, Papadimitriou DG (1996) Skeletal disorders in children with renal failure. J Pediatr Orthop 16(2):264–272
102. Blockey NJ, Murphy AV, Mocan H (1986) Management of rachitic deformities in children with chronic renal failure. J Bone Joint Surg Br 68:791–794
103. Brailsford JF (1933) Slipping of the epiphysis of the head of the femur: its relation to renal rickets. Lancet 1:16–19
104. Carbajo E, López JM, Santos F, Ordónez FA, Niño P, Rodríguez J (2001) Histologic and dynamic changes induced by chronic metabolic acidosis in the rat growth plate. J Am Soc Nephrol 12:1228–1234
105. Cattell HS, Levin S, Kopits S, Lyne ED (1971) Reconstructive surgery in children with azotemic osteodystrophy. J Bone Joint Surg Am 53(2):216–228
106. Crutchlow WP, David DS, Whitsell J (1971) Multiple skeletal complications in a case of chronic renal failure treated by kidney homotransplantation. Am J Med 50(3):390–394
107. Davids JR, Fisher R, Lum G, Von Glinski S (1992) Angular deformity of the lower extremity in children with renal osteodystrophy. J Pediatr Orthop 12(3):291–299
108. Floman Y, Yosipovitch Z, Licht A, Viskoper RJ (1975) Bilateral slipped upper femoral epiphysis: a rare manifestation of renal osteodystrophy. Isr J Med Sci 11(1):15–20
109. Goldman AB, Lane JM, Salvati E (1978) Slipped capital femoral epiphyses complicating renal osteodystrophy: a report of three cases. Radiology 126:333–339
110. Hartjen CA, Koman LA (1990) Treatment of slipped capital femoral epiphysis resulting from juvenile renal osteodystrophy. Case report. J Pediatr Orthop 10(4):551–554
111. Herring JA, Ehlrich MG (1983) Valgus knee deformity – etiology and treatment. Instructional case. J Pediatr Orthop 3(4):527–530
112. Krempien B, Mehls O, Ritz E (1974) Morphological studies on pathogenesis of epiphyseal slipping in uremic children. Virchows Arch A Pathol Anat Histol 362:129–143
113. Kirkwood JR, Ozonoff MB, Steinbach HL (1972) Epiphyseal displacement after metaphyseal fracture in renal osteodystrophy. Am J Roentgenol Radium Ther Nucl Med 115(3):547–554
114. Mehls O, Ritz E, Gilli G, Kreusser W (1978) Growth in renal failure. Nephron 21:237–247
115. Mehls O, Ritz E, Krempien B, Gilli G, Link K, Willich E et al (1975) Slipped epiphyses in renal osteodystrophy. Arch Dis Child 50:545–554
116. Nixon JR, Douglas JF (1980) Bilateral slipping of the upper femoral epiphysis in end-stage renal failure. A report of two cases. J Bone Joint Surg Br 62-B(1):18–21
117. Oppenheim WL, Shayestehfar S, Salusky IB (1992) Tibial changes in renal osteodystrophy: lateral Blount's disease. J Pediatr Orthop 12(6):774–779
118. Oppenheim WL, Fischer ST, Salusky IB (1997) Surgical correction of angular deformity of the knee in children with renal osteodystrophy. J Pediatr Orthop 17(1):41–49
119. Richardson JL (1947) Renal rickets: report of a case. J Bone Joint Surg Am 29:503–508
120. Saborio P, Krieg RJ Jr, Chan W, Hahn S, Chan JC (1998) Pathophysiology of growth retardation in chronic renal failure [*Chinese*]. Zhonghua Min Guo Xiao Er Ke Yi Xue Hui Za Zhi 39(1):21–27
121. Shea D, Mankin HJ (1966) Slipped capital femoral epiphysis in renal rickets. J Bone Joint Surg Am 48(2):349–355
122. Switzer P, Bell HM (1973) Slipping of the capital femoral epiphysis with renal rickets: a case report. Can J Surg 16(5):330–332
123. Tebor GV, Ehrlich MG, Herrin J (1983) Slippage of the distal tibial epiphysis. J Pediatr Orthop 3(2):211–215
124. Vanderhooft GA, Coleman SS (1972) Reversal of skeletal changes in renal osteodystrophy following partial parathyroidectomy and renal allotransplantation. Clin Orthop Relat Res 88:113–118

Neural

6.1 Introduction

This chapter explores the effect of peripheral nerve, spinal cord, and brain injury on growth of the physis. Also included are meningomyelocele and congenital insensitivity to pain, both of which are congenital conditions in which premature partial or complete physeal arrests occur in random physes of insensate limbs. Although poliomyelitis is an infection affecting spinal cord anterior horn cells, it is generally accepted that the limb growth deficit is due to disuse, and it is therefore discussed in Chap. 2.

The etiology of physeal growth impairment in patients with neurologic deficit is unknown, but is most likely related to diminished nerve control of the vascular supply to the physis (Chap. 1), or to disuse (Chap. 2). The precise degree to which each of these is responsible for growth impairment in each neurologic condition is difficult to measure.

The physis is generally regarded as being devoid of nerve tissue. Recent studies have challenged this assumption. In one study of 12 human bodies with an age from the 22nd gestational week to 13 months after birth, nerve fibers were found in physeal cartilage canals together with an artery and veins [2]. No myelin, Schwann cells, or mechanoreceptors were found. In a second study, nerve and vessels were found forming neurovascular complexes in the "metaepiphyseal cartilage" of the proximal humerus in newborn and 1 year old children [1]. The validity and significance of these findings have not yet been determined.

6.2 Peripheral Nerve Injury

6.2.1 Peripheral Denervation

It is generally agreed that no fibers arising from motor cells in the spinal cord terminate in bone, and fibers which have been described are derived from the sensory and the sympathetic nervous system [15].

Animal experiments have provided substantial information concerning bone growth alteration due to peripheral nerve injury. Since the efferent fibers of the spinal cord do not directly innervate the skeleton [15], the peripheral nervous system does not exert a major influence on longitudinal bone growth [10]. Paralysis of a limb interferes more with appositional growth of bones than with physeal growth [3]. Section of 3 or 4 lumbosacral motor nerve roots in rabbits and kittens caused almost complete paralysis of the hind limb, and severe atrophy of muscles, but only slight retardation of growth of the femur, and almost none of the tibia [12, 17]. The growth in length of the rat tibia continued at a normal rate following complete intrapelvic severance of the femoral, obturator, and sciatic nerves [16]. Severance of these nerves totally deprives the lower leg of motion and sensitivity, but leaves the perivascular autonomic nerves intact [16]. In a second study in growing rats unilateral sciatic neurectomy produced no difference in the longitudinal growth rate compared with the control side [18]. In a third study of unilateral sciatic nerve transection in rats, femoral and tibial lengths were no different than the control side, but the metatarsals were 3–5% shorter on the denervated side from the first week [10]. This early growth rate reduction was not sustained, suggesting that when a limb is denervated bone growth slows temporarily, and then resumes normal growth. However, section of peripheral nerves in puppies resulted in marked limb atrophy and slight shortening of limb bones [15]. In summary, there is only a minor effect on longitudinal bone growth in the denervated limb of immature animals [3].

In humans serious sciatic nerve injury can occur following the intragluteal administration of therapeutic and prophylactic agents. The injury may result from a single or repeated injections [7, 11]. Any age group is vulnerable, but the newborn and premature infants are more likely to suffer from this complication [7, 8, 11]. In addition to clinical sensory and autonomic deficit in the foot and leg, in some patients there may be retardation of leg growth (Fig. 6.1). The most notable effect is diminished growth of the foot, with resulting talipes equinovarus or calcaneovalgus [7, 8, 11]. Surgical exploration of the buttock reveals scarring in and about the sciatic nerve [7]. Postulated mechanisms of neuropathy include puncture of the nerve, ischemia of the nerve, neural damage by the injected drug, and allergic peripheral neuritis [11].

6.2.2 Brachial Plexus Palsy

Brachial plexus birth palsy (BPBP) results from fetal dystocia associated with the size, shape or position of the fetus. Spontaneous recovery occurs in 70% of patients. Those who do not recover are now often treated by brachial plexus surgical reconstruction sometime within the first 9 months of life. Hypoplasia of the affected upper extremity occurs in varying degrees in both treated and non-treated patients. Permanent BPBP causes upper limb atrophy, asymmetry, paresis, and upper limb length inequality, but no structural scoliosis or lower limb length inequality [14]. In a group of 106 patients with a mean follow-up of 13 years (range 5–32 years), the mean affected upper limb relative shortening was 6 cm (range: 1–13.5 cm) [14]. The impact of disuse was not discussed. The upper limb length discrepancy is never treated because of the neurologic deficit and functional impairment of the entire extremity.

6.2.3 Lumbar Sympathetic Ganglionectomy

In 1930, R.I. Harris proposed that under favorable circumstances, lumbar sympathectomy would diminish the relative shortness of unilateral lower extremity in patients with poliomyelitis (Sect. 2.3) [13]. Removal of vasomotor control by sympathetic ganglionectomy was theorized to sufficiently increase blood supply to the physis to induce accelerated activity. This would be advantageous in conditions where a limb is short but the physis remains intact, like poliomyelitis. Factors favorable to a good result included moderate degree paralysis, early operation (under age 6 years, if possible), the use of ganglionectomy rather than ramisection, and maintenance of the increased vascularity which follows the operation [13].

The results in humans were mixed. Increased growth occurred in less than half the patients and the amount of growth was often disappointing [13]. In addition, all experimental investigations on animals have produced no increase in leg length [4–6, 12]. In a related case, two children with Hirschprung's disease and equal leg lengths had unilateral lumbar ganglionectomy which produced significant improvement in the Hirschprung's disease and a warm lower extremity, but no change in the equal leg lengths [9].

Sympathetic ganglionectomy to increase limb length in poliomyelitis patients fell out of favor because of failure to maintain the increased vascular flow and inconsistent results. In no case was complete limb length equalization achieved and if the discrepancy was great, other procedures were needed anyway.

6.3 Spinal Cord Injury

6.3.1 Spinal Cord Traumatic Injury

A severe spinal cord contusion applied at T-10 in 7 week old rats caused disruption of the cellular organization of the physes and a 35% reduction in lower extremity growth plate width, both centrally and peripherally at 7 days post injury [29]. Due to early subject sacrifice, no subsequent data of limb length was recorded.

In children, spinal cord traumatic injury can produce lower limb average growth deficit in the order of two standard deviations from normal, and only affects

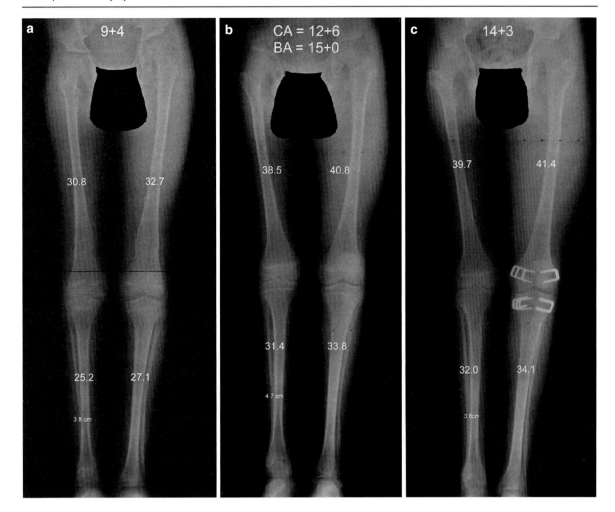

Fig. 6.1 Sciatic neuropathy with leg length discrepancy. This male was noted to "bruise" easily, bled excessively at time of circumcision, and had frequent nose bleeds. At age 9 months he was given intramuscular penicillin in the right buttock to treat a "cold", following which he was unable to move his right lower extremity. On examination at age 1 year 4 months the right lower extremity was essentially flail, there were petechiae on his shoulders, and ecchymoses on his forehead, arm and right leg. Electromyography revealed a right leg nerve palsy consistent with a proximal peripheral nerve lesion. Blood analysis resulted in a diagnosis of Glantzman's platelet deficiency. He was treated with oral iron and had no further bleeding episodes. A double upright long leg brace with no knee joint and a 90° ankle strap, worn during the day, facilitated beginning ambulation. Right drop foot and inversion (due to posterior tibial overpull) were treated by Achilles lengthening, posteromedial release, and transfer of the posterior tibial tendon to the os calcis at age 4 years 10 months. A spring wire drop foot brace was applied. His gait gradually improved, walking with the right leg abducted and externally rotated. The quadriceps could not extend the tibia when sitting, but was strong enough to maintain knee extension during gait and stance. Heel and sole shoe lifts were gradually added to the spring wire drop foot brace. Yearly scanograms beginning at age 2 years, which showed 1 cm discrepancy with 5 mm in both the femur and tibia, documented gradual increasing leg length discrepancy. (**a**) At age 9 years 4 months the right lower extremity was 3.8 cm shorter than the left; 1.9 cm in the femur and 1.9 cm in the tibia. There was compensatory right coxa valga and prominence of the lesser trochanter. Right external tibial torsion was documented by the AP orientation of the proximal tibia and external rotation of the distal tibia. There was marked soft tissue atrophy on the right. The brace was changed to a posterior leaf spring brace with a 1¼″ heel and sole lift. (**b**) At age 12 years 6 months the discrepancy was 4.7 cm, again evenly divided between femur and tibia. The bone age (BA) was 15 years 0 months. His height was 5′4″ and his father was 5′6″. Staple physeal arrest was performed on the left distal femur and proximal tibia at age 12 years 7 months. (**c**) At age 14 years 3 months the discrepancy had diminished to 3.8 cm and all physes were closed. The patient ambulated well with plastic ankle-foot orthosis and a 1 in. heel and sole lift. He was last seen at age 36 years 1 month at which time he was of a short stature, ambulating with a mild limp, wearing a plastic ankle-foot orthosis and shoe lift, and gainfully employed as an airline steward. *Note*: Since the patient had both a known buttock injection and Glantzman's platelet deficiency, it was never determined if his neurologic deficit was due to direct nerve injury from the injection, bleeding associated with the injection, or to spontaneous bleeding associated with the platelet deficiency. The bone length discrepancy in this case could be due to either the neurologic deficit or the disuse caused by the deficit. Even though he was of short stature, an earlier physeal arrest could have reduced the need for a shoe lift and its detrimental additional shoe weight

body parts distal to the neurological lesion [21]. The lower the level of cord lesion and the earlier the age of paralysis, the greater the growth deficit [21]. Since the neurologic deficit in cord trauma is usually bilateral, and the function of the extremities is reduced, no limb length treatment is usually necessary.

6.3.2 Spinal Cord Nontraumatic Injury

The most common nontraumatic spinal cord injury develops in utero and is referred to in the literature as meningomyelocele (MMC), myelomeningocele, myelodysplasia, and spina bifida. Spontaneous painless fractures of the lower extremities occur in 10–30% of patients with MMC, usually with no known history of trauma [20, 23, 26, 27, 30, 36]. Multiple fractures in a given patient are common [23], and most involve the metaphysis or diaphysis. Up to 10% of these fractures involve a physis [22, 27, 30, 36]. In addition to fractures, the physis frequently widens without a history of a specific traumatic event. The fractures and the physeal widenings are due to a combination of sensory deficiency, muscular imbalance, musculoligamentous laxity, and osteopenia. Because of the lack of sensation, injuries to physes are often mild and repetitive and not noted by the patient. The most common initial symptom is painless warm swelling near a joint. Clinically this can be mistaken for cellulitis, osteomyelitis, or septic arthritis.

Roentgenographically, the earliest abnormal physeal finding associated with MMC is widening. The physeal widening in MMC is similar to that seen in rickets, scurvy, osteomyelitis, and syphilis, and occurs in approximately 10% of patients [20, 22]. Widening is often bilateral, but can be unilateral despite symmetric lower limb paresis (Fig. 6.2a, b) [31, 34]. A roentgenogram of a contralateral asymptomatic limb may be normal, or show similar physeal widening (Fig. 6.2c) [31]. Other physes may be normal or abnormal (Fig. 6.2d). The widening has been attributed to disturbance of the normal resorption of the hypertrophic cartilage, or to secondary hyperemia causing increased growth in the germinal layer of the physis [25, 31]. Thus, vascular changes, as mentioned in Chap. 1, may be the underlying cause. On MRI the physeal widening is accompanied by irregularity at the junction with the metaphysis [32]. The widened physis may revert back to normal if weight bearing is curtailed and gradually reinstituted. These findings corroborate the mechanistic proposals for physeal changes in MMC: chronic stress or trauma to the poorly sensate limb produces micromotion at the zone of hypertrophy, producing a widened, disorganized physis, leading to epiphyseal displacement [32].

Epiphyseal displacement may occur gradually or suddenly (Fig. 6.3) [20, 22]. The distal and proximal tibia, and distal femoral physis are most frequently involved [20, 23, 24, 28, 32]. Widening of the proximal femoral physis is not commonly reported, but when present results in a high incidence of complications (premature fusion, osteonecrosis, and non-union) [36]. Most displacements occur between the ages of 2 and 10 years [22, 23, 32, 36]. The vast majority of acute displacements are fracture type 3 (Peterson classification) with a few type 2 [20, 27, 28, 36]. Physeal fractures perpendicular to the physis (Peterson type 4 and 5) have not been recorded [23]. Stripping of the periosteum may produce subperiosteal hemorrhage with subsequent new bone formation which can be massive (Fig. 6.3g, h) [19, 20, 22, 23]. This has been be mistaken for osteomyelitis or tumor [32, 35, 36]. The epiphysis is usually intact, but may be secondarily demineralized [25].

The absence of pain sensation in these patients subjects the physis to injury from daily activities such as walking, and often delays the diagnosis. These physeal injuries occur commonly following immobilization after surgery for other problems [23]. It is not uncommon for an epiphyseal displacement to occur during rehabilitation manipulations, even in experienced hands. The lesions are more frequent in non-walkers than walkers, but the consequences are more incapacitating in the latter [28].

A widened physis detected prior to patient complaint or history of trauma, as evidenced by a lack of periosteal stripping, new bone formation, or epiphyseal displacement, has a good chance of returning to normal by continuing normal activities in the patient's orthosis, but avoiding excessive use and physiotherapy [31]. Treatment of physeal widening with mild slip or angulation consists of withdrawal of weight bearing, or immobilization in splint, brace, or cast, depending on the type of physeal lesion [20, 22, 26, 32]. Prior to 1980, authors recommended complete immobilization with avoidance of weight bearing until there was clinical and roentgenographic evidence of healing [22, 36]. Authors after 1990 have recommended that the immobilization time be as short as possible [20, 23, 28]. Rigid prolonged cast immobilization predisposes these children to joint stiffness, osteoporosis, increased risk

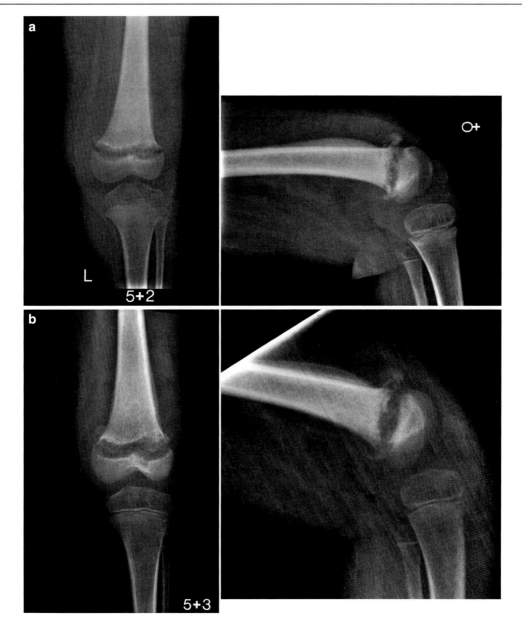

Fig. 6.2 Meningomyelocele with bilateral premature closure of distal femoral physes. This female had a low thoracic level spina bifida. She was able to propel her own wheelchair, had independent sitting posture but could not transfer on or off raised objects, could commando crawl, and walked with braces and AFOs 20 ft with a walker, but could not turn around. She had had bilateral percutaneous and open Achilles lengthenings. (**a**) At age 5 years 2 months diffuse swelling of the left knee resulted in roentgenograms which showed distal femoral physeal widening, metaphyseal new subperiosteal bone, heterotopic ossification adjacent to the physis, and soft tissue swelling about the knee and distal femur. There was no pain or history of trauma. A long leg cast with the knee in 80° flexion was applied. (**b**) At cast change on the 13th day there was crepitation and false motion at the distal femur. The physeal width was increased. The final cast was removed at 8 weeks. There was a dry 7 mm heel ulcer. The brace was readjusted and reapplied after the ulcer had healed. (**c**) At age 6 years 0 months the left distal femoral physis was narrower. Similar, but less severe changes were present on the right distal femoral physis. The proximal tibial and fibular physes were normal. (**d**) The proximal femora had normal physes. (**e**) Age 6 years 4 months. The distal right femur had less physeal widening than the left, but more subperiosteal new bone formation, suggesting epiphyseal instability. The lateral view (*right*) confirmed mild posterior epiphyseal displacement. (**f**) At age 6 years 10 months both distal femoral physes were narrower. Subperiosteal new bone formation on the right. (**g**) Age 8 years 0 months. Both distal femoral physes are in the process of closing. The proximal tibial physes are normal. (**h**) MRI at age 8 years 1 month confirmed multiple physeal bars of various sizes in both distal femora, with open tibial physes. Since the patient was no longer ambulatory no treatment was recommended. *Note*: The physis was wider on the left (**c**), but epiphyseal displacement on the right (**e**) was associated with earlier and more extensive physeal closure (**f**–**h**). The patient is presently 20 years old, is seen frequently in departments other than orthopedics, and has had no further problems requiring investigation of her lower extremities

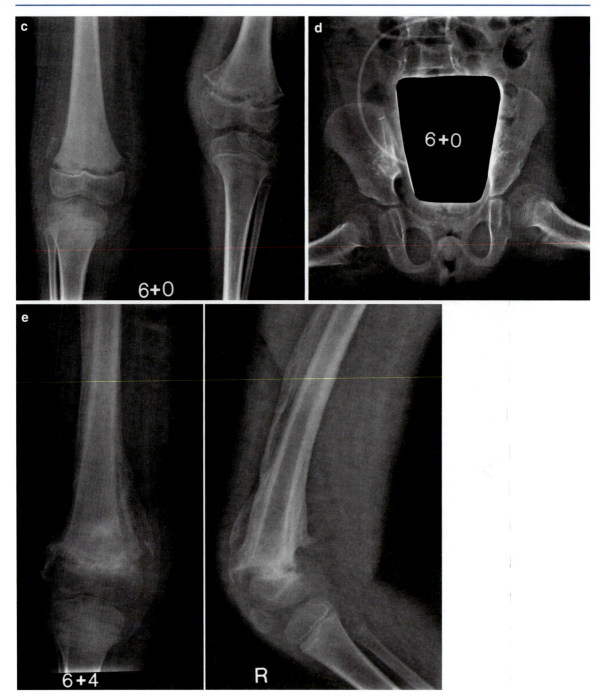

Fig. 6.2 (continued)

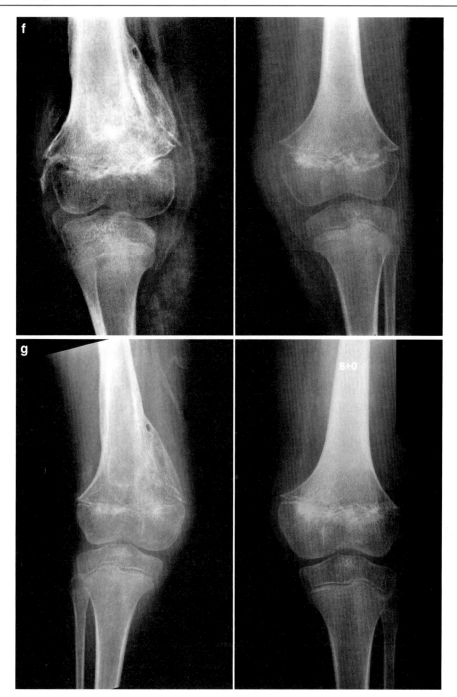

Fig. 6.2 (continued)

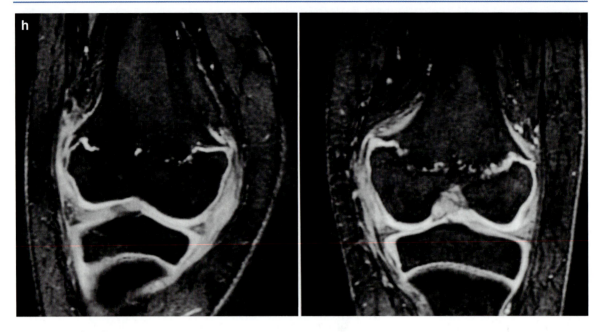

Fig. 6.2 (continued)

of subsequent fracture [31], epiphyseal displacement, and premature physeal closure, [32] and in one case life-threatening systemic hypovolemia [27]. A post cast orthosis may facilitate early weight bearing and return of function [20, 23, 28]. Significant epiphyseal displacement with instability is treated with reduction and internal fixation [20, 23, 32]. Percutaneous Kirschner wire internal fixation can be performed without anesthesia in these children, and reduces the postoperative immobilization time [23].

Healing of physeal injuries in MMC patients is generally much slower than healing of metaphyseal and diaphyseal fractures [26, 32]. In normal children, physeal fractures normally heal faster [36]. As healing progresses the widened growth plate regresses to its normal width. Most patients that were ambulatory pre-fracture regain their ability to walk [32]. Recurrent epiphyseal slipping is apparently rare, but has been reported once in the distal tibia [33]. One boy had slipping of the epiphyses of the distal femur, distal tibia, and proximal tibia, all on the right side, at two year intervals beginning at age 12 years [34]. If the physes is unprotected, premature closure may occur [26].

Some children with meningomyelocele develop ankle valgus associated with relative fibular shortening and tapering of the lateral tibial epiphysis. Since this is similar to the ankle valgus seen in other developmental conditions it is recorded in Sect. 19.3.

Fig. 6.3 Meningomyelocele with unilateral distal tibial epiphyseal displacement without physeal closure. This boy was ambulatory with short leg braces and crutches, but developed bilateral ischial decubiti at age 10 years while riding in a car on a family vacation. At age 11 years 7 months he sustained a radiator burn to the dorsum of the right foot which healed slowly over several months. (**a**) At age 12 years 1 month persistent mild swelling of the right ankle prompted a roentgenogram which was of marginal quality and showed only soft tissue swelling about the right ankle. (**b**) The distal tibial physes were normal on lateral views. (**c**) At age 12 years 3 months there was widening of the right distal tibial physis. The elevated periosteum on the anterior tibia (*right view*) suggests subperiosteal hemorrhage, possibly due to slip of the epiphysis which has returned to its normal position. (**d**) One week later ankle swelling was markedly increased. The patient had been walking against advice, but there was no other known trauma. The lateral showed posterior displacement of both right ankle epiphyses (*right*). (**e**) A closed reduction was held with a posterior plaster splint. (**f**) One week later there was beginning ossification of the subperiosteal hematoma. A cast was worn 6 weeks. (**g**) At age 12 years 5 months there was recurrent widening of the right ankle physes and marked subperiosteal new bone formation on both the distal tibia and fibula. (**h**) Lateral views showed persistent normal left ankle physes. The patient was obese and no longer ambulating. He was followed in physical therapy and other departments until age 22, and since no further orthopedic care was requested, no additional roentgenograms were made

6.3 Spinal Cord Injury

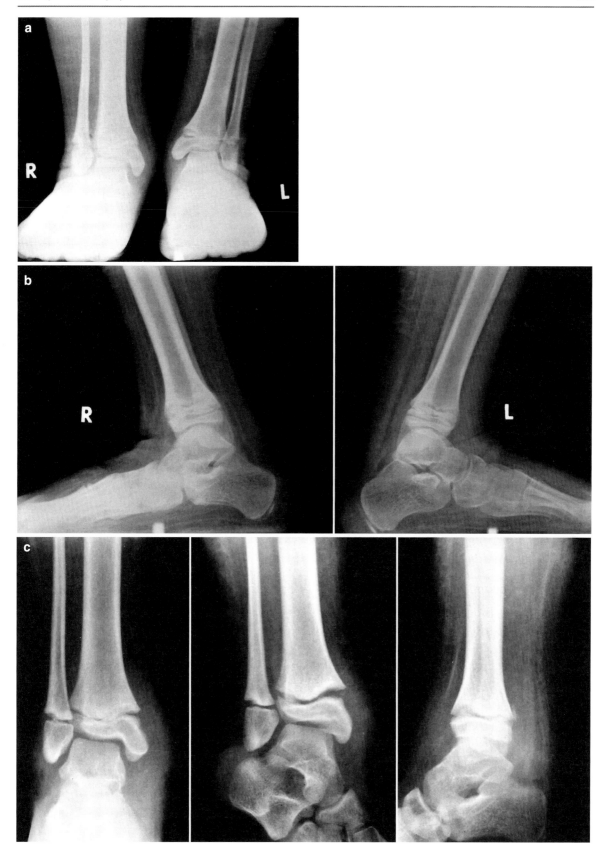

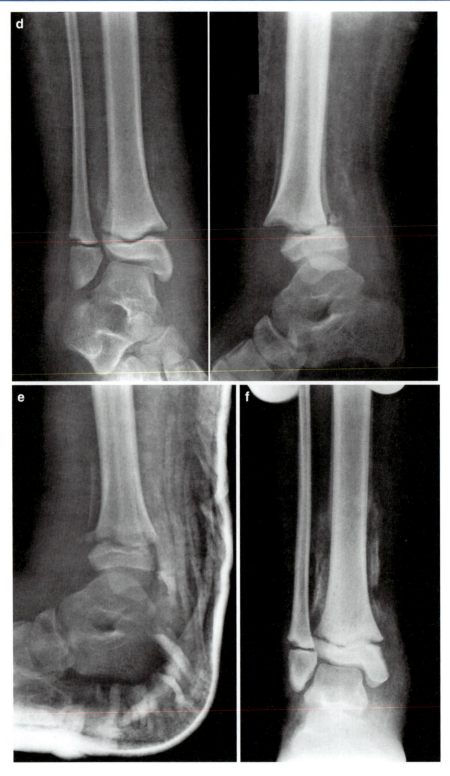

Fig. 6.3 (continued)

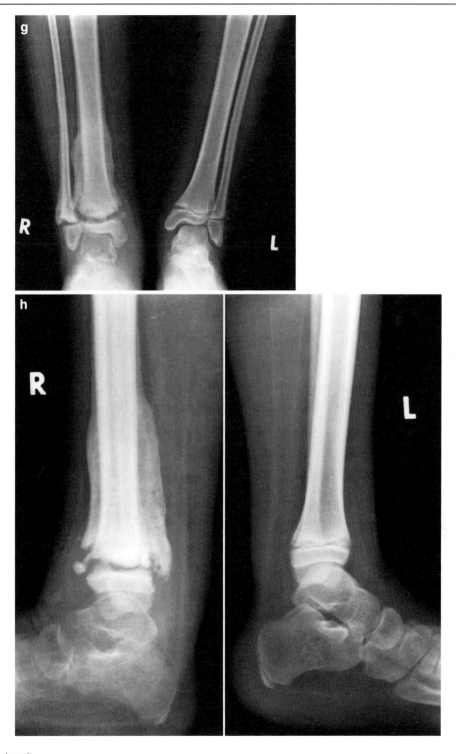

Fig. 6.3 (continued)

The most common complication of physeal injury is premature physeal arrest (Fig. 6.2f–h) which causes relative bone shortening and angular deformity [19, 20, 32, 36]. In one study, 33% of patients with physeal injury developed 1 cm or more of relative shortening, and 50% incurred more than 5% angular deformity [23]. In another study, 43% had delayed fracture union and 29% had premature physeal arrest [27]. In a third study, 5 of 9 children (56%) with widened physes developed premature physeal closure, resulting in an 8 cm femoral length discrepancy in one child [36]. Premature physeal arrest is of minor clinical significance if the patient is non-ambulatory [32].

Early recognition of physeal widening and dysfunction is obviously important. Contralateral surgical physeal arrest may be appropriate in ambulatory patients [36]. Some authors advise radiologic investigation of every unexplained lower extremity swelling [23], or yearly roentgenograms of weight bearing joints until physeal closure [22, 36].

6.4 Brain Injury

6.4.1 Physeal Growth in Hemiplegic Patients

Cerebral palsy is the result of a brain injury occurring in the perinatal period or anytime before age 5 years. Cerebral palsy significantly alters growth. The etiology of diminished growth on the affected side of hemiplegic patients remains unknown. Possible mechanisms suggested are neurotrophic alterations, vascular alterations, and disuse atrophy. None of these appears to be the sole etiology [39].

Affected children are usually smaller in stature than their unaffected peers. Limb length inequality in hemiplegia is most prominent in the upper extremity and in the distal segments [39]. The percentage of growth retardation is greatest in the radius, followed by the humerus and tibia. However, limb length inequality produces more disability in the lower extremity than in the upper extremity (Figs. 6.4 and 10.5a). The length discrepancy increases with age. Lower limb equalization by physeal arrest of the long side can be considered if a discrepancy exceeds 2 cm. In most children slight permanent relative shortening of the paretic leg

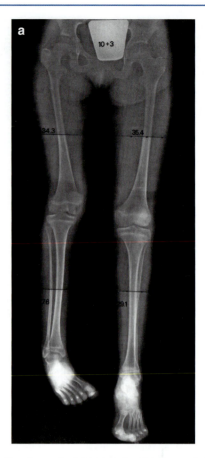

Fig. 6.4 Spastic cerebral hemiplegia with lower limb length inequality. This infant female was normal at birth. At age 1 month she was diagnosed with herpes simplex viral encephalitis. Within 6 months, diagnoses included microcephaly and right spastic hemiplegia. Right Achilles contracture was treated with surgical lengthening at age 2 years 9 months. A right lower leg orthosis with shoe lift was worn for several years. (**a**) At age 10 years 3 months a scanogram showed the right femur 1.1 cm, and the right tibia 1.5 cm shorter than the left for a total discrepancy of 2.6 cm. All physes are normal. Right adductor tenotomy, obturator neurectomy and Achilles and posterior tibialis lengthenings were done. By age 16 years her diagnosis had changed to spastic quadriparesis with greater involvement on the right, and included right hemiatrophy, seizure disorder, cataracts, and significant mental compromise. (**b**) CT scan of the head at age 16 years 9 months performed without contrast shows multiple cystic areas of low attenuation involving both of the frontal lobes and the left temporal and parietal lobes, consistent with multicystic encephalomalacia and old neonatal herpes. At age 18 years 8 months right spastic equinovarus was treated with triple arthrodesis and left equinus with Achilles lengthening. She was now residing in a total care facility. At age 21 years 11 months a pronated left flat foot was treated with triple arthrodesis and Achilles lengthening. At age 28 years 9 months she sustained a displaced right knee tibial plateau fracture treated with open reduction and internal fixation. No trauma had been witnessed and the relationship of the fracture to her known infirmities was not determined

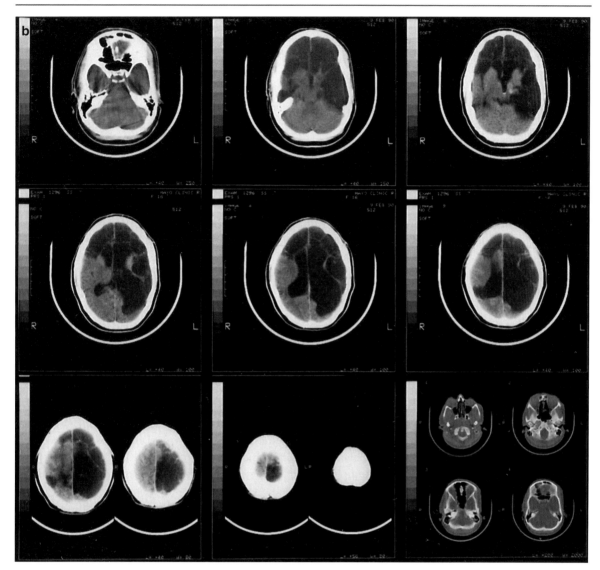

Fig. 6.4 (continued)

6.4.2 Physeal Disruption in Quadriplegic Patients

Children with spastic quadriparesis are at risk of developing fractures, spontaneously or following trivial trauma. The majority of fractures (>75%) occur in the diaphysis or metaphysis of the femur [37]. Physeal injuries are rare. Four children with 9 physeal injuries have been reported [37]. The ages ranged from 1½ to 5 years. The 9 physeal injuries were all epiphyseal displacements; 5 in the distal femur and 4 in the proximal humerus. All patients had spastic quadriparesis and were nonambulant. The epiphyseal displacements were complete, occurred spontaneously, and were not related to vigorous physical therapy or epileptic convulsion. None of the children had been subjected to surgery or immobilization. However, all four had moderate to severe malnutrition and evidence of vitamin C deficiency (Chap. 5). All four children had poor dentition, bleeding gums, irritability, and pseudoparalytic frog-leg positioning, all signs commensurate with scurvy. Roentgenograms revealed evidence of osteoporosis with thinning of the cortices along with distinctive radiological signs of scurvy. The children were treated with nutritional supplementation and ascorbic acid. No reductions were performed. The epiphyses became centered on the newly widened metaphyses and maintained that central position during the phase of remodeling. Excellent remodeling was observed even where displacement was severe. Minimal residual deformity occurred in one case. No premature physeal arrest or limb length discrepancies were noted at follow-up of 2–6 years. The authors concluded that routine dietary supplementation of vitamin C should be given to all nonambulant and potentially malnourished children [37].

A four year old child with spastic quadriparesis secondary to encephalitis at age 6 weeks developed scurvy (Sect. 5.1), and subsequent complete bilateral epiphyseal separations of the proximal humeral and distal femoral epiphyses [38]. Once the vitamin C levels were rectified the slipped epiphyses remodeled spontaneously and the child regained almost full range of motion in the shoulders and knees.

6.5 Congenital Insensitivity to Pain

Congenital insensitivity or indifference to pain (CIP) is a rare disorder defined as the absence of normal subjective and objective responses to noxious stimuli in the setting of otherwise intact central and peripheral nervous systems. There is no demonstrable anatomic, physiologic, or psychological defect in the nervous system and all parameters of the neurologic evaluation are normal, with the sole exception of failure to show the usual response to pain-producing stimuli. The disorder is present at birth and the entire body is affected. CIP presents a pattern of orthopedic complexities and complications, one of which is premature physeal arrest.

On neurologic examination, affected children have normal motor power and reflexes. Cutaneous sensation to light touch is normal; pinprick is felt, but not as pain. During childhood CIP patients often fight because they cannot feel pain [43]. While CIP is primarily a neurologic affliction, the complaints which bring the patient to a doctor are usually orthopedic problems [43, 46]. The literature pertaining to children describes spontaneous fractures, osteomyelitis, Charcot joints, cutaneous ulcers, self-inflicted injuries from biting and chewing causing scarring of the tongue, buccal musosa, and lower lip, and auto-amputation of finger tips and toe tips. The appearance of secondary centers of ossification in the distal epiphyses of hand metacarpals are felt to be due to chronic hyperemia associated with repetitive trauma [41]. The differential diagnosis is long and includes child abuse, diabetic neuropathy, syringomyelia, syphilis, leprosy, and a number of hereditary syndromes [43–46]. The three most common orthopedic manifestations of CIP are recurrent fractures, neuropathic (Charcot's) joints, and osteomyelitis [44]. These may present at any age.

Bony lesions develop through an interplay of multiple factors. These include insensitivity, repeated unappreciated trauma, obesity, abuse, personality, mental subnormality, and metabolic joint and bone disease, suggesting that environmental factors affect expression of mutant genes for inherited neuropathy [42]. The failure to establish a reasonable basis for the disease produced much theoretical speculation about the mechanism involved [44, 46]. One article reported negative family histories, and called the condition nonfamilial congenital sensory neuropathy [44]. However, two brothers with CIP were reported in one article [46], two sisters in another [48], and two reports describe subclinical neuropathy and neurogenic arthropathy in primary relatives [42, 43]. Recent investigations determined the cause of CIP to be mutations in the neurotrophic tyrosine kinase receptor type 1 gene, located on chromosome 1 (1q21-22), mentioned in the pediatric orthopedic literature for the first time in 2009 [47].

Problems pertaining to the physis are infrequently reported. A 1996 review of CIP in the world literature reported 21 patients with osteoarticular manifestations [49]. Eleven of these patients had at least one epiphyseal separation, and five had two areas of separation, the most common being the femur and tibia. The ages ranged from 2 months to 40 years. Many displacements occur without a history of a specific injury. Except for the absence of pain the physeal abnormalities are similar to those seen in stress injuries (Chap. 12). The physeal bars in the patient in Fig. 6.5 were probably caused by repeated stress injuries or fractures, which in turn were due to unappreciated and undocumented repetitive trauma.

Histologic evaluation of a roentgenographically normal distal tibial physis from a patient with CIP showed normal cell column orientation and basic tibial physeal morphology in most of the physis [45]. There was no evidence of germinal cell layer crushing, but the lateral edge showed abnormal chondrocyte orientation and morphology. Normal appearing myelinated nerves were found within the main bundles at the level of the amputation.

The key to minimizing deformity and disability due to physeal injury in CIP patients is prevention of trauma and early diagnosis [45, 46]. Some patients are intelligent and cooperative in their younger years making preventive measures possible [45]. Physeal fractures should be treated promptly, and nonoperatively if possible [46]. Optimum treatment is based on protection and prevention, but should this fail aggressive treatment is mandatory [44]. Bar excision of premature partial arrest can be successful, as noted in the proximal tibia of the patient in Fig. 6.5, but requires extremely attentive postoperative care.

Fig. 6.5 Congenital insensitivity to pain. A patient with known CIP was reported to have sustained compression fractures of both calcanei at age 3 years 8 months which were treated with short leg casts. One week after removal of the casts the patient sustained a type 2 physeal fracture of the left distal tibia which was treated closed with a long leg cast. The cast was removed at age 3 years 11 months and was followed quickly with a fracture of the proximal left tibia. (**a**) The patient was referred at age 4 years 3 months with varus deformities of the left knee and ankle. There was swelling of the left lower leg and an ulcer on the medial border of the right foot. (**b**) A scanogram shows a healing fracture of the left proximal tibial metaphysis, a left distal tibial central physeal bar, 2.2 cm left tibial relative shortening, and relative overgrowth of the left fibula. (**c**) Lateral views of the ankles show compression of the right talus (*left*) and left os calcis (*right*), and moderate cupping of the left distal tibial physis. (**d**) Tomograms confirmed a left distal tibial central physeal bar. Fearing potentially severe complications from future tibial lengthening, physeal bar excision was advised despite any record in the literature of bar excisions in previous CIP patients. (**e**) The physeal bar was excised and cranioplast was used as the interposition material. Titanium break-off wires were inserted 15 mm apart. A third marker was placed in the proximal metaphysis. A short leg cast was removed 15 days later. Within a week there was a fracture of the distal tibial metaphysis. (**f**) Three months following bar excision, the fracture through the distal tibial metaphysis was not healed and distal tibial epiphyseal displacement and the ankle varus was increased (*left*). The fracture was allowed to heal. The metal marker in the proximal tibia is shown best on the lateral view (*right*). (**g**) At age 7 years 3 months a scanogram showed the distal tibial fracture was healed, the physis was open, and the titanium markers were 33 mm apart (18 mm of new growth). The physis had grown away from the cranioplast (the radiolucent area in the metaphysis). There was a bar in the proximal left tibial physis and the tibial discrepancy had increased to 4.8 cm. The proximal tibial physis had grown a mild amount as judged from the proximal titanium marker. There was mild relative overgrowth of the left femur and of the left fibula both proximally and distally. (**h**) The proximal tibial physeal bar was confirmed on MRI. (**i**) 3D projection images derived from MR imaging data [40], revealed a central bar of 2.8 cm^2 with an irregular border. The entire physis measured 24.6 cm.^{2} The bar was 11% of the total physis. (**j**) The bar was excised and filled with cranioplast. (**k**) Two new titanium break-off wires were inserted 35 mm apart. (**l**) Eleven months later, age 8 years 2 months, the left tibia had grown 14 mm, the right 11 mm. The proximal markers were 50 mm apart, the distal 33 mm. The tibial length discrepancy was slight less at 4.5 cm. This documents that the left tibia had grown slightly more than the right in the 11 months following the proximal tibial bar excision. Distally the more proximal of the two titanium markers had come out of the bone, had migrated distally, and was no longer useful as a marker. The recurrent bar distally was reexcised and new silver clip markers placed in the epiphysis and metaphysis 23 mm apart. (**m**) At age 9 years 0 months a scanogram showed the tibial length discrepancy to be slightly less at 4.3 cm, and the proximal tibial titanium markers 58 mm apart. The two silver clip markers distally remained 23 mm apart. A rotation valgus osteotomy held with a plate and five screws was accompanied with an Achilles lengthening. This resulted in nonunion and a broken plate. (**n**) At age 9 years 5 months osteosynthesis using a compression plate and five screws was accompanied with bank chip bone grafts and osteotomy of the fibula. Subsequent incision delayed healing was treated with skin grafts by plastic surgery. (**o**) At age 10 years 4 months the osteotomy had healed. (**p**) At age 12 years 5 months the most recent metal markers were 66 mm apart proximally, 29 mm apart distally. At age 13 years 0 months physeal arrest of the right distal femur and proximal tibia were accompanied by the start of lengthening of the left tibia and fibula. (**q**) The lengthening gained 4.5 cm of length, but was complicated by infection and left a residual 10 cm length deficit. The external lengthener remained on 9 months followed by a long leg cast and eventually a PTB clamshell brace. This was later changed to a KAFO to protect the knee. The patella was removed and the patellar tendon reconstructed. (**r**) At age 17 years 10 months the patient was ambulatory. Both the proximal and distal tibial articular surfaces were abnormal. When last seen at age 18 years 8 months he was ambulating without braces or a walker. A 3 in. lift on the sole of the left shoe leveled the pelvis. There was full motion of both knees, but with occasional swelling. Note: Any surgery on patients with CIP must be considered carefully. Complications are common. Although the injuries to the tibial physes were due to stress injury or fracture, this case is included because of the rare underlying condition leading to the fractures. The arrests occurred at different ages. In this patient the proximal tibia bar excision had a positive outcome. The two bar excisions on the distal tibia produced little growth and the first was complicated by fracture which healed slowly. Osteotomy of the distal tibia at age 9 years 5 months (**n**) improved ankle alignment, but residual ankle deformity at age 17+10 (**r**) portends degenerative arthrosis in the future. This patient was referred and followed by Dr. R. P Lewallen, Billings, MT (From Borsa et al. [40], with permission and further follow-up)

6.5 Congenital Insensitivity to Pain

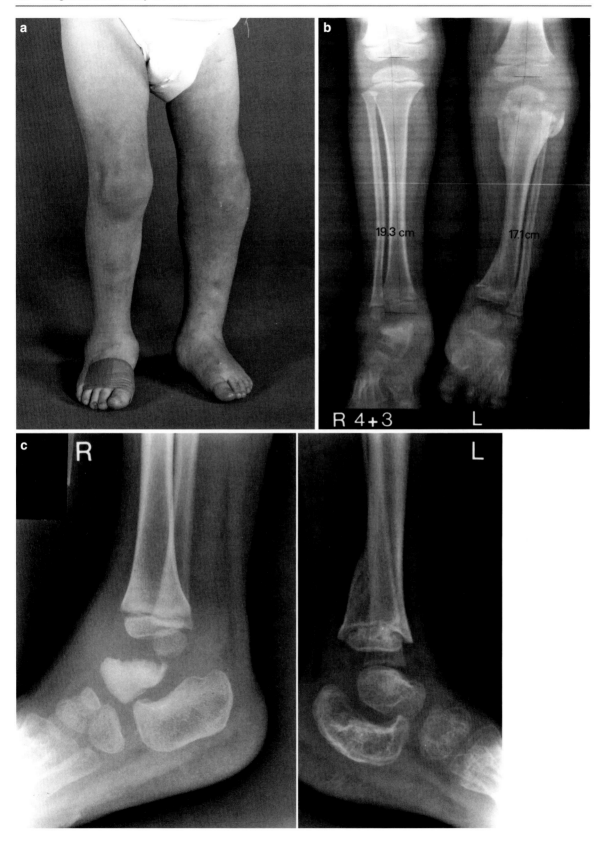

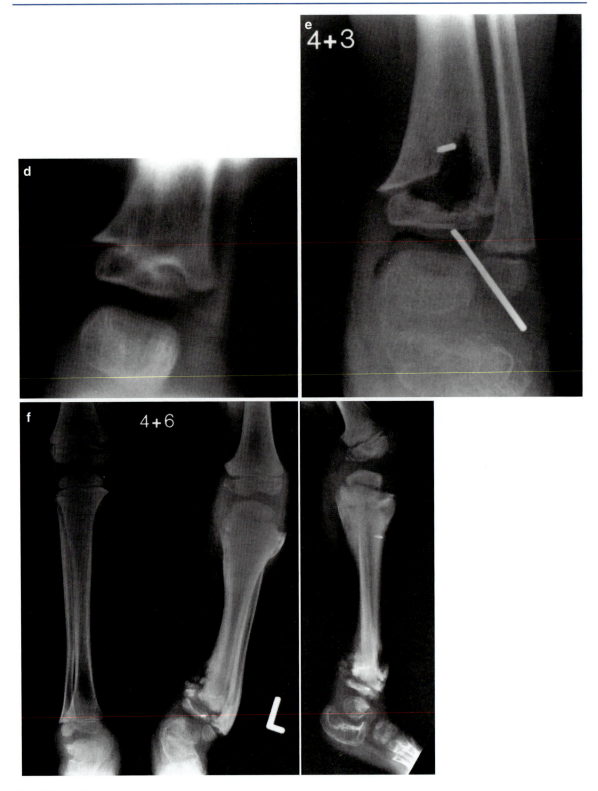

Fig. 6.5 (continued)

6.5 Congenital Insensitivity to Pain 213

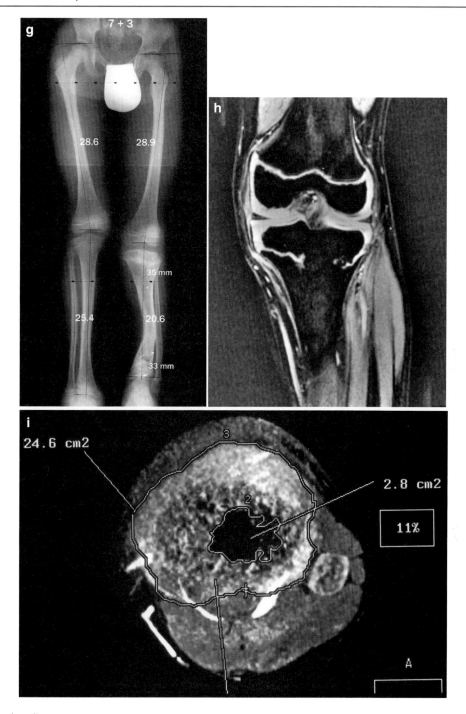

Fig. 6.5 (continued)

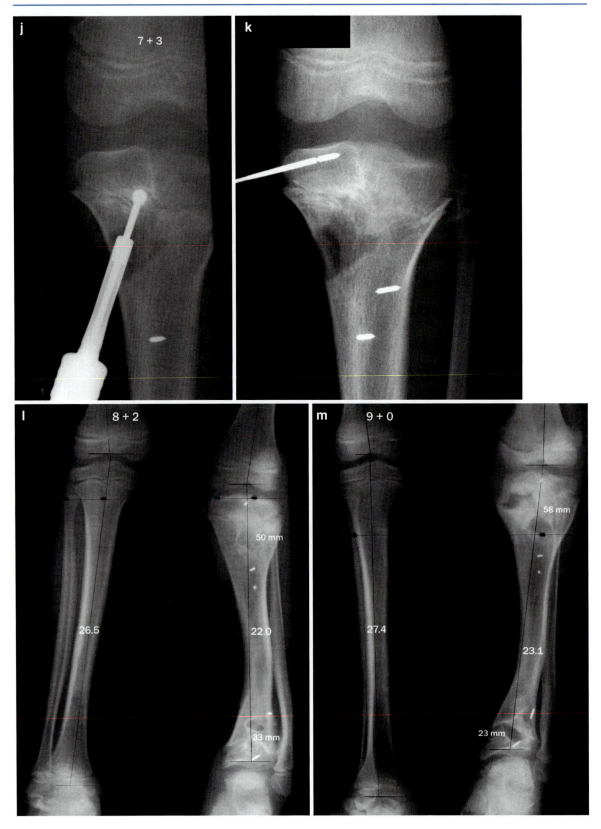

Fig. 6.5 (continued)

6.5 Congenital Insensitivity to Pain

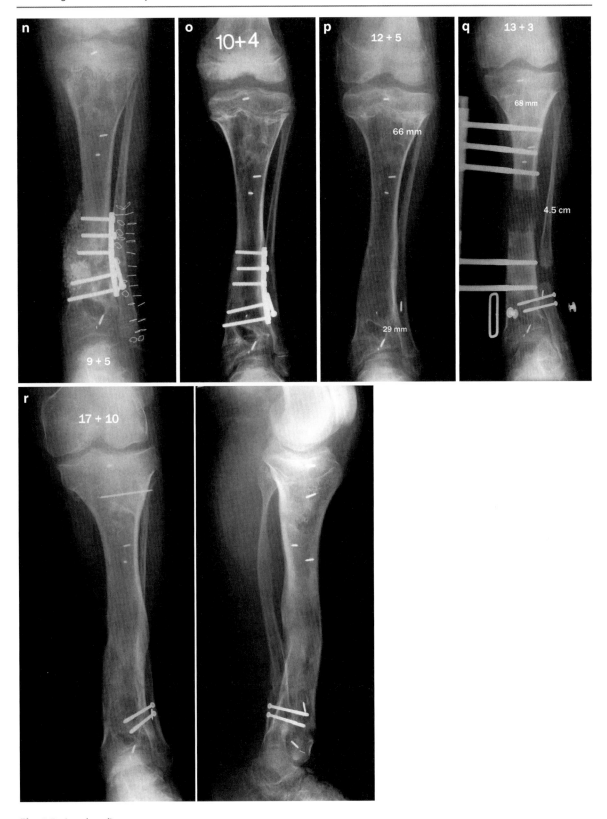

Fig. 6.5 (continued)

References

Introduction

1. Denisenko OP, Sotnikov OS, Zhukov IS, Chikhman VN (2000) Innervation of the humerus metaepiphysis in newborn and one year old children [*Russian*]. Morfologiia 118(6):44–50
2. Strange-Vognsen HH, Laursen H (1997) Nerves in human epiphyseal uncalcified cartilage. J Pediatr Orthop B 6(1):56–58

Peripheral Nerve Injury

3. Armstrong WD (1946) Bone growth in paralyzed limbs. Proc Soc Exp Biol Med 61:358–362
4. Bacq ZM (1930) The action of abdominal sympathectomy on the growth of the albino rat and the weight of the genital organs. Am J Physiol 45:601–604
5. Bisgard JD (1931) Effect of sympathetic ganglionectomy upon bone growth. Proc Soc Exp Biol Med 29:229–230
6. Bisgard JD (1933) Longitudinal bone growth: the influence of sympathetic deinnervation. Ann Surg 97:374–380
7. Combes MA, Clark WK, Gregory CF, James JA (1960) Sciatic nerve injury in infants. Recognition and prevention of impairment resulting from intragluteal injections. JAMA 173:1336–1339
8. Curtiss PH Jr, Tucker HJ (1960) Sciatic palsy in premature infants. A report and follow-up study of ten cases. JAMA 174:1586–1587
9. Fahey JJ (1936) The effect of lumbar sympathetic ganglionectomy on longitudinal bone growth as determined by the teleoroentgenographic method. J Bone Joint Surg Am 18:1042–1046
10. Garcés GL, Santandreu ME (1988) Longitudinal bone growth after sciatic denervation in rats. J Bone Joint Surg Br 70:315–318
11. Gilles FH, French JH (1961) Postinjection sciatic nerve palsies in infants and children. J Pediatr 58(2):195–204
12. Gillespie JA (1954) The nature of the bone changes associated with nerve injuries and disuse. J Bone Joint Surg 36B(3):464–473
13. Harris RI, McDonald JL (1936) The effect of lumbar sympathectomy upon the growth of legs paralyzed by anterior poliomyelitis. J Bone Joint Surg 18:35–45
14. Kirjavainen MO, Remes VM, Peltonen J, Helenius IJ, Rautakorpi SM, Vähäsarja VJ et al (2009) Permanent brachial plexus birth palsy does not impair the development and function of the spine and lower limbs. J Pediatr Orthop B 19(6):283–288
15. Ring PA (1961) The influence of the nervous system upon the growth of bones. J Bone Joint Surg 43B:121–140
16. Selye H, Bajusz E (1958) Effect of denervation on experimentally induced changes in the growth of bone and muscle. Am J Physiol 192(2):297–300
17. Troupp H (1961) Nervous and vascular influences on longitudinal growth of bone: an experimental study on rabbits. Acta Orthop Scand Suppl 51:1–78
18. Zeng QQ, Jee WSS, Bigornia AE, King JG Jr, D'Souza SM, Li XJ et al (1996) Time responses of cancellous and cortical bones to sciatic neurectomy in growing female rats. Bone 19(1):13–21

Spinal Cord Injury

19. Ahstrom JP (1965) Epiphyseal injuries of the lower extremity. Surg Clin North Am 1:119–134
20. Cuxart MD, Iborra J, Meléndez M, Pagés E (1992) Physeal injuries in myelomeningocele patients. Paraplegia 30:791–794
21. Duval-Beaupere G, Lougovoy J, Trocellier L, Lacert P (1983) Trunk and leg growth in children with paraplegia caused by spinal cord injury. Paraplegia 21(6):339–350
22. Edvardsen P (1972) Physeo-epiphyseal injuries of lower extremities in myelomeningocele. Acta Orthop Scand 43:550–557
23. Fromm B, Pfeil J, Carstens C, Niethard FU (1992) Fractures and epiphysiolyses in children with myelomeningocele. J Pediatr Orthop B 1:21–27
24. Golding C (1960) Museum pages. III Spina bifida and epiphyseal displacement. J Bone Joint Surg Br 42-B(2):387–389
25. Gyepes MT, Newbern DH, Neuhauser EBD (1965) Metaphyseal and physeal injuries in children with spina bifida and meningomyeloceles. Am J Roentgenol Radium Ther Nucl Med 95:168–177
26. Kumar SJ, Cowell HR, Townsend P (1984) Physeal, metaphyseal, and diaphyseal injuries of the lower extremities in children with myelomeningocele. J Pediatr Orthop 4:25–27
27. Lock TR, Aronson DD (1989) Fractures in patients who have myelomeningocele. J Bone Joint Surg Am 71:1153–1157
28. Medina JR (1993) Physeal lesions in the myelodysplasic patient. Mapfre Medicina 4(Suppl II):141–142
29. Morse L, Teng YD, Pham L, Newton K, Yu D, Liao WL et al (2008) Spinal cord injury causes rapid osteoclastic resorption and growth plate abnormalities in growing rats (SCI-induced bone loss in growing rats). Osteoporos Int 19:645–652
30. Quilis AN (1974) Fractures in children with myelomeningocele. Acta Orthop Scand 45:883–897
31. Roberts JA, Bennet GC, MacKenzie JR (1989) Physeal widening in children with myelomeningocele. J Bone Joint Surg Br 71(1):30–32
32. Rodgers WB, Schwend RM, Jaramillo D, Kasser JR, Emans JB (1997) Chronic physeal fractures in myelodysplasia: magnetic resonance analysis, histologic description, treatment, and outcome. J Pediatr Orthop 17:615–621
33. Stern MB, Grant SS, Isaacson AS (1967) Bilateral distal tibial and fibular epiphysial separation associated with spina bifida. Clin Orthop Relat Res 50:191–196
34. Soutter FE (1962) Spina bifida and epiphyseal displacement. Report of two cases. J Bone Joint Surg Br 44-B:106–109
35. Townsend PF, Cowell HR, Steg NL (1979) Lower extremity fractures simulating infection in myelomeningocele. Clin Orthop Relat Res 144:255–259
36. Wenger DR, Jeffcoat BT, Herring JA (1980) The guarded prognosis of physeal injury in paraplegic children. J Bone Joint Surg Am 62:241–246

Brain Injury

37. Aroojis AJ, Gajjar SM, Johan AN (2007) Epiphyseal separations in spastic cerebral palsy. J Pediatr Orthop B 16:170–174
38. Hosalkar HS, Johnston DR, Pill S, Flynn JM (2005) Multiple epiphyseal separations in a child with scurvy and cerebral palsy. Am J Orthop (Belle Mead NJ) 34:295–298
39. Staheli LT, Duncan WR, Schaefer E (1968) Growth alterations in the hemiplegic child. A study of femoral anteversion, neck-shaft angle, hip rotation, C.E. angle, limb length and circumference in 50 hemiplegic children. Clin Orthop Relat Res 60:205–212

Congenital Insensitivity to Pain

40. Borsa JJ, Peterson HA, Ehman RL (1996) MR imaging of physeal bars. Radiology 199(3):683–687
41. Caffey J (1957) Some traumatic lesions in growing bones other than fractures and dislocations: clinical and radiological features. Br J Radiol 30:225–238
42. Dyck PJ, Stevens JC, O'Brien PC, Oviatt KF, Lais AC, Coventry MB et al (1983) Neurogenic arthropathy with recurring fractures with subclinical inherited neuropathy. Neurology 33(3):357–367
43. Fath MA, Hassanein MR, James JIP (1983) Congenital absence of pain. A family study. J Bone Joint Surg Br 65: 186–188
44. Greider TD (1983) Orthopedic aspects of congenital insensitivity to pain. Clin Orthop Relat Res 172: 177–185
45. Guidera KJ, Multhopp J, Ganey T, Ogden JA (1990) Orthopaedic manifestations in congenitally insensate patients. J Pediatr Orthop 10:514–521
46. Kuo RS, Macnicol MF (1996) Congenital insensitivity to pain: orthopaedic implications. Case Report. J Pediatr Orthop B 5:292–295
47. Marik I, Kuklik M, Kuklikova D, Kozlowsk K (2009) Hereditary sensory and autonomic neuropathy type IV orthopaedic complications. J Pediatr Orthop B 18:138–140
48. Silverman FN, Gilden JJ (1959) Congenital insensitivity to pain: a neurologic syndrome with bizarre skeletal lesion. Radiology 72:176–190
49. Szöke G, Rényi-Vámos A, Bider MA (1996) Osteoarticular manifestations of congenital insensitivity to pain with anhydrosis. Int Orthop 20:107–110

Cold Injury (Frostbite)

7.1 Introduction

Frostbite is freezing of the tissues by dry cold, sometimes aided by dampness and wind [5]. Children are particularly susceptible. They often do not have the intelligence to properly protect themselves or may not appreciate the significance of numbness, an early symptom of frostbite. Complications are usually found in patients who suffer initial damage from advanced stage two or three frostbite injury [7, 8]. The skeletal abnormalities are complex and unique; only the hands and feet are affected. Cold injury in children differs from that in adults in that damage to the physis may result in growth disturbance [9, 18]. The popularity of bone banks may have given a false impression of the ability of bone and cartilage to survive extreme cold [16].

7.2 Human Involvement

Frostbite injury to the physis leads to premature fusion and abnormal growth without initial joint abnormality. Changes are manifest by irregularity, narrowing, and premature closure of physes, and eventually to irregular articular surfaces that may progress to premature degenerative arthrosis.

7.2.1 Clinical Aspects

In children, there is a striking lack of correlation between the extent of initial soft tissue injury and eventual skeletal changes. Brief exposure of the hands of very young children to temperatures of 0°–20°F (−29°C) cause second and third degree frostbite damage [3]. Longer exposure to air temperature of 8°F (−13°C) can also cause frostbite [13]. Exposure to low temperature above freezing does not cause bone damage [31]. Many patients do not seek medical attention for the initial injury. Weeks to months after the exposure the presenting complaint is joint swelling, pain, stiffness, and weakness of fingers. Subsequent loss of the fingernails occurs sometimes and is followed by nail regeneration [2, 20]. Late bony changes may not become apparent for months or years after the injury [7]. Growth of both the primary physis and the physis surrounding the secondary center of ossification are affected [7]. The physes at the distal ends of phalanges which have epiphyses, but no secondary center of ossification, are called acrophyses and are also affected [21]. Late sequelae include relative short, stubby fingers, skin redundancy, joint laxity, and mild flexion contractures [10, 15, 17, 30]. Loss of complete digits has also been recorded [13]. In cases that present late, knowledge of exposure to cold is the key to the correct diagnosis [13].

7.2.2 Imaging Evaluation

In the acute phase, roentgenography shows only soft tissue swelling and interstitial gas [18]. No bone or joint abnormalities are seen immediately after cold injury regardless of the severity of the injury [9]. Angiography reveals spasm in digital arteries without flow to the fingertips and decreased arteriovenous communications. Later, if the spasm is not reversed angiograms show digital vessels of normal caliber with tortuosity, "cork-screw-like changes," and no arteriovenous anastomoses [3, 19].

The characteristic roentgenographic osseous changes become apparent weeks to months post injury (Fig. 7.1a) [6, 8–10]. Bony changes include diffuse osteopenia with sclerosis, terminal tuft resorption, fragmentation and partial or complete disappearance of epiphyses, and premature fusion of physes [13, 18, 20, 28, 30]. The phalangeal shafts are widened. Physeal damage may occur without skin damage [1]. Initially the physes are thinned centrally [19], and there may be no obvious destruction of the epiphysis. The physis and epiphysis often have a V shape, reminiscent of similar findings in cases with vascular impairment of the central physis (cupping, Sect. 1.5) [22]. Later, premature fusion of part of the physis frequently leads to angular deformity. The affected phalanges are shorter and smaller than normal (Fig. 7.1b), and the juxta-articular bone is expanded and irregular, with a coarse cancellous spongiosa (Fig. 7.1c). The same expanded and irregular appearance is seen on the contiguous articular surface of the more proximal phalanx, where there is no secondary center of ossification [22]. Irregularity of articular surfaces may occasionally develop, predisposing to premature degenerative arthritis [1, 7, 8, 22, 25]. Bone fusion across a joint was noted in two children [28].

7.2.3 Differential Diagnosis

Differential diagnoses include epiphyseal dysplasias, premature osteoarthritis, premature physeal fusion following burns (Chap. 8), Volkmann's ischemia, a variety of dystrophies, Kirners deformity, and Thiemann's disease (usually bilateral, middle finger, and interphalangeal joints) [9, 12, 13, 15, 25].

7.2.4 Epidemiology

Frostbite in children most frequently involves the hands and is usually bilateral, but may be unilateral [2, 5, 8, 11, 14, 24, 25, 27, 28]. Necrosis of one or more physes may occur in 30% of established cases of frostbite [15]. Both genders are equally susceptible [15, 25]. Most of the affected children are less than 6 years old at the time of injury. Physes of the distal phalanges are the most commonly affected, and are always involved before the middle phalanges [1, 25]. There is a pattern of decreasing frequency from the distal to the proximal physes, except for one case where only the middle phalanx was involved [22]. Growth disturbance is most common in fingers of greatest exposure; the little, ring, and index fingers [20, 25]. In one study of 13 patients [5], the index and little fingers were involved in every frostbitten hand, the ring finger was slightly less often involved, and the middle finger was least often involved owing to its relatively protected position. In each digit, the distal phalanx was most often involved. The proximal phalanx was never involved if the distal phalanx of the same digit was also unaffected. Thumb, metacarpal, and carpal bones are rarely involved [3, 25]. The thumb is often held in the palm of the hand, is protected by the relatively large volume of tissue relative to surface area, has good circulation due to proximity of the radial artery, and therefore is rarely involved [6, 13, 15, 18, 23]. However, one study [10] recorded a patient with premature closure of all physes in one hand, distortion of the carpal anatomy, and closure of the distal radial and ulnar physes.

Fig. 7.1 A 9 year 10 month old boy sustained frostbite injury to his fingers of both hands when he pushed his bicycle home through snow in zero degree weather, gripping the steel handle bars without gloves. He was outdoors about 30 min. Upon reaching home his fingers were "blanched and white". His father rubbed his hands and placed them in cold water. Swelling of the hands "up to 3–4 times normal" occurred immediately, followed by the fingers turning red, then black. These changes subsided over the next 3 weeks. Eventually the skin of the fingers and one finger nail sloughed followed by the development of new pink skin and a new nail. The hands continued to be "sore and sensitive" and would ache intermittently. (**a**) Roentgenograms 7 months post injury were reported to show "epiphyseal sclerosis, fragmentation and destruction consistent with rheumatoid arthritis." Cortisone was given t.i.d. (dosage was in the "adult range") for 6 weeks, tapered to zero over 2 more weeks, without benefit. (**b**) At age 10 years 10 months, 1 year post injury the fingers were short and the interphalangeal joints were enlarged without tenderness or synovial swelling. The skin was normal. The grip was weak. Slight flexion of several interphalangeal joints could be passively extended to normal. (**c**) Roentgenograms revealed premature physeal closure of 11 physes of the distal and middle phalanges with malformation of epiphyses and irregularity of their articular surfaces. Roentgenograms of the feet were normal. The diagnosis of frostbite was made by combining the history, the physical examination, and the roentgenograms (From Wenzel, et al., [30] with permission)

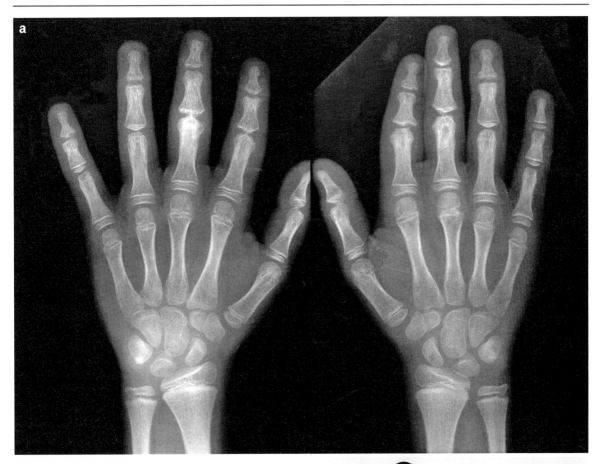
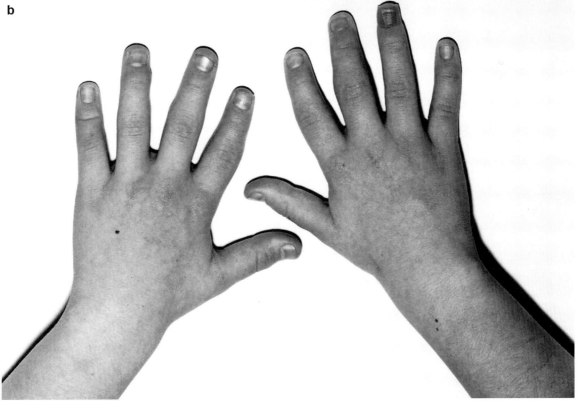

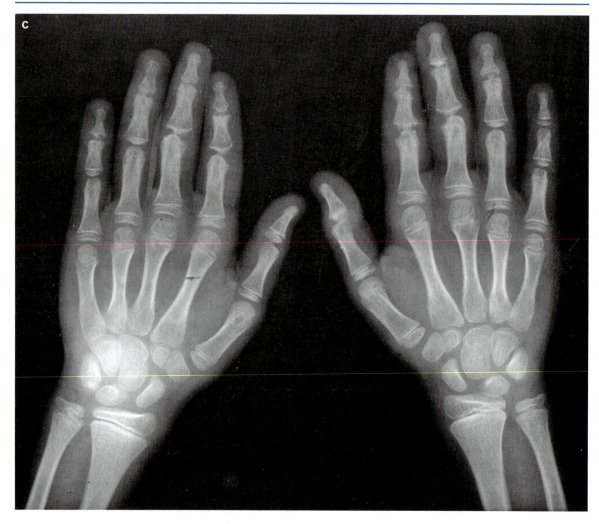

Fig. 7.1 (continued)

7.2.5 Pathological Mechanisms

Two theories of the mechanism of growth arrest secondary to frostbite have been proposed [4, 6–10, 15, 18, 20, 26]. The first is direct germinal cell chondrocyte injury due to the formation of intra- and extracellular ice crystals [3]. Since chondrocyte metabolism is largely glycolytic, this direct cellular injury may be more damaging than transient vascular insufficiency [3]. The relative absence of permanent detectable soft tissue ischemic changes supports this hypothesis [17].

The second theory is that exposure to cold causes ischemic-anoxic vascular changes which in turn result in premature physeal closure, due to vascular deficiency as described in Chap. 1. Capillaries contract just before freezing and remain closed while the extremity is frozen [5, 22]. The ischemia may also be due to temporary occlusion of circulation by freezing of blood, or to mechanical obstruction by damaged vessels [2]. Severe cold produces microvascular failure with capillary venular blood flow obstruction and massive microthrombi causing chondrocyte and osteocyte death, particularly in zones without vascular circulation [3]. During thawing, perivascular edema resulting from increased capillary wall permeability increases extracapillary pressure, further augmenting capillary stasis. Agglutination of blood cells in the small vessels further obstructs circulation [22]. One 3 year old child was noted to lack bleeding when a finger was cut 16 months after frostbite [6].

The fact that roentgenographic evidence of physeal closure first becomes evident 6–8 months following cold exposure is compatible with either hypothesis (direct chondrocyte damage or vascular damage). The fact that the arrest is often central with peripheral recovery [22], causing cupping (Sect. 1.5), favors the avascular etiology theory. The fact that isolated arrest of the peripheral physis leaving the center of physis intact (which is more likely with direct cartilage exposure to cold) has not been reported, also favors the vascular hypothesis. The vascular system also plays an important role in the recovery process following freezing injury. If recovery is to occur, it is of prime importance to maintain vascular integrity. Ogden [22] cites 13 references, both clinical and experimental, which favor the vascular hypothesis, and caused him to state that "frostbite may lead to growth retardation because of ischemia *rather than* a direct thermal effect on the physeal cartilage." The prevailing sentiment is that ischemia due to vascular occlusion plays the major role in physeal arrest [9, 29, 30].

7.2.6 Management

Supervision of young children is the best prophylaxis for frostbite. Early treatment is directed at decreasing the ischemic effects by rapid rewarming to reestablish and maintain normal blood flow [3, 10, 15]. Rapid rewarming of the frozen extremity in warm water at a temperature of 103–107°F may preserve soft tissues and reduce damage to the physis [6, 7]. In adults with frostbite intra-arterial reserpine produces dramatic subsiding of vasospasm as evidenced by angiography, relief of clinical symptoms, and healing without tissue loss [14]. Interim management includes regular follow-up, and if necessary, oral analgesics and night splints to prevent or correct angular deformities [15]. Function of the hand generally remains satisfactory without surgery. Angular deformity due to premature partial physeal arrest may be treated by surgically arresting the remaining physis, or corrective osteotomy. Soft-tissue arthroplasty, tenorrhaphy, or interphalangeal arthrodesis may be performed as indicated [3, 7, 8, 15]. The finger changes are so insidious that most children adjust, and rarely request correction of deformities or other orthopedic treatment [5, 10, 17].

7.3 Animal Research

Multiple animal experiments have been conducted on several aspects of tissue freezing. Most research has dealt only with soft tissue damage. Research that studied the effects of cold on the physis includes: degree of cold causing physeal damage [31], duration of freezing to physeal growth retardation [31–33, 36], tourniquet on the extremity at the time of freezing [32], histologic effects on both cartilage cells and vascular structures supplying the cartilage cells, [31–33, 36] and cool storage of an amputated part prior to reimplantation [37]. One study [35], harvested proximal femora from immature rabbits, froze them, subjected them to shear forces producing fracture, and studied them histologically. No statistically significant difference was demonstrated between fresh and the frozen/thawed specimens in either histologic patterns or the shear load, or stress to failure. None of these experiments determined if growth arrest was due to direct physeal cell necrosis because of the cold, or due to indirect physeal cell death because of vascular ischemia.

The similarity between the vascular lesion in frostbite and burns is marked [34].

7.4 Author's Perspective

The physeal closure which occurs following frostbite has many similarities with the physeal closure noted in vascular ischemia (Chap. 1).

References

Human Involvement

1. Beatty E, Light TR, Belsole RJ, Ogden JA (1990) Wrist and hand skeletal injuries in children. Hand Clin 6:723–728
2. Bennett RB, Blount WP (1935) Destruction of epiphyses by freezing. J Am Med Assoc 105:661–662
3. Benoit PR (1988) Thermal injuries of the growth plate. In: Uhthoff HK, Wiley JJ (eds) Behavior of the growth plate. Raven, New York, pp 119–122
4. Bigelow DR (1959) Epiphyseal fusion after frostbite (Abstr.) J Bone Joint Surg 41B(4):881
5. Bigelow DR, Ritchie GW (1963) The effects of frostbite in childhood. J Bone Joint Surg 45B(1):122–131
6. Brown FE, Spiegel SK, Boyle EW Jr (1983) Digital deformity: an effect of frostbite in children. Pediatrics 71:955–959

7. Carrera GF, Kozin F, Flaherty L, McCarty DJ (1981) Radiographic changes in the hands following childhood frostbite injury. Skeletal Radiol 6:33–37
8. Carrera GF, Kozin F, McCarty DF (1979) Arthritis after frostbite injury in children. Arthritis Rheum 22:1082–1087
9. Crouch C, Smith LW (1990) Long-term sequelae of frostbite. Pediatr Radiol 20(5):365–366
10. Dowdle JA, Kleven LH, House JH, Thompson WW (1978) Frostbite – Effect on the juvenile hand. Orthop Trans 2:13
11. Dreyfuss JF, Glimcher MJ (1955) Epiphyseal injury following frostbite. N Engl J Med 253:1065–1068
12. Florkiewiez L, Kozlowski K (1962) Symmetrical epiphyseal destruction by frostbite. Arch Dis Child 37:51–52
13. Galloway H, Suh J, Parker S, Griffths H (1991) Frostbite. Orthopedics 14:198–200
14. Gralino BJ, Porter JM, Rösch J (1976) Angiography in the diagnosis and therapy of frostbite. Radiology 119:301–305
15. Hakstian RW (1972) Cold-induced digital epiphyseal necrosis in childhood (symmetric focal ischemic necrosis). Can J Surg 15:168–178
16. Harris WR (1959) Epiphyseal fusion after frostbite (Discussion). J Bone J Surg 41B(4):881
17. House JH, Fidler MD (1988) Frostbite of the hand. In: Green DP (ed) Operative hand surgery, vol 3, 2nd edn. Churchill-Livingstone, New York, pp 2165–2174
18. Kao SCS, Smith WL (1997) Skeletal injuries in the pediatric patient. Radiol Clin North Am 35(3):727–746
19. Lindhholm A, Nilsson O, Svartholm F (1968) Epiphyseal destruction following frostbite. Report of three cases. Acta Chir Scand 134:37–40
20. Nakazato T, Ogino T (1986) Epiphyseal destruction of children's hands after frostbite: a report of two cases. J Hand Surg 11A:289–292
21. Oestreich AE (2000) Pediatric arthroses as a sequelae of enchondral damage. Examples of frostbite, Kashin-Beck disease, rat bites and other etiologies [*German*]. Radiologe 40(12):1149–1153
22. Ogden JA (2000) Injury to the growth mechanisms. In: Ogden JA (ed) Skeletal injury in the child, 3rd edn. Springer, New York, pp 178–179, 182
23. Poznanski AK (1978) Annual oration: diagnostic clues in the growing ends of long bones. J Can Assoc Radiol 29:7–21
24. Rang M (1983) Growth-plate injuries. In: Rang M (ed) Children's fractures, 2nd edn. Lippincott, Philadelphia, p 19
25. Reed MA (1988) Growth disturbances in the hand following thermal injuries in children. J Can Assoc Radiol 39:95–98
26. Selke SC (1969) Destruction of phalangeal epiphyses by frostbite. Radiology 93(4):859–860
27. Thelander HE (1950) Epiphyseal destruction by frostbite. J Pediatr 36:105–106
28. Tischler JM (1972) The soft-tissue and bone changes in frostbite injuries. Radiology 102:511–513
29. Townsend RG (1959) Epiphyseal fusion after frostbite (Discussion). J Bone Joint Surg 41B(4):881
30. Wenzel JE, Burke EC, Bianco AJ Jr (1967) Epiphyseal destruction from frostbite of the hands. Am J Dis Child 114:668–670

Animal Research

31. Bierens de Haan B, Wexler MR, Porat S, Nyska A, Teitelbaum A (1986) The effects of cold upon bone growth: a preliminary study. Ann Plast Surg 16(6):509–516
32. Bigelow DR, Hamonic MJ (1966) Effects of immersing freezing of foreleg epiphyses of growing rabbits. Int Surg 45(6):659–668
33. Blaustein A, Siegler R (1954) Pathology of experimental frostbite. N Y State J Med 54:2968
34. Crismon JM, Fuhrman FA (1947) Studies on gangrene following cold injury. VIII. The use of casts and pressure dressings in the treatment of severe frostbite. J Clin Invest 26:486
35. Lee KE, Pelker RR (1985) Effect of freezing on histologic and biomechanical failure patterns in the rabbit capital femoral growth plate. J Orthop Res 3:514–515
36. Scow RO (1949) Destruction of cartilage cells in the newborn rat by brief refrigeration, with consequent skeletal deformities. Am J Pathol 25:143–153
37. Sunagawa T, Ishida O, Ikuta Y, Yasunaga Y, Ochi M (2005) Role of simple cold storage in preventing epiphyseal growth plate impairment after replantation surgery in immature rats. J Reconstr Microsurg 21:483–489

Heat Injury (Burns)

8.1 Introduction

Five types of burns affect children: flame, hot objects, boiling water (scald), electric, and chemical. House fires are responsible for the majority of severe burns, ranking third as a cause of accidental death in children, behind motor vehicle accidents and drowning. Non-fatal burns are more frequent in children less than 5 years of age, and flame, contact with a hot surface, and water scalds are the most common causes [13]. Electrical devices which have components hot enough to produce a burn are reviewed here. Electricity involving high voltage current through the body is reviewed in Chap. 9. Burns in survivors sufficient to arrest a physis are uncommon.

8.2 Human Involvement

8.2.1 Clinical Aspects

Heat injuries that involve physes are most often in areas unprotected by clothes, such as phalanges and metacarpals of the hand [4, 12, 14, 17]. In contradistinction to cold injury, burned hands are rarely bilateral. Burns about the foot and ankle [5–7, 12] as well as burns over large areas of the limbs and trunk can result in a limb angular deformity and length discrepancy.

The most common roentgenographic finding in burned hands of children is premature physeal closure, followed by joint contractures, dislocations, amputations, joint ankylosis, and periosteal new bone formation [14]. One review of five cases in the hand [14] noted physeal arrests in all cases, but with no evidence of physeal tissue destruction. In one patient, all of the physes in the hand closed prematurely. The reviewers concluded that "the epiphyses simply seemed to develop at an accelerated rate and fuse prematurely".

In addition to random physeal arrest from direct burn, decreased overall height has been found in children who have over 40% total body surface area burn [18]. Profound decreased growth velocity was noted during postburn year 1, which slowly resolved to near normal by postburn year 3. The cause of this phenomenon remains unknown.

8.2.2 Pathological Mechanism

The mechanism causing physeal damage in severely burned limbs is not well understood [15]. Because physeal cartilage is more sensitive than articular cartilage to irradiation and cold, it may also be more sensitive to heat [12]. There may be several mechanisms:

(1) The physis may sustain direct thermal damage [3]. If the burn is deep enough to involve bone, direct heat necrosis of the physis can occur. Initially hyperemia may cause advanced physeal development, followed by premature fusion [9]. The peripheral zone of Ranvier, being more superficial, is more readily subject to the effects of heat [15]. Central closure is less likely to occur [15]. Thus, peripheral physeal closure causing an excentric bar and angular deformity is common (Fig. 8.1) [4, 12, 15].

(2) The physis is also vulnerable to prolonged ischemia secondary to burn necrosis of vessels, and from massive fluid transudation and compartment syndromes.

8.2.3 Management

Recombinant human growth hormone (rhGH) has been shown to accelerate burn wound healing, increase muscle mass, and enhance immune functions when administered during the acute postburn phase. One study of 32 children with third degree burns greater than 40% of the body, showed that rhGH given during the acute postburn phase has a long-term beneficial effect on height gain during the rehabilitation period [2]. The study lasted only 18 months post burn, and did not evaluate selected physes relative to their proximity to the burn. Whether the rhGH has a direct effect in protecting individual physes in severely burned areas is unknown.

Growing children who sustain severe burns must be carefully observed until growth is complete in anticipation of possible latent growth retardation [6, 7, 17, 19]. Partial physeal closures can be treated with arrest of the remaining physeal or osteotomy [8]. Bar excision has been proposed [8], but only one case (without follow-up) has been recorded [20]. Complete arrests can be treated with contralateral physeal arrests and bone shortening, and/or ipsilateral bone lengthening as needed and as feasible [8]. One 2 year old boy developed "burn contractures" on the lateral side of the knee and thigh from "electrical treatments" resulting in scar tissue which caused a flexion and valgus deformity of the knee [1]. Over the next 13 years he underwent 15 operations, including pedicle soft tissue grafts, four corrective osteotomies of the distal femur, and medial staple and Phemister physeal arrests. At age 14 years 7 months the limb length discrepancy of 9 cm was treated with contralateral femoral shortening. The author concluded that the diminished physeal growth posterolaterally was due to pressure applied by the scar tissue (Hueter-Volkmann Law) [1]. Total destruction and sequestion of a knee epiphysis resulted in a Van Nes rotationplasty (Fig. 4.20) in one 4 year old child [10].

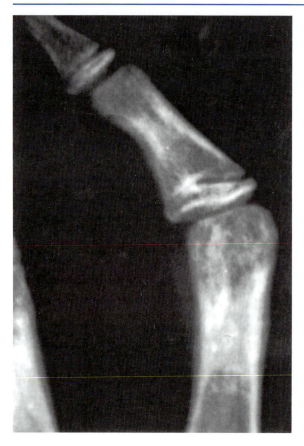

Fig. 8.1 Peripheral physeal bar in the second finger proximal phalanx in a 12 year old girl 8 years following a flame burn sustained at age 4 years. The physeal bar could be due to (a) the burn directly on the physis, (b) soft tissue scarring causing localized vascular insufficiency, or (c) scaring with tethering of ligaments, tendons, and joint capsule [Case contributed by J. de Pablos, Pamplona, Spain, with permission]

(3) Later, the restrictive or tethering effect of a contracted scar about the metaphysis and adjacent joint areas might inhibit physeal growth [1, 3, 5, 17, 19].
(4) Post burn heterotopic ossification bridging or blocking a joint may indirectly restrict physeal growth [3, 5].
(5) Burns also predispose to osteomyelitis with secondary growth arrest [7, 16].
(6) In addition, severely burned children can show growth impairment up to 3 years after the burn due to multiple factors, including disuse from immobilization, malnutrition, renal failure, and theoretically from increased production of endogenous corticosteroids and various cytokines, hypophosphatemia, and gonadal dysfunction [11]. The elbow, shoulder, and hip are particularly predisposed to this process of immobility [3].

8.3 Animal Research

There is a surprising paucity of animal experimental study correlating type, degree, and duration of heat with impairment of growth of individual physes.

One study applied burn injuries to anesthetized immature rats by immersing one hind limb in heated water (88°C) for 8 s [23]. The animals received no further treatment and no dressings were applied to the heated leg. The animals were sacrificed on day 21 post burn treatment. The longitudinal growth rate, growth plate thickness, and physeal cell production were greater in the burn-treated than in the non-burned bones. This correlated with some observations of initial acceleration of growth following burns in children, but gives no indication of the long term effects.

Another study evaluated the use of hyperthermia, as a treatment of cancer, administered alone or combined with radiotherapy in immature rats [21]. The rate at which growth stunting was caused by heat alone, or by radiation potentiated by heat, was the same. The two forms of stunting were therefore difficult to separate, although the effect of direct thermal damage was noted to occur earlier.

In a third study a small carbon resistor (7.0 × 1.5 mm) was placed in ulnar epiphyses of rabbits and connected to a 1.8 V lightweight accumulator [22]. The period of heating ranged from 4 to 31 days at a level of 70–200 mW. As the heat increased degenerative changes appeared in the physis and growth of the ulna was impaired.

8.4 Author's Perspective

It appears that the mechanism of physeal arrest from burns may be twofold. A significant burn localized near an area of a physis, resulting in peripheral partial arrest and angular deformity within a short time, is possibly due to direct damage to the peripheral physeal cartilage cells. Cases with more widespread burn that develop soft tissue scarring, contractures and total growth arrest of one or more physes over a more protracted time are more likely due to vascular impairment associated with scarring, immobility, and disuse.

References

Human Involvement

1. Ahstrom JP (1965) Epiphyseal injuries of the lower extremity. Surg Clin North Am 1:119–134
2. Ali Low JF, Jeschke MG, Barrow RE, Herndon DN (1999) Growth hormone prevents delay in height development in burned children. Proceedings, Shrine Surgeons Association Meeting, Tampa, Florida, 11–14.
3. Benoit RR (1988) Thermal injuries of the growth plate. In: Uhthoff HK, Wiley JJ (eds) Behavior of the growth plate. Raven, New York, pp 119–122
4. Bruguera JA, Alfaro C, de Pablos J (1993) Detection of physeal dysfunction by imaging techniques. Mapfre Medicina 4(suppl 2):14–23
5. Evans EB, Smith JR (1959) Bone and joint changes following burns. A roentgenographic study - preliminary report. J Bone Joint Surg 41A:785–799
6. Frantz CH, Delgado S (1966) Limb-length discrepancy after third-degree burns about the foot and ankle. Report of four cases. J Bone Joint Surg 48A:443–450
7. Gelfand DW, Law EJ, MacMillan BG (1971) The radiographic assessment of skeletal pathology in severely burned children: a review of 250 cases. In: Matter P, Barclay TL, Konickova Z (eds) Transactions of the third International Congress of research in burns. Hans Huber Publishers, Bern, pp 636–639
8. Jackson DM (1980) Destructive burns: some orthopaedic complications. Burns 7(2):105–122
9. Kao SCS, Smith WL (1997) Skeletal injuries in the pediatric patient. Radiol Clin North Am 35(3):727–746
10. Khatri B, Richard B (2000) Use of Van Nes rotationplasty to manage a burnt knee. Burns 26(1):88–91
11. Klein GL, Herndon DN, Rutan TC, Sherrard DJ, Cobern JW, Langman CB et al (1993) Bone disease in burn patients. J Bone Miner Res 8:337–345
12. Kumar D, Papini R, Tillman RM (2001) Partial growth plate fusion caused by a burn. Burns 27:664–667
13. Melhorn JM, Horner RL (1987) Burns of the upper extremity in children: long-term evaluation and function following treatment. J Pediatr Orthop 7:563–567
14. Mooney WR, Reed MH (1988) Growth disturbance in the hands following thermal injuries in children. Can Assoc Radiol J 39:91–94
15. Ogden JA (2000) Injury to the growth mechanisms. In: Ogden JA (ed) Skeletal injury in the child, 3rd edn. Springer, New York, pp 182–184, Chapter 6
16. Ogden JA (1979) Pediatric osteomyelitis and septic arthritis: the pathology of neonatal disease. Yale J Biol Med 52(5):423–445
17. Olney DB (1983) A review of the long term results of electric bar fire burns of the hand in children. Hand 15(2):179–184
18. Rutan RL, Herndon DN (1990) Growth delay in postburn pediatric patients. Arch Surg 125:392–395
19. Van Demark RE (1957) Burned hands in infants. SD J Med Pharm 10:1–3
20. Vickers DW (1980) Premature incomplete fusion of the growth plate: causes and treatment by resection (physolysis) in fifteen cases. Aust N Z J Surg 50(4):393–401

Animal Research

21. Myers R, Robinson JE, Field SB (1980) The relationship between heating time and temperature for inhibition of growth in baby rat cartilage by combined hyperthermia and x-rays. Int J Radiat Biol 38(4):373–382
22. Ring PA, Lee J (1958) The effect of heat upon the growth of bone. J Pathol Bacteriol 75(2):405–412
23. Schaffler MB, Li XJ, Jee WSS, Ho SWW, Stern PJ (1988) Skeletal tissue responses to thermal injury: an experimental study. Bone 9:397–406

Electric Injuries

9.1 Introduction

Electrical injuries produce both direct contact burns and thermal injury due to the heat generated by the resistance of tissue to the passage of the current. The damage to tissue results from heat produced by the conversion of electric energy to thermal energy in accordance with Ohms and Joules laws [6]. Direct contact with "hot" wires which cause surface burns is discussed in Chap. 8. This chapter considers the damage to deep tissues. The unique properties of electrical forces propagated through the extremities causes localized, highly variable, injury to the physis that may result in premature slowdown of growth and eventual arrest in focal areas [9]. Surprisingly little has been written about electrical injuries to bone and cartilage in children, especially those which produce delayed changes. Electrical injury resulting in physeal arrest is rare.

9.2 Electric Current

9.2.1 Clinical Aspects

Children subjected to electric current show osseous changes similar to those in adults, but may also have additional abnormalities secondary to the effect of the current on physeal cartilage [3, 10]. The epiphyseal center and physeal cartilage may be affected by the current, and the metaphyseal region remodels poorly. Permanent physeal damage has resulted in growth disturbance in children [8]. Three cases are reported in which electrical accidents resulted in extensive soft tissue burns requiring amputations of phalanges [3]. In these cases, several of the remaining phalanges showed abnormal elongation. The authors speculated that the overgrowth was secondary to chronic hyperemia resulting from the soft tissue injury and accompanying infection. Two cases of electrical injury which required below knee amputations were followed by premature physeal closure of the proximal tibial physes [10].

9.2.2 Roentgenographic Studies

Many victims of electric injury are not examined roentgenographically, perhaps because more obvious soft tissue injuries demand prompt attention. Often the first roentgenographic studies of electrically injured limbs are performed weeks, months, or years after the accident. Most of the reported late bone changes are in adults, and include bone rarefaction, mottled decalcification, fractures, and fragmentation [3]. The most complete report in children is by Ogden and Southwick [10], who report physeal thinness, severe damage, and bridging.

9.2.3 Pathological Mechanism

Multiple factors determine the effects of electric current on chondro-osseous tissue: (1) type of current, with alternating current being 3–4 times more destructive than direct current; (2) voltage, (3) amperage, (4) duration of contact with electric current, (5) the path taken through the body, (6) the resistance at the points of contact and exit, (7) points of entrance and exit, (8) atmospheric conditions, and (9) the individual's general state of health [3]. Changes specific to the physis following electrical injury may result from several possible mechanisms, most of which are not well understood [2, 10].

In a typical electrical injury, the current enters the body through the hand or wrist, traverses the arm and torso, and leaves through the legs and feet. Current density is greatest at the points of entry and exit. The skin is characteristically burned and charred at the entry area, and to a lesser extent at the exit site. Once the current enters the body, it spreads along the path of least resistance, into tissues of optimal conductivity, preferentially along neurovascular pathways. The greatest damage is produced in the tissues offering the greatest resistance. The common result is the disruption of the vascular endothelium and subsequent thrombosis. In general, bone is a poor conductor and does not carry much current; hence bone damage other than charring at the site of current entry tends to be indirect and delayed [1].

The primary damage associated with electrical injury is due to heat. During electrical accidents, tissue temperatures may momentarily reach several thousand degrees celsius or centigrade and may cause heat-induced liquefaction and necrosis of cartilage and bone. The extreme temperatures of high voltage transmission may acutely coagulate blood vessels, producing necrosis of small vessels near the physis. Electrical injury may result in cell death or may alter cellular activity either temporarily or permanently [6]. After electrical accidents, tissue repair, including callus formation, is poor. The most conspicuous damage is usually due to thermal burns, but coagulation of nearby tissues is characteristic of electrical injury.

Chronic effects include vascular disturbances with progressive thrombosis and fragility of small vessels [10]. Ischemic contractures and paralysis are frequent end stages [1]. Late bone damage is based mostly on ischemia. Extensive infarction may develop. Since the juxtaphyseal region is especially well vascularized, it is predisposed to this process.

Five experiments have been performed in attempts to either stimulate or curtail physeal growth by electrical means [2, 4, 7, 11, 12]. Experiments on rats and rabbits, attempting to accelerate growth [2, 4, 7, 12] showed either equivocal [2, 4, 12] or negative [7] results. An experiment on rabbits and dogs showed that 40 mV electrocautery, applied directly into the physis by needle for 10 seconds, demonstrated histologically proven progressive physeal narrowing and eventual closure [11]. Another study on rabbits using a high current (50 microA) delivered by a titanium electrode into a single location in the distal femoral physis caused changes in the physis volume and architecture sufficient to cause physeal arrest [5].

In summary, the mechanism of damage to the physis from electrical injury is multifactorial. The physis may be damaged directly by electrocoagulation, secondarily rendered ischemic by damage to the epiphyseal circulation, or rendered incapable of enchondral transformation by disruption of the metaphyseal circulation [10]. Electrical injuries are also frequently accompanied by infection (Chap. 3) and disuse (Chap. 2), which can negatively affect the physis. The theory that electrical current injury may result in direct alteration of physeal cell activity or death has been described [10], but apparently never studied histologically.

More basic research is needed to understand the modifications occurring in developing chondro-osseous physiology and structure as a result of electrical trauma [1, 4, 10, 12].

9.2.4 Management

Once initial resuscitative efforts have succeeded, care for most electrically injured patients centers around reconstructive surgery of soft tissue damage. Little attention has been paid to concomitant late osseous injuries. The child must be followed closely to assess skeletal growth and development. There is only one report of excision of a physeal bar due to electrical injury, and this case had no follow-up [13].

9.3 Lightning

Survival following electrical injury by lightning strike is rare, particularly in children. Reported overall lightning death rates vary in different countries from 0.2 to 1.7 per million population per year.

One survivor who subsequently developed growth arrests has been reported [14]. A 10 year 0 month old girl was struck by lightning while walking in the rain carrying an umbrella in her right hand. A younger brother walking with her died on the scene. On arrival in the emergency room, she was conscious and oriented, with normal vital signs, cardiac and respiratory function, and electrocardiogram. She sustained a third degree burn measuring 9 × 16 cm over the lateral aspect of her right upper arm, and first degree burns of the right flank and abdomen. A digital wrist watch on her right wrist was still working. There was swelling and venous congestion below both knees, with blisters involving all toes. Neurologic examination revealed paralysis and areflexia below the knees. Bilateral leg compartment syndromes confirmed by myoglobinuria and rhabdomyolysis were treated by four compartment fasciotomies 4 h after admission. Excision of the third degree burn on her right arm was treated with split skin grafts on the ninth day. She started walking on day 17 and was discharged 21 days after injury. At age 12 years 2 months, 2 years 2 months post injury she was found to have mild thoracolumbar scoliosis and bilateral knee deformities secondary to premature partial arrest of the both proximal tibial physes medially, and the right femoral physis laterally. No further follow-up was given. The authors concluded that the electric current flowed between her right shoulder and grounded through both lower limbs. They attributed the physeal injuries to be "the result of direct electrical, heat, or ischemic injury, or a combination of these factors."

A second case has also been illustrated [9]. A lateral roentgenogram of the knee of a girl struck by lightning shows enlargement of the anterior epiphysis of the distal femur causing patellofemoral irregularity. The abnormality was attributed to "damage" to the anterior distal femoral growth plate. No other details or follow-up of this case were given.

9.4 Diathermy, Microwave

Diathermy is the generation of heat in body tissues due to resistance offered by the tissues to the passage of high frequency electric currents. Short wave diathermy is the use of an oscillating electric current of high frequency. Frequencies vary from 10 million to 100 million cycles per second and wave lengths from 30 to 3 m. Ultrashort wave diathermy uses a wavelength of less than 10 m. In medical diathermy, or thermopenetration, tissues are warmed to a point short of tissue destruction. In surgical diathermy the heat is sufficient to coagulate cells and destroy tissue. These injuries are sometimes called a "burn", i.e., an electrical burn.

Extensive disturbance in bone growth has been reported following diathermy treatments in two children [19]. Both children developed deep cutaneous burns, and physeal arrests at sites other than the burns. A probable third case was recorded in a 5½ week old boy who had been treated by a chiropractor who used "electrical treatments" [15]. A severe burn on the lateral side of the knee and thigh resulted in physeal arrest of the distal femoral physis laterally. Since the arrest occurred at the site of the burn, the case is reported in detail in Chap. 8. Mention of the case is made here because the "electrical treatments" were likely diathermy. Intraoperative microwave heat treatment has been used on children with primary malignant bone tumors as an alternative to replacement by prosthesis or allografting techniques. Heating tumor-bearing bone at 50°C for 15 min resulted in separation of an adjacent epiphysis in 1 of 16 patients [18].

In rats short wave (8 m) and microwave (11 cm) diathermy applied for varying intervals of time produced partial or complete physeal destruction [19]. Diminished growth was found only in the rats where the diathermy produced soft tissue changes, such as "swelling, muscle spasm, ulceration, etc." The relative bone shortening did not necessarily parallel the extent of soft tissue injury. The abnormal histologic changes showed cystic changes, marked distortion, fibrillar degeneration, and contraction of the physis, depending on the voltage and duration of the treatment. Short wave diathermy (27.120 kilocycles for a total of 25 h) has also been used in rats to stimulate longitudinal bone growth [16]. In dogs microwave diathermy at 100 W for a total of 100 h had no effect on the rate of growth [17]. These differences in results are likely due to differences in application of the insult.

9.5 Author's Perspective

Conclusions drawn from these reports include the need to create and maintain safe electrical sources, the instruction of parents and children in their hazards, the avoidance of unnecessary exposure to lightening, and the avoidance of indiscriminate use of diathermy in children.

References

Electrical Current

1. Barber JW (1971) Delayed bone and joint changes following electrical injury. Radiology 99:49–53
2. Brighton CT, Cronkey JE, Osterman AL (1976) In vitro epiphyseal-plate growth in various constant electrical fields. J Bone Joint Surg 58A(7):971–977

3. Brinn LB, Moseley JE (1966) Bone changes following electrical injury: case report and review of literature. Am J Roentgenol Radium Ther Nucl Med 97:682–686
4. Ciombor DM, Aaron RK (1993) Influence of electromagnetic fields on endochondral bone formation. J Cell Biochem 52(1):37–41
5. Dodge GR, Bowen JR, Oh CW, Tokmakova K, Simon BJ, Aroojis A, Potter K (2007) Electrical stimulation of the growth plate: a potential approach to an epiphysiodesis. Bioelectromagnetics 28(6):463–470
6. Duffner DW (1982) Management of electroshock injury. Orthop Rev 11(5):57–66
7. Granberry WM, Janes JM (1963) The effect of electrical current on the epiphyseal cartilage: a preliminary experimental study. Proc Staff Meet Mayo Clin 38:87–95
8. Kolar J, Vrabec R (1960) Roentgenological bone findings after high tension accidents [*German*]. Fortschr Geb Rontgenstr 92(4):385–394
9. Ogden JA (2000) Injury to the growth mechanisms. In: Ogden JA (ed) Skeletal injury in the child, 3rd edn. Springer, New York, pp 176–178, 181
10. Ogden JA, Southwick WO (1981) Electrical injury involving the immature skeleton. Skeletal Radiol 6:187–192
11. Rosen MA, Beer KJ, Wiater JP, Davidson DD (1990) Epiphysiodesis by electrocautery in the rabbit and dog. Clin Orthop 256:244–253
12. Takei N, Akai M (1993) Effect of direct current stimulation on triradiate physeal cartilage. In vivo study in young rabbits. Arch Orthop Trauma Surg 112:159–162
13. Vickers DW (1980) Premature incomplete fusion of the growth plate: causes and treatment by resection (physiolysis) in 15 cases. Aust N Z J Surg 50:393–401

Lightning

14. Lim JK, Lee EH, Chhem RK (2001) Physeal injury in a lightning strike survivor. J Pediatr Orthop 21(5):608–612

Diathermy, Microwave

15. Ahstrom JP (1965) Epiphyseal injuries of the lower extremity. Surg Clin North Am 1:119–134
16. Doyle JR, Smart BW (1963) Stimulation of bone growth by short-wave diathermy. J Bone Joint Surg 45A(1):15–24
17. Granberry W, Janes JM (1963) The lack of effect of microwave diathermy on rate of growth of bone of the growing dog. J Bone Joint Surg 45A(4):773–777
18. Lu S, Wang J, Hu Y (1996) Limb salvage in primary malignant bone tumors by intraoperative microwave heat treatment. Chin Med J (Engl) 109(6):432–436
19. Wise CS, Castleman B, Watkins A (1949) Effect of diathermy (short wave and microwave) on bone growth in the albino rat. J Bone Joint Surg 31A:487–500

Compression

10.1 Introduction

The verb compress means to press together or force into less space. The noun compression is the act of compressing. The Hueter-Volkmann Law of Growth Modulation basically states that increased pressure slows bone growth and that decreased pressure or mild distraction accelerates growth. Epiphyses are located at the ends of bones, transmit weight from one bone to another, and are often referred to as *pressure epiphyses*. Apophyses are usually located on the side of the metaphysis, serve as attachments for tendons, and are called *traction epiphyses*.

The physis requires a certain physiologic pressure in order to grow normally. But little is known concerning the role of normal pressure on the physis as it relates to growth. There must be considerable differences of pressure applied to physes of the upper and lower extremities. Does the femur become longer than the humerus, and the lower leg longer than the forearm, because of weight bearing? Are the hind legs and fore legs of quadrupeds of similar length because they bear equal weight? Are the arms of some apes longer because they bear weight? Do human lumbar vertebrae grow larger than thoracic and cervical vertebrae because they are subjected to greater weight?

For the purpose of discussion in this chapter, compression is the application of abnormally increased pressure on the physis. Compression may be applied continuously (Sects. 10.2 and 10.3) or acutely (Sects. 10.4 and 10.5).

10.2 Continuous Compression – Human Involvement

Continuous increased pressure sustained over time has an inhibiting effect on growth of the physis. A physeal growth force response curve illustrates how longitudinal physeal growth responds to compression loads [9]. Beginning at zero load, mild increased loads stimulate growth. Further increases in compression suppress growth. Large compression loads stop growth.

10.2.1 Pathophysiologic Mechanism of Injury

Two theories of physeal arrest due to sustained compression have been proposed. The first theory proposes that as pressure mounts within the physeal plate the production of new cartilage cells at the germinal layer is inhibited [4, 5]. There is considerable reduction in width of the proliferating cell zone and progressive disorganization of chondrocytes within the columnar cell zone [2]. With no new cells forming, the physis becomes gradually narrower as a result of metaphyseal bone replacement of normally transformed cartilage cells.

The second theory proposes that when increased pressure across the physis is sustained, blood flow to the physis is diminished [3]. The earliest response to pressure is ischemia of the metaphyseal vasculature which reduces removal of the hypertrophic cells. As the normal germinal cells continue to proliferate, the physis widens [6] (Fig. 1.3). If the compression is continued over long periods or at increasing magnitudes, the blood supply to the epiphysis is also compromised leading to death of the germinal and proliferative cell zones (Fig 1.6) [3]. The result is physeal narrowing followed by closure.

Interference to growth is directly proportional to the magnitude and duration of the compression, and is fully reversible as long as the epiphyseal vasculature to the physis remains viable. To oppose and eventually stop growth, the compression force applied must be of the order of several hundred grams per square centimeter [3]. Unfortunately, normal forces on the physes have not been measured. Therefore it is difficult to compare the effect of forces on physeal cells with disturbances in vascularity [1].

Continuous compression may be applied actively or passively.

10.2.2 Continuous Active Compression

Active compression is the process of applying controlled, sustained, static or increasing pressure on the physis. Several examples exist.

10.2.2.1 Elastic Compression
Two metallic pins, placed parallel across the metaphysis and epiphysis, are joined externally by elastic bands [7]. This method was reported to intentionally slow growth and arrest it completely. The author declared "the arrest may take 6–12 weeks." Drawings of the surgical technique were included, but no case studies, results, or follow-up have been reported.

10.2.2.2 Asymmetric Pressure
Asymmetric pressure on the physis may result from minor bone malalignment, abnormal muscle pull, joint laxity, or the application of corrective braces or casts. This may produce angular deformity by slowing the growth on the side of compression, according to the Hueter-Volkmann law of physeal growth [5].

The best example is varus-valgus alignment of the knee. Mild varus-valgus knee malalignments are common, tend to be bilateral, and usually respond to normal pressure forces during growth to gradually produce physes and joint alignments almost perpendicular to the longitudinal axis of the bone. These normal pressure forces correct small malalignments, but makes large malalignments worse [3, 9]. Unilateral knee malalignment is usually associated with specific conditions such as metaphyseal dysplasia, infection, tumors, neuromuscular disorders, fibula hemimelia, congenital short femur, etc. These malalignments are often greater in degree and gradually progressive. Partial physeal arrests of a knee physis, for example the distal femur, may be severe enough to produce compensatory corrective asymmetric growth of the proximal tibial physis, sufficient to require osteotomy of both the femur and the tibia [8].

Hip disease involving coxa vara is often associated with genu valgum which may require corrective surgery of both the hip and the knee [10]. Blount's disease, a severe form of proximal tibial asymmetric physeal growth is often suspected to be due to asymmetric pressure (Sect. 19.2).

10.2.2.3 Muscle Pull
Alteration of normal physiologic conditions, for example muscle pull, can produce different pressure effects on growth rates and recognizable deformities. An example of increased muscle tension is recurrent vigorous muscle spasms. Spasms sufficient to apply uneven pressure on the adjacent physis have been proposed as the cause of gradual angular deformity and even slipped epiphyses in children with Satoyoski's syndrome [11].

10.2.2.4 Bone Lengthening
During surgical bone lengthening increasing tension in the non- lengthened musculotendinous structures across the adjacent joint subjects the physes to increasing pressure. There is a direct correlation between the pressure and the amount of subsequent growth [13]. Premature physeal arrest of the bone being lengthened has been attributed to this increasing pressure [14]. Femoral and tibial lengthenings less than 14% of their original length have no significant growth retardation [19]. However lengthenings which exceed 20% of their original bone length usually result in physeal arrest of the bone being lengthened [19]. One study noted only slight change of growth velocity, which was not clinically significant, if the lengthening was performed after 9 years of age [12]. Another study noted no growth inhibition of isolated femoral or tibial lengthenings in children less than 6 years of age, whereas simultaneous lengthenings of the femur and tibia or a second tibial lengthening within a year could lead to growth inhibition [15].

Patients with a congenitally short limb may be at more risk during bone lengthening because the musculo-tendinous structures are also congenitally short. One study noted a decreased growth rate of lengthened congenitally short tibiae from an average preoperative rate of 88% of normal, to an average rate of 64% of normal [17]. Thus, surgeons should consider overcorrection when lengthening congenitally short tibiae to compensate for expected growth retardation, or lengthening the tibia only near skeletal maturity to avoid post lengthening loss of correction due to growth of the contralateral tibia [17]. Children with total fibular hemimelica uniformly have complete growth retardation after tibial lengthening [18].

Four children, ages 2 to 4 years, who had 7 phalanges and 1 thumb metacarpal lengthened 2.0–3.5 cm have been reported [16]. The authors commented "where physeal plates have remained open, continuous growth has been experienced in the follow-up period." No details of the number of plates remaining open were provided.

10.2.2.5 Scoliosis

Compression of vertebral body physes on the concave side of the curve is a primary characteristic of idiopathic scoliosis. [4, 21] The rapid progress of scoliosis under gravitational forces of weight bearing, and relative control of progression of the curve by relief of this pressure (bracing and recumbency), are excellent examples of active pressure on the physis [5, 20]. The etiology of the initial malalignment to allow the uneven distribution of pressure in idiopathic scoliosis is unknown. Scoliosis following rib or chest wall resection is convex toward the side of rib resection, is related to the number of ribs resected, is progressive, and once initiated the physeal compression on the concave side occurs as in idiopathic scoliosis [22].

10.2.2.6 Kyphosis

Idiopathic kyphosis is a structural abnormality of unknown cause. Once the deformity becomes significant the increased pressure on the anterior portion of the vertebral physes accentuates the deformity. In the early stages of deformity brace treatment can be effective.

Post laminectomy kyphosis has been studied in more depth with regard to its relationship to compression. Bilateral complete vertebral laminectomy in growing children is accompanied by loss of the posterior tensile forces which resist forward flexion. The resulting kyphosis places pressure on the anterior portions of vertebral body physes which then tend to close early. As the physis continues to grow posteriorly the vertebrae become wedge shaped (Fig. 10.1) [22, 27]. Kyphosis occurs more often when the patient is young and when the laminectomy is more cephalad, in cervical and thoracic vertebrae (Fig. 10.2) [22, 24–28].

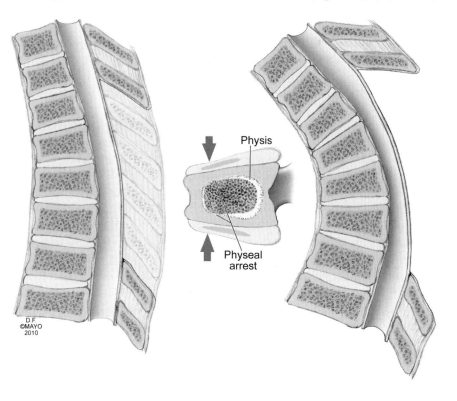

Fig. 10.1 Vertebral kyphosis secondary to anterior physis compression. *Left*: Normal growth of a vertebral body is essentially rectangular due to its global physis. *Middle* and *Right*: After multilevel laminectomy loss of the posterior supporting (tension) structures allows the pressure to shift anteriorly. Growth is inhibited anteriorly (*arrows*), but continues posteriorly resulting in vertebral body and disk wedging and kyphosis (Redrawn from Peterson [25], with permission)

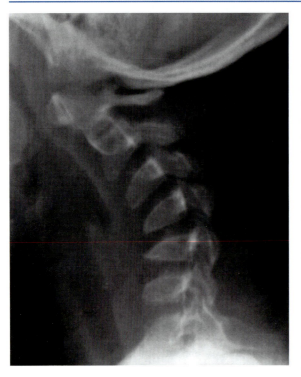

Fig. 10.2 Cervical spine kyphosis secondary to laminectomy. This boy had a normal cervical spine before laminectomy C2–C6 at age 10 years. At age 12 years 9 months the vertebral bodies are wedged anteriorly and there is mild subluxation of the facet joints (From Yasuoka et al. [27] with permission)

Laminectomy of lordotic lumbar vertebrae is much less likely to result in kyphosis [24]. Deformity may be first noted as late as 6 years post laminectomy [22, 25]. It may progress more rapidly during the adolescent growth spurt due to growth posteriorly [22, 25]. Bracing is ineffective in preventing progression of post laminectomy kyphosis [23, 25]. Surgical fusion of remaining structures (facet joints and transverse processes) with autogenous bone at the time laminectomy does not achieve as good stability as complete posterior fusion, but is frequently sufficient to prevent subsequent deformity [25]. If the deformity is significant, some combination of halo traction, anterior release and fusion, and posterior instrumentation and fusion may be necessary [23, 25–27].

Scheuermann's kyphosis, often called an osteochondrosis, is a developmental abnormality of the anterior portion of thoracic vertebral physes. The condition has many similarities to post-laminectomy kyphosis, except that brace treatment can be successful in the early stages.

10.2.2.7 Compression Force Applied to the Edge of the Physis on the Zone of Ranier

Whenever an immature hip is immobilized in wide abduction, e.g. in developmental dislocation of the hip, the acetabular labrum may press against the germinal cell layer of the physeal zone of Ranier of the femoral capital physis. Arrest of these cells laterally, along with normal growth medially causes coxa valga [29].

10.2.2.8 Slipped Capital Femoral Epiphysis

Among the many theories of etiology of slipped capital femoral epiphysis, as well as scoliosis, kyphosis, and Madelung's deformity, is one that states "a primary abnormality of the epiphyseal cartilage renders it susceptible to the effect of compression" [30].

10.2.3 Continuous Passive Compression

Passive compression is the process of rigid fixation of the epiphysis to the metaphysis, restraining the physis from growing (the "locked method"). Initially the fixation is devoid of pressure. As the germinal cells continue to multiply and expand they are "compressed" by their own increased volume.

10.2.3.1 Binding of Feet

In the not so ancient Chinese culture the feet of wealthy Chinese infant females were intentionally bound to prevent their growth. The miniature feet which were produced looked like lotus blossoms, a perceived object of beauty. Since the individual could not walk and had to be carried, bound feet were a status of wealth. The flat top talus following prolonged cast treatment for clubfoot is another example of physeal arrest due to continuous passive compression [4].

10.2.3.2 Tethering of the Physis by Soft-Tissue

Tethering of a portion of the periphery of the physis leads to angular deformity due to normal growth of the portion of the physis not tethered. It has been noted to occur in the distal femur [31, 33, 36], proximal tibia [36], distal ulna [33], and distal tibia [37]. The tether may be the periosteum [33, 36], or a fibrous band of "dense collagenous tissue" [31]. Sometimes the band appears to be limited to the metaphysis with no direct connection to the physis. These tethers are usually unilateral and the etiology is unknown. Occult trauma and a remnant of accessory muscle are speculated causes [31]. Osteotomy alone does not permanently correct the angular deformity. Surgical removal of the tether will allow the deformity to correct spontaneously, if enough growth remains [36].

With congenital absence of the fibula, the fibula is consistently replaced by a tight band of fibrous or fibrocartilaginous tissue lying posterolateral in the calf attached distally to the posterolateral aspect of the calcaneus [37]. The band is taut, firm, and inelastic and in some patients contains bits of cartilage or even bone. It is accompanied by shortening of the tibia and equinovalgus of the ankle. Excision of the band at an early age allows considerable, sometimes complete correction of the tibia.

Madelung's deformity has long been described as idiopathic physeal closure of the ulnar side of the distal radial physis in teenagers and has been called hereditary dischondrosis. It occurs more often in males than females and is twice as frequent bilaterally, usually with the same degree of severity on both sides [35]. Disagreements regarding the pathogenesis have resulted in numerous proposed etiologies [35]. Recent improvements in imaging have identified an abnormally stout ligamentous or fibrous cord-like structure attaching the ulnar side of the radial metaphysis to the lunate, sometimes called Vicker's ligament (Fig. 10.3) [32, 34, 39, 40]. Growth of the radial side of the physis results in increasing ulnar tilt of the distal radial epiphysis and articular surface. The lunate becomes wedged between the radial and ulna epiphyses [39, 40]. If the abnormal radiolunate ligament is discovered and excised before a physeal bar has formed in the radius, correction may occur spontaneously. MRI screening of young children in families with the causative gene should allow early detection of the abnormal ligament before a physeal bar and deformity appear [40]. Early excision of this ligament may have significant prophylactic potential [40]. Once a bar

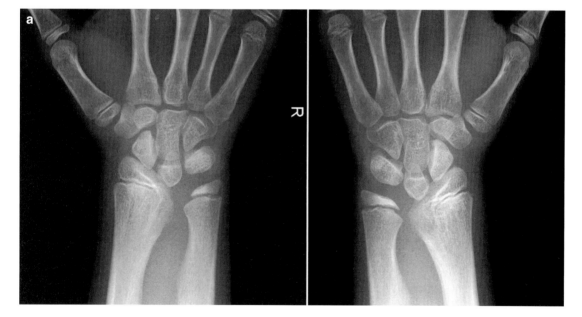

Fig. 10.3 Madelung's deformity secondary to soft tissue tether. (**a**) A 9 year 7 month old girl presented with bilateral wrist pain. Roentgenographs of both wrists show symmetric ulnar tilt of the distal radial articular surface, and a wedge shaped lunate located between the distal radio-ulnar diastasis. The ulnar side of the radial physis is not well visualized because of marked deformity of the epiphysis. There appears to be a physeal bar. (**b**) MRI shows an abnormal ligamentous structure extending from the lateral side of the distal radial metaphysis to the lunate (*arrows*) with notching of the distal radial metaphysis at the site of ligament attachment. (**c**) A more volar cut shows normal distal radial physis. (**d**) A transverse view also shows abnormality of the ulnar side of the distal radial metaphysis. (**e**) A more dorsal cut of the MRI, as well as (**b**) and (**c**) fail to show a physeal bar. *Note*: Knowledge of the pathology and sequence of events leading to premature physeal closure in Madelung's deformity would be greatly enhanced by a longitudinal case study beginning at a very early age continuing to maturity without intervening treatment. Since this would not be in the best interest of the patient such a case will be hard to find

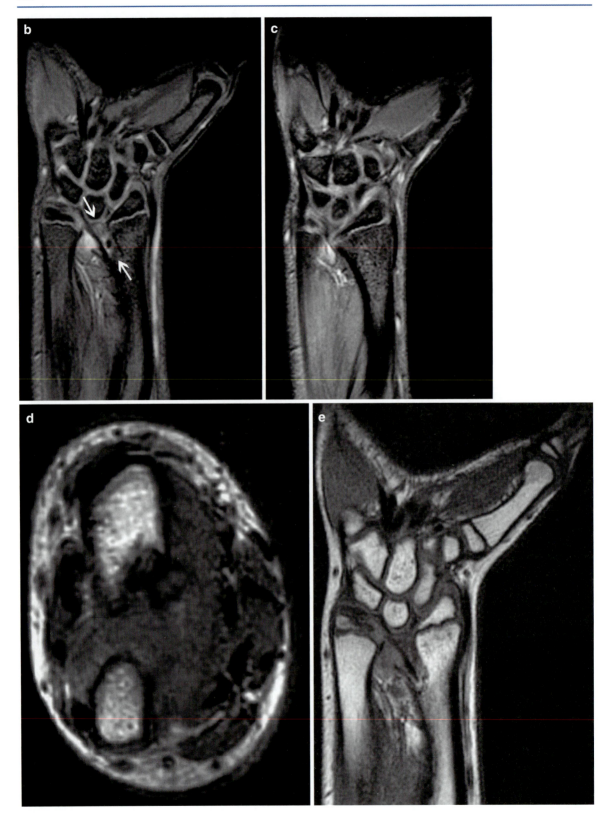

Fig. 10.3 (continued)

10.2 Continuous Compression – Human Involvement

forms, bar excision alone has been successful in restoring growth and correcting the deformity [32, 38, 40]. If the child is older and has a physeal bar, wedge resection of the bar and distracting the remaining open physis on the ulnar side will both correct the angular deformity and provide some length [34]. If deformity is discovered after closure of the entire physis, multiple procedures are available and necessary to correct the deformity [35].

10.2.3.3 Casts

Longitudinal physeal compression experienced from the use of serial casts to correct clubfoot, along with leg casts used postoperatively, has been incriminated as the cause of distal tibial premature physeal arrest [41] and may be associated with the small size of hind foot bones [42]. Disuse may be a factor (Chap. 2).

10.2.3.4 Wire Loops

Prior to the advent of staples, a wire loop constricting the physis was sometimes used to temporarily or permanently reduce growth on the longer bone [43]. Once the deformity or inequality of length was corrected the wire could be removed allowing growth to resume [43]. Wire breakage was a frequent complication (Fig. 10.4).

10.2.3.5 Staples

For over 50 years (1950–2000), the most commonly used procedure to achieve passive compression was the use of staples over the physis. When staples are first inserted they exert no pressure on the physis. The tines (legs) of the staples prevent the physis from expanding. As the germinal cells continue to multiply and expand they are compressed by their own volume. This achieves a controlled process of decelerating physeal growth [60]. The increasing force exerted by the physis against the staples is considerable. Based on deformation of staples at final examination, one study determined that the static equivalent loads exerted by the physes of the proximal tibia and distal femur were 0.5 kN per physis [52]. The estimated corresponding stress was 1 MPa. The authors concluded that successful lower limb staple hemiphyseodesis suppressed a longitudinally directed compression force on the order of body weight. Another study reported that the staples used in the 1950s "required about 450 pounds of traction to spread" [63].

Stapling is an exacting procedure [57, 58]. There is some risk involved when the technique is not precise [73]. Insertion is aided by fluoroscopy, and possibly by staples with grooved tines which are placed between wires inserted using a template [57]. To facilitate removal the surface of the staple legs should be smooth rather than rough or notched [48]. Unfortunately, smooth surface staples are also prone to extrude. The size of the staple depends on the patient age, width of the physis, and the size of the bone being operated.

Staples are used clinically in three situations; (a) to correct angular deformity, (b) to inhibit longitudinal

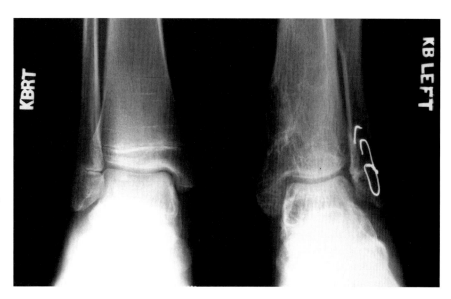

Fig. 10.4 This boy had a physeal bar excised from the left medial distal tibia at age 5 years 4 months. The bar excision was successful in reestablishing growth. At age 15 years 3 months there is slight overcorrection into ankle valgus, possibly associated with zealous use of a wire loop around the distal fibula physis. The operation was performed three times due to wire breakage (Reproduced from Peterson [44], with permission)

growth temporarily and (c) to stop longitudinal growth completely.

Correction of Angular Deformity
Angular deformity may be corrected by inserting staples over one exterior surface of the physis (hemiphyseodesis) allowing unilateral growth on the opposite side, causing a change in the angle of longitudinal growth. This is performed frequently at the knee to correct knock-knee (Fig. 4.13), bow leg, back-knee, flexion deformity, or combinations of these deformities [47–49, 53, 55–57, 59, 61, 64–66, 70, 71, 74, 76–78, 81–84]. The average age for inserting staples on one side to correct angular deformity is approximately 12 years in girls and 13 years 6 months for boys [56, 61]. The mechanical axis of the bone corrects to a physiologic range at an average of 12 months [61, 82], slightly faster in females, but is obviously dependent upon the degree of deformity and the growth rate of the child. When the deformity is corrected the staples are removed. If the child has reached maturity the staples may be left in permanently. Stapling should not be used on the shorter leg [45, 84]. Angular deformity of a bone shorter than its normal contralateral bone would be better treated by open-wedge osteotomy, which would gain a little length [79].

The advantage of stapling over permanent hemiphysiodesis to correct angular deformity is that it is an untimed procedure, can be used in younger children [53], and can be discontinued when the deformity is corrected. Restoring the mechanical axis of the bone to neutral by staples or 8-plates may improve the quality and appearance of the involved physes [89]. However, physeal behavior after staple removal is unpredictable [55]. Rebound growth following staple removal may allow recurrence of deformity and is more common in patients under 10 years of age. Stapling may be repeated for recurrent deformity [48, 70]. Staple loosening or dislocation occurs frequently in patients below age 7 years [77]. Other potential adverse outcomes include undercorrection due to premature normal closure of the entire physis, insufficient rebound of an overcorrected deformity, and progressive angular change after staple removal [55]. Hemiphyseal stapling is also used in correcting ankle (Fig. 19.4) and wrist (Fig. 19.7) angular deformities in patients with multiple hereditary osteochondromatosis (Sect. 4.2). Physes compromised by structural deficiencies, such as rickets and some skeletal dysplasias might not be expected to respond to stapling. In Blount's disease, since the medial portion of the proximal tibial physis is abnormal, stapling the lateral side will prevent progression of the tibia vara, but not correct the angular deformity [53, 71].

Temporary Inhibition of Longitudinal Growth
Stapling both sides of the physis long enough to correct bone length discrepancy, followed by timely staple removal, allows growth to resume [45, 48, 49, 58, 66, 73, 78, 80]. Growth has resumed after staple removal even in immunologically compromised patients such as juvenile idiopathic arthritis [80]. This strategy is used in young children with anticipated significant length discrepancy and eliminates some of the uncertainty in the calculation of expected future growth [49], but also introduces some unpredictability and the possibility of unwanted permanent growth cessation [73]. Difficulty in predicting growth after staple removal and in estimating growth on the opposite abnormal extremity are both troublesome [48, 49, 77]. Untoward physeal closure will probably not occur when the staple retention is limited to 2 years [46, 68]. A major limb length discrepancy may not be fully corrected within this 2 year safe period [49]. The physis begins to narrow after 36 months of staple retention in younger children [54, 60]. The germinal zone cells retain their osteogenic power for as long as 44 months [60]. However, growth is *never* resumed after 46 months of stapling [60, 73]. The most favorable time for temporary growth cessation to correct bone length discrepancy is between the bone age of 8–11 years in girls and 8–13 in boys [45]. Poor results were noted after stapling in patients less than 9 years of age [62].

The main advantage of staples is that growth may resume following staple removal. The growth resumption is usually normal for that physis [49], or there may be temporary acceleration of growth [74]. The temporary acceleration of growth may last for 8–10 months [77]. If growth resumption is excessive, recurrent length discrepancy may require repeat stapling [77]. This is less likely to occur in girls over age 12 years and boys over age 13 [77].

Permanent Cessation of Longitudinal Growth
Staples inserted on two sides of a physis on the longer leg and left permanently will cause growth of that physis to slow down and eventually cease (Fig. 6.1c) [50, 67, 68, 75]. The initial growth slow down is slow [67]. The more advanced the skeletal age at time of stapling, the more pronounced and rapid the initial growth retardation [50]. The timing of staple insertion is the key to

achieving leg length equality at maturity. This procedure is usually employed at the knee and is most beneficial in tall girls over 12 years of age and tall boys over age 13 [75]. Proximal tibial arrest with staples is usually accompanied by surgical arrest of the proximal fibular physis [75], but has been successful in older children without arrest of the proximal fibular physis [68]. Staple removal after growth has ceased is optional.

Complications from any of these three stapling strategies include misplaced staples, extrusion and breakage of staples, buried staples, failure to control growth, unwanted asymmetric growth, peroneal nerve palsy, wound infection, and loss of correction following staple removal [67, 68, 69, 75, 89, 153]. Staple deformation in which the tines splay apart, or break due to growth is not uncommon, even when up to three staples are used side-by-side [49, 51, 52]. Staple loosening and extrusion are more pronounced in children below age 10 years [50, 66, 77]. Excessive bending and extrusion of staples is prevented by using the adequate size and number of staples [48]. The unwanted complication of premature complete physeal arrest following the use of staples intended to be temporary, can be particularly disappointing. A common cause of unintended arrest is gouging the physis at time of staple removal causing a peripheral bar to form [68, 83]. This can result in the stapled longer extremity (originally usually the normal extremity) ending up being the shorter extremity (Fig. 10.5). Paralytic patients have poorer results because of compromised and unpredictable growth due to the paralysis [58].

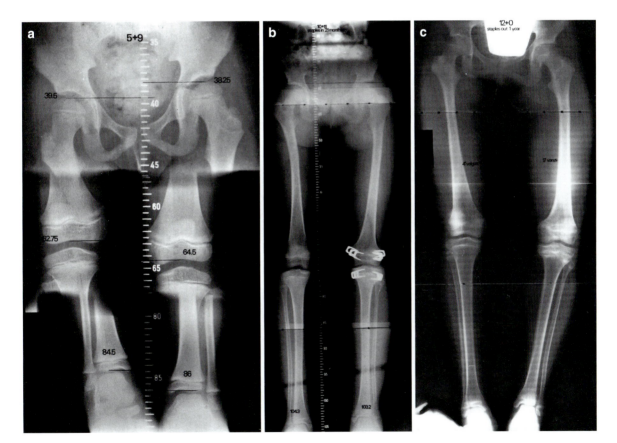

Fig. 10.5 Asymmetric growth arrest following removal of staples. This female developed spastic right hemiparesis following a skull fracture at age 4 months. Mild progressive relative shortening of the right lower extremity was first noted by the parents at age 5 years. (**a**) At age 5 years 9 months an orthoroentgenogram showed the right lower extremity 2.75 cm shorter than the left. At age 8 years 11 months the discrepancy was 3.2 cm. Staples were inserted bridging the normal left distal femur and proximal tibia physes medially and laterally at age 9 years 2 months. (**b**) Twenty-one months later, age 10 years 11 months, the leg length discrepancy was overcorrected by 1.1 cm, shorter on the left. The staples were removed 1 month later. The anticipated resumption of growth and improvement in leg length discrepancy following staple removal did not occur. (**c**) At age 12 years 0 months the left leg was 1.3 cm shorter than the right and was accompanied by 9° genu varum.

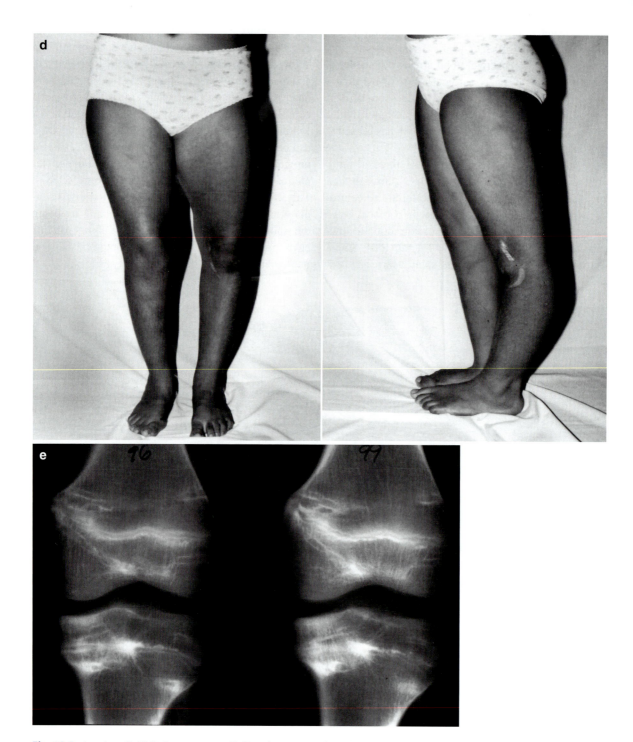

Fig. 10.5 (continued) (**d**) Left genu varum (*left*) and recurvatum (*right*) developed after staple removal. (**e**) Tomograms (two separate AP views of the left knee) confirmed physeal bars on the medial side of both the distal femur and the proximal tibia. The distance between tracts from the tines of the staples on the lateral side are increased compared with the medial side, and the angles of the holes for the tines of the staples are parallel laterally and are diverging medially. Also note growth arrest line of the distal femur with more growth present laterally than medially.

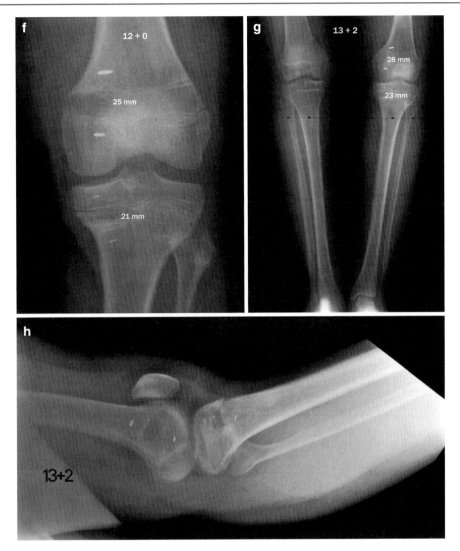

Fig. 10.5 (continued) (**f**) Bar excisions were performed on the medial side of the distal femur and proximal tibia at age 12 years 0 months. The break off titanium wires are 2.5 cm apart in the distal femur. In the proximal tibia the silver vascular clips are 2.1 cm apart. The interposition material was cranioplast. (**g**) At age 13 years 2 months the markers were only 3 mm further apart in the distal femur, 2 mm in the proximal tibia. (**h**) Knee hypertension persisted.

Fig. 10.5 (continued) (**i**) An open wedge osteotomy was performed on the proximal tibia and held with two oblique pins. (**j**) At age 13 years 9 months the osteotomy was healed and the varum and recurvatum deformities were corrected. (**k**) At age 16 years 11 months all physes were closed and the initially normal left lower extremity was 2.2 cm shorter than the palsied right lower extremity. *Note*: Since the genu varum and recurvatum occurred after staple removal it is likely that these peripheral partial physeal arrests are associated with damage to the physis at the time of staple removal. Excisions of the peripheral bars were unsuccessful in reestablishing growth. This case demonstrates the danger of using staples for temporary reversible physeal arrest. An alternative option would have been to perform permanent physeal arrest at a later age, calculated to leave the palsied leg a little shorter than the normal leg (Reproduced from Peterson [72], with permission and additional follow-up)

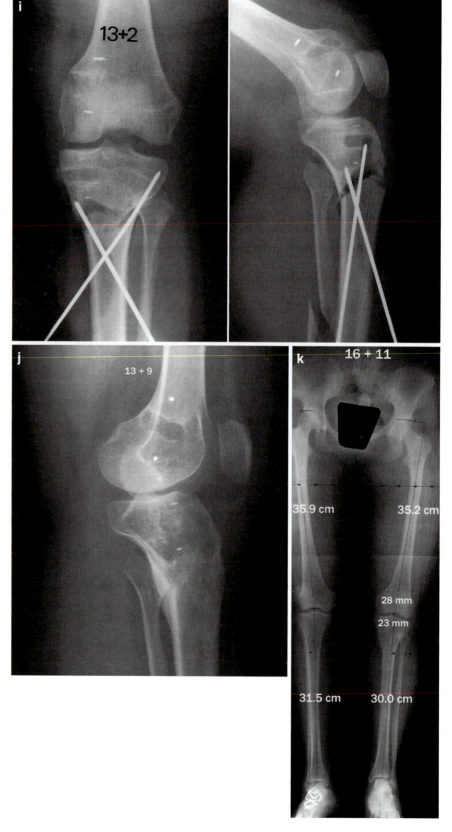

10.2.3.6 Tension Band Plate

A short non-locking plate with two holes, sometimes called an "8 plate" because it looks like an eight, was first reported in 2006 as a replacement for staples for the correction of angular deformities [90]. The waist of the plate is placed over the physis and secured with two cannulated screws, one in the epiphysis and one in the metaphysis. Usually only one plate is necessary. The concept and results are similar, if not identical to staples. The plates are placed extraperiosteally and the screws through the holes of the plate make the construct less rigid than staples. With growth, the screws diverge from each other allowing proponents of the plates to differentiate between compression (present with staples), and tension (present with the plates), and to introduce the term "guided growth" [86, 88, 89]. Nevertheless, correction of deformity occurs due to suppression of growth on the "tension" side compared with unrestricted growth on the unoperated side, just as with staples. Because of angular motion available at the plate screw junction, growth tethering takes longer than with rigid staples [85]. In one series the average age at time of insertion was 10 years 2 months, and the average duration of retention 9.5 months [85].

Eight plates are ten times more expensive than staples, but appear easier to insert, are much less likely to back out, and can be removed with less chance of damage to the edge of the physis. Another potential advantage of the 8-plate is that the screws toggle in the plate. Thus the tether is only at the periphery of the physis, which as compared with staples, may make the technique more likely to work in younger children [91]. Just as with staples, higher complication rates are observed in patients with pathologic physes [91] and 8 plates should not be used in Blount's disease [87] or pseudoachondroplasia [91]. Screw breakage has been noted [91].

In summary, 8-plates are as effective as staples for correction of angular deformity, and should be as effective for temporary reversible arrest or complete arrest of longitudinal growth.

10.2.3.7 Transphyseal Threaded Screws

Experiments on rabbits reported by Green in 1950 [135], showed that transphyseal threaded screws on the epiphysis and metaphysis produced enough anchorage to exert compression upon in the physis, gradually inhibiting growth. Forty years transpired before the screws were used for this purpose in humans. In 1992 Belle and Stevens [92] reported the insertion of a cannulated threaded screw longitudinally across the distal tibial medial malleolar physis to correct ankle valgus deformity.

The method has been used successfully at the knee to correct both varus or valgus deformity [94, 96–98, 100] and length discrepancy [96–98], as well as at the tibial medial malleolus to correct ankle valgus deformity [92, 99, 100]. The screws are placed perpendicularly or obliquely across the physis as allowed by the anatomy [98, 100]. Post operative immobilization is unnecessary. The transphyseal screws begin to exert significant growth inhibition within 6 months of insertion, and achieve maximum growth retardation over the ensuing 12 months [97]. The time lag is the result of compression building up across the physis. Growth may resume following timely screw removal allowing the procedure to be used in younger patients [93, 96–98, 100]. Recurrence of deformity may occur if the screw is removed prior to maturity. The results are similar to staples [94, 96].

Proponents of transphyseal screws site many advantages, including simplicity of technique, short operating time, rapid postoperative rehabilitation, minimal cutaneous scar, reliability, growth rate reversibility, and few complications [94, 96–98, 100].

Threaded screws are often inserted perpendicularly across the physes of patients with slipped capital femoral epiphyses to prevent further slipping (Sect. 20.2). The intended outcome in most cases is premature physeal closure. One study, however, found that the screws stabilized the epiphysis, but prevented premature physeal closure [95].

10.2.3.8 Oblique Smooth Pins

Smooth pins placed obliquely across the physis (Fig. 10.6), commonly done during fracture care, retard the physis from growing in a manner similar to staples. In general, oblique pins of small size removed in 3–4 weeks result in no detectable growth impairment. However, if left longer and physeal arrest occurs, the role of the pins may come into question (Figs. 20.1 and 20.4).

10.2.3.9 Spine Fusion

In the era before spine instrumentation, kyphosis was sometimes treated by posterior spine fusion alone. In a growing child when the fusion was unquestionably solid and fairly massive, there was no growth in the length of the fused area [101]. In some cases a slight decrease (improvement) in the kyphosis postoperatively was felt to be due to continued growth of the vertebral bodies anteriorly.

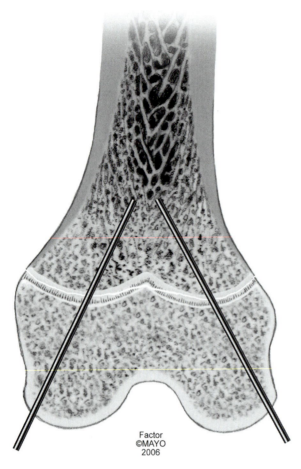

Fig. 10.6 Smooth metal pins inserted obliquely across the physis damage a few physeal cells directly and impede growth of the remaining physis (From Peterson [192], with permission)

Young skeletally immature patients with scoliosis treated by posterior spine fusion without instrumentation often developed a progressive change in spinal deformity over time. The entire fused area gradually rotated and deformed as the anterior portion of the spine continued to grow around the axis of the fusion mass causing progressive change in the spinal deformity with increasing spine curvature, rib prominence, and trunk decompensation (the crankshaft phenomenon) [102].

10.2.3.10 Ineffective Passive Compression

There are some situations in which growth of the physis overcomes the increasing compressive force. The most common example is the occasional splaying or breaking of staples placed across the physis. An example of continuing physeal growth despite even more rigid containment is shown in Fig. 10.7.

10.2.3.11 Author's Perspective

The amount of physeal arrest caused by metallic devices placed across the physis will depend on their size, number, position within the physis (peripheral vs. central), angle relative to the physis, presence or absence and size of threads, duration of retention, and possibly the type of metal (e.g. titanium) and the age of the patient. In the future, biodegradable screws with different thread size and degradation periods might find use to temporarily slow down or completely arrest physeal growth in children. Further investigation is needed.

10.3 Continuous Compression – Animal Research

10.3.1 Pathophysiologic Mechanism of Injury

When a growing physis is subjected to sustained compression, the rate and direction of its growth are modified to yield to that stress [103]. A variety of experiments performed on animals study the effect of sustained compression on the growth potential of the physis. There is significant difficulty in designing in vivo experiments to determine whether the pressure affects the physeal cartilage cells directly, or indirectly by affecting the vascular supply to the physis [107].

Proponents of pressure causing direct cell damage have noted a reduction of DNA synthesis which results in a decreased number of chondrocytes in the physis [107]. Stapled physes have shown reduction in production of lysosomal enzymes [106] and sulfates [108] along with normal glucose uptake and lactate production. Static compressive loads (10–30 N) applied for 6 weeks using an external fixator placed across rabbit proximal tibial physes caused cellular changes in the biochemical character of proteoglycans and collagens, in addition to changes in cellular and extracellular matrix architecture of the tissues [105]. Low-level compression also decreases synthetic activity and prostaglandin production by physeal cartilage in explant culture [109]. The exact etiology and implication of these changes is unknown, but they are perceived as affecting physeal cartilage cells directly and negatively.

The concept of increased pressure causing reduced growth by altering blood flow to the physis was first convincingly documented by Trueta and Trias over 50 years ago [110]. Persistent compression affects the growth

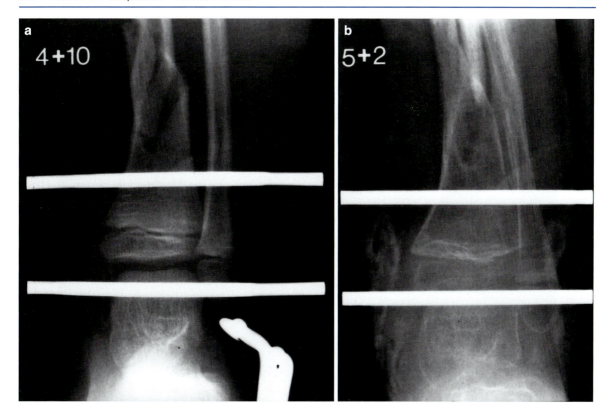

Fig. 10.7 Physeal growth overcoming rigid fixation. At a time before the advent of external fixators designed to treat extensive trauma, a 4 year 10 month old girl sustained compound comminuted fractures of the left femur and tibia, growth plate fracture of the distal femur, and ragged lacerations of most calf muscles, the medial hamstring, the popliteal artery and the posterior tibial nerve, when her leg was caught in a grain auger. The popliteal artery and posterior tibial nerve were repaired with sutures. Multiple tibial bone pieces were removed. One and one half inches of the posterior tibial artery and veins were "shredded and avulsed and no attempt was made to repair these". The wounds were debrided and packed open with furacin and dry dressings, and a Jones compression dressing with a posterior plaster splint was applied. On day nine it appeared the limb would survive. An Anderson leg lengthening apparatus was applied as a holding device in an attempt to stabilize the fractures while wound care, including skin grafting, was accomplished. This device includes two metal blocks, one proximally and one distally, each of which holds two transverse Steinmann pins at a fixed distance to each other. (**a**)The tibial shaft fractures and soft tissue injuries allowed room for only one Steinmann pin in the distal tibia. The other was placed in the talus. Neither pin included the fibula. The Anderson device allowed excellent bone immobilization and access for the multiple debridements, wound closures, and skin grafting procedures which followed. The apparatus was never lengthened. (**b**) Four months later the distal tibial physis had grown, pushing the epiphysis and the talus distally, so that the distal Steinmann pin in the talus was pulled into the joint. (**c**) Upon removal of the Anderson apparatus the tract in the talus through which the distal pin had been pulled into the joint was obvious (*arrow*). (**d**) Three months later, age 5 years 5 months, the distal tibial and fibular physes were growing well. Note growth arrest lines in the distal tibia and fibula metaphyses. (**e**) The dome of the talus also appeared to be healing well. (**f**) At age 15 years 8 months a scanogram showed the left tibia was 2 mm longer than the right despite significant differences in soft tissue mass. All physes were closed. (**g**) At age 24 years 4 months the gait was normal, but there was limited motion and pain with stress in the left ankle. The joint is narrow and has early degenerative arthrosis. At age 29 years 11 months left ankle and subtalar surgical arthrodesis were combined with tenotomy of the flexor hallucis longus. (**h**) At age 30 years 8 months the left ankle fusion was healed in good position. (**i**) The metal was removed at age 30 years 10 months. When last seen at age 39 years 5 months the patient had children ages 19, 17, and 12 years. Her left leg felt "tired" after walking 100 yards or so, and she used a wheelchair while shopping in large grocery stores. She had handicapped parking. *Note*: The most troublesome long lasting complication in this case was degenerative arthrosis of the ankle secondary to deformity caused by the distal tibial physis overcoming rigid restraint. This case documents the ability of a physis to overcome a strong compressive force. The lesson to be learned is to avoid placing a rigid external fixator across a physis of a child for more than a brief period.

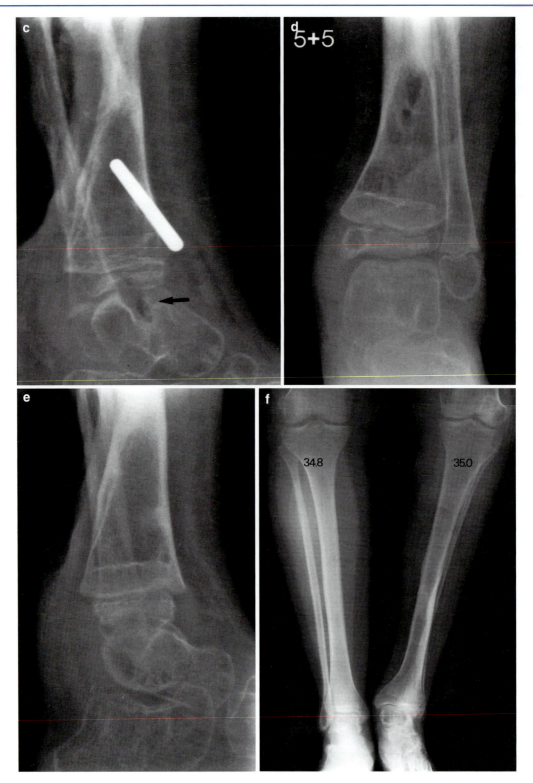

Fig. 10.7 (continued)

10.3 Continuous Compression – Animal Research

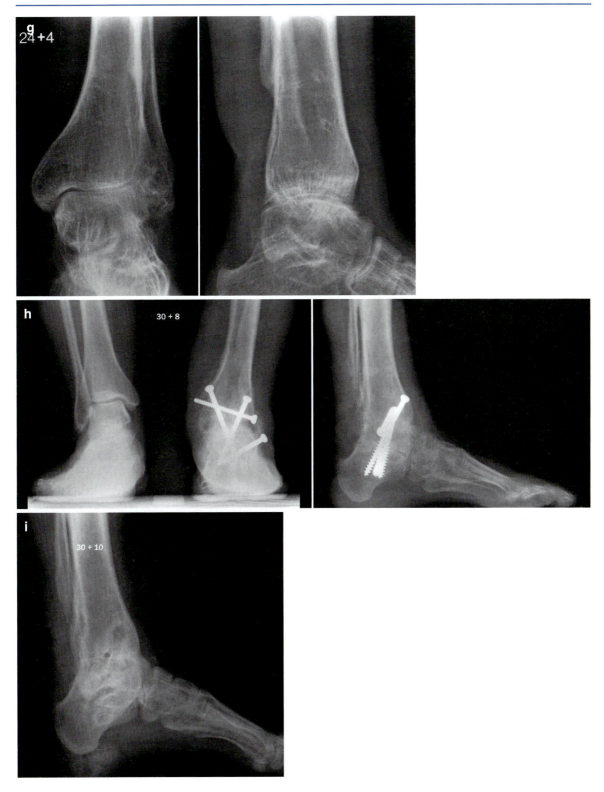

Fig. 10.7 (continued)

plate by interference with the blood flow, and hence the nutrient supply, on one or both sides of the physis. The earliest response to pressure is an increased thickness in the physis [104]. This early effect is histologically identical to that seen with ischemia of the metaphyseal vasculature. Trueta and Trias concluded that increased pressure caused a decrease of metaphyseal blood supply reducing removal of hypertrophic zone cells. Normal germinal production and cell division both combined to produce widening of the physis. Pressure continued over longer periods or at increased magnitudes caused the blood supply on the epiphyseal side to also be compromised, leading to death of germinal cell layer chondrocytes, and narrowing of the physis. The formation of bony bridges during compression is the result of vascular invasion of the injured area of the physis, as anastomoses are established between the epiphyseal and metaphyseal vessels [111]. Interference to growth is directly proportional to the magnitude and duration of compression, and is fully reversible as long as the epiphyseal vasculature to the physis is still viable [110].

10.3.2 Histologic Studies

Compression of the physis affects both the morphology and function of the chondrocytes [121]. A gradual decline in cell division is followed by the appearance of degenerate chondrocytes, distorted columns, and reduced physeal height [106, 111]. The greatest changes are noted in the proliferative zone [111]. Although Trueta and Trias noted initial widening of the physis [110], other authors have noted only narrowing, particularly a reduction in the proliferative and hypertrophic zone heights [103, 112]. Physes at which growth has ceased show complete disappearance of all cartilage cells [113].

10.3.3 Amount of Compression

Pressure does not inhibit growth by an all-or-nothing law. Longitudinal growth suppression caused by axial loading of the physis is proportional to the magnitude of the load [115]. As pressure increases growth diminishes [111].

Some authors feel that extremely mild forces can inhibit or modify physeal growth [109]. Furthermore, there is no sign that there is a threshold below which pressures are ineffective. Stresses from a plaster cast, positional stresses, and even gravitational and muscle stresses are sufficient to affect it [121]. Rabbit proximal tibial growth was stopped completely by a pressure of body weight multiplied by 1.3–2 [120].

Other studies conclude that only an extreme increase in pressure leads to an inhibition of longitudinal growth [112, 119]. The physis can bear, without damage, a much higher degree of pressure than is affected under normal physiologic conditions, such as muscle pull or weight bearing [112, 119]. Bone growth in calves takes place as rapidly when the animal is grazing as when it is lying down at night [119]. The amount of compression to produce complete physeal arrest in calves was calculated to be "equal, roughly to three times body weight" [119]. Forces greater than 17–30 N cause cell damage and rapid cessation of physeal growth [114, 115]. In another study growth ceased at compression forces which were expressed as "approximately 3 kg per epiphyseal disc or 15 g per mm [2] cross-sectional area of the disc or 15 mg per column of cartilage cells" [113]. In addition, the physis is a resilient structure and has good potential to recover when compression ceases [111, 115].

Within certain (low) limits, physeal growth can be stimulated by either an increase or a decrease of dynamic loading [116]. The amount and kind of loading are the important factors to accelerate physeal growth [116].

10.3.4 Duration of Compression

One study found that sustained stress inhibited physeal growth more than cyclic stress [117]. However, another study showed that static loads inhibit physeal growth, whereas cyclic loads stimulate growth [103]. Static compressive loads of 10 and 30 N applied to rabbit proximal tibial physes using an external fixator showed no changes after 2 weeks. After 6 weeks the physes had shorter, disorganized chondrocyte columns, loss of lamellar patterning in adjacent collagen, and markedly different collagen fibrils [105]. Calf proximal tibial physes temporarily arrested for 6 months by spring tension devices resumed growth after removal of the devices [118]. This 6 month arrestment in the immature calf was judged to be equivalent to 3–4 years in the human.

10.3.5 Direction of Pressure Applied

Constant longitudinal pressure applied perpendicular to and in the center of the physis inhibits longitudinal growth. Caudad vertebrae of growing rats compressed for 4 weeks grew only 52–68% of control rates [123, 124]. Excentric longitudinal pressure can cause angular deformity. The rate of growth on the compressed side is reduced, the noncompressed side continues to grow [121]. Pressure applied to one side of the rabbit proximal tibial physis caused an angular deformity of 90° [120]. Removal of asymmetrically applied loading allows a return to normal growth [122]. Reversing the asymmetrically applied load corrects the deformity, suggesting that growth is not necessarily permanently affected by asymmetric loading [122]. Transverse pressure on the epiphysis with a corresponding opposite direction on the metaphysis causes bending of the cartilage columns in the direction of the force on the epiphysis, but no diminution of growth at least initially [121]. Likewise, torsional pressure will produce rotational deformities of the growing physis [121]. The ease with which torsional or angular deformities are produced in growing bones varies inversely with the diameter of the physis. The smaller the physis, the greater its plasticity [121].

10.3.6 Periosteal Tether

The periosteum attaches directly and firmly into the zone of Ranvier at each end of developing bone. Bone grows in length by apposition at the physis, whereas periosteum grows interstitially like skin. The periosteum is like an elastic stocking sliding over the surface of the bone as the bone grows in length. The periosteum is strong and subjects the physis to significant forces [126]. When the periosteal tension is increased the bone grows a little slower, and when the tension is reduced the bone grows a little faster [33, 125]. Periosteal division even reverses, to some extent, the effects of growth slowdown of a physis under mechanical compression [126].

A 24-gauge wire suturing the periosteum to bone near the distal ulnar physis in 3 week old rabbits resulted in progressive angular growth deformity over the 3 months of observation [33]. The maximum deformity was 30°. The apex of the deformity was at the site of tethering. Growth was not significantly affected when the procedure was performed in old immature rabbits. This experiment corroborated the concept of periosteal tethering in humans proposed by Beaty and Barrett [31].

10.3.7 Staples

Animal studies are particularly beneficial in obtaining histologic findings after different durations of staple retention. The effect of stapling is a direct pressure inhibition of the proliferating stage of the epiphyseal growth [133]. The germinal cells continue maturation, but the metaphyseal vascular channels progressively invade the degenerating hypertrophic cells, the palisading cells, and eventually the germinal cell layer, gradually thinning the physis until eventual arrest occurs [133].

When staples were placed over two sides of proximal tibial physes of rabbits, longitudinal growth gradually stopped during the first postoperative week [128, 129]. The physis was largely preserved, but extremely thin, and considerable cellular derangement occurred. If the staples are removed within 2–6 weeks growth generally started again [128, 129, 131], unless the staples were inserted subperiosteally [127]. From 3 to 4 weeks onwards, growth did not resume. In dogs, growth resumed following staple removal after varying lengths of time, but the new growth was not as rapid as the normal rate of growth [130]. When removing the staples there is a possibility of mechanically injuring the physis which may hinder the function of the physis [130].

Staples or wires inserted on one side of the physis in rabbits, dogs and cats prevented growth on that side [130]. Growth on the opposite side was also retarded, but to a lesser degree. The restraining force is exerted on the entire physis, less on the non-restrained side [130]. Thus, there was a diminution of total bone length by staples inserted on one side. This effect has not been noted nor measured in humans. Staples placed on the medial side of the distal femoral physis in rabbits producing genu varum, induced an opposite angulation in the proximal tibial physis [129]. However, no growth rate changes were noted in the distal femoral physis when the proximal tibial physis was stapled [129, 131].

In canine puppies unilateral clamping of one or more vertebrae by staples created a compression force sufficient to cause a lateral spine curvature in 6–8 weeks [132]. The additional characteristics that developed, secondary curves and torsional changes in thoracic, were similar to scoliosis seen in children. When the staples were removed early the scoliosis corrected spontaneously. The curves of cases stapled for a longer duration did not correct spontaneously, but could be corrected by reinserting the staples on the convex side of the curve. The authors cautioned that the staples be placed without damage to the physis.

10.3.8 Transphyseal Threaded Screws and Pins

In 1950 Green reported that metal screws placed perpendicularly across the physis of rabbits produced enough anchorage on the two sides of the physeal plate to cause compression of the physis and gradual inhibition of growth [135]. A single threaded metallic pin, 1/4 or 5/32 in. diameter, inserted across the center of the distal femoral physis in dogs caused gradual narrowing of the entire physis and subsequent complete arrest in all 17 cases [134]. The gauge of the threads of the pins or screws must be sufficient to mechanically fix the metaphysis to the epiphysis.

In an attempt to determine the appropriate number of pins in the treatment of slipped capital femoral epiphysis, one or two Asnis screws (Howmedica, Rutherford, NJ) were placed across the proximal femoral physes of calves and tested on a hydraulic test machine [136]. Double pin fixation yielded only a 33% increase in stiffness as compared to a single pin. Resistance to further slip was not proportional to the number of pins. The stiffness of neither the double or single screw fixation approximated that of the intact physis. Single screw fixation for slipped epiphysis was recommended because the small gains in stiffness with a second screw did not offset the risk of complication.

10.3.9 Crossed Smooth Metallic Pins

Two smooth pins placed diagonally across the physis (Fig. 10.6) of rabbits and dogs caused no growth impairment if removed immediately, approximately 20% growth reduction if left in 21 days, and complete arrest if left in situ permanently [137]. Single pins placed perpendicularly across physes caused approximately 50% retardation of growth. There was evidence of compensatory growth from the non-restricted physis at the opposite end of the bone. Two crossed pins placed diagonally excentrally on one side of the distal radial physis of dogs caused angular deformity and growth slowdown [137]. In this experiment the arrest on only one side of the physis to correct angular deformity also retarded growth on the opposite side of the same physis to a lesser degree, thereby causing some, usually minor, relative shortening of the bone compared with the contralateral normal bone. This was not precisely measured and apparently is not troublesome in humans since no author reporting correction of angular deformity by partial physeal arrest in humans has mentioned concurrent relative shortening. Pins placed in the diaphysis caused no growth loss. Removal of metal devices from the vicinity of the physis may cause damage to the plate itself or to the vascular circulation of the plate causing unintended arrest.

Two smooth 5/64 in. Kirschner wires crossed in the center of the proximal tibial physis of a rabbit caused little or no inhibition of growth [133]. "The wires either separated or the epiphysis continued to grow, leaving the crossed wires behind in the metaphysis."

10.3.10 Biodegradable Screws and Crossed Pins

Interest in biodegradable screws and pins so far has been primarily to internally fix physeal fractures. The intent is to produce fracture stabilization while the implant biodegrades, followed by normal growth of the physis. However, biodegradable screws or crossed pins could potentially be used to intentionally arrest the physis. The absorption time would need to take long enough to assure arrest. The advantage of using a biodegradable implant for either fracture treatment or intentional physeal arrest would be the lack of need to remove the implant.

The disappearance of a single smooth polyglactin 910 or polydioxanone (PDS) 3.2 mm diameter rod across the distal femoral physis of rabbits, and its replacement by a cancellous bone bridge, resulted in a growth disturbance 6 weeks after implantation similar to that of a drill hole of equal bone [141, 142]. However, the pressure of growth was able to break the implant allowing regeneration of the physis in the area between the broken ends of the implant. The insertion of similar 2.0 mm rods caused no permanent growth disturbance [141].

Polydioxanone (PDS) pins, 1.3 mm in diameter, placed across the central portion of the proximal tibial physes caused "significant" osseous bridge formation of the physis in 7 of 10 rabbits [144]. However, the implants biodegraded "almost completely" in 3 months and caused no growth disturbance.

When Polyglycolide (PGA) rods were inserted into distal femoral 3.2 mm drill holes in rabbits and 2.0 mm in rats, physeal arrest and significant shortening was seen only in the control group (drill hole without biodegradable rod) [143]. The drill holes filled with PGA rods did not promote physeal arrest.

Temporary physeal arrest was achieved in rabbits by inserting a 4.5 mm diameter absorbable polyglycolide (Sp-PGA) screw perpendicularly across the femoral greater trochanteric physis [139]. The screws were macroscopically visible at 1 month, their shape was lost at 2 months, and growth resumed at 3 months. A second report by the same authors stated that the screws maintained their morphology at 1 month preventing the formation of a bone bridge [138]. Two months postoperatively peripheral degradation of the screw permitted the formation of bone tissue from the periphery of the hole giving rise to small marginal bone bridges. Three months postoperatively greater degradation of the screw was accompanied by more physeal growth and no permanent bone bridge formed.

The use of biodegradable pins and screws to cause temporary or permanent physeal arrest by compression and then biodegrade needs more investigation.

10.3.11 Absorbable Filament

Metal screws inserted transversely into one side of the distal femoral metaphysis and epiphysis in rabbits connected by an absorbable filament achieved unilateral closure of the physis by compression producing angular deformity [140]. Although the biodegradable tether dissolves, the metal screws remain in place. This procedure is similar to the application of an eight plate; the absorbable filament replacing the plate. There are no reports of use of this method in humans.

10.3.12 Surgical Bone Lengthening

Distraction osteogenesis adversely affects the physes of bones being lengthened, functionally and histomorphogenically [145, 147, 149]. Lee, et al. [146], postulated "that pressure exerted on the articular surface during bone lengthening compresses the cartilage growth plates. The possibility of changes of the blood vessels, however, cannot be ruled out." Immature rabbit bones lengthened from 10 to 20% of their original length resulted in no physeal growth changes [2, 145–147]. When lengthened more than 30% of the original length growth retardation occurred and persisted until skeletal maturity [2, 146]. Resistance to lengthening is greater in the tibia-fibula than in the femur because of tighter musculotendinous units [2]. Concomitant Achilles lengthening significantly reduces the compressive force and preserves the proximal tibial physis architecture and growth potential [148]. Bone shortening had no effect on physeal growth in rabbits [149].

10.3.13 Spine Fusion

Posterior spine fusion of dogs resulted in loss of growth of the posterior vertebral elements [150]. As the vertebral bodies continued to grow anteriorly lordosis developed, and there was decreased growth in the overall length of the fused area.

10.3.14 Tensioned Soft Tissue Grafts

In dogs tensioned connective tissue grafts placed across the distal femoral and proximal tibial physes to represent the anterior cruciate ligaments caused significant valgus deformity in the distal femur and significant varus deformity in the proximal tibia [151]. There was no radiographic or histologic evidence of physeal bar formation. The observed deformities were felt to be a result of an alteration of physeal growth due to compression from the excessively tensioned transphyseal graft reconstruction, and not a result of premature physeal closure. More details of tensioned grafts in the repair of anterior cruciate ligament rupture are recorded in Sect. 20.4.5.

10.3.15 Compensatory Growth

Growth cessation by stapling the proximal tibial physes of rabbits resulted in stimulation of the distal tibial physis [128, 131]. Similarly, growth cessation by stapling the distal tibial physes in dogs resulted in stimulation of the proximal tibial physis [130]. No change of growth was noted in the distal femur. The additional growth contribution made by the unstapled physis is never sufficient to compensate for the loss of the growth in the stapled physis.

10.4 Acute Compression – Human Involvement

10.4.1 The Concept

A single instantaneous longitudinal blow to a bone sufficient to compress the physeal cartilage without observable damage to the bone is an interesting concept. If it exists it is very rare. The concept of sudden physeal compression without fracture was first proposed in 1958, separately by Cassidy [153] and Brashear [152].

Cassidy stated "A forceful thrust in the long axis of the bone will displace the epiphysis only slightly, but the crushing force on the germinal zone of the epiphyseal plate may cause complete or partial growth arrest. The x-ray may indicate little damage, but the end result may be disastrous. The prognosis must be guarded until adequate growth at the involved epiphyseal plate has been observed. The resulting angular and/or linear deformity may prove to be great" [153]. Cassidy is ambiguous by stating that the epiphysis will displace "only slightly," while the x-ray indicates "little damage." No such case or drawing was illustrated and no attempt was made to classify the "injuries".

Brashear stated that post traumatic knee angular deformities were "clinically suspected" to be due to a localized crushing injury of the subepiphyseal cartilage bone plate "without a demonstrable definite fracture" [152]. A drawing was illustrated (Fig. 10.8), but no illustrative case, patient series, or relative frequency was given. Brashear contradicted himself in the last sentence of the summary where he stated, "Distracting, transverse shearing, and rotational forces tend to produce defects in the cartilage plate; compression forces usually result in damage to the bony portions." Brashear proposed a classification of physeal fractures (Fig. 10.9) by adding the crushing injury to the classification previously described by Aitken. Brashear's classification of four types was never used by any other author.

In 1963 Salter and Harris (S-H) [157] published an article entitled "Injuries Involving the Epiphyseal Plate" which included the crushing injury of Cassidy and Brashear. Cassidy's article was listed in the references, but not cited in the manuscript. Brashear's article was neither referenced nor cited. It is worth repeating Salter and Harris' entire discussion of their type 5 injury, for what it states and does not state.

> This relatively uncommon injury results from a very severe crushing force applied through the epiphysis to one area of the epiphyseal plate. It occurs in joints which move in one plane only, such as the ankle or the knee. A severe abduction or adduction injury to a joint that normally only flexes or extends is likely to produce crushing of the epiphyseal plate, which may separate. Displacement of the epiphysis is unusual under these circumstances, and the first roentgenogram gives little indication of the seriousness of the injury; indeed, the injury may be dismissed as a sprain. [157]

This description states quite clearly that (a) the injury is due to compression of the physis, (b) that it occurs only in uniaxial joints which allow only flexion and extension, such as the knee, ankle, elbow, and phalanges, and that (c) only "one area" of the physis is involved (Fig. 10.10), excluding any injury in which the entire physis closes. It also strongly implies that no

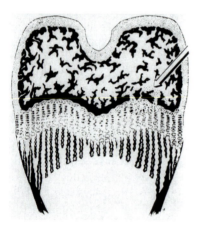

Fig. 10.8 Brashear used this drawing to illustrate his Type IV fracture. The accompanying caption stated: "Localized injury to the subepiphyseal cartilage bone plate (*arrow*) possibly the result of a longitudinal compression force" (From Brashear [152], with permission)

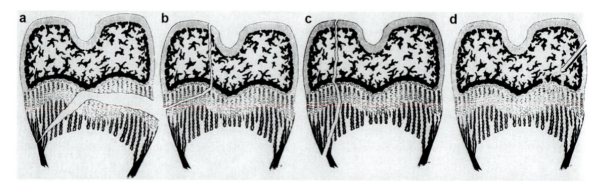

Fig. 10.9 Classification of physeal fractures proposed by Brashear. Types A, B, and C were Aitken's types 1, 2 and 3 (From Brashear [152], with permission)

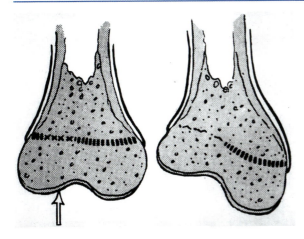

Fig. 10.10 Salter-Harris type V epiphyseal plate injury: *Left*, crushing of the physis; *Right*, premature closure (Reproduced from Salter and Harris [157], with permission). In the figure on the right the absence of growth on one side, with continued growth on the other, has caused angular deformity of the bone. Note that bone structure, contours and volume of the epiphysis are changed little, if at all, and the articular surface of the epiphysis is unchanged

fracture occurs since the roentgenogram at the time of injury is normal.

Salter and Harris included two case illustrations, one of the proximal tibia and one of the distal tibia. Each is a single roentgenographic AP view taken an unspecified time after injury and shows angular deformity. Any original views taken at the time of injury are not shown. Salter was challenged at several meetings to show the original normal roentgenograms of these two cases, but never did so, despite lecturing extensively and publishing on the subject three more time over a time span of 29 years [154–156]. In the proximal tibial case the epiphysis has significant deformity and the entire physis is closed (Fig. 10.11). Articular surface abnormalities suggest it is more likely the result of a S-H type 4 fracture than a compression injury (Fig. 10.12). None of Salter's articles showed a patient series or relative frequency of physeal fractures. In

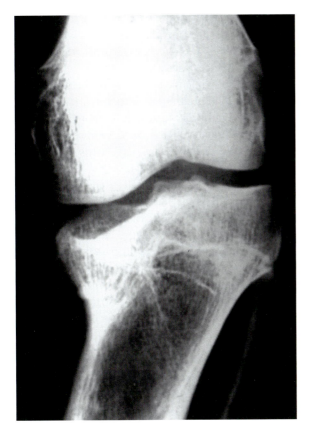

Fig. 10.11 This roentgenogram from Salter and Harris' 1963 article was captioned "Fig. 30: Four years after Type V injury involving medial portion of the left upper tibial epiphysis" (Reproduced from Salter and Harris [157], with permission)

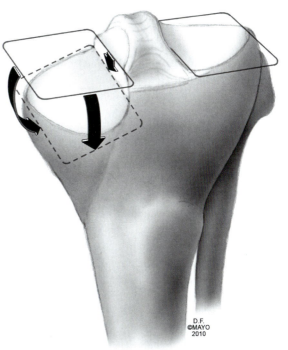

Fig. 10.12 This drawing of the roentgenogram in Fig. 10.11 shows the plane of the articular surface of the medial tibial condyle (*dotted line square*) is displaced distally (*straight arrow*), and angled in both the coronal and sagittal planes (*curved arrows*) relative to the articular surface of the normal lateral condyle. Normally, and following a S-H type 5 injury, the articular surfaces of the medial and lateral condyles are in the same plane (*solid line squares*). This incongruity of the articular planes should not occur following a S-H type 5 injury and would most likely occur following a displaced, incompletely reduced, medial S-H type 4 fracture

addition, the original S-H article illustrated the histology of physeal fractures type 1–4 in rabbits, but not the type 5 injury [157].

In 1988 Salter [156] added that the injury is "very rare", that "there is no gross disturbance of anatomy," and that "the epiphysis does not separate so the diagnosis is seldom obvious, either clinically or radiographically." In this article, as well as in his 1974 [154] and 1992 [155] articles, Salter remained silent on the possibility of the physeal crush injury involving the entire physis, or occurring simultaneously with fracture elsewhere in the same bone. In deference to the type 5 injury Salter and Harris [157] and Salter [154–156] consistently used the word "*injuries*" rather than fracture in describing their classification. This suggests they recognized that by including the compression injury, their classification was one of injuries rather than fractures. However, their classification does not begin to include all injuries to the physis, as recorded in this textbook.

10.4.2 The Compression Concept Challenged

In 1981 the existence of an acute compression type 5 injury was questioned [159] because: (1) at the time there were no reports of type 5 injury in the upper extremity where physeal fractures are the most common (70%); (2) all SH type 5 cases illustrated up to that time involved complete rather than partial physeal arrest, as required by S-H, and which one would expect from an abduction or adduction force; (3) none of the reported cases illustrated a normal roentgenogram at the time of injury; and (4) most of the reported patients underwent treatment for associated fractures, including skeletal traction and prolonged immobilization, which, in themselves, are known to cause growth disturbance (Chap. 2).

Criteria were suggested to prove the existence of the compression injury: (a) normal roentgenograms in at least two planes taken at the time of injury; (b) no treatment; and (c) subsequent roentgenograms showing partial closure of the physis [159]. Since this challenge in 1981, no such case has yet appeared in the literature. There have been several reports of injuries suspected to be S-H type 5. In almost all of these cases there have been associated non-physeal fractures with subsequent treatment, often with prolonged immobilization in either traction or cast. In the cases with accompanying fracture of the diaphysis or metaphysis it is interesting to speculate whether the physeal compression occurs a nanosecond before the fracture or simultaneously with the fracture. When would the force change from compression to torsion or an oblique mode to cause the fracture? It seems unlikely that compression would occur after the fracture since any longitudinal force would then be dissipated at the fracture site.

The controversy over the existence of the S-H type 5 "crushing" injury has generated both support and opposition. Much of the controversy is due to different interpretations of the S-H concept.

10.4.3 Clinical Support for the S-H Type 5 Compression Injury Concept

A diaphyseal bone fracture in an older child is occasionally accompanied by closure of one of its physes or a physis of an adjacent bone. This occurs occasionally at the knee with fractures to the diaphysis of either the tibia [164–166] or the femur [164]. The diaphyseal fractures are usually oblique or spiral. Discounting traction pins through or near the proximal tibial physis [162, 164, 166], the cause of the premature closure is unknown, but is suspected to be from compression sustained at the time of injury. While the possibility of central or complete physeal closure from an acute compression injury cannot be totally discounted, it is more likely that compressive trauma would cause peripheral physeal injury as specified by Salter and Harris [157], with resultant angular deformity [164, 165].

One 10 year old female pedestrian was struck on the lateral side of the knee by the bumper of a car moving at high speed [171]. The roentgenograms showed a "flake fracture" at the lateral edge of the distal femoral condyle and "indisputable evidence of compression of the left lateral femoral condyle and signs of contusion of the bone adjacent to the growth plate." An AP valgus stress view, also taken at the time of injury, showed flattening of the lateral condyle which "clearly demonstrates that a compression of the lateral femoral condyle had occurred." Thus this patient had multiple fractures in the epiphysis with the likelihood of fragments pushing into the physis as noted by Ogden [199]. But was the subsequent lateral physeal closure due to compression of the physis, fracture across the physis, or vascular compromise?

A 13 year old girl whose lateral proximal tibial physis was closing was regarded to have a S-H type 5 injury despite no history of injury (and thus no initial roentgenogram), no angular deformity, and no tibial length discrepancy [169].

The ankle of a 6 year old boy was injured in an automobile accident [172]. "Within a year" partial closure of the distal tibial physis (a bar) was accompanied by varus deformity. No roentgenogram from the time of injury was shown.

At the wrist four papers support the S-H type 5 compression concept [160, 161, 173, 174], despite the fact that the wrist is a multiaxial joint. Four of the five reported cases had fractures of the distal radial metaphysis [160, 161, 173] and one had fracture extension to the physis [161] (Peterson type 1 physeal fracture [201]). All five cases were treated in cast, and three had complete closure of the distal radial physis [160, 161, 174]. These cases did not meet S-H criteria of being in a hinge joint, or of having asymmetric closure. Of the two cases with partial closure [161, 173] one was a Peterson type 1 physeal fracture [201], and the other was struck on the dorsum of the wrist with a rubber ball [160], and therefore did not have an axial crushing injury.

Two S-H type 5 injuries have been suspected in the distal ulna [163, 167]. A 10 year old girl fell, sustaining a torus (incomplete) fracture of the distal radial metaphysis [163]. A short arm cast was worn 3 weeks. At age 16 ulnar relative shortening was accompanied with ulnar bowing of the distal radius and all physes were closed. The original injury roentgenogram was not shown. A 13 year old boy fell playing basketball, sustaining an injury of his wrist which was thought to be a "sprain." [167] He was not medically examined at the time of injury. One and a half years later growth arrest of the distal ulna (2.9 cm shorter) was accompanied with ulnarward bowing of the radius. In both cases longitudinal compression on the distal ulnar physis would be unlikely since the distal ulna does not articulate directly with the carpus.

A comminuted fracture of the distal epiphysis and metaphysis of the fifth metatarsal was reported as a S-H type 5 injury [168]. Although this fracture was likely caused by compression, the marked comminution of both the epiphyseal and metaphyseal bone make it a comminuted S-H type 4 fracture.

Since none of the above published cases adhere to the few and straight forward S-H precepts, it is interesting to speculate which of these cases, if any, Salter and Harris would have included in their injury classification.

In 1997 a "broad interpretation" of the S-H type 5 injury was proposed [170]. "A Salter-Harris type V injury should include non-displaced injury about the growth plate with resulting premature physeal arrest in which there *was* or *was not* an associated fracture of the metaphysis or diaphysis, or both not otherwise identifiable as a Salter II-IV injury." This interpretation seemingly excludes displaced injury about the physis, but nevertheless would expand the compression concept considerably. The inclusion of "non-displaced injury about the growth plate" could be problematic, as this could be interpreted by some to include injury due to vascular deprivation, disuse, infection, tumor, heat, cold, radiation, etc. No subsequent article has endorsed this "broad interpretation."

10.4.4 Alternative Mechanisms

Several authors have attempted to explain the phenomenon of late, otherwise unexplained physeal closure following trauma by theories other than compression of the physis. Blount [176] observed that hyperemia following a shaft fracture in an older child causes initial bone growth acceleration, followed by early epiphyseal closure resulting in relative shortening.

While reviewing fractures of the distal femoral physis in 1960, Neer reported "the instances of late premature closure of the ossification centers seen in this study are presumably based upon injury of blood supply and nutrition, rather than crushing and immediate death of the proliferating cells" [177].

In 1967 Barnhart [175] reported a case of fracture of the tibial diaphysis which developed premature closure of the proximal tibial physis. He discounted the proximal tibial traction pin and subsequent cast immobilization as causes, and speculated that "a wrenching or twisting disturbance may be the mechanism of injury in these patients." The article did not cite Salter and Harris and made no mention of compression.

Siffert in 1980 stated "the mechanism of growth arrest in Type V involvement has not been clarified as to whether it is direct crush, vascular damage, unrecognized central fracture through the cancellous bone, or all three" [180].

In 1981 Peterson and Burkhart [159] speculated that premature physeal closure following diaphyseal fracture may be the result of decreased blood supply to the physis due to arterial damage, shunting of the major portion of the vascular supply to the healing fracture, immobilization, or disuse (Fig. 10.13). Central or

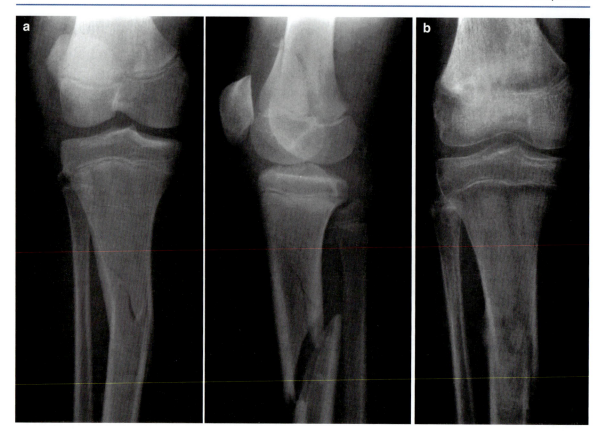

Fig. 10.13 Complete physeal arrest about the knee following tibial diaphyseal fracture. A 14½ year old boy was injured in a motorcycle accident. (**a**) There is an oblique mildly comminuted fracture of the tibial diaphysis and an undisplaced Peterson type 5 (S-H type 4) physeal fracture of the distal femoral physis. The treatment was "casting until healing had occurred". (**b**) Two months after the injury the fractures were healing, but there was a pronounced area of bone lysis in the metaphysis adjacent to each of the three knee physis which are all narrower than on (**a**). He regained full painless knee motion and function. (**c**) Two years 4 months after injury, age 16 years 10 months, there was relative shortening of both the right femur and tibia. (**d**) A scanogram showed the right femur 2.3 cm and the tibia 3.0 cm shorter than the left. Note the proximal right fibular physis is also closed and has not overgrown the tibia. The left femur was surgically shortened 5.0 cm. (**e**) At age 18 years 9 months the patient was normally active and asymptomatic. The knee height discrepancy remains, but the body alignment is improved. (**f**) The femoral shortening was healed and the metal was subsequently removed. *Note*: Although this case is similar to several in the literature supporting a compression mechanism of injury, the following factors mitigate against it: (1) the oblique fracture of the tibia (**a**) suggests a transverse, possibly rotation force, rather than compression, (2) the uniform area of bone lysis on the metaphyseal side of all three physes in the early healing phase (**b**) is more compatible with a vascular change than compression of the physis, (3) uniform complete (rather than partial) closure of all three physes, and (4) premature closure of the proximal fibular physis, the epiphysis of which does not articulate with the femur and therefore is not subjected to longitude pressure. (**a**, **b**, and **d**) reproduced from Burkhart and Peterson [158, 159], with permission and additional follow-up)

10.4 Acute Compression – Human Involvement

Fig. 10.13 (continued)

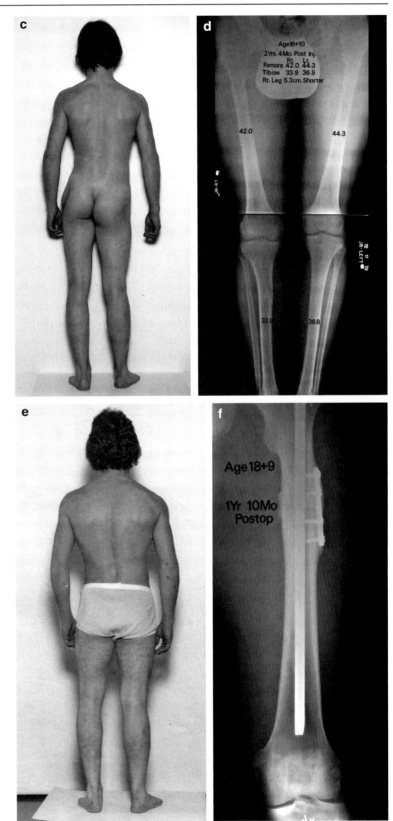

complete closure is more easily explained by vascular deprivation (Chap. 1) than compression.

In 1990 Ogden [179] reviewed 79 childhood distal radial and ulna post traumatic gross specimens and proposed a microtrauma concept. Seven distal ulnar and two distal radial physes showed histologic evidence of incomplete transverse fractures only a millimeter across extending through different zones of the physis causing microscopic damage to the juxta subchondral end-plate. Radiographic corroboration was not evident. These were compared with specimens of known physeal ischemia. Ogden concluded that the microscopic changes evident in this study support the concept that undetectable ischemic damage was the primary etiologic factor for growth arrest following roentgenographic negative injury. Thus microtrauma with focal damage to the vascularity of a small segment of the epiphyseal cartilage and germinal zones appears to be a plausible mechanism of formation of these osseous striations. In 2000, Ogden [178] illustrated a distal femur torus fracture case accompanied more distally with a focal area of physeal displacement not visible radiographically which "is likely to disrupt the vascular supply, rather than 'crush' the cartilage cells."

10.4.5 Clinical Opposition to or Evidence Against the S-H Type 5 Compression Injury Concept

Most reported series of physeal fractures at all sites, as well as at individual sites, record no S-H type 5 fractures [192]. Those that do, usually do not discuss or illustrate the type 5 cases.

In 1978 Hunter and Hensinger [186] reported an 11 year old girl who fell from a moving tractor, sustaining a comminuted fracture of the proximal femoral diaphysis and was treated in a spica cast 5½ months. She subsequently developed premature complete closure of the ipsilateral distal femur, proximal tibial, and distal tibial physes. They concluded that "some generalized vascular or neural disturbance seems to be the most reasonable explanation for the monomelic growth arrest."

In 1982 Wahl noted that cartilage tissue is more capable of resisting pressure forces than bone tissue [203].

In 1983, Mercer Rang, Salter's associate, stated "Even when everyone agreed on the nature of the type-V injuries, they were considered rare. Now, there is much to be said for retiring the term altogether. Bone bridging should be regarded as a *complication* of any growth-plate injury and not as a special type of injury" [194].

In 1984 Ogden et al. [191]. subjected six neonatal stillborn pelvic and femoral units to compression or traction forces until the proximal femoral head–great trochanter epiphysis separated from the metaphysis. Histologic examination showed that the fracture propagated across the entire composite physis as a S-H type 1 growth mechanism injury. The principal level of cellular disruption was the junction between the hypertrophic cell columns and the primary spongiosa of the metaphysis. In two cases "there was no crushing of the germinal zone, but rather propagation of the fracture into the epiphysis, splitting the germinal zone away from the epiphyseal blood supply." There was "complete absence of crushing of the cellular components of the germinal zone, which would support the recent suggestion that this is not the true mechanism of a type 5 physeal injury." They concluded that "localized vascular injury (i.e., microscopic disruption of the epiphyseal vessels to the physis) may occur if an infant sustains a pattern of injury similar to our experimental human model."

In 1985 Connolly, et al. [184]. reported an 11 year old girl with a torus fracture of the distal radial metaphysis followed by complete closure of the distal radial physis. They concluded that "blunt trauma apparently affected epiphyseal circulation sufficiently to halt growth of the entire radial plate." Compression was not mentioned and the article by Salter and Harris was not cited. This case is almost identical to that shown by Abram and Thompson [160], who attributed the premature closure to compression. This disparity emphasizes the ambiguity of the S-H type 5 injury.

Herring and Birch [185] surmised a vascular explanation for distal tibial fracture with subsequent significant progressive angular deformity which corrected spontaneously.

In 1988 Letts [187] wrote, "The integrity of the perichondrium and perichondrial ring adds considerable stability to the epiphyseal plate" and "protects the growth plate from compression forces." "The more elastic cartilage cells appear to withstand compression better than metaphyseal bone trabeculae. Fracturing first occurs in the metaphyseal region during a compression injury." "Continued compressive forces may result in the metaphyseal bone being forced up into

Table 10.1 Distribution of physeal fractures at all anatomic sites by type (Salter-Harris classification [156])[a]

Year	Author[b]	Type 1	2	3	4	5	Unclassified	Total
1933	Bergenfeldt	23	251	19	13	–	4	310
1970	Rogers	7	89	9	12	1		118
1977	Oh[c]	34	92	19	17	0		162
1979	Mbindyo	18	42	4	5	2		71
1986	Worlock	30	121	5	15	0		171
1987	Chadwick	1	56	2	25	0	13	97
1987	Mizuta	30	257	23	42	1		353
1990	Mann[c]	210	483	143	102	5		943
1994	Peterson	126	510	104	62	0	149	951
	Total	479	1901	328	293	9	166	3176
	Percentage	15.1	59.9	10.3	9.2	0.3	5.2	100.0

[a]Incidence series of type at only one anatomic site not included
[b]Most articles have more than one author
[c]Includes only humerus, radius, ulna, femur, tibia, and fibula
Reproduced from Peterson [192] with permission

the growth plate resulting in damage to all layers of the epiphyseal plate." The latter scenario was depicted in a drawing by Ogden [199, 200], and would be visible roentgenographically.

In 1990 Beals [181] reported three children, ages 11, 11 and 13 years, two with fractures of the femoral diaphysis and one with compound fractures of both the femur and tibia. Treatment consisted of a combination of skeletal traction, spica cast and brace. In the patient with fractures of both the femur and tibia, premature arrest of distal femur was attributed to direct trauma, while no etiology was suggested for premature closure of the proximal femur, proximal tibia, and distal tibial physes on the same side. In the discussion, Beals noted that the physeal premature closure was unusual and does not appear related to the severity of injury. He mentioned both decreased and increased vascular flow following fracture, but favored Blount's hypothesis [176] by stating "It is possible that premature physeal closure in this age group is related to general hyperemia following fracture." Beals made no mention of compression and did not cite Salter and Harris.

Ogden and co-authors [182], while reporting wrist injuries in 1990, concluded "the type 5 injury probably arises from vascular disruption, rather than from direct compression injuries." In 1993 Ogden [189] and Ogden et al. [190], examined tissue from traumatic limb avulsions of 57 children and stated "the unique opportunity to observe the potential effects of excessive pressure on the physis confirmed the concept of Peterson and Burkhart that direct crushing of the germinal zone, as originally proposed by Harris and Salter, probably does not occur, even in the presence of significant pressure related changes within other areas of the epiphysis." In 2000 he went further by stating that longitudinally applied force " is likely to disrupt the vascular supply, rather than 'crush' the cartilage cells," and concluded that the "pure compression injury pattern (mechanism) does not exist." [188]

In 2000 a study aimed to assess physeal fractures of the pediatric knee by MR imaging was reported [183]. The authors performed MR imaging on 315 consecutive pediatric traumatic knee injuries and found 9 S-H physeal fracture types 1–4, but no type 5 injuries.

In the largest and only population based study of physeal fractures, 953 physeal fractures were identified and there were no S-H type 5 compression injuries [193]. Distribution of physeal fractures by type, using the S-H classification has been accumulated from series which include all bones (Table 10.1). The 9 S-H type 5 compression injuries comprised 0.3% of 3,176 physeal fractures. Few of the nine recorded cases were illustrated, none included initial normal roentgenograms, and none met all S-H criteria. Similar findings occur when examining case series of physeal fractures at each anatomic site [192].

Records at Mayo Clinic Rochester include over eight million individual patients, most registering multiple times, and the diagnosis of S-H type 5 injury has yet to be made.

10.4.6 New Classifications

Multiple physeal fracture classifications appeared after those of Brashear (1958) and S-H (1963). The new classifications were created because of either inability to document a compression injury [196, 197, 201, 204] to be more pathophysiologic [202], to more closely correlate with mechanism of injury, for simplicity, and more direct implication for treatment, [195, 197, 198, 203] to more closely correlate with prognosis [172, 196, 197] or to add new types [199–201]. Of these new classifications only those of Ogden [199, 200] and Specht [172], include the compression injury, and Ogden subsequently concluded that *"the type 5 compression injury does not exist."* [188, 190] The most recent classification of physeal fractures, published in 1994 [201], was created because in a population based study of 954 physeal fractures there were two previously unclassified physeal fractures and no Brashear type 4 or S-H type 5 compression injuries.

10.5 Acute Compression – Animal Research

Several animal experiments have been performed in an attempt to learn more about the pathology and pathomechanisms of acute compression on the physis. These studies favor either direct compression of the germinal cells or compression/disruption of the vascular supply as the cause of subsequent physeal arrest. There are shortcomings in any animal study. Conclusions are based on circumstantial evidence because it is impossible to histologically document an acute injury, the chronic lesion, and the subsequent growth disturbance in the same animal [206].

10.5.1 Animal Studies Supporting the Compression Concept

In 1992 Mendez, et al. [206], subjected both hind limbs of 5 week old rats to acute combined valgus and compressive forces. Fifteen rats were studied immediately and 31 rats at 4 months post injury. In the group of 15 rats examined immediately, 23 tibiae were subjected to compression and seven left as controls. Twelve limbs subjected to a lighter compression force had no gross or radiographic abnormalities of the proximal epiphyseal-physeal-metaphyseal area. In 11 limbs subjected to greater weight all femurs fractured upon impaction. Seven of these limbs demonstrated microscopic hematomas that separated columns of chondrocytes in the proliferating cartilage. Nuclei lost their normal affinity for hemotoxylin and a dropout of nuclei in individual chondrocytes was more evident in the proliferating zone than in the resting and maturing zone. In the group of 31 rats examined at 4 months post injury, only one tibia of each rat was subjected to compression, the other tibia serving as a control. None had roentgenographic abnormality of the physis at time of injury, though all 14 in the greater weight group sustained fracture of the diaphysis at the time of impact. Four had valgus deformity associated with a histological fibro-osseous bridge across the lateral half of the physis. The remaining 27 physes were histologically normal. There was a "trend toward there being a greater proportion of tibial valgus deformities in hind limbs sustaining concomitant femoral shaft fractures." The authors also noted that "this lesion was induced traumatically by the application of forces including, but probably not limited to compression", and concluded that "certainly the relationships among mechanical, metabolic, and circulatory factors in this process require further study in order to alter the retrospective nature of this diagnosis."

In 1994 Johnson, et al. [205]. histologically analyzed 13 naturally occurring physeal fractures from 6 traumatized dogs, which were euthanized at the request of their owners. In one dog a wavy appearance (distortion) of the cells in the columnar zone of the distal ulnar physis was suspected to be a S-H type V injury, despite no change noted in individual cells, and no documentation of growth arrest since the animal had been euthanized immediately after the fracture.

10.5.2 Animal Studies Refuting the Compression Concept

In 1959 Brashear published a study in rats [207] which essentially refuted the compression theory he proposed in 1958 [152]. In the rat study varus forces were produced at the knee "until a snap was heard." "Roentgenograms were made with the extremity in the deformed position. A Brashear type 1 (S-H and Peterson type 2) fracture was produced in each instance (Fig. 10.9a). The deformity was then reduced." "No attempt was made to immobilize the extremity." This study included histologic analysis of only his type 1 fracture. Brashear concluded that the injury resulted in compression on the side of the external force and distraction on the side opposite the external force (Fig. 10.14). "On the distraction side the fracture line passed through the zone of hypertrophic cartilage. On the compression side it either involved the metaphyseal bone or resulted in a grinding injury to the deeper layers of the epiphyseal cartilage." This 1959 article [207] did not mention his type 4 injury (Figs. 10.8 and 10.9) published the year before [152].

In 1984 Moen and Pelker [210] tested machined specimens of calf femoral and tibial physes in different modes of loading. Compressed specimens failed through the zone of provisional calcification and the metaphyseal trabeculae. This study attempted to eliminate the affect of physeal topography and the perichondral ring. The authors "could find no evidence to support the theory that the Salter-Harris V growth arrest fractures occur from excessive compression to the germinal layer."

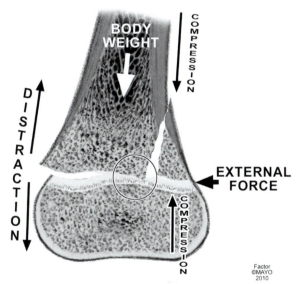

Fig. 10.14 Brashear type 1 fracture (S-H type 2) depicting an external transverse force resulting in internal compression and distraction forces (Redrawn from Brashear [152, 207], with permission). When physeal arrest occurs following this fracture it is invariably at the point where the metaphysis impacts and "grinds" (Brashear's term) the physis (*circle*, added by the present author). There is no case in the literature that shows subsequent arrest on the compression side between the metaphyseal fragment attached to the epiphysis, and the epiphysis

In 1989 Greco, et al. [208]. reported the results of an in vitro study assessing the metabolic response of growth plate cartilage explants to mechanical stress. Cultured explants were exposed to two types of stress: (a) single high compressive force, and (b) multiple low-compressive forces. Their findings suggested that too high a force, even acting for a short time, may result in permanent injury of growth plate cartilage. They "hypothesized that there might be an unknown pathogenetic mechanism of the S-H fifth-type physeal injury."

In 1991 Ogden [211] stated that "pure compression probably is not the mechanism of injury in type V fractures, as was originally proposed. When we tried to create type V fractures in the laboratory using compression, all we succeeded in doing is to crush both the epiphyseal and metaphyseal bone: the growth plate is intact." He went on to say subsequent growth arrest "must be considered each time we see a patient with a severe injury, particularly around the knee. But again, we need to think in terms of what is happening in these injuries microscopically."

In 2005 the proximal femora of calves were subjected to repeated mechanical impacts [209]. "The results showed that the areas most susceptible to trauma were the layers of immature bone located underneath the epiphyseal zone and underneath the growth plate. The authors conclude that blood vessels in these areas are highly vulnerable to mechanical damage, and the resulting impairment of blood flow to the femoral head leads to the development of Perthes disease in children."

10.6 Author's Perspective

The acute compression physeal injury is a theoretical hypothesis that begs for confirmation. It is difficult to conceptualize how germinal cartilage cells residing in a relatively soft cartilage matrix, can be "crushed" to death without fracture of the hard bony container in which they are encased. When reporting clinical cases most authors have used the compression injury concept as a "wastebasket" for premature physeal closure not explained by any other obvious cause. This unwittingly stifles investigation into other, perhaps more plausible, mechanisms of premature physeal closure. More research on the subject is needed.

References

Continuous Compression, Human Involvement: Pathophysiologic Mechanisms of Injury

1. Ehrlich MG (1998) Overview. Effects of distraction and compression on growth plate function. In: Buckwalter KA, Ehrlich MG, Sandell LJ, Trippel SB (eds) Skeletal growth and development: clinical issues and basic science advances. American Academy Orthopaedic Surgeons, Rosemont, pp 513–515
2. Forriol F, Shapiro F (2005) Bone development. Interaction of molecular components and biophysical forces. Clin Orthop 432:14–33
3. Lefebvre J, Benacerraf R (1968) Pressure forces and pathology of the metaphysis. [French]. Ann Radiol 11(5–6): 336–340
4. Siffert RS (1977) The effect of trauma to the epiphysis and growth plate. Skeletal Radiol 2:21–30
5. Siffert RS (1966) The growth plate and its affections. J Bone Joint Surg 48A:546–563, and AAOS Instr Course Lect 19, Chapter 5: 26–40, 1973
6. Trueta J (1958) The influence of growth on the sequelae of bone and joint injuries (abstr). J Bone Joint Surg 40B:154

Continuous Active Compression: Elastic Compression

7. Boggiano HF (1985) Knee epiphysiodesis. Comments. In: Orthopedic Surgery. Elastic compression. Guynes, El Paso, Texas, pp 457–460

Asymmetric Pressure

8. Beck A, Kundel K, Ruter A (1997) Significance of correction growth of opposite physes in the surgical correction of deformity following epiphyseal injury around the knee joint. Knee Surg Sports Traumatol Arthrosc 5(1):38–41
9. Frost HM (1997) Biomechanical control of knee alignment. Some insights from a new paradigm. Clin Orthop 335: 335–342
10. Shim JS, Kim HT, Mubarak SJ, Wenger DR (1997) Genu valgum in children with coxa vara resulting from hip disease. J Pediatr Orthop 17(2):225–229

Muscle Pull

11. Ikegawa S, Nagano A, Satoyoshi E (1993) Skeletal abnormalities in Satoyoshi's syndrome: a radiographic study of eight cases. Skeletal Radiol 22(5):321–324

Bone Lengthening

12. Hope PG, Crawfurd EJP, Catterall A (1994) Bone growth following lengthening for congenital shortening of the lower limb. J Pediatr Orthop 14(3):339–342
13. Pennecot GF, Hermann S, Pouliquen JC (1983) The effects on the growth plate of progressive lengthening of the tibia. Rev Chir Orthop 69:623–627
14. Price CT, Carantzas AC (1996) Severe growth retardation following limb lengthening: a case report. Iowa J Orthop 16:139–146
15. Sabharwal S, Paley D, Bhave A, Herzenberg JE (2000) Growth patterns after lengthening of congenitally short lower limbs in young children. J Pediatr Orthop 20(2): 137–145
16. Seitz WH, Froimson AI (1995) Digital lengthening using the callotasis technique. Orthopedics 18(2):129–138
17. Shaprio F (1987) Longitudinal growth of the femur and tibia after diaphyseal lengthening. J Bone Joint Surg 69A(5): 684–690
18. Sharma M, MacKenzie WG, Bower JR (1996) Severe tibial growth retardation in total fibular hemimelica after limb lengthening. J Pediatr Orthop 16(40):438–444
19. Viehweger E, Pouliquen JC, Kassis B, Glorion C, Langlais J (1998) Bone growth after lengthening of the lower limb in children. J Pediatr Orthop B 7(2):154–157

Scoliosis

20. Arkin AM (1952) Prophylaxis of scoliosis. J Bone Joint Surg 34A(1):47–48
21. Farkas A (1954) The pathogenesis of idiopathic scoliosis. J Bone Joint Surg 36A:617–653
22. Peterson HA (1994) Iatrogenic spinal deformities. In: Weinstein SL (ed) The pediatric spine: principles and practice, chapter 29. Raven Press Ltd., New York, pp 651–654

Kyphosis

23. Otsuka NY, Hey L, Hall JE (1998) Postlaminectomy and postirradiation kyphosis in children and adolescents. Clin Orthop 354:189–194
24. Papagelopoulos PJ, Peterson HA, Ebersold MJ, Emmanuel PR, Choudhury SN, Quast LM (1997) Spinal column deformity and instability after lumbar or thoracolumbar laminectomy for intraspinal tumors in children and young adults. Spine 22(4):442–451
25. Peterson HA (1985) Spinal deformity secondary to tumor, irradiation, and laminectomy. In: Bradford DS, Hensinger RN (eds) The pediatric spine, chapter 19. Thieme Inc., New York, pp 273–285
26. Seller K, Jager M, Kramer R, Krauspe R, Wild A (2004) Occurrence of a segmental kyphosis after laminectomy of C2 for an aneurysmatic bone cysts – course and treatment strategy. [German]. Z Orthop Ihre Grenzgeb 142(1): 83–87
27. Yasuoka S, Peterson HA, Laws ER, MacCarty CS (1981) Pathogenesis and prophylaxis of postlaminectomy deformity of the spine after multiple level laminectomy: difference between children and adults. Neurosurgery 9(2): 145–152
28. Yasuoka S, Peterson HA, MacCarty CS (1982) Incidence of spinal column deformity after multilevel laminectomy in children and adults. J Neurosurg 57:441–445

Zone of Ranvier

29. Campbell P, Tarlow SD (1990) Lateral tethering of the proximal femoral physis complicating the treatment of congenital hip dysplasia. J Pediatr Orthop 10(1):6–8

Slipped Capital Femoral Epiphysis

30. Rennie AM (1960) The pathology of slipped upper femoral epiphysis. A new concept. J Bone Joint Surg 42B(2):273–279

Continuous Passive Compression Tethering of the Physis by Soft-Tissue

31. Beaty JH, Barrett IR (1989) Unilateral angular deformity of the distal end of the femur secondary to a focal fibrous tether. J Bone Joint Surg 71A(3):440–445
32. Cook PA, Yu JS, Wiand W, Lubbers L, Coleman CR, Cook AJ 2nd et al (1996) Madelung deformity in skeletally immature patients: morphologic assessment using radiography, CT and MRI. J Comput Assist Tomogr 20(4):505–511
33. Haasbeek JF, Rang MC, Blackburn N (1995) Periosteal tether causing angular growth deformity: report of two clinical cases and an experimental model. J Pediatr Orthop 15(5):677–681
34. Murphy MS, Linscheid RL, Dobyns JH, Peterson HA (1996) Radial opening wedge osteotomy in Madelung's deformity. J Hand Surg 21A(6):1035–1044
35. Nielsen JB (1977) Madelung's deformity. A follow-up study of 26 cases and a review of the literature. Acta Orthop Scand 48:379–384
36. Poul J, Straka M (2003) Periosteal tethers of growth plate – focal fibrocartilaginous dysplasia. [Czech]. Acta Chir Orthop Traumatol Cech 70(3):182–186
37. Thompson TC, Straub LR, Arnold WD (1957) Congenital absence of the fibula. J Bone Joint Surg 39A(6):1229–1237
38. Vickers DW (1984) Langenskiold's operation (physiolysis) for congenital malformations of bone producing Madelung's deformity and clinodactyly (abstr). J Bone Joint Surg 66B:778
39. Vickers D (1998) Madelung's deformity. In: Cooney WP, Linscheid RL, Dobyns JH (eds) The wrist. Diagnosis and operative treatment, chapter 41, vol 2. Mosby, St. Louis, Missouri, pp 966–981
40. Vickers D, Nielsen G (1992) Madelung deformity: surgical prophylaxis (physiolysis) during the late growth period by resection of the dyschondrosteosis lesion. J Hand Surg 17B(4):401–407

Casts

41. Ahstrom JP (1965) Epiphyseal injuries of the lower extremity. Surg Clinics No America 1:119–134
42. Segev E, Yavor A, Ezra E, Hemo Y (2009) Growth and development of tarsal and metatarsal bones in successfully treated congenital idiopathic clubfoot: early radiographic study. J Pediatr Orthop B 18:17–21

Wire Loops

43. Hass SL (1945) Retardation of bone growth by a wire loop. J Bone Joint Surg 27(1):25–36
44. Peterson HA (1980) Operative correction of post-fracture arrest of the epiphyseal plate. Case report with ten-year follow-up. J Bone Joint Surg 62A(6):1018–1020

Staples

45. Blount WP (1971) A mature look at epiphyseal stapling. Clin Orthop 77:158–163
46. Blount WP, Brockway A et al (1963) End-result of sixty-two stapling operations (discussion). J Bone Joint Surg 36A(5):1069–1070
47. Blount WP (1958) Stapling is the method of choice to treat linear and angular epiphyseal deformities (abstr). J Bone Joint Surg 40B:154–155
48. Blount WP, Clarke GR (1949) Control of bone growth by epiphyseal stapling. A preliminary report. J Bone Joint Surg 31A(3):464–478, Reprinted in Clin Orthop 77: 4–17, 1971
49. Brockway A, Craig WA, Cockbell BR Jr (1954) End-result study of sixty-two stapling operations. J Bone Joint Surg 36A(5):1063–1070
50. Bylander B, Hansson LI, Selvik G (1983) Pattern of growth retardation after Blount stapling: a roentgen stereophotogrammetric analysis. J Pediatr Orthop 3(1):63–72
51. Bylander B, Selvik G, Hansson LI, Aronson S (1981) A roentgen stereophotogrammetric analysis of growth arrest by stapling. J Pediatr Orthop 1(1):81–90
52. Bylski-Austrow DI, Wall EJ, Rupert MP, Roy DR, Crawford AH (2001) Growth plate forces in the adolescent human knee: a radiographic and mechanical study of epiphyseal staples. J Pediatr Orthop 21(6):817–823
53. Castañeda P, Urquhart B, Sullivan E, Haynes RJ (2008) Hemiepiphysiodesis for the correction of angular deformity about the knee. J Pediatr Orthop 28(2):188–191
54. Cherry JC (1952) Epiphysial arrest by stapling (abstr). J Bone Joint Surg 34B:328
55. Cho TJ, Choi IH, Chung CY, Yoo WJ, Park MS, Lee DY (2009) Hemiepiphyseal stapling for angular deformity correction around the knee joint in children with multiple epiphyseal dysplasia. J Pediatr Orthop 29(1):52–56
56. Degreef I, Moens P, Fabry G (2003) Temporary epiphysiodesis with Blount stapling for treatment of idiopathic genua valga in children. Acta Orthop Belg 69(5):426–432
57. Eidelman M, D'Agostino P (2005) Hemiepiphysiodesis around the knee by percutaneously guided and grooved staple. J Pediatr Orthop B 14:434–435
58. Frantz CH (1971) Epiphyseal stapling: a comprehensive review. Clin Orthop 77:149–157
59. Fraser RK, Dickens DRV, Cole WG (1995) Medial physeal stapling for primary and secondary genu valgum in late childhood and adolescence. J Bone Joint Surg 77B(5):733–735
60. Goff CW (1967) Histologic arrangements from biopsies of epiphyseal plates of children before and after stapling. Correlated with roentgenographic studies. Am J Orthop Surg 9(5):87–89

61. Guarniero R, Malheiros Luzo CA, Cárdenas Arena E, Pugas Leiva T (1998) Correction fo knee angular deformities by physeal stapling and epiphysiodesis. In: de Pablos J (ed) The immature knee. Masson, SA, Barcelona, pp 328–332
62. Guest KE (1959) Epiphysial retardation by stapling (abstr). J Bone Joint Surg 41B:215
63. Harsha WN (1957) Effects of trauma upon epiphyses. Clin Orthop 10:140–147
64. Howorth B (1971) Knock knees. With special reference to the stapling operation. Clin Orthop 77:233–246
65. Kramer A, Stevens PM (2001) Anterior femoral stapling. J Pediatr Orthop 21(6):804–807
66. Krauspe R, Raab P, Wild A, Vispo-Seara JL, Richter A (1998): Temporary stapling of the growth-plate according to blount for the treatment of axial deformities and leg-length discrepancies. In: de Pablos (ed) Surgery of the growth plate, chapter 32. Ediciones Eregon, S.A., Madrid, pp 267–274
67. May VR Jr, Clements EL (1965) Epiphyseal stapling: with special reference to complications. South Med J 58:1203–1207
68. McGibbon KC, Deacon AE, Raisbeck CC (1962) Experiences in growth retardation with heavy vitallium staples. J Bone Joint Surg 44B:86–92
69. Menelaus MB (1991) Growth plate arrest. In: Menelaus MB (ed): The management of limb inequality, chapter 6. Churchill Livingstone, London, pp 71–94
70. Mielke CH, Stevens PM (1996) Hemiepiphyseal stapling for knee deformities in children younger than 10 years: a preliminary report. J Pediatr Orthop 16(4):423–429
71. Park SS, Gordon JE, Luhmann SJ, Dobbs MB, Schoenecker PL (2005) Outcome of hemiepiphyseal stapling for late-onset tibia vara. J Bone Joint Surg 87A(10):2259–2266
72. Peterson HA (2001) Physeal injuries and growth arrest. In Beaty JH, Kasser JR (eds) Rockwood and wilkins' fractures in children, chapter 5, 5th ed. Lippincott Williams and Wilkins, Philadelphia, pp 91–138
73. Pilcher MF (1962) Epiphyseal stapling: thirty-five cases followed to maturity. J Bone Joint Surg 44B:82–85
74. Pistevos G, Duckworth T (1977) The correction of genu valgum by epiphysial stapling. J Bone Joint Sug 59B(1):72–76
75. Poirier H (1968) Epiphysial stapling and leg equalization. J Bone Joint Surg 50B(1):61–69
76. Pritchard AE (1957) Epiphysial stapling in idiopathic knock-knee (abstr). J Bone Joint Surg 39B(3):581
77. Raab P, Wild A, Seller K, Krauspe R (2001) Correction of length discrepancies and angular deformities of the leg by Blount's epiphyseal stapling. Eur J Pediatr 160:668–674
78. Rydholm U, Brattström H, Bylander B, Lidgren L (1987) Stapling of the knee in juvenile chronic arthritis. J Pediatr Orthop 7(1):63–68
79. Scheffer MM, Peterson HA (1994) Opening-wedge osteotomy for angular deformities of long bones in children. J Bone Joint Surg 76A(3):325–334
80. Skyttä E, Savolainen A, Kautiainen H, Lehtinen J, Belt EA (2003) Treatment of leg length discrepancy with temporary epiphyseal stapling in children with juvenile idiopathic arthritis during 1957–99. J Pediatr Orthop 23(3):378–380
81. Stevens PM, Maguire M, Dales MD, Robins AJ (1999) Physeal stapling for idiopathic genu valgum. A preliminary series using a tension bond plate. J Pediatr Orthop 19(5):645–649
82. Stevens PM, Murdock LE (1996) Hemiepiphyseal stapling for post traumatic tibial valgus in children. J Bone Joint Surg 78B(Supp 1):78
83. Volpon JB (1997) Idiopathic genu valgum treated by epiphyseodesis in adolescence. Int Orthop (SICOT) 21:228–231
84. Zuege RC, Kempken TG, Blount WP (1979) Epiphyseal stapling for angular deformity at the knee. J Bone Joint Surg 61A(3):320–329

Tension Band Plate

85. Burghardt RD, Herzenberg JE, Standard SC, Paley D (2008) Temporary hemiepiphyseal arrest using a screw and palte device to treat knee and ankle deformities in children: a preliminary report. J Child Orthop 2:187–197
86. Klatt J, Stevens PM (2008) Guided growth for fixed knee flexion deformity. J Pediatr Orthop 28(6):626–631
87. Schroerlucke S, Bertrand S, Clapp J, Bundy J, Gregg FO (2009) Failure of orthofix eight-plate for the treatment of Blount disease. J Pediatr Orthop 29(1):57–60
88. Stevens PM (2007) Guided growth for angular correction. A preliminary series using a tension band plate. J Pediatr Orthop 27(3):253–259
89. Stevens PM, Klatt JB (2008) Guided growth for pathological physes. Radiographic improvement during realignment. J Pediatr Orthop 28(6):632–639
90. Stevens PM, Pease F (2006) Hemiepiphysiodesis for post-traumatic tibial valgus. J Pediatr Orthop 26(3):385–392
91. Wiemann JM, Tryon C, Szalay EA (2009) Physeal stapling versus 8-plate hemiepiphysiodesis for guided correction of angular deformity about the knee. J Pediatr Orthop 29(5):481–485

Transphyseal Threaded Screws

92. Belle RM, Stevens PM (1992) Medial malleolar screw epiphysiodesis for ankle valgus. Orthop Trans 16:655
93. Davids JR, Valadie AL, Ferguson RL, Bray EW III, Allen BL Jr (1997) Surgical management of ankle valgus in children: use of a transphyseal medial malleolar screw. J Pediatr Orthop 17(1):3–8
94. De Brauwer V, Moens P (2008) Temporary hemiepiphyseodesis for idiopathic genua valga in adolescents. Percutaneous transphyseal screws (PETS) versus stapling. J Pediatr Orthop 28(5):549–554
95. Guzzanti V, Falciglia F, Stanitski CL, Stanitski DF (2003) Slipped capital femoral epiphysis: physeal histologic features before and after fixation. J Pediatr Orthop 23(5):571–577
96. Khoury JG, Tavares JO, McConnell S, Zeiders G, Sanders JO (2007) Results of screw epiphysiodesis for the treatment of limb length discrepancy and angular deformity. J Pediatr Orthop 27(6):623–628
97. Métaizeau J, Wong-Chung J, Bertrand H, Pasquier P (1998) Percutaneous epiphysiodesis using transphyseal screws (PETS). J Pediatr Orthop 18(3):363–369
98. Nouh F, Kuo LA (2004) Percutaneous epiphysiodesis using transphyseal screws (PETS). J Pediatr Orthop 24(6):721–725
99. Shah HH, Doddabasappa SN, Joseph B (2009) Congenital posteriomedial bowing of the tibia: a retrospective analysis of growth abnormalities in the left. J Pediatr Orthop B 18:120–128
100. Stevens PM, Belle RM (1997) Screw epiphysiodesis for ankle valgus. J Pediatr Orthop 17(1):9–12

Spine Fusion

101. Johnson JTH, Southwick WO (1960) Bone growth after spine fusion. J Bone Joint Surg 42A(8):1396–1412
102. Richards BS (1998) The effects of growth on the scoliotic spine following posterior spinal fusion. In: Buckwalter JA, Ehrlich MG, Sandell LJ, Trippel SB (eds) Skeletal growth and development: clinical issues and basic science advances, chapter 33. American Academy of Orthopaedic Surgeons, Rosemont, pp 577–587

Continuous Compression

Animal Research
Pathophysiologic Mechanism of Injury

103. Alberty A, Peltonen J, Ritsilä V (1993) Effects of distraction and compression on proliferation of growth plate chondrocytes. Acta Orthop Scand 64(4):449–455
104. Bowden WG, Etherington P, Winlove CP, Murray D, Urban JPG (1999) Effect of load on nutrient delivery to the growth plate measured electrochemically (abstr). J Bone J Surg 81B: 51, Supp II
105. Bries A, Jacquet R, McBurney D, Lowder E, Landis WJ, Horton WE, et al. (2010): A study in vivo of the effects of a static compressive load on the proximal tibial physis in rabbits. Am Acad Pediatr Section on Orthop, Spring Newsletter, p 14
106. Ehrlich MG, Mankin HJ, Treadwell BV (1972) Biochemical and physiological events during closure of the stapled distal femoral epiphyseal plate in rats. J Bone J Surg 54A:309–322
107. Farnum CE, Wilsman NJ (1998) Effects of distraction and compression on growth plate function. In: Buckwalter JA, Ehrlich MG, Sandell LJ, Trippel SB (eds) Skeletal growth and development: clinical issues and basic science advances, chapter 30. Am Acad Orthop Surg, Rosemont, pp 517–530
108. Herwig J, Schmidt A, Matthiab HH, Kleemann H, Buddecke E (1987) Biochemical events during stapling of the proximal tibial epiphyseal plate in pigs. Clin Orthop 218:283–289
109. Mankin KP, Zaleske DJ (1998) Response of physeal cartilage to low-level compression and tension in organ culture. J Pediatr Orthop 18(2):145–148
110. Trueta J, Trias A (1961) The vascular contribution to osteogenesis. IV. The effect of pressure upon the epiphysial cartilage of the rabbit. J Bone Joint Surg 43B:800–813

Histologic Studies

111. Arriola F, Forriol F, Cañadell J (2001) Histomorphometric study of growth plate subjected to different mechanical conditions (compression, tension and neutralization): an experimental study in lambs. Mechanical growth plate behavior. J Pediatr Orthop B 10(4):334–338
112. Gelbke H (1951) The influence of pressure and tension on growing bone in experiments with animals. J Bone Joint Surg 33A(4):947–954
113. Sijbrandij S (1963) Inhibition of tibial growth by means of compression of its proximal epiphysial disc in the rabbit. Acta Anat 55:278–285

Amount of Compression

114. Bonnel F, Peruchon E, Baldet P, Dimeglio A, Rabischong P (1983) Effects of compression on growth plates in the rabbit. Acta Orthop Scand 54:730–733
115. Ohashi N, Robling AG, Burr DB, Turner CH (2002) The effects of dynamic axial loading on the rat growth plate. J Bone Miner Res 17(2):284–292
116. Simon MR (1978) The effect of dynamic loading on the growth of epiphyseal cartilage in the rat. Acta Anat 102(2): 176–183
117. Stokes IAF, Aronsson DD, Dimock AN, Cortright V, Beck S (2006) Endochondral growth in growth plates of three species at two anatomical locations modulated by mechanical compression and tension. J Orthop Res 24:1327–1334
118. Strobino LJ, Colonna PC, Brodey RS, Leinbach T (1956) The effect of compression on the growth of epiphyseal bone. Surg Gynecol Obstet 103(1):85–93
119. Strobino LJ, French GO, Colonna PC (1952) The effect of increasing tensions on the growth of epiphyseal bone. Surg Gynecol Obstet 95(6):694–700
120. Sybrandy S (1963) Compression of the epiphysial plate of the tibia in rabbits. J Bone Joint Surg 45B:432

Direction of Pressure Applied

121. Arkin AM, Katz JF (1956) The effects of pressure on epiphyseal growth. J Bone Joint Surg 38A(5):1056–1076
122. Mente PL, Aronsson DD, Stokes IAF, Iatridis JC (1999) Mechanical modulation of growth for the correction of vertebral wedge deformities. J Orthop Res 17(4):518–524
123. Stokes IA, Mente PL, Iatridis JC, Farnum C, Aronsson DD (2002) Enlargement of growth plate chondrocytes modulated by sustained mechanical loading. J Bone Joint Surg 84A(10):1842–1848
124. Stokes IAF, Spence H, Aronsson DD, Kilmer N (1996) Mechanical modulation of vertebral body growth. Implications for scoliosis. Spine 21(10):1162–1167

Periosteal Tether

125. Houghton GR, Rooker GD (1979) The role of the periosteum in the growth of long bones. An experimental study in the rabbit. J Bone Joint Surg 61B(2):218–220
126. Wilson-MacDonald J, Houghton GR, Bradley J, Morscher E (1990) The relationship between periosteal division and compression or distraction of the growth plate. An experimental study in the rabbit. J Bone Joint Surg 72B(2): 303–308

Staples

127. Aykut US, Yazici M, Kandemir U, Gedikoglu G, Aksoy MC, Cil A, Surat A (2005) The effect of temporary hemiepiphyseal stapling on the growth plate. A radiologic and

immunohistochemical study in rabbits. J Pediatr Orthop 25(3):336–341
128. Christensen NO (1973) Growth arrest by stapling. An experimental study of longitudinal bone growth and morphology of the growth region. Acta Orthop Scand Suppl 151:1–71
129. González-Herranz J (1998) Growth cartilage arrest with staples. Experimental study. In: de Pablos (ed) Surgery of the growth plate, Chapter 6. Ediciones Eregon, S.A., Madrid, pp 33–53
130. Haas SL (1948) Mechanical retardation of bone growth. J Bone Joint Surg 30A(2):506–512
131. Hall-Craggs ECB, Lawrence CA (1969) The effect of epiphysial stapling on growth in length of the rabbit's tibia and femur. J Bone Joint Surg 51B(2):359–365
132. Nachlas IW, Borden JN (1951) The cure of experimental scoliosis by directed growth control. J Bone Joint Surg 35A(1):35–45
133. Siffert RS (1956) The effect of staples and longitudinal wires on epiphyseal growth an experimental study. J Bone Joint Surg 38A(5):1077–1088

Transphyseal Threaded Metallic Screws and Pins

134. Campbell CJ, Grisolia A, Zanconato G (1959) The effects produced in the cartilaginous epiphyseal plate of immature dogs by experimental surgical traumata. J Bone Joint Surg 41A(7):1221–1242
135. Green WT (1950) Restriction of bone growth. Discussion. J Bone Joint Surg 32A:350
136. Karol LA, Doane RM, Cornicelli SF, Zak PA, Haut RC, Manoli A II (1992) Single versus double screw fixation for treatment of slipped capital femoral epiphysis: a biomechanical analysis. J Pediatr Orthop 12(6):741–745

Crossed Smooth Metallic Pins

137. Haas SL (1950) Restriction of bone growth by pins through the epiphyseal cartilaginous plate. J Bone Joint Surg 32A: 338–343

Biodegradable Screws, Crossed Pins, and Filaments

138. Gil-Albarova J, Fini M, Gil-Albarova R, Melgosa M, Aldini-Nicolo N, Giardino R, Seral F (1998) Absorbable screws through the greater trochanter do not disturb physeal growth. Rabbit experiments. Acta Orthop Scand 69(3):273–276
139. Gill-Albarova J, Giardino R, Seral F (1997) Epiphyseodesis by using absorbable screws. An experimental study in rabbits. J Bone Joint Surg 79B(Supp II):164
140. Gil Albarova R, Gil Albarova J, Garrido Lahiguera R, Melgosa Gil M (2001) An experimental model for hemiepiphysiodesis by using absorbable polymers [Spanish]. Mapfre Medicina 12(2):117–121
141. Mäkelä A, Vainiopää S, Vihtonen K, Mero M, Helevirta P, Törmälä P, Rokkanen P (1989) The effect of a penetrating biodegradable implant on the growth plate. An experimental study on growing rabbits with special reference to polydioxanone. Clin Orthop 241:300–308
142. Mäkelä A, Vainiopää S, Vihtonen K, Mero M, Laiho J, Törmälä P, Rokkanen P (1987) The effect of a penetrating biodegradable implant on the epiphyseal plate: an experimental study on growing rabbits with special regard to polyglactin 910. J Pediatr Orthop 7(4):415–420
143. Österman K, Alberty A, Paavolainen P, Ritsilä V (1993) Physeal reaction to a penetrating biodegradable rod. An experimental study in rats and rabbits. Mapfre Medicina 4(Supl II):143–145
144. Otsuka NY, Mah JY, Orr FW, Martin RF (1992) Biodegradation of polydioxanone in bone tissue: effect on the epiphyseal plate in immature rabbits. J Pediatr Orthop 12(2):177–180

Surgical Bone Lengthening

145. Ginsburg GM, Reynolds RAK, Franzino SJ, Antonelli DJ, Forsteain MA (1999): An indirect method of measuring intra-articular and intraphyseal forces during femoral lengthening: a lamb model (abstr). AAOS Annual Meeting, Anneheim, CA, Feb 6, 1999
146. Lee DY, Chung CY, Choi IH (1993) Longitudinal growth of the rabbit tibia after callotasis. J Bone Joint Surg 75B(6):898–903
147. Lee SH, Szöke G, Simpson H (2001) Response of the physis to leg lengthening. J Pediatr Orthop B 10(4):339–343
148. Sabharwal S, Harten RD, Sabatino C, Yun JS, Munjal K (2005) Selective soft tissue release preserves growth plate architecture during limb lengthening. J Pediatr Orthop 25(5):617–622
149. Wilkinson JA (1967) Experimental bone growth (abstr). J Bone Joint Surg 49B:583

Spine Fusion

150. Coleman SS (1968) The effect of posterior spine fusion on vertebral growth in dogs. J Bone Joint Surg 50A(5): 879–896

Tensioned Soft Tissue Grafts

151. Edwards TB, Greene CC, Baratta RV, Zieske A, Willis RB (2001) The effect of placing a tensioned graft across open growth plates. A gross and histologic analysis. J Bone Joint Surg 83A(5):725–734

Acute Compression

Human Involvement
The Concept

152. Brashear HR (1958) Epiphyseal fractures of the lower extremity. South Med J 51:845–851

153. Cassidy RH (1958) Epiphyseal injuries of the lower extremities. Surg Clinics No Am 38:1125–1135
154. Salter RB (1974) Injuries of the ankle in children. Orthop Clinic No Am 5(1):147–152
155. Salter RB (1992) Injuries of the epiphyseal plate. In: Instructional Course Lectures, chapter 37, vol 41. AAOS, Park Ridge, pp 351–359
156. Salter RB (1988) Salter-Harris classification of epiphyseal plate injuries. In: Uhthoff HK, Wiley JJ (eds) Behavior of the growth plate. Raven, New York, pp 97–103
157. Salter RB, Harris WR (1963) Injuries involving the epiphyseal plate. J Bone Joint Surg 45A(3):587–621

The Concept Challenged

158. Burkhart SS, Peterson HA (1979) Fractures of the proximal tibial epiphysis. J Bone Joint Surg 61A(7): 996–1002
159. Peterson HA, Burkhart SS (1981) Compression injury of the epiphyseal growth plate: fact or fiction? J Pediatr Orthop 1(4):377–384

Clinical Support for the S-H Type 5 Compression Injury Concept

160. Abram LJ, Thompson GH (1987) Deformity after premature closure of the distal radial physis following a torus fracture with a physeal compression injury. Report of a case. J Bone Joint Surg 69A(9):1450–1453
161. Aminiam A, Schoenecker PL (1995) Premature closure of the distal radial physis after fracture of the distal radial metaphysis. J Pediatr Orthop 15(4):495–498
162. Bowler JR, Mubarak SJ, Wenger DR (1990) Tibial physeal closure and genu recurvatum after femoral fracture: occurrence without a tibial traction pin. Case report. J Pediatr Orthop 10:653–657
163. Collado-Torres F, Zamora-Navas P, De La Torre-Solis F (1995) Secondary forearm deformity due to injury to the distal ulnar physis. Acta Orthop Belg 61(3):242–244
164. Hresko MT, Kasser JR (1989) Physeal arrest about the knee associated with non-physeal fractures in the lower extremity. J Bone Joint Surg 71A(5):698–703
165. Keret D, Mendez AA, Harcke HT, MacEwen GD (1990) Type V physeal injury: a case report. J Pediatr Orthop 10(4):545–548
166. Morton KS, Starr DE (1964) Closure of the anterior portion of the upper tibial epiphysis as a complication of tibial-shaft fracture. J Bone Joint Surg 46A(3):570–574
167. Nelson OA, Buchanan JR, Harrison CS (1984) Distal ulnar growth arrest. J Hand Surg 9A(2):164–171
168. Pozarny E, Kanat IR (1987) Epiphyseal growth plate fracture: Salter and Harris type V. J Foot Surg 26(3):204–209
169. Sato T, Shinozaki T, Fukuda T, Watanabe H, Aoki J, Yanagawa T, Takagishi K (2002) Atypical growth plate closure: a possible chronic Salter and Harris type V injury. J Pediatr Orthop B 11:155–158
170. Schoenecker PL (1997) Letter to the editors. J Pediatr Orthop 17(1):127
171. Skak SV (1989) A case of partial physeal closure following compression injury. Arch Orthop Trauma Surg 108:185–188
172. Specht EE (1974) Epiphyseal injuries in childhood. Am Fam Physician 10:101–109
173. Tang CW, Kay RM, Skaggs DL (2002) Growth arrest of the distal radius following a metaphyseal fracture: case report and review of the literature. J Pediatr Orthop B 11(1):89–92
174. Valverde JA, Albiñana J, Certucha JA (1996) Early post-traumatic physeal arrest in distal radius after a compression injury. J Pediatr Orthop B 5(1):57–60

Alternative Mechanisms

175. Barnhart J (1967) Premature closure of the proximal tibial epiphysis following fracture of the tibial shaft. South Medical J 60(3):317–320
176. Blount WP (1955) Fractures in children. Williams and Wilkins, Baltimore, p 132
177. Neer CS (1960) Separation of the lower femoral epiphysis. Am J Surg 99:756–761
178. Ogden JA (2000) Injury to the growth mechanisms. In: Skeletal injury in the child, chapter 6. Springer-Verlag, New York, pp172-177
179. Ogden JA (1990) Transphyseal linear ossific striations of the distal radius and ulna. Skeletal Radiol 19:173–180
180. Siffert RS (1980) Injuries to the growth plate and the epiphysis, chapter 5. AAOS Instr Course Lect 29: 62–72

Clinical Opposition to or Evidence Against the S-H Type 5 Compression Injury

181. Beals RK (1990) Premature closure of the physis following diaphyseal fractures. J Pediatr Orthop 10(6):717–720
182. Beatty E, Light TR, Belsole RJ, Ogden JA (1990) Wrist and hand skeletal injuries in children. Hand Clin 6(4):723–738
183. Close BJ, Strouse PJ (2000) MR of physeal fractures of the adolescent knee. Pediatr Radiol 30:756–762
184. Connolly JF, Eastman T, Huurman WW (1985) Torus fracture of the distal radius producing growth arrest. Fracture of the month. Nebr Med J 70:204–207
185. Herring JA (1987) Whither the bar. Instructional case. J Pediatr Orthop 7(6):722–725
186. Hunter LY, Hensinger RN (1978) Premature monomelic growth arrest following fracture of the femoral shaft. J Bone Joint Surg 60A(6):850–852
187. Letts RM (1988) Compression injuries of the growth plate. In: Uhthoff HK, Wiley JJ (eds) Behavior of the growth plate. Raven, New York, pp 111–118
188. Ogden JA (2000) Injury to the growth mechanisms. In: Skeletal injury in the child, Chapter 6, 3rd edn. Springer-Verlag, New York, pp 147–208
189. Ogden JA (1993) The pathology of growth plate injury. Mapfre Medicina 4(Suppl II):8–14
190. Ogden JA Ganey T, Light TR, Southwick WO (1993) The pathology of acute chondro-osseous injury in the child. Yale J Biol Med 66:219–233

191. Ogden JA, Lee KE, Rudicel SA, Pelker RR (1984) Proximal femoral epiphysiolysis in the neonate. J Pediatr Orthop 4(3):285–292
192. Peterson HA (2007) Epiphyseal growth plate fractures. Springer, Heidelberg, p 914
193. Peterson HA, Madhok R, Benson JT, Ilstrup DM, Melton LJ III (1994) Physeal fractures: part 1. Epidemiology in Olmsted county, Minnesota, 1979–1988. J Pediatr Orthop 14:423–440
194. Rang M (1983) Injuries of the epiphysis, the growth plate, and the perichondrial ring. In: Children's fractures, Chapter 2, 2nd edn. JB Lippincott Company, Philadelphia, pp 10–25

Alternative Classifications

195. Boissevain ACH, Raaymakers ELFB (1979) Traumatic injury of the distal tibial epiphysis. An appraisal of forty cases. Reconstr Surg Trauma 17:40–47
196. Bylander B, Aronson S, Egund N, Hansson LI, Selvik G (1981) Growth disturbance after physial injury of distal femur and proximal tibia studied by roentgen stereophotogrammetry. Arch Orthop Trauma Surg 98:225–235
197. Chadwick CJ, Bentley G (1988) Chadwick and bently classification of distal tibial growth plate injuries. In: Uhthoff HK, Wiley JJ (eds) Behavior of the growth plate. Raven, New York, pp 105–110
198. Dias LS, Tachdjian MO (1978) Physeal injuries of the ankle in children. Classification. Clin Orthop 136:230–233
199. Ogden JA (1981) Injury to the growth mechanisms of the immature skeleton. Skeletal Radiol 6:237–253
200. Ogden JA (1988) Skeletal growth mechanism injury patterns. In: Uhthoff HK, Wiley JJ (eds) Behavior of the growth plate. Raven, New York, pp 85–96
201. Peterson HA (1994) Physeal fractures: part 3. Classification. J Pediatr Orthop 14:439–448
202. Shapiro F (1982) Epiphyseal growth plate fracture-separations. A pathophysiologic approach. Orthopedics 5(6):720–736
203. Wahl VD (1982) Epiphyseal injuries in childhood and their classification [German]. Zbl Chirurgie 107:1281–1286
204. Von Laer L (1981) Klinische aspekte zur einteilung kinderlicher frakturen, insbesondere zu den traumatischen läsionen der wachstumsfuge [German]. Unfallheilkunde 84:229–236

Acute Compression

Animal Research
Studies Supporting the Compression Concept

205. Johnson JM, Johnson AL, Eurell JC (1994) Histological appearance of naturally occurring canine physeal fractures. Vet Surg 23(2):81–86
206. Mendez AA, Bartal E, Grillot MB, Lin JJ (1992) Compression (Salter-Harris type V) physeal fracture: an experimental model in the rat. J Pediatr Orthop 12(1):29–37

Studies Refuting the Compression Concept

207. Brashear HR (1959) Epiphyseal fractures. A microscopic study of the healing process in rats. J Bone Joint Surg 41A(6):1055–1064
208. Greco F, de Palma L, Specchia N, Mannarini M (1989) Growth-plate cartilage metabolic response to mechanical stress. J Pediatr Orthop 9(5):520–524
209. Kandzierski G, Karski T, Czerny K, Kisiel J, Kalakucki J (2005) In-vitro mechanical impacts on claves' proximal femurs: significance of mechanical weakening of the femoral head in the etiology of perthes disease in children. J Pediatr Orthop B 15(2):120–125
210. Moen CT, Pelker RR (1984) Biomechanical and histological correlations in growth plate failure. J Pediatr Orthop 4(2):180–184
211. Rang M, Armstrong P, Crawford AH, Kasser JR, Ogden JA (1991) Symposium: management of fractures in children and adolescents – part I. Contemp Orthop 23(5):517–548

Distraction

11.1 Introduction

Controlled, slow, symmetric distraction of the physis, also known as *chondrodiatasis*, is a method of bone lengthening in children. When distraction results in separation of the physis, it is termed epiphysiolysis, or more correctly *physiolysis*. *Hemichondrodiatasis* refers to asymmetric distraction of the physis to correct angular deformity. Ring [3] is frequently cited as the first to explore the therapeutic potential of physeal distraction, despite the earlier writings of Gelbke [1] and Smith and Cunningham [4]. Zavyalov and Plaskin [5, 6] were the first to record its use in humans. Interest in physeal distraction in humans has gradually increased and has stimulated considerable animal research, much of which is recorded here.

Distraction of the physis does not appear to occur in nature or as a traumatic event. Its complications are therefore entirely iatrogenic. It is included in this text because the phyeal injury incurred during distraction usually results in growth arrest. The effects of distraction lengthening of bone (the diaphysis or metaphysis) on the physis are discussed in Chap. 10. Distraction of a physis containing a physeal bar has been reported in depth in the text book "Epiphyseal Growth Plate Fractures" (Chapter 34) [2], and is not repeated here.

11.2 Human Involvement

Zavyalov and Plaskin [5] noted physiolysis serendipitously when 9 of 15 children undergoing surgical bone lengthening (callotasis) were noted to have elongation of the physis of 2–7 cm. They felt distraction physiolysis was superior to callotasis because it involved less trauma and accelerated bone regeneration. Physeal growth continued after lengthening in three cases followed 1–1½ years.

In humans, physeal distraction is performed primarily for conditions other than trauma [7, 11, 13, 16, 17, 33, 36, 42, 44, 46–48, 50, 53, 54], and is said to be "well-tolerated, and relatively painless" [17, 23]. Mechanical distraction of post traumatic elbow stiffness in children has not resulted in any widening of physes or separation of epiphyses [30].

11.2.1 The Procedure

Steinmann pins are placed in the bone to be lengthened in the coronal plane parallel to each other and perpendicular to the long axis of the bone. In the diaphysis two pins are used, one more proximal than the other. In the epiphysis, one to three (usually two) pins are placed in the same transverse plane parallel to the articular surface. A lengthener is attached to the pins parallel to the long axis of the bone to avoid lateral or angular displacement of the epiphysis during distraction. Any mechanical bone distractor can be used [19]. The Orthofix Dynamic Axial Fixator (Orthofix S.R.L, Verona, Italy) with an articulated body and detachable lengthener, is ideal for this procedure [7, 8, 12, 16, 17, 22, 48, 50]. The Wagner [11, 19–22, 24, 54], Ilizarov [5, 12, 32, 42–44, 46, 47, 53, 54], and other devices [9, 10, 13–15, 25, 26, 29, 36, 39, 41, 44, 45, 49, 52] have also been used. Most devices are rigid, threaded, turnbuckle distraction devices.

Distraction begins on the first postoperative day at a rate of 0.25 mm two to four times per 24 h and should not exceed 1 mm per day [7, 8, 16, 17, 25, 46, 47, 52, 54].

A low rate of distraction maintains physeal viability and reduces the potential for bar formation. Ambulation with crutches is allowed the day after the fixator is applied and weight bearing is gradually increased until the limb is bearing full weight [8, 16, 52]. Or weight bearing is forbidden until the cortex is adequately developed to support the weight of the body, which in one study averaged 7–8 months [45]. Sometime during the lengthening, the epiphysis usually detaches from the metaphysis, a feature noted by sudden local pain. After one or two days of rest, the lengthening is restarted at a rate up to 1.25 mm a day in divided increments. Angulation adjustments can be made incrementally. Limb alignment is checked clinically and roentgenographically every 20–40 days and the lengthening is continued until the desired effect is achieved [7, 8, 17].

When distraction is complete, the fixator is tightened (locked) and the distractor is removed. Dynamic loading on the bone is gradually increased by gradually loosening the locking screws. The fixation device should be maintained until the lengthened gap has healed, as evidenced by completely formed cortical bone 2 mm in thickness [52], but not so long as to create a compressive force and promote closure of the growth plate [13]. The profuse blood supply of the physis (Fig. 1.1) augments its healing. The duration the fixator remains on the patient is variable, depending on the site, rate of lengthening, amount lengthened, and age of the patient, but in general is "several months" [23]. When there is clear roentgenographic evidence of uniform ossification, the fixator is removed [8]. After the fixator is removed, application of a protective cast is optional [52]. Guidelines for additional protection of a recently distracted physis have not been determined.

Theoretically, distraction is applicable to any physis. However, at the distal femur the wires or screws in the epiphysis cross the intraarticular space. This creates a risk for infection and possibly a delay in consolidation due to synovial fluid mixing with the hematoma. In addition, there is often substantial decrease in knee motion [46, 47]. At the distal tibia complications due to alteration of the anatomical relationship between the length of the tibia and fibula are increased [46, 47]. Both proximal and distal tibial physeal distractions should be accompanied by osteotomy of the fibula [5, 11].

Psychological resistance to the procedure and its duration has caused some clinicians to require preoperative psychiatric screening to assess the patient's capacity to successfully complete the procedure [44].

11.2.2 Results

Distraction of minor intensity maintained below the strain tolerance of cartilage provokes a mechanical deformation of the physis [52]. Low incremental physeal distraction may avoid both physiolysis and growth arrest [18]. Under such conditions, the main roentgenographic and histologic change is physeal widening caused by ischemia of the metaphyseal capillaries interfering with removal of degenerating cells, while proliferation of cells in the germinal layer continues. This physeal widening is usually a minor part of the overall bone lengthening [52].

A fixed rate of distraction of as little as 0.25 mm twice daily is likely to result in physiolysis [38]. One group, using a distraction rate of 0.25 mm twice a day noted physiolysis, but no premature growth arrest in all 40 patients, despite performing the physiolysis in the operating room in 14 of those children [54]. The distal femoral physis of an 8 year old girl also remained open after lengthening 0.5 mm/day [18]. Two years later a second physeal distraction achieved significant additional length. Thus, when the physis remains open, the procedure can be repeated [18].

If a significant increase in length is required close to skeletal maturity, lengthening of the physis must be rapid to avoid bar reformation, and a fracture of the physis (physiolysis) is inevitable [40, 41, 52]. When the epiphysis separates from the metaphysis (after an average of 10 days distraction in two studies [37, 46, 47], with a range from 4 to 33 days [11, 15, 38, 39, 42, 52]), there is a sudden increase in pain [11, 37, 46, 47, 52], accompanied by a sudden reduction in the peak distraction force [40]. In order to avoid this painful episode two groups performed the physiolysis in the operating room under roentgenographic control at the time of apparatus application [45, 54]. At the time of physiolysis the ruptured metaphyseal vessels cause a hematoma between the epiphysis and metaphysis contained by the periosteum which is stretched, but not broken. This is the site of the new bone formation within the lengthened area [46, 47, 52]. Bone formation at the site of distraction may be periosteal in origin, rather than apposition from the metaphyseal side [48]. The fracture separation is confirmed roentgenographically by widening between the metaphysis and epiphysis, and histologically by an irregular fracture separation between the hypertrophic physeal layer and the zone of provisional calcification [39, 41]. Ultrasonic studies reveal a "window" in the bone adjacent to the plate containing areas of increased echogenicity, in keeping with the appearance of microfractures of the physis [37].

The amount of force required to distract the physis varies considerably between patients and physes, varying all the way from 250 to 800 N [14, 15, 37–41] with a mean peak distraction force of 0.258 N per square mm of physis [14]. Younger patients experience physiolysis earlier and with less force than older patients [37]. The force to cause separation is greater for the distal femur than for the tibia. However, when the force per unit area is considered, the values are similar for the distal femur, proximal and distal tibia, suggesting no difference in physeal strength of these three physes [14, 37]. Nor do the undulating contours of the distal femoral physis increase the force required to separate it [14]. The maximum distraction force which can be applied across a pre-adolescent physis without causing separation is approximately 0.150 N/mm^2 [14, 38].

Closure of physes undergoing distraction correlate closely with the skeletal age of the patient at the time of distraction [36]. In children with skeletal age less than 9 years the physis often remains open after distraction (Fig. 11.1), and growth may continue until maturity. In children with skeletal age from 9 to 11 years the physis often will stay open for 2–4 years, but will ossify earlier before maturity. In children with skeletal age over 12 years the physis usually closes during the distraction, and increasing discrepancy resumes until maturity. The authors concluded that the decisive factor influencing physeal closure associated with physeal distraction is the skeletal age of the patient [36].

Chondrodiatasis is most effective for bone length inequalities of 10% or less [7]. Along with physiolysis, lengthenings of 5–10 cm are common [36, 45, 51] and have been used to gain up to 36% of the original bone length in non-achondroplastic patients, and up to 64.5% in achondroplastic patients [16, 17, 25, 52]. The mean duration of lengthening is approximately 1 month per centimeter lengthened [46, 47]. In one study the healing index for the distal femur was 38.1 days/cm and for the proximal tibia 35.7 days/cm [54]. In another typical series the average period of distraction was 5.25 months, and the fixators were left in situ for four more months to allow consolidation of the lengthened segment [25].

Rapid physeal distraction is sometimes used to gain length prior to excision of a metaphyseal malignant tumor (Sect. 4.3). This gain in length allows enbloc excision of the tumor with preservation of the epiphysis and a margin of the metaphysis.

Hemichondrodiatasis has been used to correct angular deviations of up to 30° [12, 23, 35, 42, 49]. External control of the correction can be maintained until the bone has consolidated. If used only for correction of angular deformity the external fixator may be removed earlier and alignment maintained with a cast [49]. However, loss of correction occurs if the distractor is removed too early [12]. Hemichondrodiatasis has been performed at the knee, ankle, wrist and thumb [34, 35, 49]. At the knee it has been used to correct Blounts' disease [9, 12, 21, 24, 28, 29, 34, 35, 43], and genu varum associated with bone dysplasias [31]. The bone dysplasia children were very young (ages 3–7 years), were followed 3–11 years, and no adverse effects on the physis were indentified [31]. However, in a series of 12 children ages 11–14.5 years, all developed premature complete closure of the distracted physis [12]. The angular correction can be combined with lengthening, either concurrently or before or after the lengthening [22, 43]. Over lengthening 2–3 cm in anticipation of premature physeal arrest following the angular correction has proven beneficial in some cases, as the limbs were equal in length at the end of growth [43, 53]. Complications of hemichondrodiatasis are typically less without concurrent lengthening, but similar to chondrodiatasis when accompanied with lengthening.

The benefits of physeal distraction must be weighed against the costs. The advantages include rapid single surgery, only pin site incisions and scars, no need for osteotomy, bone grafts or internal fixation, short hospitalization, early post surgical joint motion and ambulation, the potential to achieve significant length, minimal likelihood of nonunion, and the possibility of retaining some post lengthening growth potential [16, 19, 20, 22–24, 31, 32, 38, 42, 45]. The child is able to walk, attend school, and enjoy many normal activities while the fixator is in place [16].

The disadvantages include the discomfort, inconvenience, and duration of the fixator, financial concerns, and complications. There are many potential complications [7, 11, 16–20, 22, 23, 25–27, 36, 38, 42, 44, 45, 51, 52, 54]. These include fixator failures, failed epiphyseal separation, pin tract infections, peroneal nerve deficit, fractures through the lengthened physis, hematoma in the fracture gap obstructing healing, subluxation/dislocation of the knee joint, joint stiffness, knee flexion contracture, early fusion of the osteotomized fibula, proximal and distal fibular dislocation, bending of the newly formed bone (Fig. 11.1), post-immobilization fatigue fracture, and most commonly premature physeal closure. The premature physeal closure, combined with continued contralateral growth, may result in recurrent limb length discrepancy.

In summary, chondrodiatasis has the potential to gain considerable length. Avoiding physeal arrest is most likely when the rate of distraction is low and performed in a young child. However, if a young child does develop arrest, the problem of length deficit following the distraction is compounded since there is then no opportunity for a second distraction, and arresting the contralateral physis only maintains the status quo. Therefore, many authors advise that the method

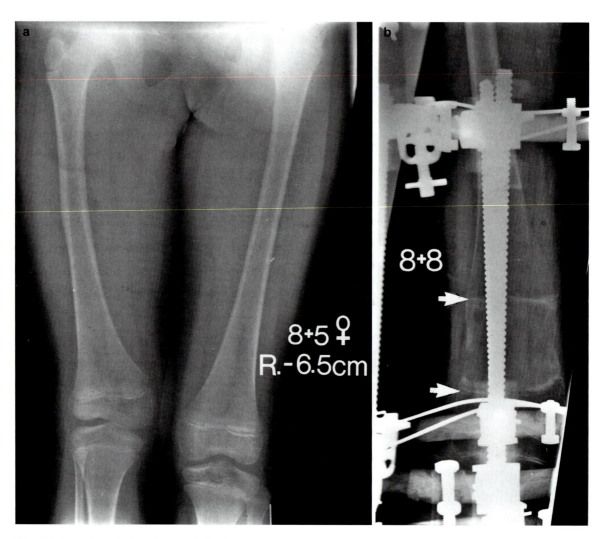

Fig. 11.1 Post physeal distraction angular bending. (**a**) A congenitally short right femur in an 8 year 5 month old girl was 6.5 cm shorter than the left. (**b**) Ninety-five days after beginning distraction (age 8 years 8 months) the physis had lengthened over 6 cm (*arrows*). New bone is forming but there is a paucity of cortical bone. The lengthening device was removed 5 days later and a spica cast applied. (**c**) Shortly thereafter posterior angulation of the lengthened bone was noted. The cast was removed 150 days (21.5 weeks) after beginning lengthening. (**d**) Ten months after beginning lengthening, age 9 years 3 months, the posterior angulation deformity measured 59°. (**e**) Fifteen months after beginning lengthening, age 9 years 8 months, the angular deformity measured 73°. (**f**) Closing wedge corrective osteotomy was performed. The physis appears open. *Note*: this angular deformity is most likely due to the tension of knee flexor muscles on immature lengthened bone with a weak cortex. (Case contributed by Dr. Peter Damjanov, Plovdiv, Bulgaria, reproduced from Peterson [2], with permission)

11.2 Human Involvement

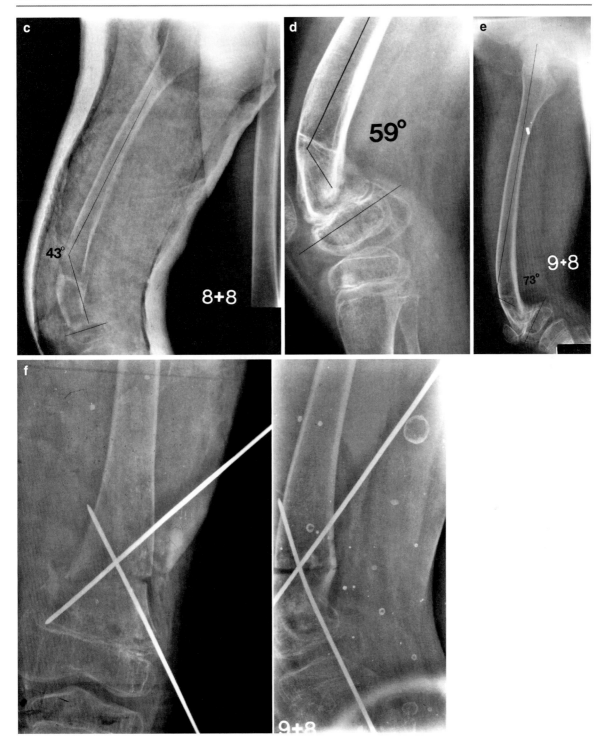

Fig. 11.1 (continued)

should be used only in adolescents near skeletal maturity [8, 11, 19, 20, 23, 26, 27, 33, 38, 41, 44–47, 50–53, 74, 87].

11.3 Animal Research

Early attempts to distract the physis in animals by springs or piston cylinders gave equivocal results [79, 84, 98]. Better and more reproducible results occur with rigid, threaded, turnbuckle devices, like those ultimately used on humans. Insertion of one or more pins transversely across an epiphysis does not affect growth of the physis [64], as long as the pin does not involve the physis.

During the initial distraction period the physis widens, accompanied by elongation of the perichondrium and metaphyseal periosteum [65]. The epiphyseal arteries enlarge, suggesting increased nutritional demands of the physis. There is a lack of agreement on the underlying cause of the physeal widening. The histological response to different distraction loads in animals is unpredictable [89, 100]. Some investigators have noted that low magnitude or slow rate distraction forces stimulate cell proliferation in the germinal or proliferative zone of the physis [60, 62, 76, 81, 101, 102], resulting in increased growth [106], with an increase in length of up to 36% [104]. Another study found that "the growth increase was associated with hyperplasia and hypertrophy of the plate, as well as an increased rate of cell division" [99]. Intermittent distracting forces at 10–14 day intervals revealed that the physeal widening was due to elongation of the cartilage cells [4]. All of these findings are in keeping with the law of tension stress which states that tissues subjected to slow steady traction become metabolically active, a phenomenon characterized by the stimulation of both proliferative and biosynthetic (anabolic formation of chemical substances) cellular functions which results in histogenesis [108].

Others, however, feel that distraction does not stimulate germinal cell production, but actually inhibits it [61, 69, 80]. These authors propose that the apparent increase in growth plate thickness results from metaphyseal ischemia and inhibition of enchondral ossification (as shown on Fig. 1.3) resulting in accumulation of cells in the columnar and hypertrophic layers [61, 67, 69, 76]. A second possibility is that cellular proliferation is unaffected by distraction and that in both chondrodiatasis and physiolysis there is an alteration of blood supply, either increased blood flow or metaphyseal ischemia [72]. Trueta showed that a decrease in pressure across the physis caused an increased metaphyseal blood flow which caused early closure of the physis [107]. A third possibility is that chondrodiatasis does not produce any significant changes in the percentages of cells *or* the blood supply to the physis, but rather stretches the matrix passively [71]. Gradually increasing tensile loading across the physis causes elongation of the collagen fibers in the cartilage matrix, while the sleeve of supporting perichondrium remains intact [66]. Regardless of the underlying mechanism, there is an elongation of the zones of proliferating cells and hypertrophic cell columns [57, 58, 68, 69, 99], as well as an increase in matrix production [80] or passive stretching of the matrix [71].

Using low distraction rates (e.g. 0.5 mm qd), passive elongation of the physis occurs without fracture [17, 68, 89, 90, 99, 101, 102]. This lengthening causes no hemorrhage [68] and no discomfort [3]. The individual chondrocyte heights differ little from controls [105]. With no physeal separation, arrest may not occur. However, histologic damage to the physis occurs with increasing frequency at increasing loads. Thus, significant damage can occur with loads even less than those needed to cause disruption of the physis [96]. The amount of chondrodiatasis that can be produced without physiolysis relates directly to the size and weight of the bone [67], by inference to the area of the physis. One study, however, concluded that bone growth is not stimulated by chondrodiatasis, and that any increase in length more than the normal growth was due to physeal separation [88]. When the physis stayed open after lengthening the post distraction growth rates were equal to contralateral controls [95].

As distraction forces increase, chondrodiatasis is inevitably accompanied by sudden physiolysis within the hypertrophic chondrocyte zone or zone of provisional calcification [3, 18, 45, 55, 57–59, 63, 65, 68, 69, 73, 75, 80, 85–87, 89–93, 100, 102, 103]. This is somewhat determined by age since older physes are thinner but stronger than younger physes which are thicker and weaker [109]. In one study growth plate failure correlated with rabbit weight, femoral length, and physis surface area [78], all of which are age related. These age-dependent increases in tensile strength do not result merely from physeal enlargement or conformational changes and may explain why physeal distraction used clinically has produced varied and somewhat unpredictable results [78].

The fracture line is not necessarily confined to a single histologic zone of the physis, but typically does not involve the germinal cell layer [3, 96]. This is essentially Salter-Harris type 1 fracture (Peterson type 3 [2]). Near skeletal maturity separation of the physis requires more force and some physeal fractures are type 2 [91]. With separation there is defective metaphyseal capillary filling and marked enlargement of the epiphyseal vessels which may indicate increased nutrition demands of the physis [56]. Any significant increase in length is due to distraction of the fracture gap [80]. The ensuing hematoma is usually contained within a stretched (but not broken) periosteum, enhancing the repair process [3, 52, 86, 92]. Osteoblasts of the inner layer of the periosteum produce the first new bone, forming a cylinder of bone encircling the region of physeal lengthening [91]. At consolidation, the distraction area is composed of lamellar trabecular bone and partly woven bone [91]. This is an area of weakness is prone to subsequent fracture [3].

All these seemingly conflicting reports reflect the inherent difficulty in predicting physeal behavior during and after chondrodiatasis in experimental animals. They appear to suggest that single rate of distraction may not be appropriate for all situations [53]. Acoustic emission technology has been used in an attempt to detect impending physeal failure thereby allowing the distraction to be curtailed prior to physiolysis [97]. Definitive results and recommendations have not been published.

In some animal experiments physiolysis has been followed by normal physeal growth in some of the animals [3, 45, 90–93]. Maintenance of growth appears to depend on the integrity of the germinal cell layer, which is usually unaffected by the separation [3]. Studies using double banding with tetracycle were inconclusive in determining post distraction physeal growth [63]. Indomethacin impeded bone bridge formation across the separated physis in some rabbits [55]. Usually, however, the majority, often all, of the animals have developed substantial growth retardation and premature arrest [45, 73–75, 77, 80–82, 86, 87, 99, 103]. The gain in length at the end of distraction rarely equals the expected gain, due to mechanical problems and to early physeal arrest combined with continuing growth of the normal contralateral bone [3, 75, 82, 103].

Several additional observations unrelated to each other have been made. The effect of physeal distraction is enhanced by circumferential division of the metaphyseal periosteum [110]. Distraction of apophyses in puppies did not increase enchondral bone growth; on the contrary, it had the same effect as compression which was inhibition of longitudinal growth [1]. Distraction increased synthetic activity and prostaglandin production by physeal cartilage in explant culture over a 24 h period [83].

Hemichondrodiatasis has been used to produce angular deformity in sheep [91, 94]. The physis was not separated. After removal of the device, angular deformities of up to 20° corrected spontaneously. When the induced angle exceeded 20° correction was poor.

Complications of chondriatasis in animals include pain, reduced weightbearing, muscular hypertrophy, fractures through the newly lengthened bone, non-union at the site of lengthening, permanent loss of joint motion, and premature physeal arrest [3, 82, 103]. Pin tract infections are common, usually heal following pin removal, but can result in chronic osteomyelitis [73].

Chondrodiatasis in animals can be summarized by stating that the response to controlled distraction of the physis is dependent upon the level of force used, the rate of distraction, and the maturity of the physis [78, 101, 109]. The lower the distraction force and speed, the greater the short-term and long-term viability of the growth cartilage [70]. To evaluate both chondrodiatasis and physiolysis, the following variables are manipulated in an effort to optimize results: magnitude of the force applied, rate of distraction, duration of distraction, continuous versus intermittent distraction, timing of distraction relative to the remaining normal growth potential of the particular physis (the age of the animal), and use of additional experimental perturbations, such as electromagnetic stimulation to enhance the effect [72].

11.4 Author's Perspective

When treating bone length inequality, consideration of chondrodiatasis is primarily dependent on the child's age and the amount of length needed. The surgeon must weight the advantages and disadvantages of the distraction process against the need for additional possible procedures, e.g., bone lengthening or shortening, contralateral physeal arrest, osteotomy, etc. Since physiolysis has the potential to result in premature physeal arrest, and since the precise amount to be lengthened is difficult to estimate in a young child, chondrodiatasis is best done near completion of growth. In the older child physeal distraction may be included in the list of bone length equalization procedures, and for some it may be the preferred method.

References

Introduction

1. Gelbke H (1951) The influence of pressure and tension on growing bone in experiments with animals. J Bone Joint Surg 33A(4):947–954
2. Peterson HA (2007) Epiphyseal growth plate fractures. Springer, Heidelberg, p 914
3. Ring PA (1958) Experimental bone lengthening by epiphyseal distraction. Br J Surg 46:169–173
4. Smith WS, Cunningham JB (1957) The effect of alternating distracting forces on the epiphyseal plates of calves; a preliminary report. Clin Orthop 10:125–130
5. Zavyalov PV, Plaskin IT (1968) Distraction epiphyseolysis in prolongation of the lower limb in children [Russian]. Khirurgiia (Mosk) 44:121–124
6. Zavyalov PV, Plaskin IT (1967) Elongation of crural bones in children using a method of distraction epiphysiolysis [Russian]. Vestn Khir Grekova 103:67–82

Human Involvement

7. Aldegheri R, Trivella G, Lavini F (1989) Epiphyseal distraction. Chondrodiatasis. Clin Orthop 241:117–127
8. Aldegheri R, Trivella G, Lavini F (1989) Epiphyseal distraction. Hemichondrodiatasis. Clin Orthop 241:128–136
9. Aparisi T, Olerud S (1981) Leg lengthening by distraction epiphysiolysis. Acta Orthop Scand 52:439
10. Bensahel H, Huguenin P, Briard JL (1983) Transepiphyseal lengthening of the tibia. Apropos of a case [French]. Rev Chir Orthop Reparatrice Appar Mot 69(3):245–247
11. Bjerkreim I (1989) Limb lengthening by physeal distraction. Acta Orthop Scand 60(2):140–142
12. Canadell J, de Pablos J (1992) Correction of angular deformities by physeal distraction. Clin Orthop 283:98–105
13. Connolly JF, Huurman WW, Lippiello L, Pankaj R (1986) Epiphyseal traction to correct acquired growth deformities: an animal and clinical investigation. Clin Orthop 202:258–268
14. Crawfurd EJP, Jones CB, Dewar ME, Aichroth PM (1987) Distraction forces in children undergoing epiphyseal leg lengthening. Orthop Trans 11:302–303
15. Crawfurd EJP, Jones CB, Dewar ME, Aichroth PM (1987) The force required to rupture the epiphysis in children undergoing epiphyseal leg lengthening (abstr). J Bone Joint Surg 69B:496
16. De Bastiani G, Aldegheri R, Renzi Brivio L, Trivella G (1986) Chondrodiatasis-controlled symmetrical distraction of the epiphyseal plate. Limb lengthening in children. J Bone Joint Surg 68B(4):550–555
17. De Bastiani G, Lavini F, Trivella G, Renzi Brivio L (1988) Epiphyseal distraction: chondrodiatasis and hemichondrodiatasis. In: Uhthoff HK, Wiley JJ (eds) Behavior of the growth plate. Raven, New York, pp 195–199
18. de Pablos J (1993) Biology of bone lengthening by means of physeal distraction. Mapfre Med 4(suppl II):77–82
19. de Pablos J (1998): Bone lengthening by physeal distraction. In: de Pablos J (ed) Surgery of the growth plate, Chapter 29. Ediciones Ergon, S.A., Madrid, pp 250–257
20. de Pablos J (1993) Bone lengthening by physeal distraction. Mapfre Medicina 4(Supp II):179–185
21. de Pablos J, Alfaro J, Barrios J (1997) Treatment of adolescent Blount disease by asymmetric physeal distraction. J Pediatr Orthop 17(1):54–58
22. de Pablos J, Cañadell J (1998) Correction of angular deformities by physeal distraction. In: dePablos J (ed) Surgery of the Growth Plate. S.A. Madrid, Ediciones Ergon, pp 308–322
23. de Pablos J, Cañadell J (1993) Correction of angular deformities by physeal distraction. Mapfre Med 4(supl II):231–238
24. de Pablos J, Franzreb M (1993) Treatment of adolescent tibia vara by asymmetrical physeal distraction. J Bone Joint Surg 75B(4):592–596
25. Emery RJH, Jones CB, Aichroth PM, Dewar M (1987) Early experience with epiphyseal distraction in the management of limb length discrepancy (abstr). J Bone Joint Surg 69B:154
26. Foster BK (1988) Interpositional and distractional physiolysis: clinical results. In: Uhthoff HK, Wiley JJ (eds) Behavior of the growth plate. Raven, New York, pp 243–246
27. Franke J, Hein G, Simon M, Hauch S (1990) Comparison of distraction epiphyseolysis and partial metaphyseal corticotomy in leg lengthening. Int Orthop 14(4):405–413
28. Ganel A (1997) Hemichondrodiatasis in Blount's disease. Letter to the editors. J Pediatr Orthop 17:828
29. Ganel A, Heim M, Farine I (1986) Asymmetric epiphyseal distraction in treatment of Blount's disease. Orthop Rev 15(4):237–240
30. Gausepohl T, Mader K, Pennig D (2006) Mechanical distraction for the treatment of posttraumatic stiffness of the elbow in children and adolescents. J Bone Joint Surg 88A(5):1011–1021
31. Givon U, Schindler A, Ganel A (2001) Hemichondrodiastasis for the treatment of genu varum deformity associated with bone dysplasias. J Pediatr Orthop 21(2):238–241
32. Grill F (1984) Distraction of the epiphyseal cartilage as a method of limb lengthening. Case report. J Pediatr Orthop 4(1):105–108
33. Hamanishi C, Tanaka S, Tamura K (1992) Early physeal closure after femoral chondrodiatasis. Loss of length gain in 5 cases. Acta Orthop Scand 63(2):146–149
34. Hamanishi C, Tanaka S, Tamura K, Fujio K (1990) Correction of asymmetric physeal closure. Rotatory distraction in 3 cases. Acta Orthop Scand 61(1):58–61
35. Ishkanian J (1993) Hemichondrodiatasis: asymmetric slow physeal distraction. Mapfre Med 4(Supl II):239–244
36. Janovec M, Jochymek M (1993) The state of the human growth plate two and more years after physeal distraction. Mapfre Med 4(Supl II):190–195
37. Jones CB, Aichroth PM, Dewar ME (1985) Gradual distraction of the epiphysial growth plate: a human study of the forces generated and early effects on the growth plate (abstr). J Bone Joint Surg 67B:843–844
38. Jones CB, Dewar ME, Aichroth PM, Crawfurd EJ, Emery R (1989) Epiphyseal distraction monitored by strain gauges. J Bone Joint Surg 71B:651–656

39. Kenwright J, Cunningham JL (1998): In-vivo mechanical response of the human growth plate to distraction close to skeletal maturity. In: dePablos J (ed). Surgery of the growth plate, Chapter 31. Ediciones Ergon, S.A., Madrid, pp 261–263
40. Kenwright J, Cunningham JL (1993) In-vivo mechanical response of the human growth plate to distraction close to skeletal maturity. Mapfre Med 4(Supl II):188–189
41. Kenwright J, Spriggins AJ, Cunningham JL (1990) Response of the growth plate to distraction close to skeletal maturity. Is fracture necessary? Clin Orthop 250:61–72
42. Langlois V, Laville JM (2005) Physeal distraction for limb length discrepancy and angular deformity [French]. Rev Chir Orthop Reparatrice Appar Mot 91(3):199–207
43. Monticelli G, Spinelli R (1984) A new method of treating the advanced stages of tibia vara (Blount's disease). Italian J Orthop Traumatol 10(3):295–303
44. Monticelli G, Spinelli R (1981) Distraction epiphysiolysis as a method of limb lengthening. III. Clinical applications. Clin Orthop 154:274–285
45. Monticelli G, Spinelli R (1981) Limb lengthening by epiphyseal distraction. Int Orthop 5(2):85–90
46. Monticelli G, Spinelli R, Forte R, Lorio L (1998) Leg lengthening by distraction epiphysiolysis. In: de Pablos J (ed) Surgery of the growth plate, Chapter 30. Ediciones Ergon, S.A., Madrid, p 334
47. Monticelli G, Spinelli R, Forte R, Lorio L (1993) Leg lengthening by distraction epiphysiolysis. Mapfre Med 4(Supl II):186–187
48. Nakamura K, Nagano A, Tobimatsu H, Kurokawa T (1988) Tibial lengthening by epiphyseal distraction. J Jpn Assoc 62(1):37–41
49. Patel MR, Moradia VJ (1995) Correction of an angular deformity of the thumb in a juvenile by epiphyseal distraction. J Hand Surg 20A(2):258–260
50. Sharrard SW, Aldegheri R, Trivella G (1985) Limb lengthening by chondrodiatasis (abstr). J Pediatr Orthop 5:613
51. Siffert RS (1987) Lower limb-length discrepancy. Current concepts review. J Bone Joint Surg 69A(7):1100–1106
52. Spinelli R (1988) Bone lengthening through physeal distraction-separation. In: Uhthoff HK, Wiley JJ (eds) Behavior of the Growth Plate. Raven, New York, pp 201–208
53. Valdivia GG, Fassier F, Hamdy RC (1998) Chondrodiatasis in a patient with spondyloepimetaphyseal dysplasia using the ilizarov technique: successful correction of an angular deformity with ensuing ossification of a large metaphyseal lesion. A case report. Int Orthop (SICOT) 22:400–403
54. Zarzycki D, Tesiorowski M, Zarzycka M, Kacki W, Jasiewicz B (2002) Long-term results of lower limb lengthening by physeal distraction. J Pediatr Orthop 22(3):367–370

Animal Research

55. Ahn et al (1989) Experimental study of distraction epiphysiolysis–rabbit model (abstr). J Pediatr Orthop 9:107–125
56. Alberty A (1993) Effects of physeal distraction on the vascular supply of the growth area: a microangiographical study in rabbits. J Pediatr Orthop 13:373–377
57. Alberty A, Peltonen J (1993) Proliferation of the hypertrophic chondrocytes of the growth plate after physeal distraction. An experimental study in rabbits. Clin Orthop 297:7–11
58. Alberty A, Peltonen J, Ritsilä V (1990) Distraction effects on the physis in rabbits. Acta Orthop Scand 61(3):258–262
59. Alberty A, Peltonen J, Ritsilä V (1993) Effects of distraction and compression on proliferation of growth plate chondrocytes. A study in rabbits. Acta Orthop Scand 64(4):449–455
60. Apte S, Kenwright J (1988) An autoradiographic study of chondrocyte proliferation in the distracted growth plate. J Bone Joint Surg 70B:850
61. Apte SS, Kenwright J (1994) Physeal distraction and cell proliferation in the growth plate. J Bone Joint Surg 76B:837–843
62. Arriola F, Forriol F, Cañadell J (2001) Histomorphometric study of growth plate subjected to different mechanical conditions (compression, tension and neutralization): an experimental study in lambs. Mechanical growth plate behavior. J Pediatr Orthop B 10(4):334–338
63. Ashworth MA (1979) Femoral lengthening by distal epiphyseal distraction. A feasibility study on rabbits. Orthop Trans 3:155
64. Cavanagh SP, Pho RWH, Pereira B (1990) A quantitative analysis of growth plate behavior following slow epiphyseal distraction: an epiphyseal study in the immature rabbit (abstr). J Bone Joint Surg 72B:1106
65. Connolly JF, Huurman WW, Pankaj R (1982) Long-term effect of physeal distraction (abstr). Orthop Trans 8:267
66. Connolly JF, Huurman WW, Ray S (1979) Physeal distraction treatment of fracture deformities. Orthop Trans 3:231–232
67. Connolly J, Shindell R, Lippiello L, Guse R (1988) Prevention and correction of growth deformities after distal femoral epiphyseal fractures. In: Uthoff HK, Wiley JJ (eds) Behavior of the growth plate. Raven, New York, pp 209–215
68. De Bastiani G, Aldegheri R, Renzi Brivio L, Trivella G (1986) Limb lengthening by distraction of the epiphyseal plate. A comparison of two techniques in the rabbit. J Bone Joint Surg 68B(4):545–549
69. de Pablos Jr J, Cañadell J (1990) Experimental physeal distraction in immature sheep. Clin Orthop 250:73–80
70. de Pablos J, Villas C, Canadell J (1986) Bone lengthening by physial distraction. An experimental study. Int Orthop (SICOT) 10(3):163–170
71. Elmer EB, Ehrlich MG, Zaleske DJ, Polsky C, Mankin HJ (1992) Chondrodiatasis in rabbits: a study on the effect of transphyseal bone lengthening on cell division, synthetic function, and microcirculation in the growth plate. J Pediatr Orthop 12:181–190
72. Farnum CE, Wilsman NJ (1998) Effects of distraction and compression on growth plate function. In: Buckwalter JA, Ehrlich MG, Sandell LJ, Trippel SB (eds) Skeletal growth development, Chapter 30. Am Acad Orth Surgeons, Rosemount, pp 517–531
73. Fishbane BM, Riley LH Jr (1978) Continuous transphyseal traction: experimental observations. Clin Orthop 136:120–124
74. Fjeld T, Steen H (1990) Growth retardation after experimental limb lengthening by epiphyseal distraction. J Pediatr Orthop 10:463–466
75. Fjeld TO, Steen H (1988) Limb lengthening by low rate epiphyseal distraction. An experimental study in the caprine tibia. J Orthop Res 6(3):360–368
76. Forriol F, Shapiro F (2005) Bone development. Interaction of molecular components and biophysical forces. Clin Orthop 432:14–33
77. Foster BK, Rozenbilds MAN, Yates R (1986) Further results of distraction physeolysis in a sheep model (abstr). J Bone Joint Surg 68B:333

78. Guse RJ, Connolly JF, Alberts R, Lippiello L (1989) Effect of aging on tensile mechanical properties of the rabbit distal femoral growth plate. J Orthop Res 7(5):667–673
79. Harsha WN (1962) Distracting effects placed across the epiphyses of long bones. A study in experimental animals. JAMA 179(10):132–136
80. Kenwright J, Apte S (1998) Physeal distraction: Review of experimental evidence. What is the response of the cells on the growth plate? In: de Pablos J (ed) Surgery of the growth plate, Chapter 9. Ediciones Ergon, S.A., Madrid pp 70–74.
81. Kenwright J, Apte S, Kershaw CJ (1990) Biologic responses of the normal and bridged physis to distraction. Acta Orthop Scand 61(Suppl 237):64
82. Letts RM, Meadows L (1978) Epiphysiolysis as a method of limb lengthening. Clin Orthop 133:230–237
83. Mankin KP, Zaleske DJ (1998) Response of physeal cartilage to low-level compression and tension in organ culture. J Pediatr Orthop 18(2):145–148
84. Marsh HO, Adas E, Laroia K (1961) An experimental attempt to stimulate growth by a distracting force across the lower femoral epiphysis. Am Surgeon 27:615–618
85. Moen CT, Pelker RR (1984) Biomechanical and histological correlations in growth plate failure. J Pediatr Orthop 4(2):180–184
86. Monticelli G, Spinelli R (1981) Distraction epiphysiolysis as a method of limb lengthening. I. Experimental study. Clin Orthop 154:254–261
87. Monticelli G, Spinelli R, Bonucci E (1981) Distraction epiphysiolysis as a method of limb lengthening. II. Morphologic investigations. Clin Orthop 154:262–273
88. Nakamura K, Matsushita T, Okazaki H, Nagano A, Kurokawa T (1991) Attempted limb lengthening by physeal distraction. Continuous monitoring of an applied force in immature rabbits. Clin Orthop 267:306–311
89. Noble J, Diamond R, Stirrat CR, Sledge CB (1982) Breaking force of the rabbit growth plate and its application to epiphyseal distraction. Acta Orthop Scand 53:13–16
90. Noble J, Sledge CB, Walker PS, Diamond R, Stirrat C, Sosman JL (1978) Limb lengthening by epiphysial distraction (abstr). J Bone Joint Surg 60B(1):139–140
91. Peltonen J (1989) Bone formation and remodeling after symmetric and asymmetric physeal distraction. J Pediatr Orthop 9(2):191–196
92. Peltonen J, Alitalo I, Karaharju E, Helio H (1984) Distraction of the growth plate. Experiments in pigs and sheep. Acta Orthop Scand 55:359–362
93. Peltonen J, Kahri A, Karaharju E, Alitalo I (1988) Regeneration after physeal distraction of the radius in sheep. Acta Orthop Scand 59(6):675–680
94. Peltonen JI, Karaharju EO, Alitalo I (1984) Experimental epiphyseal distraction producing and correcting angular deformities. J Bone Joint Surg 66B:598–602
95. Pereira BP, Cavanagh SP, Pho RWH (1997) Longitudinal growth rate following slow physeal distraction. The proximal tibial growth plate studied in rabbits. Acta Orthop Scand 68(3):262–268
96. Poliakoff SJ, Jones CB, Bright RW (1990) Histological and mechanical observations of experimental tension epiphysiolysis (abstr). J Bone Joint Surg 72B:737–738
97. Poliakoff SJ, Miller RK, Jones CB, Bright RW (1990) Physeal distraction using acoustic emission monitoring: an in vitro study (abstr). J Bone Joint Surg 72B:737
98. Porter RW (1978) The effect of tension across a growing physis. J Bone Joint Surg 60B(2):252–255
99. Sledge CB, Noble J (1978) Experimental limb lengthening by epiphyseal distraction. Clin Orthop 136:111–119
100. Spriggins AJ (1987) Effects of distraction loads on the growth plate of the tibia: an experimental study. Orthop Trans 11:413–414
101. Spriggins AJ, Bader DL, Cunningham JL, Kenwright J (1989) Distraction physiolysis in the rabbit. Acta Orthop Scand 60(2):154–158
102. Spriggins AJ, Kenwright J (1986) Effects of distraction epiphysiolysis on the proximal tibial epiphysis of rabbits (abstr). J Bone Joint Surg 68B:840–841
103. Steen H, Fjeld TO, Rønningen H, Langeland N, Gjerde NR, Bjerkreim I (1987) Limb lengthening by epiphyseal distraction: an experimental study in the caprine femur. J Orthop Res 5:592–599
104. Stokes IAF, Aronsson DD, Dimock AN, Cortright V, Beck S (2006) Endochondral growth in growth plates of three species at two anatomical locations modulated by mechanical compression and tension. J Orthop Res 24:1327–1334
105. Stokes IA, Mente PL, Iatridis JC, Farnum CE, Aronsson DD (2002) Enlargement of growth plate chondrocytes modulated by sustained mechanical loading. J Bone Joint Surg 84A(10):1842–1848
106. Stokes IA, Spence H, Aronsson DD, Kilmer N (1996) Mechanical modulation of vertebral body growth. Implications for scoliosis progression. Spine 21(10):1162–1167
107. Trueta J (1958) The influence of growth on the sequelae of bone and joint injuries (abstr). Int Surg 40B:154
108. Wang H, Li M, Wu Z, Zhao L (2007) The deep fascia in response to leg lengthening with particular reference to the tension-stress principle. J Pediatr Orthop 27(1):41–45
109. Williams JL, Do PD, Eick JD, Schmidt TL (2001) Tensile properties of the physis vary with anatomic location, thickness, strain rate and age. J Orthop Res 19:1043–1048
110. Wilson-McDonald J, Houghton GR, Bradley J, Morscher E (1990) The relationship between periosteal division and compression or distraction of the growth plate. An experimental study in the rabbit. J Bone Joint Surg 72B(2):303–308

Stress 12

12.1 Introduction

The term *stress injury* used in this chapter connotes increased repetitive force to of the physis, rather than a technical bioengineering definition. It results in pain, widening and irregular margins of the physis, and premature or delayed closure of the physis. It occurs in the physes of both epiphyses and apophyses. The terms "overuse injury" [2, 4, 6, 15, 21], "chronic physeal injury" [9, 16], "repetitive physeal injury" [7], "stress reaction" [21], and "stress fracture" [1, 5, 30] have also been used for this condition. Stress injuries of the physis should not be confused with stress fractures of the metaphysis or diaphysis in adolescents [3]. There has been no animal research on the physeal stress injury.

The physes of both epiphyses and apophyses usually handle the stresses of daily living well. Apophyses are the site of muscle attachments. Stress injuries of apophyses are common, particularly at the distal humeral medial epicondyle (little leaguer's elbow), the proximal anterior tibial tubercle (Osgood-Schlatter lesion), and the calcaneal apophysis (Seaver disease). These stress injuries are generally regarded as being the result of repetitive traction on the apophysis and are sometimes known as "traction apophysitis". Since apophyses produce no longitudinal bone length, stress injuries of the apophyses are not reported here.

Stress injuries to physes of epiphyses, which lie at right angles to long bones, may be the result of repetitive *compression*, *distraction*, *torsion*, or *shear* forces, and are discussed here separately from Chapters 10 and 11 because the insulting force is applied intermittently over a long period of time, may be a combination of forces, and the precise force is often unknown. Stress injuries of the physes of the distal radius and ulna, proximal humerus, proximal ulna, and proximal tibia are discussed separately at length in the book "Epiphyseal Growth Plate Fractures, Peterson HA: Springer, Heidelberg, 2007, pp 914, 2007 [8], and are not repeated here.

12.2 Mechanism of Injury

Stress injury occurs when forces applied over time exceed the ability of the physis to repair itself. The forces represent repetitive subfracture loading. The constant anatomic feature found initially in all stress injuries is widening of the physis. The increased width may be of the entire physis or a part of it. The cause of the physeal widening is not entirely clear. It may be multifactorial. The pathophysiology of growth-plate widening is more likely a result of metaphyseal injury than of growth plate injury [25]. The most plausible explanation seems to be that repetitive microtrauma in the zone of provisional calcification in the metaphysis, or at the junction of the provisional and hypertrophic zones (Fig. 12.1), disrupts the blood supply interfering with mineralization of the hypertrophied chondrocytes. In the absence of being turned into bone the hypertrophic zone enlarges (widens) as the germinal cells continue to divide and grow. A reaction very similar to stress injury also occurs following loss of the metaphyseal blood supply, as noted in Figs. 1.3 and 1.4. In both cases the initial roentgenogram is normal in the intial stages.

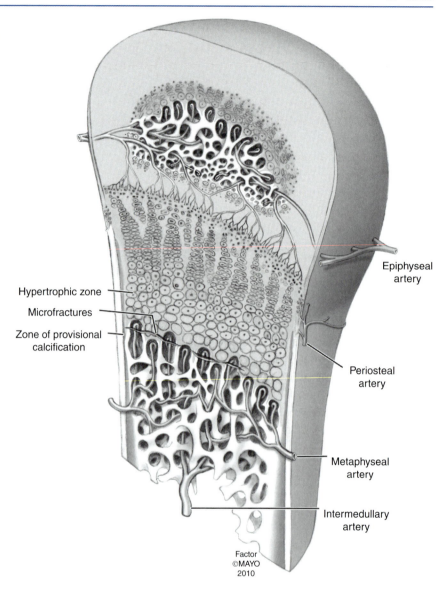

Fig. 12.1 Micro trauma in the zone of provisional calcification or its junction with the hypertrophic zone prevents ossification and allows cells in the hypertrophic zone to accumulate. The physis widens. Compare with Fig. 1.2

There is strong correlation between the orientation of the physis and related stress patterns [13]. The greater part of most physes of epiphyses lie at right angles to principal compressive forces and are constantly subjected to pure compression between epiphysis and diaphysis [13]. When the forces are repetitive and excessive there may be micro fractures of the physis or adjacent metaphysis as described above and in Chapter 10.

Distractive forces (tensile stress) on the physes of epiphysis are not common in activities of daily living. However, the repetitive distraction which occurs in some sports, could also cause microfractures across the physis, or metaphysis, producing physeal widening, just as in continuous distraction described in Chapter 11.

Physeal widening may also be associated with shear or torsional forces. Although intermittent repetitive forces have not been tested on animals, a study on rats showed that shearing stresses created interstitial cracks between or within specific cell layers (zones) at as low as 50% of the energy necessary to cause overt physeal fracture [10]. These cracks appeared in all layers of the physis, but were most common in the hypertrophic zone. Subsequent growth in the germinal zone resulted in widening of the growth plate. Thus the initial roentgenograph was normal, but 2–3 weeks later physeal widening occurred. These changes do not fit the criteria of any fracture type in classifications, but might be considered a "forme fruste" of a Salter-Harris type 1 or Peterson type 3 physeal fracture [8].

Controversy over the type of the stress is greatest at the distal radial epiphysis where the stress from gymnastics is thought to be due to distraction, compression, torsion, or shear by various authors [8]. Competing in the floor exercise, vault, pommel horse, and beam produces repetitive compression, torsion, or shear forces, while competing in the high bar, uneven parallel bars, and rings produces distractive forces [9, 12]. Most competitors do all events available for their gender. Dowel grips or hand guards used during swings on the high bar and uneven bars allow greater distraction forces to act across the wrist without a measurable increase in forearm activity [9, 11, 12]. When the distal ulna is also involved, it is difficult to implicate compression since the ulna does not articulate with the carpus.

Most sports require certain patterns of activity that result in special risks to different parts of the body [16]. The inciting activity determines whether the lesion is unilateral (throwing and racket sports) or bilateral (gymnastics and running). Some lesions, may be unilateral or bilateral depending on the nature of the activity causing the stress.

12.3 Evaluation

Stress injuries become manifest by pain localized to the site of the involved physis. Clinical examination reveals painful limitation of extremes of joint motion and tenderness localized to the level of the physis [9, 21]. Occasionally the pain is reproduced by manual traction [9]. Because stress injuries involve repetitive forces over time, this injury occurs almost exclusively in actively training adolescent athletes. The pain develops during training and becomes more intense as workouts and competition progress. Elite athletes are more prone to the injury. Initially the pain is relieved by rest. As training progresses the pain persists after workouts. The male: female ratio of stress injuries in adolescents 9:1 [24], which is in accordance with the more rapid growth rate and increase in body weight in the male [14], as well as differences in activity and participation numbers in each sport.

Since microfractures in the metaphyseal-physeal junction are not visible roentgenographically, stress injuries are first visualized by irregularity and sclerosis of the adjacent metaphysis and widening of the physis without displacement of the epiphysis (Fig. 12.2a, b) [22]. This produces a picture similar to rickets and thus the condition has also been called "pseudorickets" [20]. The roentgenographic widening within the physeal cartilage has similarities to both compression and distraction injuries (Chapters 10 and 11). The appearance is similar to the Salter-Harris type 1 and Peterson type 3 fractures, except for one type 2 injury noted in the proximal tibia of a runner [1]. This type 2 fracture was thought to represent rotational or shear stress and bolsters the microfracture concept of mechanism of injury. Widening of the physis is progressive, may eventually be accompanied by fragmentation of the metaphysis [23] or epiphysis [6], and in some cases progresses to premature or delayed physeal closure.

MR imaging has demonstrated physeal widening with irregularity of the bordering metaphysis [16, 17, 20], suspicious of metaphyseal ischemia. Other than the physeal widening no other abnormalities of the physis itself have been identified [25]. Horizontal linear high signal intensity striations in the metaphysis adjacent to the physis without cortical interruption are thought to be impending fractures [25].

Stress injuries of physes predominate in the upper extremity. The most common physeal sites:

Distal radius, sometimes accompanied by the distal ulna – gymnast's wrist (discussion and 31 references presented in Peterson [8], Chapter 10A)

Proximal humerus – little leaguer's shoulder (discussion and 16 references presented in Peterson [8], Chapter 17C)

Proximal ulna (discussion and 14 references presented in Peterson [8], Chapter 22A)

Proximal tibia – catcher's knee (discussion and 2 references presented in Peterson [8], Chapter 20A)

Less common epiphyseal sites are the distal femur in runners [5, 22] soccer [17], and place kickers [16], the distal fibula in runners [22], the distal humerus in baseball [21], the distal ulna in breakdancers [19], and the thumb distal phalanx in piano players [15]. The mechanism producing the lesion at these sites and from these activities is often unclear, and could be associated with any combination of compression, distraction, torsion, or shear forces [13, 21].

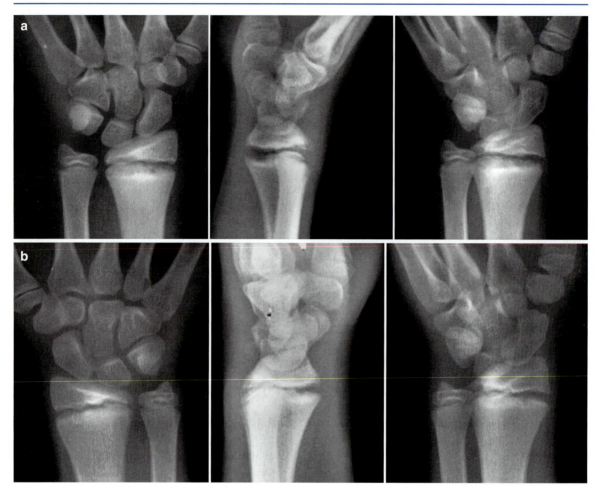

Fig. 12.2 Stress injury and reinjury of the distal radius. This actively growing 12 year 6 month old elite female gymnast complained of right wrist pain, most apparent after exertion. She trained 4 h, 5 days a week. There had been progressive reliance on dowel grips for uneven bar routines. (**a**) Right wrist physeal widening, irregularity, and marginal sclerosis (wrists are supinated on the AP and oblique views). (**b**) Left wrist; similar less marked findings. Asymptomatic. The physis is more wide on the volar side (*middle*). The ulna is not involved. (**c**) A right short arm cast was worn 3 weeks followed by a modified activity program with no improvement. Gymnastics was then discontinued for 3 months. (**d**) At age 12 years 9 months, the pain was gone and the physeal anatomy was markedly improved (left wrist on left, right wrist on right). Limited gymnastic activity was allowed. Dowel grips were again used. (**e**) At age 13 years 0 months the pain had returned and the physes of both wrists showed increased widening, irregularity, and marginal sclerosis. A period of complete abstinence from gymnastic activity and avoidance of dowel grips allowed eventual return to her preinjury level of competition. (**f**) Right wrist at age 13 years 11 months; the pain had returned accompanied by recurrent increased physeal widening. (**g**) Right wrist at 16 years 10 months; the wrists were asymptomatic and the physes were closing (From Ruggles et al. [12] with permission)

12.3 Evaluation

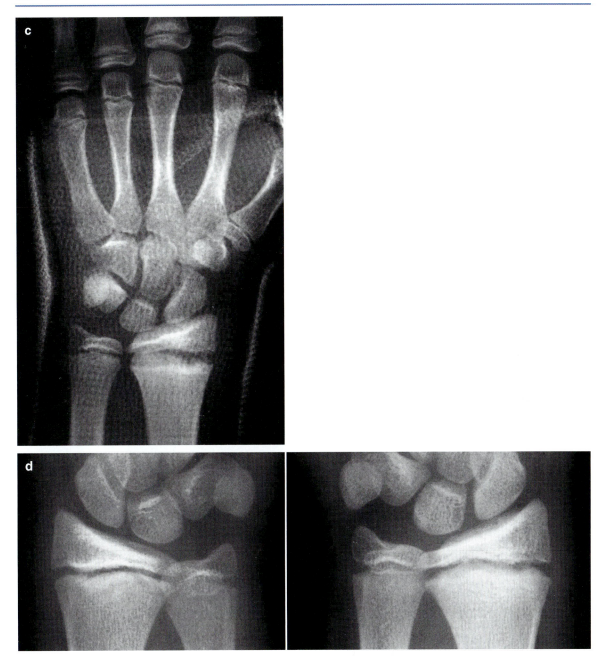

Fig. 12.2 (continued)

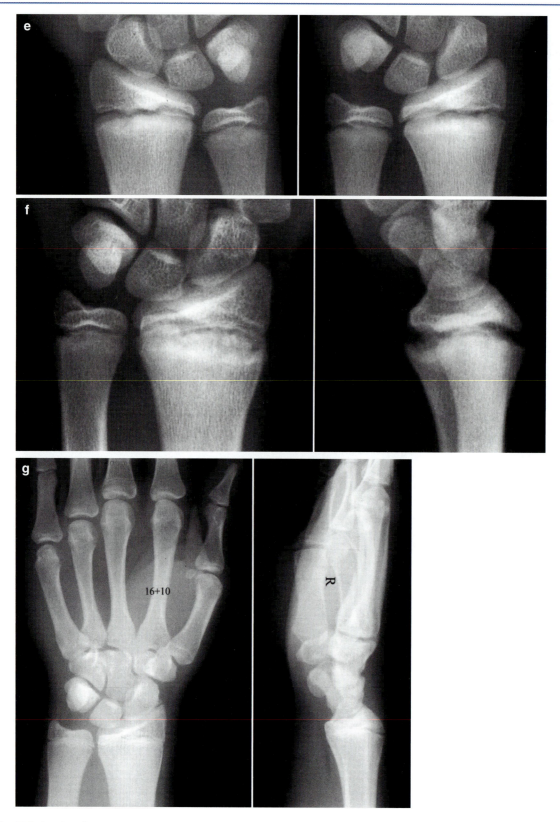

Fig. 12.2 (continued)

12.4 Management

Prevention is the foremost treatment for stress injuries [21]. Coaches knowledgeable in proper sporting techniques, training regimens, equipment, and rules, should be able to prevent most of these injuries. When stress injuries occur the treatment is symptomatic and consists of complete, but temporary cessation of the activity responsible for the injury. The application of a cast is one way to provide symptomatic relief, ensure rest, and prevent the patient from continuing the activity (Fig. 12.2c) [12]. Initially the anatomic changes in the physis are completely reversible (Fig. 12.2d). It may take up to 6 months for the patient to become asymptomatic and the physis to revert to normal. When properly diagnosed and treated stress injuries of physes usually heal uneventfully, just like stress fractures of bone [3]. Most subjects improve with rest and are able to return to their sport. However, continued activity may result in overall growth slowdown and eventually premature partial or complete cessation of the physis [16].

12.5 Complications

When patients return to active training too soon or too vigorously, the condition returns (Fig. 12.2e–f). In cases with longstanding symptoms, implying continuance of the activity, premature physeal arrest may occur. The physeal arrest is usually complete, resulting in cessation of growth. Usually the children are adolescents with little growth remaining and the growth arrest causes minor length discrepancy. However, early closure of the distal radial physis may result in relative overgrowth of the ulna (positive ulnar variance [4, 22]) which might require surgical arrest or shortening of the distal ulna, bilaterally if necessary [26, 27].

Partial arrest occurs less commonly, but has resulted in altered radiocarpal articular angle deformities similar to Madelung deformity (Fig. 10.3a). [4, 16, 18, 27–29, 31] Surgical physeal arrest of the distal radial and ulnar growth plates have been used to prevent progression of these Madelung-like deformities. There are no reports of bar excision for partial physeal arrest due to stress injuries.

Nonunion of the proximal ulnar physis due to persistence of activity has been treated by surgical osteosynthesis [6, 30].

12.6 Author's Perspective

Stress injuries are totally preventable by coaches' knowledge concerning appropriate training schedules, techniques, and equipment. For the physician, counseling when and how to return to training can be the most difficult feature of this injury, especially with aspiring athletes who have goals encouraged by parents and coaches. The physician's recommendations may be contrary to the wishes of the patient, parents, and coaches. The physical well-being of the patient is the physician's primary concern; remain firm.

References

Introduction

1. Cahill BR (1977) Stress fracture of the proximal tibial epiphysis: a case report. Am J Sports Med 5(5):186–187
2. Caine DJ, Linder KJ (1985) Overuse injuries of growing bones: the young female gymnast at risk? Phys Sports Med 13:51–64
3. Devas MB (1963) Stress fractures in children. J Bone Joint Surg Br 45:528–541
4. Gill TJ, Micheli LJ (1996) The immature athlete: common injuries and overuse syndromes of the elbow and wrist. Clin Sports Med 15(2):401–423
5. Godshall RW, Hansen CA, Rising DC (1981) Stress fractures through the distal femoral epiphysis in athletes. A previously unpublished entity. Am J Sports Med 9:114–116
6. Maffulli N, Chan D, Aldridge MJ (1992) Overuse injuries of the olecranon in young gymnasts. J Bone Joint Surg Br 74:305–308
7. Ogden JA (2000) Repetitive physeal injury. In: Ogden JA (ed) Skeletal injury in the child, 3rd edn. Springer, New York, pp 406–407, Chapter 12
8. Peterson HA (2007) Epiphyseal growth plate fractures. Springer, Heidelberg, p 914
9. Yong-Hing K, Wedge JH, Bown CVA (1988) Chronic injury to the distal ulnar and radial growth plates in an adolescent gymnast: a case report. J Bone Joint Surg Am 70: 1087–1089

Mechanism of Injury

10. Bright RW, Richmond V, Burstein AH, Elmore SM (1974) Epiphyseal-plate cartilage. A biomechanical and histological analysis of failure modes. J Bone Joint Surg Am 56:688–703
11. Neal RJ, Kippers V, Plooy D, Forwood MR (1995) The influence of hand guards on forces and muscle activity during giant swings on the high bar. Med Sci Sports Exerc 27(11):1550–1556
12. Ruggles DL, Peterson HA, Scott SG (1991) Radial growth plate injury in a female gymnast. Med Sci Sports Exerc 23(4):393–396

13. Smith JW (1962) The relationship of epiphysial plates to stress in some bones of the lower limb. J Anat 96:58–78

Evaluation

14. Alexander CJ (1976) Effect of growth rate on the strength of the growth plate-shaft junction. Skeletal Radiol 1:67–76
15. Attkiss KJ, Buncke HJ (1998) Physeal growth arrest of the distal phalanx of the thumb in an adolescent pianist: a case report. J Hand Surg Am 23(3):532–535
16. Caine D, DiFiori J, Maffuli N (2006) Physeal injuries in children's and youth sports: reasons for concern? Br J Sports Med 40:749–760
17. Connolly SA, Connolly LP, Jaramillo D (2001) Imaging of sports injuries in children and adolescents. Radiol Clin North Am 39(4):773–790
18. DiFiori JP, Caine DJ, Malina RM (2006) Wrist pain, distal radial physeal injury, and ulnar variance in the young gymnast. Am J Sports Med 34(5):840–849
19. Gerber SD, Griffin PP, Simmons BP (1986) Break dancer's wrist. Case report. J Pediatr Orthop 6(1):98–99
20. Liebling MS, Berdon WE, Ruzal-Shapiro C, Levin TL, Roye D Jr, Wilkinson R (1995) Gymnast's wrist (pseudorickets growth plate abnormality) in adolescent athletes: findings on plain films and MR imaging. AJR Am J Roentgenol 164:157–159
21. Podestra L, Sherman MF, Bonamo JR (1993) Distal humerus epiphyseal separation in a young athlete: a case report. Arch Phys Med Rehabil 4:1216–1218
22. Rogers LF, Poznanski AK (1994) Imaging of epiphyseal injuries. Radiology 191:297–308
23. Roy S, Caine D, Singer KM (1985) Stress changes of the distal radial epiphysis in young gymnasts. Am J Sports Med 13(5):301–308
24. Segesser B, Morscher E, Goesele A (1995) Lesions of the growth plate caused by sports stress. Review [German]. Orthopade 24(5):446–456
25. Shih C, Chang C, Penn I, Tiu C, Chang T, Wu J (1995) Chronically stressed wrists in adolescent gymnasts: MR imaging appearance. Radiology 195(3):855–859

Complications

26. Albanese SA, Palmer AK, Kerr DR, Carpenter CW, Lisi D, Levinsohn EM (1989) Wrist pain and distal growth plate closure of the radius in gymnasts. J Pediatr Orthop 9(1):23–28
27. Bak K, Boeckstyns M (1997) Epiphysiodesis for bilateral closure of the distal radial physis in a gymnast. Scand J Med Sci Sports 7:363–366
28. Brooks TJ (2001) Madelung deformity in a collegiate gymnast: a case report. J Athl Train 36:170–173
29. Vender MI, Watson HK (1988) Acquired Madelung-like deformity in a gymnast. J Hand Surg Am 13(1):19–21
30. Wilkerson RD, Johns JC (1990) Nonunion of an olecranon stress fracture in an adolescent gymnast. A case report. Am J Sports Med 18:432–434
31. Zlotolow DA, Bennet C (2008) Athletic injuries of the hand and wrist. Review article. Current Orthop Practice 19(2):206–211

Irradiation

13.1 Introduction

Radiation is the energy and *irradiation* is the process. There is a noun form and a verb form for each. The x-ray tube and the isotope radiate energy, and the patient is being irradiated. In common usage, however, the words radiation and irradiation are frequently used interchangeably.

Roentgen made his historic discovery in 1895. Perthes [10] may have been the first to document the inhibition of bone growth due to radiation when in 1903 he noted that 1 day old chicken wings irradiated on one side grew less than the non-irradiated side. Radiation used as therapy for a variety of conditions began in earnest in the 1920s. Although multiple complications were noted immediately, Desjardins [3] may have been the first to record retardation of growth in a child.

13.1.1 Radiation Terminology

External radiation is given in many forms, for example x-rays, gamma rays, protons, or fast neutrons [14]. Internal radiation is given in the form of alpha or beta particles of bone-seeking radionuclides [14]. The original unit used for measuring dose was the *rad* (radiation absorbed dose, often abbreviated as *r*). One rad is the absorbed energy equivalent of 100 ergs/g of tissue. Today the more commonly used unit of measurement is the *gray* (Gy); 1 Gy = 100 rad = 100 cGy.

Through the years many types of therapeutic radiation have been used, including high-voltage, super-voltage, ortho-voltage, mega-voltage, cobalt teletherapy, brachytherapy, etc. Although there is no fundamental difference in the histology of lesions produced by any form of radiation [12, 14], these differences make comparisons between reports difficult. For example, ortho-voltage irradiation is more likely to cause physeal arrest than mega-voltage irradiation delivered by modern linear accelerators [4, 81, 102, 108]. This is because ortho-voltage (200–250 kV) is absorbed more readily by bone and cartilage than energies in the mega-voltage range. Thus ortho-voltage equipment (used until the 1950s) has been replaced by higher energy machines in modern radiation oncology departments, and its use should be discouraged in all but the most extraordinary circumstances when treating children [5, 7].

13.1.2 Radiation Effects

The effects of ionizing irradiation are the same for normal and pathologic tissue. The exact mechanism by which irradiation causes disordered bone growth is uncertain. Irradiation can affect growth in four ways. First is a direct effect on the physeal cartilage which is a radiosensitive tissue. The action of irradiation affects all phases of physeal activity and is solely destructive. The cell at most risk is the cell with the greatest proliferative potential [14]. The most sensitive tissues are the immature dividing chondroblasts in the germinal and proliferative zones (Fig. 1.2). Radiation may cause arrest of cell division or immediate cell death [14], preventing normal endochondral maturation. The specific energy of the x-ray beam determines the degree of growth retardation. Second, the fine arterioles supplying the physis are also sensitive and susceptible to the untoward effect of irradiation, resulting in indirect injury to the physis (Fig. 1.2) [2, 5, 48, 87, 100, 113]. Pathophysiologically this is called vascular fibrosis [6, 84].

Even minor influences on the vascular supply may be important in this relatively hypoxic tissue structure [4]. Third, damage of endocrine organs can alter growth negatively [15]. Fourth, muscle atrophy as a result of irradiation develops a poliomyelitis-like disuse phenomenon [5], as discussed in Chap. 2. The fact that there are numerous accounts of growth being significantly reduced only to resume later, could occur with each of these mechanisms. Most authors who comment on the mechanism of injury due to irradiation state that it is due to reduction of the reproductive integrity of chondrocytes, or to vascular damage resulting in reduced blood flow. Histologic descriptions of irradiated physes in children are few [68, 91], and do not determine the precise mechanism of injury. All physes, in the extremities, the head and the trunk, are at risk.

Variables which determine the extent of physeal damage induced by radiation therapy include: (a) the quantity of radiation delivered (including both dose per treatment and total dose), (b) the intervals between exposures (called fractionation) and the length of time over which irradiation occurs, (c) the age and stature velocity of the patient at the time of therapy, (d) the site to which the radiation is delivered and the growth potential of that site, (e) the size of the physis and the amount of soft tissues the radiation must traverse to reach the physis (called the volume treated), (f) the field size, and (g) the concomitant use of chemotherapy of which some agents are radiosensitizers or radioprotectorants. Diet and general metabolic activity are modifying factors [14].

All investigations emphasize high dosage as the major factor for physeal arrest. "Massive" dose delivery is very detrimental to the physis. Fractionation of the total dose and extension of the interval between exposures allow tissue recuperation, and greatly lessens the amount of growth retardation [16, 20]. The advents of chemotherapy and mega-voltage irradiation have lowered the dosage requirements for curative irradiation [4]. This along with an awareness to shield the physis, when possible, has reduced the overall risk of growth arrest. Unfortunately, the physes cannot always be protected during irradiation. If a portion of a physis must be treated to adequately cover a tumor, it may be better to include the entire physis, in an attempt to avoid angular deformity [3].

The age of the patient is extremely important. The more rapid the cell turnover, the greater is the effect of radiation. Thus the effect of irradiation on the physis is greatest at times of rapid growth; early childhood and adolescence. The tissues of neonatal children are decidedly more embryonal in type, and consequently more radiosensitive than in older children. Also, younger patients have longer growing time causing greater length discrepancy. Differences in capacity for growth may explain variations in reaction when two bones, such as the tibia and femur, are exposed simultaneously [7, 16].

Because of these variables it is difficult to accurately estimate a dose-effect relationship on the physis. The damaging doses of x-rays for bones of an infant and a child have been roughly estimated to be 25% and 50%, respectively, of the erythema doses for an adult [16]. A radiation dose as low as 400 cGy can produce growth retardation, and as the dose increases, so does the extent of cellular damage [6]. The minimum tolerance dose associated with a 5% complication rate for growth impairment occurring within 5 years after treatment has been stated to be 800 cGy for children under 3 years and 1,400 cGy for older children using conventional 200 cGy /day, 1,000 cGy/week fractionation [1]. However, the dose-effect relationship may increase rapidly between 15 and 30 Gy [4]. Doses of 2,000 cGy usually produce growth changes [7, 28]. Twenty-five Gy (2,500 cGy) is often considered the critical dose to cause growth arrest, but this will depend on the variables mentioned previously. The upper level of amount of radiation which the physis will tolerate without untoward effects has not been established [7, 19].

13.1.3 Side Effects and Complications

There are many widespread and undesirable effects of radiation on many different normal structures in the body, including bone. The greatest threat is the development of sarcoma in the long term survivor. Although the incidence is relatively low, the problem remains a real one. Close long-term follow-up of all patients is indicated since sarcoma has appeared as long as 30 years after treatment [12].

Combining chemotherapy with mega-voltage irradiation has lowered the dose requirements for curative irradiation [36]. However, the effects of some chemotherapy agents, such as actinomycin-D, glucocorticosteriods, adriamycin, cyclophosphamide, and methotrexate may sensitize the irradiated physis, causing enhanced bone growth retardation [4, 5, 8].

Scoring systems and predictive guidelines of late effects have been proposed in an effort to improve finding growth related sequelae earlier [4, 11, 13].

However, these efforts to devise a consistent system for scoring late effects are hampered by the multiplicity of factors that influence the severity of treatment related effects [4].

The medical literature and the annals of law courts record many instances where irradiation in childhood resulted in a degree of disability that could never have been matched by the untreated disease. Thus, benign disease is now rarely treated by irradiation [12, 100]. However, in malignant disease radiation therapy can be life-saving, and treatment should not be denied because of risk of growth related deformity [2, 7, 105, 113]. Triple therapy, consisting of surgery, irradiation, and chemotherapy, used in varying combinations and sequences, can be effective. Pediatric orthopedists, pediatric radiation oncologists, pediatric oncologists, and pediatric endocrinologists must cooperate closely to determine the optimal management strategy and follow-up [4].

13.2 Diagnostic Irradiation

Although under certain circumstances diagnostic x-rays directed to a fetus in utero may result in an increased risk of leukemia, there is no evidence that diagnostic roentgenography of children is a hazard to growth [14]. There are no reports of physeal retardation or arrest from the use of diagnostic irradiation [17], even when full body films, scanograms, tomograms or CT scans are taken repeatedly over prolonged periods, for example in patients with scoliosis, developmental dislocation of the hip, growth plate injuries, fracture management, clubfeet, etc.

Radionuclide bone scans are a common diagnostic tool frequently used in children. Bone seeking radioactive agents accumulate in higher concentrations in physeal cartilage than in surrounding bone. Following injection of a bone seeking agent (^{99m}Tc-EHDP), radioactivity in the growth complexes of the distal femur and proximal tibia in a series of children 4–16 years of age was measured [18]. The dose to the growth plate was found to range from 0.8 to 4.7 rad when adjusted to an administered activity of 200 uCi/kg, compared to approximately 0.6 rad to the adult skeleton. Nevertheless, adverse effects on the physis from the use of such scans has not been reported.

The use of fluoroscopy has been implicated for partial physeal arrest in one case [17]. Fluoroscopy was used during the removal of a darning needle from the medial side of the left knee of a 5 year old boy in 1941. The operation lasted "about one hour"; the duration of fluoroscopy was not recorded. One month later a bulbous eruption appeared on the medial side of the knee, and the skin of the entire knee region acquired a dark color. The extremity grew normally for 10 years when genu varum (7° distal femur, 4° proximal tibia) was noted during a period of rapid growth. Roentgenograms showed open physes with "irregularity" of the medial proximal tibial physis. Teleangiectasia and hyperpigmentation persisted on the medial side of the knee. The author concluded that abnormal growth of both the distal femur and proximal tibia were due to the irradiation received 10 years earlier. An osteotomy was planned when growth was complete.

13.3 Therapeutic Irradiation; Extremities

The effect of therapeutic irradiation on enchondral cartilage (the physis) is the slowdown or arrest of chondrogenesis. Relative bone shortening is, therefore, a frequent complication of therapeutic irradiation in children from any cause (Table 13.1). Along with the shortening there is usually a decrease in shaft diameter

Table 13.1 Pathologic conditions of the extremities treated by irradiation with subsequent physeal disturbance

Benign
Hemangioma (soft tissue) [24, 25, 28, 37, 41, 43, 65]
Hemangioma (bone) [66]
Hemangio-endothelioma [27]
Langerhans cell histiocytosis [37]
Giant cell tumor [39]
Cutaneous nevus (finger) [20]
Eosinophilic granuloma [9]
Malignant
Ewing's sarcoma [5, 12, 22, 26, 30, 33, 35, 36, 78, 100]
Rhabdomyosarcoma [29, 33, 36]
Synovial cell sarcoma [23, 32, 33]
Non-Hodgkins lymphoma [31, 36]
Soft tissue sarcoma (type unspecified) [12, 21]
Soft tissue sarcoma (extraosseous Ewings) [32]
Osteogenic sarcoma [3]
Fibrosarcoma [33]
Epitheliod sarcoma [19]
Angiosarcoma [41]
Neurofibrosarcoma [12]
Undifferentiated embryonal sarcoma [29]
Hodgkin's disease [29]
Vascular nevo-carcinoma of skin [40]

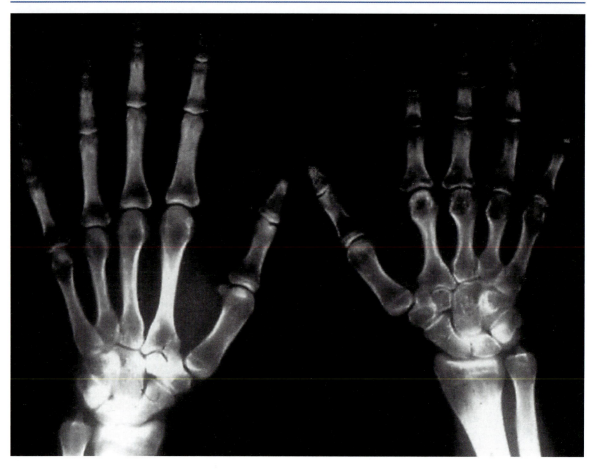

Fig. 13.1 Irradiation of the hand. A hemangioma on the dorsum of the hand of a girl was irradiated at age 7 years. Radiation type, dose, and duration are unknown. In adulthood all right phalanges and metacarpals are shorter than the left. For this degree of relative shortening the physeal arrests must have been sudden and complete. Note normal joint width and contours, suggesting little damage to articular cartilage (Case contributed by Dr. J DePablos, Pamplona, Spain, with permission)

and cortical thickness. Hyaline cartilage (the articular surface) is relatively insensitive to radiation [16], and joints within the irradiated field continue to appear and function normally (Fig. 13.1) [2, 24].

The response of the physis to irradiation is variable. Some physes show diminished growth (relative to the contralateral nonirradiated physis) with subsequent resumption of normal growth, and a resultant net loss that does not worsen with time [30]. The capacity of the physis and its blood supply to recover is remarkable [14]. Surviving clones of chondroblasts eventually repopulate the physis, with recovery being indirectly proportional to the radiation dose applied [169]. Some physes show diminished growth and may remain open for considerable time (years) before closing prematurely [24]. Some develop physeal widening resembling rickets [12, 22, 32], which either persists or reverts to normal width and resumption of normal growth. Some develop widening with eventual slipping of the epiphysis (see following section). Some develop physeal widening and mild cupping (Fig. 13.2a–c), but with no growth and gradual relative bone shortening (Fig. 13.2d). This widening is possibly due to vascular damage in the metaphysis (as shown in Fig. 1.3) [5]. Some irradiated physes develop benign osteochondromata (exostoses), which by themselves reduce longitudinal growth (see following section). In some cases the relative shortening is sufficient to require amputation (Fig. 13.2i–k) [21, 24, 34].

Thus, although the response of the physis to irradiation is variable, the consistent result is reduction of growth with relative bone shortening. On occasion

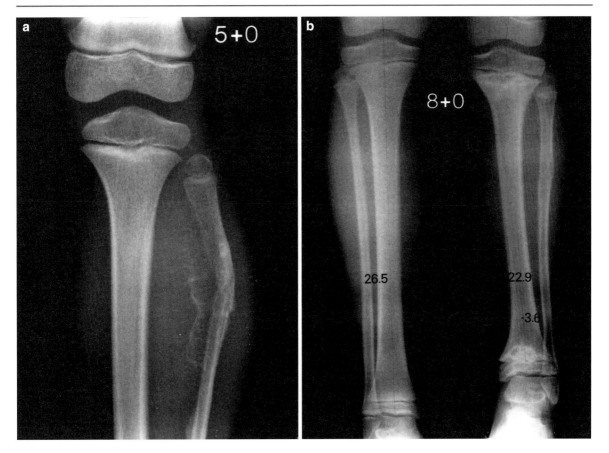

Fig. 13.2 Irradiation in a girl with Ewing's sarcoma of the fibula, causing tibial physeal closure. (**a**) A 5 years 0 month female had Ewing's sarcoma of the proximal left fibula, diagnosed by open biopsy. Metastasis to the lung was confirmed by open thoracotomy biopsy. The patient received radiation of 5,000 cGy to the left leg in 24 fractions over 8 weeks, and 1,500 cGy to the lungs in 12 fractions over 2 weeks. (**b**) At age 8 years 0 months the patient was tumor free but had increasing tibial length discrepancy (3.6 cm). There had been no growth of the left tibia or the fibula. (**c**) At age 9 years 0 months the tibial physes are open, but the distal physis had mild cupping. Although no bar could be identified, the central portion of each physis was excised and filled with cranioplast in hope of resuming growth. (**d**) At age 9 years 9 months the length discrepancy had increased to 6 cm. and there had been no growth between silver clips inserted at time of bar excision in both the proximal and distal epiphyses and metaphyses. Surgical physeal arrest of the right tibia and fibula was not done because of the desire to maintain one normal extremity, maintaining normal body height in the face of several unknowns in the abnormal extremity. Tibial and fibular lengthening with a Wagner distracter was undertaken. (**e**) Both the tibia and fibula were lengthened 51 mm over 52 days and held with a plate and screws. (**f**) The lengthenings failed to unite resulting in non-unions; the left tibia was now 8.6 cm shorter than the right. (**g**) At age 11 years 1 month the pseudarthrosis was excised, stabilized with a Rush rod, and bone grafted. (**h**) The tibia and fibula united, but at age 15 years 0 months the left tibia was 12.2 cm shorter than the right. All physes were closed and there had been no growth from either bar excision. Genu valgum was 7° on the right, 15° on the left. All physes were closed. (**i**) The patient ambulated with a 4 ½ in. shoe lift which accentuated genu valgum and ankle varum. The patient requested amputation. (**j**) A Syme ankle disarticulation was combined with removal of the Rush rod and distal femoral varus osteotomy. (**k**) At age 16 years 2 months the left femur was 1.3 cm shorter than the right, the tibia 12.2 cm, for a total limb length discrepancy of 13.5 cm. The patient became a good prosthesis wearer and was normally active with no evidence of disease when last seen at age 19 years 3 months. Since there were no surgical physeal arrests of the normal leg her standing height was normal. This case has many lessons. Better shielding should have prevented damage of the distal tibial physis. Irradiated physes may completely stop growing without developing a roentgenographic bar. Bar excision is ineffectual because the remaining irradiated physis has no growth potential. Lengthening of irradiated diaphyseal bone is prone to develop non-union. Physeal arrest of the normal right tibia at a younger age would have reduced the patient's height and produced significant femoral-tibial length disproportion. Amputation may be the best solution for extreme shortening secondary to irradiated physes (Updated from Peterson [34], with permission)

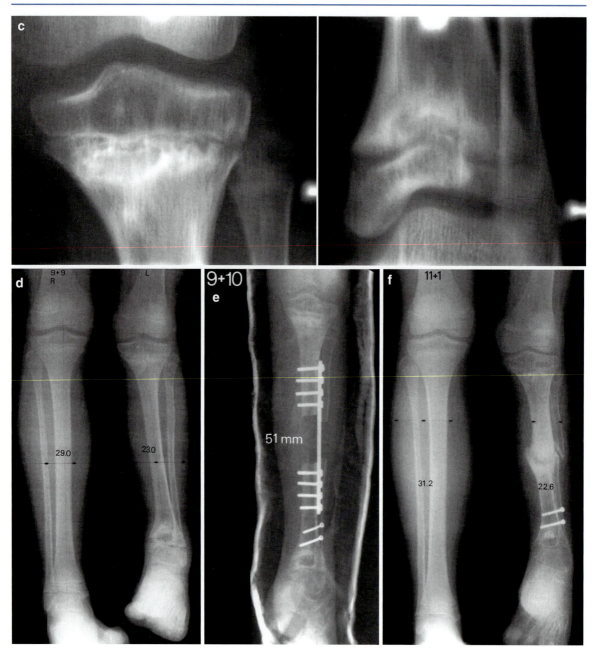

Fig. 13.2 (continued)

13.3 Therapeutic Irradiation; Extremities

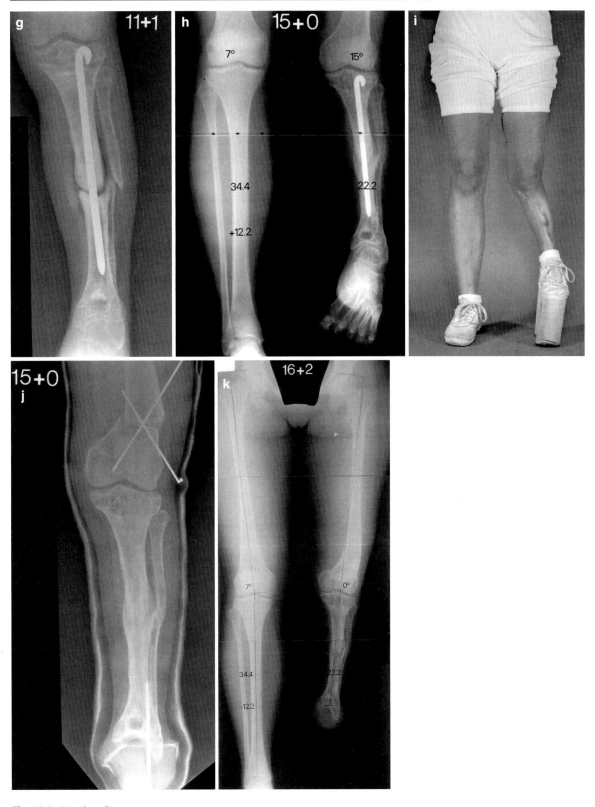

Fig. 13.2 (continued)

Table 13.2 Variables which affect growth following irradiation

Year	Author	Patient age	Diagnosis	Part irradiated	Radiation dose	Duration radiation	Total dose	Relative shortening
1937	Siegling [39]	12 years	Benign giant cell	Dist femur		"Several months"	3,800 cGy	0
1950	Franz [24]	3 weeks	Hemangioma	Entire leg	200–400 cGy	5 months	1,800 cGy	10 in.
1991	Goldwein [5]	6 years	Ewing's sarcoma	Prox tibia			6,000 cGy megavoltage	2.5 cm
		11 years	Ewing's sarcoma	Prox tibia			5,000 cGy orthovoltage	9 cm
1993	Irwin [29]	8 months	Rhabdomyo sarcoma	Prox femur	45 Gy	26 fractions 36 days	130 cGy	"Measurable"

This sample of reports emphasizes the problem of comparing cases. There are significant differences in effects due to variables such as patient age, tumor irradiated, body part irradiated, and the dose, duration, and type of irradiation. The youngest patient had the least amount of radiation, but had the greatest relative shortening. However, the 11 year old who received 5,000 cGy orthovoltage to the proximal tibia had greater relative shortening than the 6 year old who received 6,000 cGy megavoltage to the proximal tibia. The 56 year time span between articles also allows for differences in the type and administration of the radiation, and the accompanying use of various chemotherapies

partial peripheral arrest causes angular deformity [41], sometimes sufficient to require epiphysiodesis of the remaining physis [23] or corrective osteotomy (Fig. 13.2i, j) [19, 20, 31].

13.3.1 Dose and Age Effects

Bone growth retardation resulting from irradiation is subject to multiple variables, the foremost of which are the dose and the patient age [5, 12, 20, 29]. The greater the dose and the younger the age, the greater the effect. At a younger age growth plates are more susceptible to irradiation, but also have a greater potential for recovery [19]. A radiation dose of as low as 400 cGy can produce growth retardation, which may be reversible. As the dose increases and the doses accumulate, so does the extent of physeal damage. A total surface dose of 1,500–2,500 cGy, divided over a period of 6–8 weeks, with single doses of 300–800 cGy appears to cause no growth disturbance [43]. Permanent structural cellular changes sufficient to impair growth may begin with doses as little as 2,000 cGy in young children [5, 19]. However, most children who receive doses lower than 3,000 cGy have minor growth impairment (but a greater chance of tumor recurrence) [36]. In general, the threshold of irradiation that will cause complete physeal arrest in any location is 3,000 cGy in a young child and is 4,000 cGy in an older child. Growth arrest uniformly occurs with physeal irradiation of 4,500 cGy or greater [36]. Doses of 5,000 cGy or greater reliably ablate the primary tumor, but are associated with greater morbidity [9, 36]. However, the variables mentioned in the introduction make dose-effect predictions difficult (Table 13.2). As an example, a dose of as little as 130 cGy protracted over 26 fractions (5 cGy per fraction) in a 12 month old child resulted in measurable leg length discrepancy and maldevelopment at 7 years follow-up [29]. One study [25] concluded that the dose of irradiation was a more important factor than the age.

13.3.2 Physes Involved

Physes of the extremities with recorded growth arrest from irradiation are listed on Table 13.3. Irradiation of the upper extremity is more acceptable [30], probably because loss of length is less critical than in

Table 13.3 Physes damaged following therapeutic irradiation of the extremities in humans

Distal femur [8, 12, 19–21, 24, 30–32, 36, 39, 40, 65]
Proximal tibia [8, 12, 19, 21, 24, 30, 32, 36, 65, 100]
Distal tibia [21, 24, 40, 65, 99]
Proximal femur [29, 37]
Proximal humerus [3, 22]
Metacarpal [28, 33]
Finger phalanges [20, 28]
Distal radius [66]
Proximal radius [30]

the lower extremity. In older children the effects of irradiation are less detrimental [30], because there is less growth remaining. If an entire lower extremity of an infant is irradiated, the length discrepancy and limb atrophy at maturity may be sufficient to require amputation [21, 24, 34].

13.3.3 Side Effects

Numerous deleterious effects other than growth arrest have been recorded from irradiation to the physis (Table 13.4). Some of these deleterious effects in themselves can reduce vascularity to the physis, resulting in growth impairment. These abnormalities, along with the risk of secondary malignancies, combined with improved multidrug chemotherapy, have caused a reduction in the use of irradiation of extremity lesions, especially for Ewing's sarcoma [30, 36]. However, improved survival rates may result in more long-term morbidity such as growth arrest [30], which will require closer evaluation of the survivors.

The desirable effect of compensatory overgrowth of a normal physis proximal or distal to an impaired physis, which often occurs following growth arrest due to physeal fracture, has not been reported in humans following post irradiation physeal closure. Compensatory overgrowth did not occur in the cases presented in Figs. 13.2 and 13.3. It has been reported in animals (Sect. 13.9.6).

13.3.4 Multimodality Therapy

Multimodality therapy, consisting of surgery, chemotherapy and radiation, has become the standard of care for a number of life-threatening childhood malignancies. A serious, complication of this strategy in children is the impairment of bone growth, resulting in limb shortening. Of these therapies it appears the radiation plays the most prominent part producing physeal arrest.

Current strategies to reduce the effects of radiation on bone growth and subsequent stunting are limited to minimizing the radiation dose given directly to the major growth-contributing physis in the involved bone, or excluding this area from the treatment field. However, this is not always possible without also excluding essential tumor volume from the field of irradiation and thus seriously compromising therapy. Radioprotectant drugs have been evaluated in animal trials, in an effort to lessen the effects of limb shortening by irradiation (Sect. 13.9.9).

13.3.5 Management

The best prevention of physeal damage is to use judicious irradiation protocols and optimal shielding [35, 36, 38]. Follow-up until skeletal maturity is needed to assess limb length inequality. Extensive operative procedures are indicated to preserve or restore function, if life expectancy is reasonable [42]. Lower limb length discrepancies can be treated by shoe lifts on the short side, or properly timed epiphyseodesis [33] or bone shortening on the normal long side. There is a report of unsuccessful bar excision for partial physeal closure following irradiation [34] and no reports of success. My own experience was unrewarding (Fig. 13.2). Excision of a physeal bar secondary to irradiation may be unsuccessful due to the fact that the remaining physeal cartilage around the bar is not normal. Surgical lengthening of irradiated

Table 13.4 Deleterious clinical side effects of irradiation therapy to extremities, other than physeal arrest, SCFE, osteochondroma, and secondary malignancy

Soft tissue atrophy [20, 33, 36]
Fibrosis [12, 33, 38]
Impaired mobility and extremity function [12, 33, 38]
Muscle atrophy [3, 8, 33]
Osteoporosis [3, 37]
Telangiectasia [3, 20]
Edema [33, 38]
Flexion contracture [40]
Pigmented skin [3]
Skin scars [42]
Skin atrophy [40]
Bone weakness [36]
Fracture [33]
Osteonecrosis [38]
Peripheral nerve injury [33]
Hair loss [36]
Soft tissue swelling [37]
Vasculitis with thrombosis [33]

bone is hazardous because of the adverse effects of radiotherapy on callous formation and should be avoided (Fig. 13.2d–g) [31]. Healthy non-irradiated bone contiguous to irradiated bone can be safely lengthened [26]. In extreme situations, amputation and limb prosthesis may provide the best functional outcome (Fig. 13.2h–j) [3, 21, 24, 34].

13.3.6 Slipped Epiphyses

Irradiation of the upper thigh, pelvis, and lower abdomen that includes the femoral heads may result in slipped capital femoral epiphysis (SCFE). The majority of reported cases have been in children 4 years or less when treated, and were given doses exceeding 2,500 cGy (Table 13.5). The proposed mechanism of action for slipping is that the irradiation injures the germinal and proliferation cell zones and their vascular supply, causing arrest of chondrogenesis [4, 48]. These two effects act synergistically to delay maturation of the physis, causing widening and structural weakness in the physis and its matrix. In addition, irradiation of the gonads may alter the hormonal balance to decrease the strength of the physis [46].

Physeal widening occurs in the zone of hypertrophy (Fig. 1.2), and the slippage usually occurs between the zone of hypertrophy and zone of provisional calcification. In the matrix the findings include a change of chemical properties and a loss of cohesion on histologic sections [58]. Physeal widening may be present for several years before the slipping occurs (Fig. 13.3a–d). One case was first noted to slip 13 years after irradiation [52]. The structural defects in the physis, along with the stress of weight bearing, combine to allow slipping of the physis [58]. This is enhanced by the gradual change of the proximal femoral physis from horizontal to a more oblique plane, which along with increasing body weight causes more sheer stress with increased activity [58]. Thus, as the strength of the physis decreases, the stress on the physis increases.

There are multiple differences between irradiated and non-irradiated hips which develop SCFE. The incidence of slipping following irradiation is significantly higher than slipping in non-irradiated children. The subsequent slipping occurs at a younger age than expected [58, 60]. The peak discovery age for post irradiation SCFE is 11 years of age [44]. The peak ages for SCFE in non-irradiated children is 13–14 years in boys and 11–12 years in girls [51]. Slips have been recorded following irradiation of the pelvis undertaken for a variety of causes. Because of this variety the gender distribution of the slips is equal (Table 13.5) [53], whereas SCFE in non-irradiated children is more common in males (approximately 2–1). Children with post-irradiation slips are usually thin (median weight 10th percentile), in contrast to children with typical SCFE who are usually obese (50% of both males and females have weights at or above the 95th percentile for their age) [53]. There are no data concerning race for SCFE following irradiation. In one study [46] of 48 irradiated children, 60% had bilateral slips. If only one hip is irradiated, only that hip slips [52]. The slips are usually first noted years after the irradiation (Table 13.5), yet the majority of slips are mild compared with non-irradiated SCFE [60].

In one typical study [58] of 50 irradiated patients under 15 years of age, 83 proximal femoral physes were at risk. All patients received intensive chemotherapy prior to and after abdominal irradiation. Eight physes (9.6%) in five patients (10%) developed slipping. Children under age 4 at the time of irradiation were at higher risk; 7 of 15 physes (47%) developed slipping. Most slippages were noted between 8 and 10 years of age, 5–7 years post irradiation. No slippage occurred in patients who received doses below 2,500 cGy (25 Gy).

Patients given chemotherapeutic agents that are radiosensitizers are at increased risk to develop SCFE [45, 48]. Children with growth hormone deficiency who have undergone chemo and radiotherapy for leukemia are at even more risk [50]. One of 13 patients developed SCFE despite being given intraoperative high-dose-rate brachyotherapy which was used to decrease the dose of external beam radiotherapy [55]. In addition to SCFE, aseptic necrosis of femoral heads and radiation-induced sarcoma have been recorded [52].

In many instances post irradiation SCFE is a preventable complication. The femoral heads and acetabula should be shielded from the treatment fields when their inclusion is not crucial to the treatment of the underlying disease [56, 57, 60]. Judicious use of primary or secondary blocking systems can limit or eliminate the dose to open femoral physes in most cases [58]. Conversely, increasing survival rates may cause more cases to be seen in the future [46, 61].

Since SCFE in early stages usually has no pain, regular examination of the hips is necessary. Early slip may be detected clinically by an increase in external rotation accompanied by reduction in internal rotation and abduction, as well as a tendency for the hip to externally rotate as it is flexed. Serial roentgenograms following irradiation have been advocated to detect early physeal widening [52, 60], which is present before the clinical signs.

The treatment of SCFE due to irradiation is surgical fixation of the epiphysis (Fig. 13.3e–g) [4, 44–46, 54, 55, 60, 105]. After pinning, the physis often fuses slowly, but satisfactorily, and there are no wound healing problems as might be expected with irradiated tissues [46]. If the physis is widened and irregular and the bone adjacent to the physis is sclerotic (a pre-slip), prophylactic pinning may be indicated even in the absence of a visible slip [4, 44, 45, 59]. This is particularly appropriate for the side opposite a confirmed slip, if both hips were irradiated. If the child is young at the time of slip diagnosis, for example 10 years or less, surgical epiphyseodesis of the greater trochanter [57] should also be considered. Patients with very severe slippage, more than 60°, may require osteotomy and osteoplasty [4]. Keep in mind that the complications of total hip arthroplasty in previously irradiated bone are also much higher than in non-irradiated bone (Cabanela ME, Personal communication). Close observation instead of surgery may be appropriate for older children with a widened physis and no slip. One boy, 14 years old at time of irradiation and chemotherapy, and 15 years 3 months at the time widening of the physis was first noted, was observed and went on to normal physeal closure [58].

Proximal humeral epiphyseal growth retardation and slipping also occurs as a sequela of irradiation [47, 49]. Since stress on the proximal humeral epiphysis is less than on the proximal femur, higher radiation doses are required to cause slipping. As in SCFE, the younger the child, the more severe the consequences. Contrary to SCFE due to other causes only unilateral cases have been recorded (since only one side has been irradiated).

13.3.7 Osteochondroma (Exostosis)

An osteochondroma is an abnormal bony protuberance capped with cartilage. Benign osteochondromas were first noted to develop on the surface of the metaphysis adjacent to the physes within the irradiation treatment field in 1950 [24], and have since been found to occur following irradiation for either benign or malignant conditions [37, 41, 62–66, 95, 121]. As the physis grows away from the metaphysis, the osteochondroma when first noted may be located on the metaphysis well away from the physis [63], or even on the diaphysis [62]. Post irradiation exostoses characteristically are first noted years after irradiation (3–30 years) [63, 65]. Since routine post irradiation roentgenograms are usually not obtained, the time of discovery is variable. No exostoses have been found in irradiated children outside the fields of radiation [63, 65].

The precise mechanism of development of radiation-induced osteochondromas is unknown [12, 63]. They are roentgenographically and histologically identical to those that arise spontaneously [9]. The pathogenesis has been speculated to be a failure of differentiation of the reserve cell layer of the physis combined with a persistence of undifferentiated cartilage in the metaphysis where it may develop into either endochrondoma or osteochondroma [65]. In this context it may not represent a true neoplasm, but simply a perversion of normal growth [63]. Most, but not all, of the patients have received supplemental chemotherapy. There are no reports of osteochondromas developing in irradiated adults.

Most radiation-induced osteochondromas have been reported in patients who received local doses of

Table 13.5 Postirradiation slipped femoral capital epiphysis

Year	Author[a]	Diagnosis	Gender	Age at irradiation (years)[b]	Total tumor dose (cGy)	Days of Rx	Chemotherapy[c]	Age at SCFE (years)[b]	Side	Interval (years)
1962	Rubin [105]	Neuroblastoma	F	1	5,130	28	–	9	R/L	8
1977	Wolf [61]	Neuroblastoma	F	2	2,850	26	–	7	L	5
		Rhabdosarcoma		3.5	5,400	41	–	9	L	5.5
		Non-Hodgkin's lymphoma	M	4	4,000	28	–	11	L	7
		Hodgkin's disease	M	10	3,950	41	–	11	R/L	1
		Hodgkin's disease	F	10	4,000	28	MOPP	14	L	4
1979	Dickerman [48]	Rhabdomyosarcoma	M	4	5,940	53	V,A,C	7	L	3
1979	Ryan [56]	Neuroblastoma	F	2	2,850	21	V,C	7.5	L	5.5
		Ryabdosarcoma	M	6.5	6,000	49	V,A,C	9	L	2.5
1980	Chapman [46]	Wilm's	F	3	3,000	26	–	12	R/L	9
		Wilm's	F	3	3,000	29	–	11	L/R	8
		Yolk sac tumor	F	3	3,000	27	V,A,C	7	R/L	4
		Rhabdomyosarcoma	M	3	3,000	27	A	12	R	9
		Neuroblastoma	M	3	3,000	35	–	12	R	9
1981	Libshitz [52]	Rhabdomyosarcoma		2.5	3,000			11.5	L	9
		Rhabdomyosarcoma	M	7	4,000			11.5	L	4.5
		Ewing's		9.5	5,500			11		1.5
1981	Silverman [58]	Rhabdomyosarcoma	M	1.5	6,125	35 fr	V,A,C	9	R	7.5
		Rhabdomyosarcoma	M	3	5,280	–	V,A,C	6.5	L	3.5
		Malig. Lymphoma	M	3.5	2,800	16 fr	V,P,M	6.5	R/L	3
		Rhabdomyosarcoma	M	4	5,940	36 fr	V,A,C	5.5		1.5
		Rhabdomyosarcoma	M	14	5,041	28 fr	V,A,C	15		1
1981	Wiss [60]	Rhabdomyosarcoma	F	1.5	4,400	35	V,A,C	6.5	R/L	5
		Rhabdomyosarcoma	F	3	4,250	42	V,A	7	R/L	4
		Neuroblastoma	M	5.5	4,000	42	V,C	9.5	R/L	4
		Hodgkin's disease	M	8	4,550		–	10	R/L	2
1981	Walker [59]	Rhabdomyosarcoma	M	1.5	6,500	35 fr	V,A,C	7.5	R/L	6
		Non-Hodgkin's lymphoma	M	2.5	2,800	16 fr	VPMC-6	8	R/L	5.5
1983	McAfee [54]	Rhabdomyosarcoma	F	8.5	8,000	20	Yes	12.5	R	4
		Undiff. sarcoma	F	13	4,000	21	Yes	20	R	7
1985	Barrett [44]	Embry. sarcoma	M	5	3,800	25	Yes	14	R	9
		Rhabdomyosarcoma	F	6	4,500	35	Yes	9	R	3
1987	Sabio [57]	Rhabdomyosarcoma	M	2.5	5,900	36	V,A,C	8.5	R/L	6
		Hodgkin's disease	M	4	3,500	20	MOPP	8	R/L	4

13.3 Therapeutic Irradiation; Extremities

Year	Author	Diagnosis	Sex	Age	Dose		Chemo		R/L	
1994	Fletcher [121]	Leukemia	M	0.5	1,200	3	Yes	9	–	8.5
1998	Loder [53]	Undiff sarcoma	F	1	5,600	60	Yes	6	R/L	5
		Rhabdomyosarcoma	F	1.5	5,940	38	Yes	5	R	3.5
		Rhabdomyosarcoma	F	1.5	3,040	28	Yes	14.5	R/L	13
		Rhabdomyosarcoma	F	2	4,100	–	Yes	10	L	8
		Ewing's	M	2	4,500	30	Yes	7.5	R/L	5.5
		Rhabdomyosarcoma	F	3	4,960	28	Yes	13	L	10
		Ewing's	M	4	6,000	42	Yes	9.5	R	5.5
		Rhabdomyosarcoma	F	4.5	3,500	28	Yes	6	L	1.5
		Wilm's	F	7.5	1,000	7	Yes	14.5	L	7
		Rhabdomyosarcoma	F	8.5	5,500	48	Yes	13	R/L	4.5

[a] Most articles have more than one author; see References
[b] Age to the closest half year
[c] Chemotherapy may occur prior to or after irradiation. *A* Actinomycin D, *C* Cyclophosphomide, *M* Methotrexate, *P* Prednosone, *V* Vincristine
MOPP Nitrogen mustard, Oncovine (vincristine), Prednisolone, Procarbizine, *VPMC-6* Vincristine, Prednisone, Methotrexate, Cyclophosphonate, G-MP

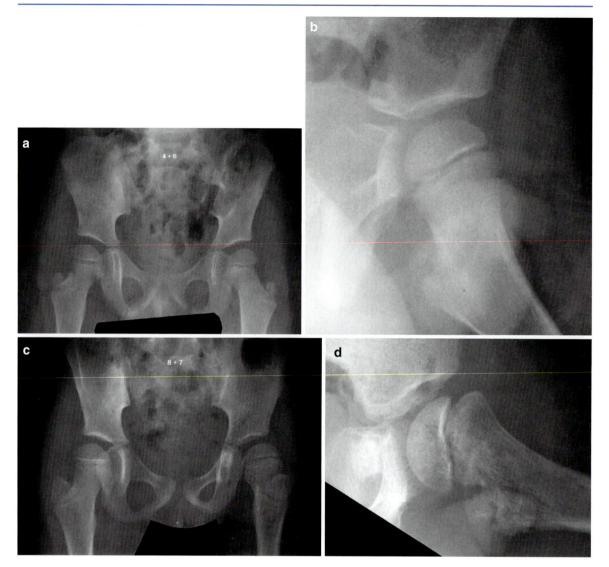

Fig. 13.3 Radiation-induced SCFE. (**a**) At age 4 years 6 months this boy had left hip pain. The bone structure was normal. The pubis and ischia were symmetrically equal in size and shape. (**b**) Oblique view showed a normal proximal femoral physis and triradiate cartilage. At age 4 years 10 months a rhabdomyosarcoma was surgically removed from the left buttock, followed by radiation and chemotherapy. The hip joint was in the irradiation field. Mild relative left femoral shortening developed gradually. (**c**) At age 8 years 7 months the patient was normally active with only a slight short leg limp. Roentgenograms showed left hip external rotation, widening of the physis, less height of the epiphysis, and smaller pubic and ischium bones on the left than on the right. Scanogram showed the left femur 13 mm shorter than the right. (**d**) An oblique view at the same time as (**c**) showed posterior slip of the epiphysis. (**e**) A scanogram at age 9 years 8 months showed the femoral length discrepancy had increased to 1.9 cm. At age 10 years 9 months the hip was pinned in-situ. (**f**) At age 11 years 8 months the femoral discrepancy was 2.4 cm on scanogram. The left ischium and pubis were smaller than the right and the left triradiate cartilage was indistinct. (**g**) Oblique view at same time as (**f**), 11 months post operative, showed no further slip of the epiphysis. The physis remains open. The patient developed radiation-induced osteogenic sarcoma, and died at age 14 years 3 months of respiratory failure

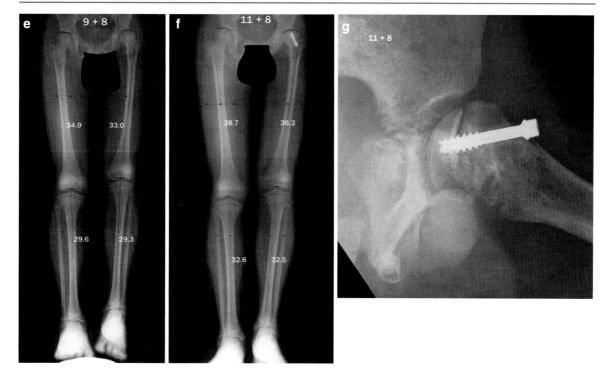

Fig. 13.3 (continued)

1,500–5,500 cGy (15–55 Gy) [63, 121], administered between ages 13 months and 12 years of age [63]. In Murphy and Blount's three cases [65] the total irradiation ranged from 1,600 to 6,425 cGy, but they noted a case from the German literature of a 1 week old child given a single dose or 125 cGy, who was later found to have an osteochondroma. Although there is a direct association of irradiation and exostoses, there is no way to exclude the possibility of spontaneous occurrence [63].

The frequency of osteochondromas following radiation therapy is 6–24% [62–64, 121], compared with <1% in non-irradiated children [63]. Any open physis is vulnerable 65], including the spine and ribs [63, 91]. Younger patients are at greater risk [121]. Exostoses which occur in non-irradiated patients are usually multiple. Osteochondromas found after irradiation are usually singular, though if multiple physes are included within the irradiated field, any physis may have an exostosis [65, 121]. In an exception, three post irradiation exostoses were found on one proximal tibia, and two on an iliac crest of another child [63]. When osteochondromas occur on multiple physes, "extreme" relative limb shortening may be present [65].

The incidence of malignant transformation of naturally occurring non-irradiated solitary exostoses varies from 1% to 7% [12], and that of patients with multiple hereditary osteochondromata (MHO) is somewhat greater [65]. Most radiation induced bone malignancies are associated with higher radiation doses than those generally responsible for osteochondromas [63]. Malignant transformation of irradiation-induced osteochondromas was initially thought to be non-existent [7, 12, 65], but in 1967 [95] a low-grade chondrosarcoma was reported in a femoral osteochondroma

12 years after the bone was irradiated during infancy. Since it is so uncommon, no article has suggested prophylactic surgical removal of a post-irradiation osteochondroma for fear of later malignant transformation. Nevertheless, longer surveillance of postirradiation exostoses is appropriate.

13.3.8 Intentional Physeal Retardation of Extremity Physes

Irradiation of normal lower extremity physes has been used to intentionally inhibit growth. In a 1941 report [67], three children ages 5–8 years, with length discrepancies from 1¼ to 3½ in., were given total doses of 1,600–2,400 cGy to both the anterior and posterior aspects of the knee of the normal longer leg over a period of 12–28 months. In each child growth was retarded, but not stopped. When growth resumed, the final discrepancy was reduced by 2 in. in one child, and increased by one-fourth and three-fourths inch in the other two. Without the irradiation these discrepancies would have increased to a greater extent in all three children. The author concluded that "bone growth can be deterred by roentgen irradiation".

A second report [68], also in 1941, records intentional irradiation used to equalize leg lengths in four children. Roentgen therapy of 2,656 cGy given on four consecutive days to a 6 year old girl, and 4,300 cGy given divided doses to an 8 year old girl and an 11 year old boy produced physeal closure. But 1,992 cGy and 672 cGy given 6 months apart to a 3 year old girl failed to cause arrest. The author concluded that around 3,000 cGy given in one fractionated series will produce epiphyseal closure. The fractionation of the dose can be arranged as best suited to produce tanning, but not epidermitis.

Despite the validity of the concept, intentional growth retardation by irradiation did not pass the experimental stage, probably because it required prolonged treatment, was not easy to control, and had potential side effects. This is a dangerous enterprise, and any perceived advantage over operative epiphysiodesis should be carefully scrutinized [154].

13.4 Therapeutic Irradiation; Head and Neck

Irradiation of the head can produce craniofacial growth abnormalities causing, in some cases, functional deformity. There is a strong correlation between age and radiation doses and the degree of dentofacial development [12, 73, 74].

Children with intracranial tumors [69, 70, 72, 100, 101, 105], acute lymphoblastic leukemia [71, 74, 100, 101], and nasopharyngeal carcinoma [75], treated by external irradiation to the head may receive incidental irradiation to the pituitary-hypothalamic axis, reducing the levels of growth hormone which in turn may depress or abolish further bone growth [5, 72]. Six of seven patients (86%) <15 years of age at the time of cranial irradiation in one study became growth hormone deficient [70]. None of these six became taller in adulthood than the 50th percentile for their gender. They had received from 2,300 cGy (for a 6 year old), to 4,300 cGy for a 12 year old, over 4–6 weeks. Children 12 years old or older who receive irradiation to the head, have minor growth retardation, if any. Children who have had cranial irradiation and are in prolonged remission with a decreased growth velocity may benefit from a 6 month trial of growth hormone [71].

Similar effects may occur in children who receive irradiation to the thyroid gland, suppression of which can impede normal bone growth [5, 69].

13.5 Therapeutic Irradiation; Trunk

Therapeutic irradiation of the trunk may expose physes of vertebrae, ribs, scapulae, and pelvis, which in turn may produce spine deformity, stature loss [12, 87], hypoplasia of ribs [7, 12, 76, 78, 81, 87, 102, 108, 110, 111] scapulae [8, 87], and pelvic bones, [6, 7, 9, 12, 78, 81, 105, 108–111, 115] acetabular dysplasia [6, 12, 105], irregular ossification of proximal femoral epiphyses with associated SCFE (discussed in Sect. 13.3), and impaired growth of the proximal femur (7 of 32 patients in one series [36]).

Soft tissues of the trunk in the irradiated field are also subject to deleterious outcomes similar to those on extremities as listed on Table 13.4. In addition there may be agenesis of the breast [8, 95], pulmonary dysfunction [110, 111], periocarditis [110], radiation nephritis [110], gonadal dysfunction [110], hepatic dysfunction [110], and visceral involvement. Chronic irradiation enteritis may be manifested by intestinal obstruction, fistulae, perforation, and hemorrhage. Any intestinal problem that occurs postoperatively in a scoliosis patient who has received radiation treatment, must be differentiated from cast syndrome or spinal traction syndrome. Irradiated bowel is ischemic, and necrosis with spontaneous perforation can only be avoided with early diagnosis and surgical intervention [106]. Muscle scarring and shortening may also produce a soft tissue contracture causing or contributing to spinal deformity.

13.5.1 Stature Loss

Vertebral bodies have physes which grow axially by endochondral ossification similar to the physes of long bones (Fig. 13.4) [99]. These vertebral physes react to the negative effect of therapeutic irradiation the same as long bone physes. Irradiation of the entire immature vertebra results in a smaller than normal vertebral body with reduction of longitudinal height (platyspondylia) [6, 9, 100]. Children whose trunks are irradiated have shorter adult stature than those who are not irradiated [107]. Compared to a normal population, there is a modest reduction in median final standing height, a marked reduction in final sitting height, and no apparent effect on subischial leg length. Thus, the measurement of sitting height compared with standing height is necessary to document the full effect of irradiation on the growing spine [100, 112].

The five most important factors in determining adult stature in irradiated children are: (1) radiation dose and fractionation, (2) number of vertebrae exposed, (3) age of the patient and stature velocity at time of treatment, (4) adjunctive chemotherapy, and (5) the interaction of genetic or familial background with the first four factors. The dose required to retard axial growth is approximately 2,500 cGy or more [12, 84]. This is well documented in the shorter stature of one 3 year old monozygotic twin who received 2,420 cGy over a period of 21 days [87].

13.5.2 Spine Deformity

Irradiation of a portion of the vertebral physes results in angular growth producing spine deformity. Conditions of the trunk treated by irradiation which included the axial skeleton and resulted in subsequent spine deformity are listed on Table 13.6.

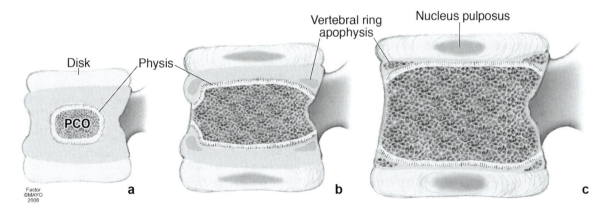

Fig. 13.4 Anatomy of a vertebral body. At birth (**a**) the primary center of ossification (*PCO*) is round and is surrounded by its physis. As the physis grows the PCO becomes cuboid (**b**) and later rectangular (**c**), growing longitudinally from the superior and inferior physes. Secondary centers of ossification associated with the physes never develop in humans, but do in some animals (From Peterson [99], with permission)

Table 13.6 Conditions of the trunk treated by irradiation which included the axial skeleton with subsequent spine deformity

A. *Intraabdominal*

Wilms tumors (nephroblastoma) [7, 12, 77–89, 91, 92, 94, 96–98, 102–108, 111, 115]

Neuroblastoma [7, 9, 12, 78, 79, 85, 87–92, 94, 95, 105, 106, 110, 112]

Hodgkins disease [78, 88, 100, 101, 106]

Non-Hodgkins lymphoma [78, 106]

Sarcoma [88, 106]

Embryonic carcinoma [88]

Embryonal adenocarcinoma [76]

Embryoma [91]

Retinoblastoma [94]

Lymphoma [88]

Renal teratoma [115]

B. *Intrathoracic/mediastinal*

Ganglioneuroblastoma [95, 117]

Ganglioneurolemoma [95]

Neuroblastoma [95]

C. *Intraspinal*

Medulloblastoma [105, 113]

D. *Soft tissue*

Acute leukemia [94, 100, 101]

Rhabdomyosarcoma [92, 94]

Malignant mesenchyma [94]

Embryonal cell sarcoma [94]

Neurofibrosarcoma [94]

Hepatoma [94]

Hemangiosarcoma [94]

Hemangioma [91]

Metastatic teratoma [92]

Nevoectodermal tumor [92]

Many cases of post irradiation spine deformity resemble those of idiopathic scoliosis and are a combination of scoliosis and kyphosis, called kyphoscoliosis. Numerical measurements to separate or classify the dominant deformity have not been developed. Although some articles emphasize scoliosis [76, 85, 105] or kyphosis [92, 103, 114], they are discussed here together in general terms. Scoliosis due to irradiation was first documented in the German literature in 1949 [82], and in the English literature in 1950 [76].

13.5.3 Etiology and Natural History of Spine Deformity

The amount of irradiation received by different portions of the vertebral body and the amount of growth remaining in the nonirradiated portion determine the subsequent deformity. Irradiation of a portion of a vertebra inhibits growth of that portion, promoting progressive axial spine deformity as the remaining portion of the vertebra grows. When irradiation involves a lateral portion of the body, the maximum inhibition of vertebral growth plate growth and loss of height will occur laterally, producing scoliosis concave toward the side of irradiation (Fig. 13.5a–e) [103]. Most authors have not defined scoliosis, but those that do usually included any curve >10° (Cobb method) [7, 78, 88]. Although structural changes are common, symptoms or dysfunction are infrequent. A functional classification for scoliosis based on symptomatology has been

Fig. 13.5 A girl with a right Wilms' tumor treated by nephrectomy and irradiation developed scoliosis controlled by a brace (all frontal images are posterior-anterior projections). (**a**) Age 1 year 2 months; preoperative roentgenogram of the lumbar spine and pelvis. Bone structures are normal; note the straight spine and symmetry of vertebrae, particularly the pedicles. At the time of right nephrectomy the tumor was found to extend outside the kidney. (**b**–**d**) Scout roentgenograms taken on the 14th, 15th, and 19th postoperative days to aid in determining portals for radiation therapy. The primary treatment field (x) lay lateral to the spine, but a portion of the spine was included within the area to be irradiated, as determined by these scout films. Presumably, the portals were altered to exclude or include the entire spine after these scout films were made. However, a second scout film was not recorded before radiation therapy, and a portion of spine may still have been included in the irradiation field. Mild left lumbar scoliosis in these views could be positional or related to the operative wound. Radiation dosage was 1,975 cGy in 12 doses over 20 days. (**e**) At age 2 years 0 months, 8 months after irradiation, there is left lumbar scoliosis, minimal vertebral rotation, pedicle size discrepancy, and asymmetry of each vertebra (vertebral body shape is irregular, and the height of each vertebral body is less on the right side than on the left). A Milwaukee brace with a single left lumbar pad was worn for 16 months. (**f**) At age 3 years 6 months the spine was satisfactorily aligned. The Milwaukee brace was changed to a body jacket at age 6 years 3 months. (**g**) At age 7 years 8 months the curve is mild and there is significant size increase in the structures of the right side of the vertebrae. The body jacket was continued until age 14 years 9 months. (**h**) Age 15 years 8 months. Residual left lumbar scoliosis measures 21°. (**i**) The patient is normally active but has occasional low back pain, possibly related to residual thoraco-lumbar kyphosis (48°). Note anterior wedging of lumbar vertebral bodies 1, 2, and 3. Note: The thoracolumbar kyphosis is the result of impairment of growth of the physes of the vertebral bodies with normal growth of the posterior elements which have apophyses, none of which have horizontally oriented physes. Was the improvement of the lumbar scoliosis due to post-irradiation resumption of growth, or to the wearing of a brace for more than 12 years. Was the brace necessary? Would the outcome have been different without the brace? (From Peterson [98], with permission and additional follow-up)

13.5 Therapeutic Irradiation; Trunk

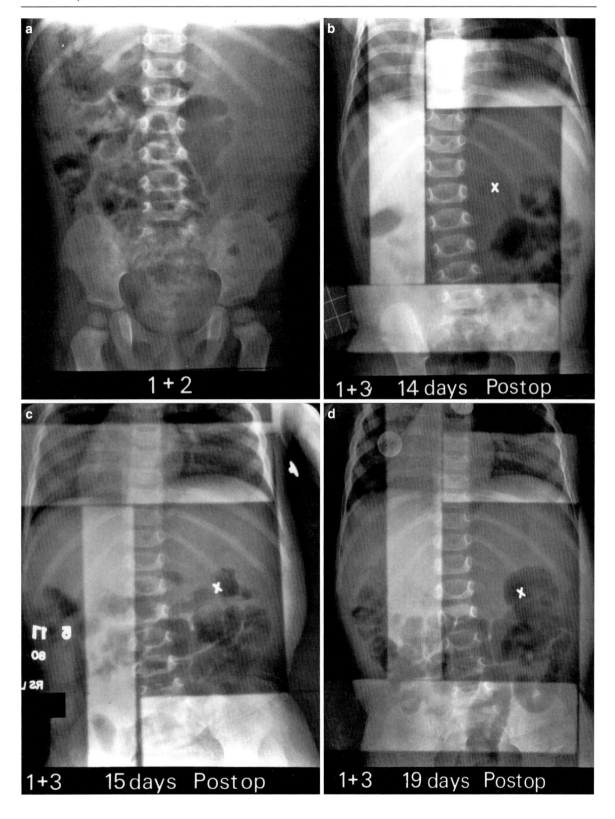

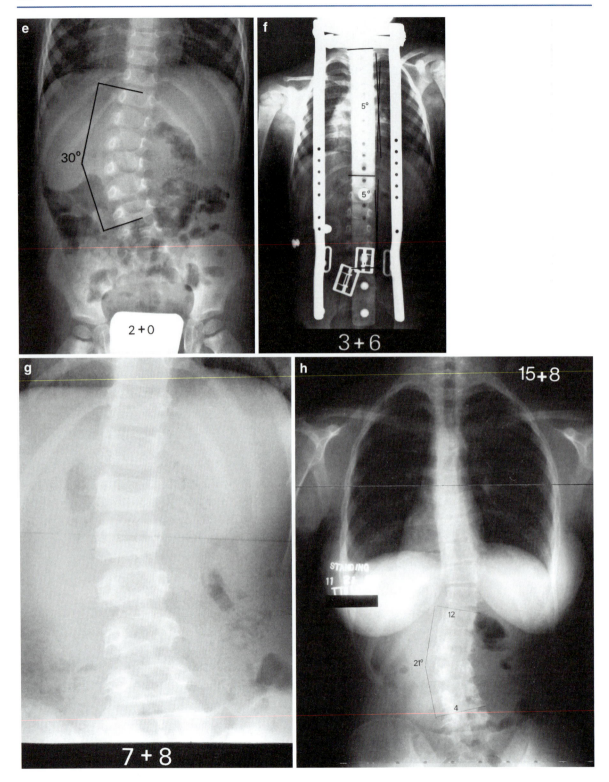

Fig. 13.5 (continued)

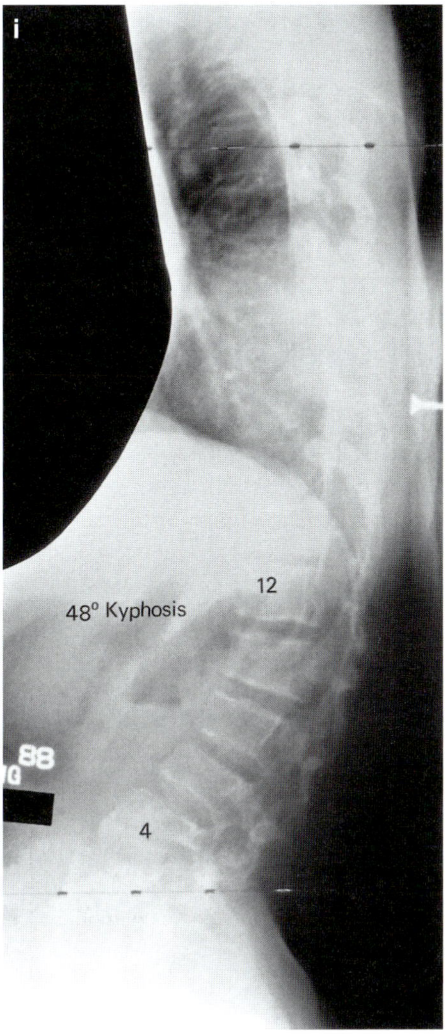

was irradiated [12, 91, 103, 113], or as a temporary scoliosis that improves when growth resumes if only a lateral portion of the body was irradiated (Fig. 13.5h) [95–97]. Vertebral growth that resumes after irradiation is disordered and associated with abnormal roentgenographic findings [101]. Doses of 2,000–3,000 cGy or more will cause permanent inhibition of physeal growth and contour irregularity, manifest first as irregularity or scalloping of vertebral end plates with diminished axial height, or as abnormalities with anterior or flat-beaked vertebral bodies, and later as partial growth arrest causing spine deformity [89–91, 93, 100, 108]. There is a correlation between the amount of irradiation and severity of curvature. Of 81 patients irradiated for Wilm's tumor, those that received <2,600 cGy had no spine deformity [104]. Patients who had a mean average dose of 3,150 cGy had deformities of <25°, and patients who had >3,600 cGy had curves in excess of 25° [103]. The degree of growth inhibition is related to the age of the child as well as the dose. The greatest growth retardation occurs when irradiation is received during periods of most active bone growth, i.e., under 6 years of age and during puberty [100, 101]. The most severe changes occur in patients 2 years of age or younger at the time of irradiation [91].

Roentgenographic architectural changes in vertebrae can be recognized as early as 6 months after irradiation [12]. Early changes are characterized by vertebral endplate irregularity, followed by vertebral growth arrest lines such as "a bone within a bone " appearance, vertebral contour abnormalities, and symmetric or asymmetric failure of vertebral development [12, 89, 91, 105]. The sclerotic lines of "a bone within a bone" indicate impaired growth followed by resumption of growth, but are not unique to irradiation, occurring with severe illness of any kind, congenital syphilis, lead poisoning, phosphorus medication, etc [113].

There is a paucity of histologic data from irradiated vertebrae in children. In one study [91], vertebrae of 11 children showed non-specific growth retardation manifest by decreased thickness and activity of the proliferative cartilage, and the deposition of a thin bony plate on its under surface, similar to a growth arrest line. These children had received between 360 and 2,680 cGy and all had died within 5 months of irradiation. Areas of cartilage degeneration were greater in patients receiving higher dose of irradiation.

Some spine deformities become more obvious and progress more rapidly during the adolescent growth

Fig. 13.5 (continued)

developed. When irradiation is confined to the anterior portion of the vertebral growth plate, kyphosis occurs [103]. Irradiation confined to the posterior aspects of vertebrae producing lordosis is relatively rare [113].

Depending upon the age and radiation dose and sequence there can be a temporary cessation of growth, with a resumption of the normal rate thereafter and a resultant net loss of spine height that does not worsen with time (Fig. 13.5e–h) [8, 100]. An accumulated dose of 1,000 cGy does not produce detectable inhibition of vertebral growth, irrespective of the patient's age [91]. An intermediate dose (1,000–2,000 cGy) may produce a temporary or inhibiting dose in a young child. This will manifest as transverse growth arrest lines or a "bone within a bone" if the entire vertebra

period [85, 86, 89]. Kyphotic curves (Fig. 13.5i) tend to progress after the adolescent growth spurt while mild and moderate scoliotic curves do not [81, 103]. When growth gradually ceases, the progression of mild to moderate deformity decreases, and the curve eventually stabilizes. Severe curves, however, continue to progress even after the patient attains skeletal maturity and need to be observed indefinitely. Spinal deformity may occur later in life in patients with spinal tumors who received radiation therapy many years previously.

Spinal deformity in patients who have received irradiation is not always caused by physeal damage of the vertebra. The deformity may be due to soft-tissue fibrosis and contracture [89, 113], rib and iliac hypoplasia, or as a result of the tumor or the surgery. Some of these factors may be present in Wilms' tumor patients who develop deformity, but did not receive radiation. In one study [80], Wilm's tumor patients treated with radiation developed scoliosis seven times more often (35 of 57) than did those who did not receive radiation (5 of 53). The five who were not irradiated support this point. In neuroblastoma the spinal deformity can be intrinsic, such as tumor involvement of the vertebrae or paralysis from spinal cord invasion or compression, or extrinsic, such as extraosseous soft tissue fibrosis and contracture, laminectomy, or asymmetric spinal irradiation [90]. Post irradiation kyphosis is usually rigid due to the vertebral structural changes and dense scarring of the paraspinal soft tissues [103].

In summary, the severity of spine deformity correlates primarily with the radiation dose, the patient age, and the length of follow-up [89].

13.5.4 Incidence of Spine Deformity

The incidence of spinal deformity following irradiation of the spine is reported to be 9–100% [10, 78, 79, 89, 91, 94, 110]. This wide range is a product of the variables of dose, age, amount of spine exposure, the inconsistent definition of scoliosis or kyphosis, and the length of follow-up. Mayfield [89, 90] reported a 50–80% incidence of spine deformity in children given radiation for Wilms' tumor and neuroblastoma, but the majority of these deformities were minimal requiring no treatment. Riseborough [104] reported 70%, but only 25% of the patients had curves >25°. The incidence of post irradiation kyphosis is much less than that of scoliosis [103] and has been reported to be 26%
in Wilm's tumor and 16% in neuroblastoma [90]. The kyphosis is most frequently located in the thoracolumbar region (Fig. 13.5i) [89, 103]. When both scoliosis and kyphosis occur, the major deformity is usually kyphosis (Fig. 13.5h–i) [89, 103].

The statistics have been gathered mainly from children who received radiation therapy for abdominal neoplasms such as Wilms' tumor and neuroblastoma (Table 13.6). The vertebral epiphyseal plate is more sensitive to radiation than is the Wilms' tumor. Neuroblastoma patients may undergo laminectomy, itself a precursor of spinal deformity [98], making the amount of spinal deformity caused by irradiation difficult to assess. Surgery for tumors that do not involved the spine leaves the vertebral column intact. Thus, it is possible to study the effects of irradiation alone on the adjacent bony structures. In one study [77], 16 patients who had nephrectomy for Wilms' tumor were reevaluated 13–26 years later (mean 17 years). All but one had irradiation. Some degree of scoliosis was present in all patients except the one who had not received irradiation. Scoliosis was the only symptomatic sequela for these patients.

In recent years the incidence of significant sequelae is lower and manifestations are fewer than those reported in previous decades. This reduction in skeletal complications may be attributed to appropriate field selection, the shielding of physes, and decreased total irradiation doses, the latter aided by improvements in chemotherapy.

13.5.5 Prophylaxis

Most cases of spinal deformity following irradiation can be avoided by excluding vertebrae from the field to be irradiated. This is not always possible. If the spine cannot be excluded from the field to be irradiated, inclusion of the entire width of the vertebra will diminish the wedging effect of partial epiphyseal damage [12, 83, 91, 117]. However, overlapping the spine to include the entire vertebral body may not completely prevent an asymmetrical radiation effect or the physis because of a rapid fall-off of dosage at the periphery of the field [87, 89, 103, 105, 115]. This was confirmed in a study of 31 children, all of whom received irradiation of the entire vertebrae [102]. Eighteen (58%) developed scoliosis "of varying degrees" and four (13%) developed kyphosis. In addition, every effort should be made to exclude the iliac crests, acetabulae, and femoral heads from the treatment field, since hypoplasia of these structures promotes compensatory scoliosis secondary to leg length discrepancy and pelvic tilt [105].

The difference between orthovoltage and megavoltage was well demonstrated in one study [102] which showed that of 10 patients who received orthovoltage (median 2,890 cGy), 8 (80%) had scoliosis, 5 (50%) lower rib deformity, 2 (20%) kyphosis, and 3 (30%) required orthopedic intervention, whereas of 21 patients receiving megavoltage (median 3,000 cGy) no child developed scoliosis >20°, or required orthopedic intervention. In another study [108], more severe changes were seen following orthovoltage therapy as compared with megavoltage.

13.5.6 Treatment

All children who have received therapeutic irradiation of the neck, chest, or abdomen should be observed closely for spinal deformity. The initial vertebral changes occur 6 months to 2 years after irradiation, but the deformity may not become manifest until years later. Because scoliotic changes generally take at least 5 years to manifest and kyphotic curves may continue to progress after the adolescent growth spurt, continued follow-up of survivors through and beyond puberty until the deformity has stabilized, is recommended [81, 88–90, 97–99, 103].

Mild, transient scoliotic curves of <20° may be associated with the effects of surgery, such as absence of a kidney or soft-tissue scar of the abdominal wall, rather than vertebral malformation. If vertebral changes are evident or if the scoliosis or thoracolumbar kyphosis is noted to progress above 20°, bracing should be instituted (Fig. 13.5e–f) [89, 116]. A brace will not correct kyphosis, but may serve primarily as a holding device during growth [89, 104]. Bracing is less effective for post irradiation kyphosis and for patients with soft tissue contractures contributing to the deformity [89, 103, 104]. Bracing can be expected to prevent progression of deformity in only 50%, the remaining frequently require spinal fusion [89].

Most children requiring surgery, initially received spinal irradiation in excess of 3,000 cGy (orthovoltage) [89]. If curve progression continues in spite of adequate bracing, and exceeds 40° for scoliosis [89] or 35° for kyphosis [103], spinal fusion with or without instrumentation may be undertaken irrespective of the patient's age. Delay only allows further progression and makes correction and fusion more difficult. The placement of a distraction rod without fusion, but with periodic lengthening of the rod with growth can be difficult because of the poor quality of the irradiated bone, and it would be ineffectual if there was no growth on half of several vertebral bodies. The bone substance in post irradiated patients is poor, and successful arthrodesis may not be achieved following a single operation even with adequate amounts of iliac bone grafting. Bone for grafting should be taken from the iliac wing of the non-irradiated side if possible [103]. Reexploration of the fused area within 6 months, adding more autogenous iliac bone and continuing the immobilization in a cast an additional 6 months, has been suggested [89]. Patients with severe deformity and marked scar contracture may benefit from preoperative halo-femoral distraction to stretch the contracted skin, fascia, and subcutaneous tissue [89]. Soft-tissue release prior to institution of traction may be necessary to achieve maximal benefit from the traction. Two-stage anterior and posterior fusion would be appropriate for many of these patients.

The majority of children requiring treatment for radiation induced spinal deformity have a kyphotic deformity. A single posterior fusion in these children will not be enough [89]. Patients with significant rigid kyphosis require combined two-stage anterior release and fusion and posterior fusion to obtain maximum correction of the deformity and to diminish the chance of pseudarthrosis [89, 92, 103, 104, 116].

The complication rate following spine surgery for post irradiation deformity is higher than in patients with idiopathic deformity [104]. Healing is delayed [116]. Of six Wilm's tumor patients treated by spinal fusions in one study [85], three repeat fusions were done because of pseudarthrosis, broken rods, and rod pull-out. Of 7 patients with neuroblastoma 12 repeat spinal fusions were performed due to pseudarthrosis, broken rods and infections; two developed paraplegia [85]. This experience caused the authors to subsequently recommend early and extensive combined two-stage, long anterior and posterior fusions for kyphosis over 35°, and posterior fusion with instrumentation and extensive bone grafting for scoliosis over 35°. The post operative infection rate is also higher in post irradiation patients, 23% in one study [103], due to debilitation of post irradiated tissues. Postoperative immobilization by cast and brace is longer than for a patient with a nonirradiation deformity and is frequently 1 year [103, 116].

13.5.7 Osteochondroma

Benign exostosis similar to those seen in the multiple familial form occur on vertebrae, ribs, scapula, and ileum with greater frequency in children whose physes have been irradiated, than in the normal population [12, 81, 91, 110, 111]. Much of the discussion of post irradiation osteochondromas in extremities (Sect. 13.3.7) is applicable to the trunk. Of 28 patients with Wilm's tumor and neuroblastoma who survived 3 years or more, 5 (18%) developed osteochondromas in the irradiated field [7]. The sites included the clavicle, 12th rib, and proximal humerus. Two patients had multiple exostoses. In another study [80] of 680 Wilm's patients all treated with irradiation, osteochondromas occurred ten times more frequently in irradiated fields (17 of 486 or 3.5%), than in non-irradiated fields (2 of 680 or 0.3%). In a third study [91], 5 of 34 patients (15%) irradiated for a variety of conditions developed exostoses on the ribs and ileum that did not differ from naturally developing exostoses.

13.5.8 Correction of Spine Deformity by Irradiation

Correction of scoliosis by treating with radium or other gamma rays to the convexity of the curve has been suggested [118]. There are no reports of this being done in children.

13.6 Therapeutic Irradiation; Total Body

Generally, total body irradiation (TBI) is given in a single dose of 10 Gy or in multiple (fractionated) doses for a total of 12–14 Gy [121]. Children with leukemia who undergo TBI may have reduced growth of both the spine and extremities, as a direct effect on the physes as well as on the thyroid gland and gonads [119, 122]. These children respond to treatment with growth hormone with an increase in height velocity that is adequate to restore a normal growth rate, but not to "catch up" [122]. TBI given prior to bone marrow transplant is the major contributor to growth impairment in long term survivors [120]. The most important factors are irradiation dose, fractionation, age, and dose of chemotherapy.

In one study of six survivors who received TBI before age 8 years, all six children had marked short stature (height 10th–50th percentile for age), five had osteochondromas, two had short fourth metacarpals, and one had SCFE [121]. The five patients with osteochondromas had a total of 19 osteochondromas, all on the extremities. None of these patients had a family history of MHO. Younger patients are at greater risk.

Monkeys given 750–900 cGy TBI showed 11% growth inhibition. Doses <750 cGy showed no growth inhibition [123]. The authors concluded that "in view of the close similarity between monkeys and man, irradiation of children of doses >750 cGy may carry a strong risk of subsequent growth retardation".

13.7 Nuclear Irradiation

Little is known of the sensitivity of the human physis exposed to external ionizing radiation of various dosages. In Hiroshima and Nagasaki it was possible to study large numbers of individuals of all ages who had been so exposed. The atomic bombs were detonated in 1945. Approximately 4,000 surviving children exposed in Hiroshima were examined in 1951, 1952 and 1953, and compared with a similar group of children who moved into Hiroshima after 1945 [124]. The exposed children were smaller in stature and matured later than those in the control group. Children within 1,500 m of the hypocenter were smaller and matured later than those outside this hypocenter, and those who had severe acute radiation symptoms lagged behind those who did not have these complaints.

Children exposed as a fetus in utero were also found in 1973 to have delayed physeal closure, 6–7 months later in boys and 8–9 months later in girls, compared to published results for other Japanese and American children [125]. There was no correlation between the exposure dose to the mother and the time of physeal closure in the children.

In 1954 inhabitants of the Marshall Islands were accidentally exposed to radiation from experimental detonation of a large nuclear device over Bikini Atoll [126]. An unpredicted shift in wind caused deposition of significant amounts of fallout on three nearby islands. Retardation in both statural growth and skeletal maturation occurred in exposed children compared to non-exposed children. The retardation was greatest among children 12–18 months old at time of exposure. There were no differences in the growth patterns of children born subsequently to exposed parents.

It is unknown if the small stature, or the delayed physeal closure, was due to intrinsic growth plate dysfunction, endocrine dysfunction, or nutritional deficit. Vascular capillaries were noted to have significant morphologic changes in atomic bomb subjects [127], and this could also be a cause of growth changes in these individuals.

13.8 Nuclear Imaging

Bone scintigraphy is a low-radiation procedure which depends on bone metabolism, and is therefore particularly applicable to changes occurring in the physes [130]. It is performed with a variety of radionuclides, most often Tc^{99m}. After the radionuclide is injected into the body it accumulates in areas of increased vascularity or rapid growth. Bone scans in children show increased radionuclide uptake in physeal cartilage. The procedure is most useful in children to identify areas of the skeleton where vascularity or osteogenesis is disturbed [129–131]. As expected, there is a normal slow decrease in physeal activity in subjects over 16 years of age [128]. In rabbits the accumulation ratio for the radionuclide is a more sensitive index of the effect of radiation than the rate of growth [132]. Thus, scintigraphy could be advantageous for the early detection of the influence of irradiation on the physis in humans [132].

There are no reports of the nuclear imaging itself causing physeal damage or growth disturbance.

13.9 Experimental Irradiation; Extremities

There is a plethora of irradiation based experiments concerning growth on a variety of animals (Table 13.7). Quantitative relationships between the vulnerability to damage by irradiation of specific tissues in various animal species have not been studied extensively.

Table 13.7 Animals used in experiments to determine the effect of irradiation on the growth of extremities

Rats [2, 133, 134, 139, 141–145, 147, 149, 150, 152, 157, 158, 160–165, 168, 169, 173, 174, 181–185]
Rabbits [133–135, 140, 153, 156, 159, 166, 167, 170–173, 176, 178, 187, 189]
Mice [138, 146, 151, 155, 177, 179]
Dogs [136, 137, 154, 176, 188]
Chickens [133]

There are unexplained species differences in sensitivity [12, 138], and mechanisms of bone growth vary in detail between different species [2]. Chickens are less radiosensitive than rabbits, and both are less sensitive than dogs and goats [133]. In addition, different physes in the same animal react differently to irradiation [133]. Difference in physis size may be a factor.

Comparing animals and humans, there is no evidence to suggest any *qualitative* difference from the effects of irradiation, but detailed accounts are lacking. A comparative study of the *quantity* of dose required to produce physeal change between man and animals does not yet exist. In dogs and rats, severe disturbances of growth were elicited in long bones by single roentgen treatments with dosages far lower than those delivered to the spine of humans [91]. Skin erythema and epilation doses in rabbits and other animals are approximately 2.5 times higher than those in man [133]. Also, since the growing time in animals is short, radiosensitivity of the physis decreases rapidly with the age of the animal [133], possibly in a more linear fashion than in humans. Until it is shown that similar doses produce similar tissue response independent of the species, or until a unit or scale is devised which can serve as a common denominator for local tissue effects in all animal forms, safe and effective irradiation dosage in man can only be determined empirically.

Nevertheless much has and can be learned concerning growth by experimental irradiation of immature animals. Experiments relating to growth may be grouped according to the intent of the experiment and include (1) the effect of radiation dose, fractionation, and age of the animal, (2) the histologic result of irradiation, (3) the oxygen effect, (4) the local hormonal effect, (5) the abscopal effect, (6) compensatory growth, (7) targeted radiotherapy, (8) intra-articular therapy, and (9) the use of radioprotectants. Some animal experiments address more than one of these issues, but the reports that follow are grouped by the most prominently addressed issue.

13.9.1 The Effect of Radiation Dose, Fractionation and Age

Definitive dose-response relationships and fractionation effects on growth have been demonstrated in several animal species [134–155]. The amount of growth retardation and eventual bone shortening is directly related to dose [133, 138, 139, 144, 147, 148, 150, 151, 153–155]. The greater the dose the greater the effect. Dividing the total dose into multiple smaller doses (fractionation) and increasing the time between doses reduces growth deficits [141–143, 155, 159]. There are also dose-time relationships, with greater changes at higher doses, and changes which lessen with time [136, 137]. Recovery from growth retardation is dependent primarily on dose and age [147], the smaller the dose and the younger the animal the better the recovery [146]. There is a linear relationship of the amount of radiation required to produce physeal arrest to the age of the animal treated [147, 149, 152]. Dose was judged to be a greater factor than age in one study [146].

13.9.2 The Histologic Result

The effects of irradiation on growth plate chondrocytes are not well understood [156–176]. The physes is a very radiosensitive tissue and the effects of irradiation are solely destructive, never stimulatory [157, 159]. Histologic changes are recorded in several studies, and are dependent on interrelated factors such as dose, age, and interval after irradiation [133, 138, 156–176]. Alterations in the physis are prompt [174]. There is an almost immediate drop in matrix water, followed by diminution in the caliber and number of blood vessels [164, 165]. Congestion in the vascular buds adjacent to the matrix is followed by disorganization of the chondrocytes, as early as 1 day post irradiation [162, 164]. Immature cartilage cells have the highest radiosensitivity [167]. Mitosis is almost completely inhibited during the first few hours after irradiation [138], and decreased cell proliferation is followed sequentially by bizarre cartilage cells, marked variation size and shape of cells, empty lacuane, and decreased growth [158, 160].

The histologic changes are directly related to the magnitude of dose [176]. Irradiation with a low dose (1,000 cGy or less) causes changes in cell mitosis of physeal chondrocytes in 24 h, followed by swelling of the cells in the hypertrophic zone and nuclear pyknosis in the germinative and proliferative areas at 1–3 days [175], disorganization of the columnar arrangement at 7 days, reduced thickness of the physis at 14 days, revascularization in the germinative layer at 21 days, incomplete development of the proliferative area at 28 days, and signs of regeneration in all layers at 30–90 days, depending on the dose. Recovery of the physis from irradiation injury is noted by the appearance of clones of dividing cells [169]. Restoration of growth is associated with the proliferative activity and production of extra cellular matrix by chondrocytes as they expand in volume, but not in numerical density [168]. If no physeal bar forms, the injured portions of the cartilage may be pushed aside by adjacent normal unirradiated cartilage growing into the irradiated area from the side [170, 171, 173]. More marked changes are recorded using 1,500–2,000 cGy [169]. Doses higher than 2,000 cGy cause complete interruption of physiologic activity in the zone of chondroblastic activity which is rarely reestablished. The changes include marked variation in the size and shape of cells, empty lacunae, and loss of orderly columnar orientation of cells [158]. The consistent result is premature closure [145]. A single dose of 6,000–20,000 r to the distal radial or ulnar physis of rabbits provoked foci of changes characteristic of those found in Ollier's disease [172].

Articular cartilage, in comparison with physeal cartilage, suffers very little radiation damage in humans [158]. Minor degenerative changes were found histologically in articular cartilage of irradiated dog knees and wrists [154]. The articular cartilage was less thick than controls, but the cartilage was normal grossly, and the animals showed no functional impairment. Could articular cartilage be less prone to radiation damage than physeal cartilage because it is less vascular?

13.9.3 Oxygen Effect

The "oxygen effect" is the increase in radiosensitivity caused by increased oxygen in tissues [177–180]. When hypoxia is induced in a rabbit extremity by the application of a tourniquet, growth plate changes from irradiation are minimal [178]. Conversely, the administration of oxygen, with or without pressure, makes anoxic radioresistant tumor cells more sensitive to irradiation [177]. Oxygen given in hyperbaric conditions significantly increases radiosensitivity of the physis. Mice tibiae irradiated under hyperbaric condition (three atmospheres) of pure oxygen were 3.7% shorter than controls [177]. When basic fibroblastic growth factor (bFGF) is given with hyperbaric oxygen, the radiation effects on bone growth are reduced [179].

13.9.4 Local Hormonal Effect

The study of hormonal changes within irradiated physes is in its infancy [181, 182]. A limited number of growth factors and cytokines may play a role in growth plate proliferative and hypertrophic chondrocyte recovery following irradiation [182]. The expression of both parathryoid hormone and the Indian hedgehog are decreased in irradiated rat physes [181].

13.9.5 Abscopal Effect

The abscopal effect of irradiation is that which is evident at a distance from the irradiated area within the same organism [183, 184]. In rats 400 cGy to the entire hind limb retards growth of the bones directly irradiated; 800 cGy to the entire limb retards growth to the bones directly irradiated, and abscopally also retards general skeletal and somatic growth; 800 cGy to only one knee retards the growth of those bones, but has no abscopal effect on skeletal growth elsewhere [184]. No similar abscopal effect has been noted in humans.

When the vascular systems of two rats are joined together (parabiosis), the shielded partner sustained no abscopal deleterious irradiation effects [183]. However, the bone growth deficit in the irradiated rat was reduced by shielding its parabiotic partner. This suggests that the irradiation effect on bone growth is a result, at least in part, of hormonal imbalance rather than solely the consequence of the effects of radiation.

13.9.6 Compensatory Overgrowth

The physis is a radiosensitive tissue and the effects of irradiation are solely destructive, never stimulatory [157, 159, 185, 186]. Rabbits given 2–5% of the skin erythema dose showed no stimulation of bone growth [159]. In dogs and rats, when the growth of one physis of a long bone is retarded as a result of irradiation, the physis at the other end of the bone showed acceleration in growth [154, 185, 186]. This has not been reported in humans, and did not occur in cases Figs. 13.2 and 13.3.

13.9.7 Targeted Radiotherapy

Targeted radiotherapy using 153SmEDTMP is currently under investigation for possible use in treatment of human cases of osteosarcoma [187, 188]. In immature rabbits the highest uptake was found in the metaphysis, followed by the epiphysis, and the physis [187]. The conclusion was that the physis can be irradiated from multiple areas, which could increase the expression and degree of radiation damage. The arrest of one physis of paired bones, such as the radius and ulna, allows asynchronous growth of the adjacent physis [188].

13.9.8 Intra-Articular Radiotherapy

The intra-articular injection of radioactive erbium 169 and yttrium 90 is used clinically for synovial ablation [189]. In immature rabbits these beta emitters slow down bone growth in proportion to the amount of radioactivity injected [189]. If the joint had been previously damaged by inflammatory arthritis the effect of the radiation on bone growth is reduced.

13.9.9 Radioprotectants

Certain substances, given alone or in combination, may protect the physis from radiation damage [190–206]. A sample of these investigations is listed in the bibliography. The investigations have been carried out on rats [190–198, 202–206], chickens [200, 201] and rabbits [199]. Hopefully these investigations will lead to reduction of irradiation damage to the physes of humans.

13.10 Experimental Irradiation; Head, Neck and Trunk

Although whole body irradiation to the fetal and neonatal rat and mouse result in stunted growth, irradiation limited to the head of neonatal rats produces stunting of body weight, with essentially no effect on bone growth [212]. Pathologic changes occur in brain neurons, neuralgia, blood vessels and choroid plexus, but skeletal maturation proceeds normally, thyroid and adrenal histology is normal, and gonadal maturation occurs in pace with controls. The well known endocrine mechanisms are not responsible for growth stunting [212].

Structural scoliosis can be produced in rabbits by irradiating the vertebrae asymmetrically. The resulting unequal bone growth yields wedging of the vertebral bodies with the lesser height toward the irradiated side. A single dose of 1,000 cGy is required to induce definite wedging in the spines of young rabbits [207, 208]. Radium needles or seeds placed alongside the spines of young rabbits and goats produced the same effect [208, 210]. Doses of 350 cGy or less have no effect on spine growth [208].

The beneficial effect of both fractionation and the oxygen effect, as described in Sect. 13.9 concerning extremities, also occur in the spine. In rat tail vertebrae oxygen acts as a dose-modifying agent with respect to the sparing effect of dose fractionation [209].

Attempts to correct scoliosis by irradiating vertebrae of goats was not achieved because by the time a curvature was produced, the animals were fully grown and the physis was too mature to react sufficiently to radiation [211].

13.11 Conclusions

1. Diagnostic irradiation does not cause premature physeal arrest.
2. Therapeutic irradiation confined to the diaphysis of bone has no effect on longitudinal growth, providing the physes are protected from direct irradiation.
3. The action of therapeutic irradiation of physeal cartilage is solely destructive. The result is dependent on many factors:
   (a) The greater the radiation dose, the greater the effect.
   (b) Fractionation of the total dosage, and protraction of the interval between sessions greatly lessens the effect.
   (c) The more immature the physis (the younger the age), the greater the effect.
4. The roentgenographic results of irradiation on the physis are variable and include:
   (a) No change in width.
   (b) Physeal widening with continuous growth (normal or slower than normal).
   (c) Physeal widening with temporary cessation of growth followed by resumption of growth.
   (d) Physeal widening which persists, but produces no growth.
   (e) Physeal widening with subsequent narrowing, closure, and loss of growth.
   (f) Physeal narrowing, closure, and loss of growth (partial or complete).
5. Excision of a physeal bar due to irradiation results in no growth, probably because the remaining roentgenographically normal looking physis has no growth potential.

13.12 Author's Perspective

The pathophysiology of irradiation of the physis is a bit puzzling. All histologic studies report prompt cell changes in the most immature cells. If cells in the germinal cell zone die, the normal vascular invasion from the metaphysis should cause rapid narrowing, obliteration and closure of the physis (Fig. 13.1). However, the physis rarely closes immediately after irradiation. Instead, the physis either retains its normal thickness or widens a small amount. The mild widening often persists, but no growth occurs. This indicates that both the process of cell formation and cell division on the epiphyseal side, and the vascular invasion on the metaphyseal side, come to a halt more or less simultaneously. The hypertrophic zone is not removed by the metaphyseal vessels. This suggests the role of vascular damage on the metaphyseal side is more important than previously suspected.

Physeal growth abnormalities due to irradiation are somewhat predictable and are related to a number of specific factors, many of which are within control of physicians. It is imperative that the condition to be irradiated, and the modality and dose of radiation, be chosen with care. Appropriate positioning of the part to be irradiated, and shielding of the unintended body parts, are of vital concern. My experience with excision of physeal bars and lengthening of bone previously subjected to irradiation, as documented in Fig. 13.2, caused me to delete these procedures as treatment options in subsequent patients with irradiated bones.

Children with cancer suffer the greatest long term harm from conventional radiation therapy since their organs adjacent to the tumor are still developing. Because the newly developed proton pencil beam therapy can be adjusted precisely to the size and shape of a tumor, it is especially effective for treating children with anatomically complex tumors located adjacent to critically sensitive organs, such as the physis. Proton beam therapy is the future of radiation therapy.

References

Introduction

1. Cooper RA (1975) Professional self-evaluation and continuing education program for radiation therapy. In: Radiation biology and radiation pathology syllabus. American College of Radiology, Chicago, pp 213–214
2. Dawson WB (1968) Growth impairment following radiotherapy in childhood. Clin Radiol 19:241–256
3. Desjardins AU (1930) Osteogenic tumor: growth injury of bone and muscular atrophy following therapeutic irradiation. Radiology 14:296–307
4. Eifel PJ, Donaldson SS, Thomas PRM (1995) Response of growing bone to irradiation: a proposed late effects scoring system. Int J Radiat Oncol Biol Phys 31(5):1301–1307
5. Goldwein JW (1991) Effects of radiation therapy on skeletal growth in childhood. Clin Orthop 262:101–107
6. Katz LD, Lawson JP (1990) Radiation induced growth abnormalities. Skeletal Radiol 19(1):50–53
7. Katzman H, Waugh T, Berdon W (1969) Skeletal changes following irradiation of childhood tumors. J Bone Joint Surg 51A(5):825–842
8. Littman PS, D'Angio GJ (1979) Growth considerations in the radiation of children with cancer. Ann Rev Med 30:405–415
9. Mitchell MJ, Logan PM (1998) Radiation-induced changes in bone. Radiographics 18:1125–1136
10. Perthes G (1903) Uber den Einfluss der Röentgenstrahlen auf epitheliale Gewebe, insbesondere auf das carcinom [German]. Arch Klin Chir 71:955–1000
11. Ramuz O, Bourhis J, Mornex F (1997) Late effects of radiation on mature and growing bone [French]. Cancer Radiother 1(6):801–809
12. Rutherford H, Dodd GD (1974) Complications of radiation therapy: growing bone. Semin Roentgenol 9(1):15–27
13. Teft M (1972) Radiation effect on growing bone and cartilage. Front Radiat Ther Oncol 6:289–311
14. Vaughn J (1968) The effects of skeletal irradiation. Clin Orthop 56:283–303
15. Wang JC, Chang WP, Wang JD (1999) The effects of excessive radiation exposure on the growth of children. Chinese J Public Health 18(1):3–12
16. Warren S (1943) The effects of radiation on normal tissues. Arch Path 35:304–353

Diagnostic Irradiation

17. Langenskiöld A (1953) Growth disturbance appearing 10 years after Roentgen ray injury. Acta Chir Scand 105(5):350–352
18. Thomas ST, Gelfand MJ, Kereiakes JG, Ascoli FA, Maxon HR, Saenger EL, Feller PA, Sodd VJ, Paras P (1978) Dose to the metaphyseal growth complexes in children undergoing ^{99m}Tc-EHDP bone scans. Radiology 126:193–195

Therapeutic Irradiation: Extremity

19. Ackman JD, Rouse L, Johnston CE II (1988) Radiation induced physeal injury. Orthopedics 11(2):343–349
20. Bisgard JD, Hunt HB (1936) Influence of Roentgen rays and radium on epiphyseal growth of long bones. Radiology 26:56–64
21. Blount WP (1960) Unequal leg length. In: Instructional course lectures, vol 17. CV Mosby Co, St. Louis, pp 218–245
22. DeSmet AA, Kuhns LR, Fayos JV, Holt JF (1976) Effects of radiation therapy on growing long bones. AJR Am J Roentgenol 127:935–939
23. Fletcher DT, Warner WC, Neel MD, Marchant TE (2004) Valgus and varus deformity after wide-local excision, brachytherapy and external beam irradiation in two children with lower extremity synovial cell sarcoma: case report. BMC Cancer 4:57
24. Frantz CH (1950) Extreme retardation of epiphyseal growth from roentgen irradiation. A case study. Radiology 55:720–724
25. Gonzalez DG, Breur K (1983) Clinical data from irradiated growing long bones in children. Int J Radiat Oncol Biol Phys 9(6):841–846
26. González-Herranz P, Burgos-Flores J, Ocete-Guzmán JG, López-Mondejar JA, Amaya S (1995) The management of limb-length discrepancies in children after treatment with osteosarcoma and Ewing's sarcoma. J Pediatr Orthop 15:561–565
27. Gratzek FR, Holstrom EG, Rigler LG (1945) Post-irradiation bone changes. Am J Roentgenol Radium Ther 53:62–70
28. Hildebrand H (1950) Radiation damage of bone (abstract). Year Book of Radiology. p 459
29. Irwin CJR, Thomson E, Plowman PN (1993) Case report: paediatric radiotherapy – the avoidance of late radiation to the growing hip. Br J Radiol 66:369–374
30. Lewis RJ, Marcove RC, Rosen G (1977) Ewing's sarcoma – functional effects of radiation therapy. J Bone Joint Surg 59A:325–331
31. Matsubara H, Tsuchiya H, Sakurakichi K, Yamashiro T, Watanabe K (2005) Distraction osteogenesis of a previously irradiated femur with malignant lymphoma: a case report. J Orthop Sci 10:430–435
32. Mullen LA, Berdon WE, Ruzal-Shapiro C, Levin TL, Fountain KS, Garvin JH (1995) Soft-tissue sarcomas: MR imaging findings after treatment in three pediatric patients. Radiology 195:413–417
33. Paulino AC (2004) Late effects of radiotherapy for pediatric extremity sarcomas. Int J Radiat Oncol Biol Phys 60(1):265–274
34. Peterson HA (2001) Physeal injuries and growth arrest. In: Beaty JH, Kasser JR (eds) Rockwood and Wilkins' fractures in children, 5th edn. Lippincott Williams & Wilkins, Philadelphia, Chapter 5, pp 106
35. Prindull G, Jurgens N, Jentsch F (1985) Radiotherapy of non-metastatic Ewing sarcoma. J Cancer Res Clin Oncol 110(2):127–130
36. Robertson WW Jr, Butler MS, D'Angio GJ, Rate WR (1991) Leg length discrepancy following irradiation for childhood tumors. J Pediatr Orthop 11:284–287
37. Roebuck DJ (1999) Skeletal complications in pediatric oncology patients. Radiographics 19:873–885
38. Scarborough M, Zlotecki R (1999) Late effects of radiation after the treatment of musculoskeletal tumors. Curr Opin Orthop 10(6):481–484
39. Siegling JA (1937) Lesions of the epiphyseal cartilages about the knee. Surg Clin North Am 17:373–379
40. Stevens RH (1935) Retardation of bone growth following roentgen irradiation of an extensive nevo-carcinoma of

the skin in an infant four months of age. Radiology 25: 538–544
41. van Nes CP (1967) Disturbances of skeletal growth after irradiation [Abstr]. J Bone Joint Surg 49B:798
42. Wagner J (1981) Radiation injuries of the locomotor system [German]. Archiv fur Chirurgie 355:181–185
43. Weishaar J, Koslowski K (1959) The problem of bone growth in cases of haemangiomata localized in the vicinity of the epiphysis [German]. Strahlentherapie 108(2):173–202

Slipped Epiphyses

44. Barrett IR (1985) Slipped capital femoral epiphysis following radiotherapy. J Pediatr Orthop 5(3):268–273
45. Berard J, Brunat-Mentigny M, Cocchi P, Naouri A (1985) Slipped capital femoral epiphysis after radiotherapy for pelvic tumor in infancy. Report on five new cases [French]. Chir Pediatr 26(3):163–166
46. Chapman JA, Deakin DP, Green JH (1980) Slipped upper femoral epiphysis after radiotherapy. J Bone Joint Surg 62B(3):337–339
47. Dey HM, Spencer RP (1988) Asymmetrical humeral head activity after therapeutic irradiation. Clin Nucl Med 13(9):681
48. Dickerman JD, Newberg AH, Moreland MD (1979) Slipped capital femoral epiphysis (SCFE) following pelvic irradiation for rhabdomyosarcoma. Cancer 44:480–482
49. Edeiken BS, Libshitz HI, Cohen MA (1982) Slipped proximal humeral epiphysis: a complication of radiotherapy to the shoulder in children. Skeletal Radiol 9(2):123–125
50. Frisch J (1997) Pharmacovigilance: the use of KIGS (Pharmacia and Upjohn International growth database) to monitor the safety of growth hormone treatment in children. Endocrinol Metab Suppl 4(B):83–86
51. Kelsey JL (1973) Epidemiology of slipped capital femoral epiphysis: a review of the literature. Pediatrics 51(6): 1042–1050
52. Libshitz JI, Edeiken BS (1981) Radiotherapy changes of the pediatric hip. AJR Am J Roentgenol 137(3):585–588
53. Loder RT, Hensinger RN, Alburger PD, Aronsson DD, Beaty JH, Roy DR, Stanton RP, Turker R (1998) Slipped capital femoral epiphysis associated with radiation therapy. J Pediatr Orthop 18(5):630–636
54. McAfee PC, Cady RB (1983) Endocrinologic and metabolic factors in atypical presentations of slipped capital femoral epiphysis. Clin Orthop 180:188–197
55. Nag S, Tippin D, Ruymann FB (2001) Intraoperative high-dose-rate brachytherapy for the treatment of pediatric tumors: the Ohio State University experience. Int J Radiat Oncol Biol Phys 51(3):729–735
56. Ryan BR, Walters TR (1979) Slipped capital femoral epiphysis following radiotherapy and chemotherapy. Med Pediatr Oncol 6(4):279–283
57. Sabio H, Sussman M, Levien M (1987) Postradiation slipped capital femoral epiphyses (SCFE). J Surg Oncol 36(1): 45–47
58. Silverman CL, Thomas PRM, McAlister WH, Walker S, Whiteside LA (1981) Slipped femoral capital epiphyses in irradiated children: dose, volume and age relationships. Int J Radiat Oncol Biol Phys 7:1357–1363
59. Walker SJ, Whiteside LA, McAlister WH, Silverman CL, Thomas PR (1981) Slipped capital femoral epiphysis following radiation and chemotherapy. Clin Orthop Relat Res 159:186–193
60. Wiss DA, Reid B (1981) Slipped capital femoral epiphysis following pelvic irradiation for malignant tumors in children, effect on growth plate. Orthop Rev 10(3):105–111
61. Wolf EL, Berdon WE, Cassady JR, Baker DH, Freiberger R, Paviov H (1977) Slipped femoral capital epiphysis as a sequela to childhood irradiation for malignant tumors. Radiology 125(3):781–784

Osteochondroma

62. Cole ARC, Darte JMM (1963) Osteochondromata following irradiation in children. Pediatrics 32:285–288
63. Jaffe N, Ried HL, Cohen M, McNeese MD, Sullivan MP (1983) Radiation induced osteochondroma in long-term survivors of childhood cancer. Int J Radiat Oncol Biol Phys 9:665–670
64. Libshitz HI, Cohen MA (1982) Radiation induced osteochondromas. Radiology 142(3):643–647
65. Murphy FD, Blount WP (1962) Cartilaginous exostoses following irradiation. J Bone J Surg 44A:662–668
66. Pogrund H, Yosipovitch Z (1976) Osteochondroma following irradiation. Case report and review of the literature. Isr J Med Sci 12(2):154–157

Intentional Physeal Retardation of Extremity Physes

67. Judy WS (1941) An attempt to correct asymmetry in leg lengths by roentgen irradiation. A preliminary report. Am J Roentgenol Radium Ther 46:237–240
68. Spangler D (1941) The effect of x-ray therapy for closure of epiphyses: preliminary report. Radiology 37:310–315

Therapeutic Irradiation; Head and Neck

69. Fromm M, Littman P, Raney RB, Nelson L, Handler S, Diamond G, Stanley C (1986) Late effects after treatment of twenty children with soft tissue sarcomas of the head and neck. Cancer 57:2070–2076
70. Harrop JS, Davies TJ, Capra LG, Marks V (1976) Hypothalamic-pituitary function following successful treatment of intracranial tumors. Clin Endocrinol 5:313–321
71. Romshe CA, Zipf WB, Miser A, Miser J, Sotos JF, Newton WA (1984) Evaluation of growth hormone release and human growth hormone treatment in children with cranial irradiation-associated short stature. J Pediatr 104: 177–181
72. Shalet SM, Beardwell CG, Aarons BM, Pearson D, Morris Jones PH (1978) Growth impairment in children treated for brain tumors. Arch Dis Child 53:491–494

73. Shelton DW (1977) Late effects of condylar irradiation in a child: review of the literature and report of case. J Oral Surg 35(6):478–482
74. Sonis A, Tarbell N, Valachovic R, Gelber R, Schwenn M, Sallen S (1990) Dentofacial development in long-term survivors of acute lymphoblastic leukemia. A comparison of three treatment modalities. Cancer 66:2645–2652
75. Tan BC, Kunaratnam N (1966) Hypopituitary dwarfism following radiotherapy for nasopharyngeal carcinoma. Clin Radiol 17:302–304

Therapeutic Irradiation; Trunk

76. Arkin AM, Pack GT, Ransohoff NS, Simon N (1950) Radiation-induced scoliosis; a case report. J Bone Joint Surg 32A:401–404
77. Barrera M, Roy LP, Stevens M (1989) Long-term follow-up after unilateral nephrectomy and radiotherapy for Wilms' tumor. Pediatr Nephrol 3(4):430–432
78. Butler MS, Robertson WW Jr, Rate W, D'Angio GJ, Drummond DS (1990) Skeletal sequelae of radiation therapy for malignant childhood tumors. Clin Orthop 251: 235–240
79. Donaldson WF, Wissinger HA (1967) Axial skeletal change following tumor dose radiation therapy (abstract). J Bone Joint Surg 49A:1469–1470
80. Evans AE, Norkool P, Evans I, Breslow N, D'Angio GJ (1991) Late effects of treatment for Wilms' tumor. Cancer 67:331–336
81. Heaston DK, Libshitz HI, Chan RC (1979) Skeletal effects of megavoltage irradiation in survivors of Wilms' tumor. AJR Am J Roentgenol 133:389–395
82. Hildebrand H (1949) Beitrag zur Strahlenschädigung des Knochens. Fortschr. a. d. Geb. Röntgenstrahlen 72:107–111 (Abstract in Year Book of Radiology 1950, p 459)
83. Jaffe N, McNeese M, Mayfield JK, Riseborough EJ (1980) Childhood urologic cancer therapy related sequelae and their impact on management. Cancer 45(7 Suppl): 1815–1818
84. Kao SCS, Smith WL (1997) Skeletal injuries in the pediatric patient. Radiol Clin North Am 35(3):727–746
85. King J, Stowe S (1982) Results of spinal fusion for radiation scoliosis. Spine 7(6):574–585
86. Lemerle J (1982) Complications and sequelae of the treatment of Wilms' tumor. Renal tumors: proceedings of the first international symposium on kidney tumors. Prog Clin Biol Res 100:119–121
87. Lyons AR, Grebbell FS, Nevin NC (1973) Growth impairment following irradiation in one of a pair of monozygotic twins. Clin Radiol 24:370–375
88. Mäkipernaa A, Heikkilä JT, Merikanto J, Marttinen E, Siimes MA (1993) Spinal deformity induced by radiotherapy for solid tumors in childhood. A long-term follow up study. Eur J Pediatr 152:197–200
89. Mayfield JK (1979) Postradiation spinal deformity. Orthop Clin North Am 10(4):829–844
90. Mayfield JK, Riseborough ED, Jaffe N, Nehme ME (1981) Spinal deformity in children treated for neuroblastoma. The effect of radiation and other forms of treatment. J Bone Joint Surg 63A(2):183–193
91. Neuhauser EBD, Wittenborg MH, Berman CZ, Cohen J (1952) Irradiation effects of roentgen therapy on the growing spine. Radiology 59(5):637–650
92. Otsuka NY, Hey L, Hall JE (1998) Postlaminectomy and postirradiation kyphosis in children and adolescents. Clin Orthop 354:189–194
93. Parker RG, Berry HC (1976) Late effects of therapeutic irradiation on the skeleton and bone marrow. Cancer 37:1162–1171
94. Pastore G, Antonelli R, Fine W, Li FP, Sallan SE (1982) Late effects of treatment of cancer in infancy. Med Pediatr Oncol 10:369–375
95. Perez CA, Vietti T, Ackerman LV, Eagleton MD, Powers WE (1967) Tumors of the sympathetic system in children: an appraisal of treatment and results. Radiology 88:750–760
96. Perra JH (2001) Iatrogenic spinal deformities. In: Weinstein SH (ed) The pediatric spine: principles and practice, 2nd edn. Lippincott Williams & Wilkins, Philadelphia, Chapter 26, pp 491–504
97. Peterson HA (1994) Iatrogenic spinal deformities. In: Weinstein SL (ed) The pediatric spine: principles and practice. Raven Press, New York, Chapter 29, pp 651–654
98. Peterson HA (1985) Spinal deformity secondary to tumor, irradiation, and laminectomy. In: Bradford DS, Hensinger RM (eds) The pediatric spine. Thieme Inc., New York, Chapter 19, pp 273–285
99. Peterson HA (2007) The spine. In: Peterson HA (ed) Epiphyseal growth plate fractures. Springer, Heidelberg, Chapter 28, pp 797–805
100. Probert JC, Parker BR (1975) The effects of radiation therapy on bone growth. Radiology 114:155–162
101. Probert JC, Parker BR, Kaplan HS (1973) Growth retardation in children after megavoltage irradiation of the spine. Cancer 32:634–639
102. Rate WR, Butler M, Robertson W, D'Angio GJ (1988) Later orthopedic effects in Wilms' tumor treated with abdominal radiation (abstract). Radiat Oncol Biol Phys 15(Suppl 1):206
103. Riseborough EJ (1977) Irradiated induced kyphosis. Clin Orthop 128:101–106
104. Riseborough EJ, Grabias SL, Burton RI, Jaffe N (1976) Skeletal alterations following irradiation for Wilms' tumor. J Bone Joint Surg 58A:526–536
105. Rubin P, Duthie RB, Young LW (1962) The significance of scoliosis in postirradiated Wilms's tumor and neuroblastoma. Radiology 79(4):539–559
106. Shah M, Eng K, Engler GL (1980) Radiation enteritis and radiation scoliosis: intestinal obstruction following spinal fusion. N Y State J Med 80(10):1611–1613
107. Silber JH, Littman PS, Meadows AT (1990) Stature following skeletal irradiation for childhood cancer. J Clin Oncol 8:304–312
108. Smith R, Davidson JK, Flatman GE (1982) Skeletal effects of orthovoltage and megavoltage therapy following treatment of nephroblastoma. Clin Radiol 33(6): 601–613

109. Strauss J, Connolly LP, Drubach LA, Treves ST (2003) Pelvic hypoplasia after radiation therapy. Clin Nucl Med 28(10):847–848
110. Thomas PRM, Griffith KD, Fineberg BB, Perez CA, Land VJ (1983) Late effects of treatment for Wilms' tumor. Int J Radiat Oncol Biol Phys 9(5):651–657
111. Vaeth JM, Levitt SH, Jones MD, Holtfreter C (1962) Effects of radiation therapy in survivors of Wilms' tumor. Radiology 79:560–568
112. Wallace AU, Shalat SM, Morris-Jones PH, Swindel R, Gattamanenci HR (1990) The effect of abdominal irradiation on growth in boys treated for Wilms' tumor. Med Pediatr Oncol 18:441–446
113. Ward HWC (1965) Disordered vertebral growth following irradiation. Br J Radiol 38:459–464
114. Warner Jr WC (2006) Radiation kyphosis. In: Morrissy RT, Weinstein SL (eds) Lovell and Winter's pediatric orthopaedics, 6th edn, Chapter 20, pp 819–820
115. Whitehouse WM, Lampe I (1953) Osseous damage in irradiation of renal tumors in infancy and childhood. Am J Roentgenol Radium Ther Nucl Med 70:721–729
116. Winter RB (1978) Postirradiation spinal deformity. In: Lovell WW, Winter RB (eds) Pediatric orthopedics. JB Lippincott Co., Philadelphia, pp 646–647
117. Zajchuk R, Bowen TE, Seyfer AE, Brott WH (1980) Intrathoracic ganglioneuroblastoma. J Thorac Cardiovasc Surg 80(4):605–612

Correction of Spine Deformity by Irradiation

118. Engel D (1968) Can juvenile scoliosis be corrected by circumscribed radium-irradiation of the spine? Med Hypotheses 19(2):161–168

Therapeutic Irradiation; Total Body

119. Cohen A, Duell T, Socie G, Van-Lint M, Weiss M, Tichelli A, Rovelli A, Apperley JF, Ljungman P, Kolb HJ (1999) Nutritional status and growth after bone marrow transplantation (BMT) during childhood: EBMT late-effects working party retrospective data. Bone Marrow Transplant 23(10):1043–1047
120. Cohen A, Rovelli R, Zecca S, Van-Lint MT, Parodi L, Grasso L, Uderzo C (1988) Endocrine late effects in children who underwent bone marrow transplantation: review. Bone Marrow Transplant 21(Suppl 2):64–67
121. Fletcher BD, Crom DB, Krance RA, Kun LE (1994) Radiation-induced bone abnormalities after bone marrow transplantation for childhood leukemia. Radiology 191(1):231–235
122. Papdimitriou A, Uruena M, Hamill G, Stanhope R, Leiper AD (1991) Growth hormone treatment of growth failure secondary to total body irradiation and bone marrow transplantation. Arch Dis Child 66(6):689–692
123. Sonneveld P, van Bekkum DW (1979) The effect of whole-body irradiation on skeletal growth in rhesus monkeys. Radiology 130(3):789–791

Nuclear Radiation

124. Miller RW (1956) Delayed effects occurring within the first decade after exposure of young individuals to the Hiroshima atomic bomb. Pediatrics 18:1–18
125. Russell WJ, Keehn RJ, Ihno Y, Hattori F, Kogure T, Imamura K (1973) Bone maturation in children exposed to the A-bomb in utero. Radiology 108:367–374
126. Sutow WW, Conard RA, Griffith KM (1965) Growth status of children exposed to fallout radiation on Marshall Islands. Pediatrics 36:721–731
127. Tsuya A, Wakano Y, Otake M (1971) Capillary microscopic observation on the superficial minute vessels of atomic bomb survivors, 1956–1957. Radiat Res 46:199–216

Nuclear Imaging

128. Guillet J, Guillet C, Blanquet P (1982) Radionuclide assessment of skeletal growth and maturation (160 bone scans in patients aged 0 to 21 years). Ann Pediatr 29(3):189–192
129. Mandell GA (1998) Nuclear medicine in pediatric orthopedics. Semin Nucl Med 28(1):95–115
130. Mandell GA (1999) Nuclear medicine in pediatric musculoskeletal imaging. Semin Musculoskelet Radiol 3(3):289–315
131. Murray IP (1980) Bone scanning in the child and young adult. Part I. Skeletal Radiol 5(1):1–14
132. Ohtake H, Sakai Y, Morita S, Bussaka Y, Kikuchi S, Okinaga T, Oshibuchi M, Umezaki N (1986) An experimental study of the effects of radiation on growing bone by bone scintigraphy. Kurume Med J 33:143–148

Experimental Irradiation; Extremities

133. Engel D (1938) An experimental study of the action of radium on developing bones. Br J Radiol 11(132):779–803

Effect of Radiation Dose, Fractionation and Age

134. Alheit H, Baumann M, Thames HD, Geyer P, Kumpf R, Hermann T (1998) Fractionation effect on radiation-induced growth retardation of tibia in rabbits and rats. Acta Oncol 37(2):151–158
135. Aronson AS, Gustafsson M, Selvik G (1976) Bone growth in the rabbit after irradiation. Acta Radiol Diagn 17(6):838–844
136. Barnhard HJ, Davis ME, Kamp GH (1963) Effects of roentgen radiation on growing bone. Radiology 80:306–308
137. Barnhard HJ, Geyer RW (1962) Effects of x-radiation on growing bone. A preliminary report. Radiology 78:207–214
138. Blackburn J, Wells AB (1963) Radiation damage to growing bone: the effect of x-ray doses of 100 to 1,000 r on mouse tibia and knee joint. Br J Radiol 36:505–513
139. Cohn SH, Gong JK (1953) Effect of 2,000 roentgens local x-irradiation on the growth of rat bone. Growth 17(1):7–20
140. D'Angio GJ, Jung J, Wright KA, Cohen J (1964) Disturbance in bone growth produced by 32.5 MEV. Electron irradiation of young rabbit limbs. Am J Roentgenol Radium Ther Nucl Med 91:1132–1137

141. Eifel PJ (1986) Decreased bone growth arrest with hyperfractionated irradiation in weanling rats. Int J Radiat Oncol Biol Phys 12(Suppl 1):180
142. Eifel PJ (1988) Decreased bone growth arrest in weaning rats with multiple radiation fractions per day. Int J Radiat Oncol Biol Phys 15(1):141–145
143. Eifel PJ, Sampson CM, Tucker SL (1990) Radiation fractionation sensitivity of epiphyseal cartilage in a weaning rat model. Int J Radiat Oncol Biol Phys 19(3):661–664
144. Engstrom H, Jansson JO, Engstrom C (1983) Effect of local irradiation on longitudinal bone growth in the rat. A tetracycline labeling investigation. Acta Radiol Oncol 22(2):129–133
145. Gall EA, Lingley JR, Hilcken JA (1940) Comparative experimental studies of 200 kilovolt and 1000 kilovolt roentgen rays. Am J Pathol 16:605–618
146. Gonzalez DG, van Dijk JDP (1983) Experimental studies on the response of growing bones to x-ray and neutron irradiation. Int J Radiat Oncol Biol Phys 9(5):671–677
147. Hinkel CL (1942) The effect of roentgen rays upon the growing long bones of albino rats. I. Quantitative studies of the growth limitation following irradiation. AJR Am J Roentgenol 47(3):439–457
148. Jacobsson M, Jonsson A, Albrektsson T, Turesson I (1985) Alterations in bone regenerative capacity after low level gamma irradiation. A quantitative study. Scand J Plastic Reconstr Surg 19(3):231–236
149. Kolar J, Babicky A (1961) Different susceptibility of growth cartilage in bones to radiation. Cesk Rentgenol 15(4):251–255
150. Margulies BS, Horton JA, Want Y, Damron TA, Allen MJ (2006) Effects of radiation therapy on chondrocytes in vitro. Calcif Tissue Int 78(5):302–313
151. Masuda KM, Reid O, Hunter N, Withers HR (1990) Bone growth retardation induced by single and multifractionated irradiation. Radiother Oncol 18(2):137–145
152. Phillips RD, Kimeldorf DJ (1966) Age and dose dependence of bone growth retardation induced by x-irradiation. Radiat Res 27:384–396
153. Regen EM, Wilkins WE (1936) The effect of large doses of x-rays on the growth of young bone. J Bone Joint Surg 18:61–68
154. Reidy JA, Lingley JR, Gall EA, Barr JS (1947) The effect of roentgen irradiation on epiphyseal growth. II. Experimental studies upon the dog. J Bone Joint Surg 29:853–873
155. Wells AB (1969) The effect of acute and fractionated doses of X rays on the growth of the mouse tibia. Br J Radiol 42:364–371

The Histologic Result

156. Argüelles F, Gomar Jun F, Garcia A, Esquerdo J (1977) Irradiation lesions of the growth plate in rabbits. J Bone Joint Surg 59B:55–88
157. Barr JS, Lingley JR, Gall EA (1943) The effect of roentgen irradiation on epiphyseal growth. AJR Am J Roentgenol 49:104–115
158. Baserga R, Lisco H, Cater DB (1961) The delayed effects of external gamma irradiation on the bones of rats. Am J Pathol 39:455–472
159. Brooks B, Hillstrom HT (1933) Effect of roentgen rays on bone growth and bone regeneration. An experimental study. Am J Surg 20:599–614
160. Dameron TA, Horton JA, Nagui A, Margulies B, Strauss J, Grant W, Farnum CE, Spadaro JA (2004) Decreased proliferation precedes growth factor changes after physeal irradiation. Clin Orthop 422:233–242
161. Engstrom H, Magnusson BC, Turesson I (1983) Effect of 50 kV irradiation on enzyme activities of growing rat bone. A histopathologic and enzyme histochemical investigation. Acta Radiol Oncol 22(1):65–70
162. Furstman LL (1972) Effect of radiation on bone. J Dent Res 51:596–604
163. Gunsel E (1953) Irradiation injury in growing bones [German]. Strahlentherapie 91(4):595–601
164. Hinkel CL (1943) The effect of irradiation upon the composition and vascularity of growing rat bones. AJR Am J Roentgenol 50(4):516–526
165. Hinkel CL (1943) The effect of Roentgen rays upon the growing long bones of albino rats. II. Histopathological changes involving endochondral growth centers. AJR Am J Roentgenol 49(3):321–348
166. Hiranuma H, Jikko A, Iwamoto M, Fuchihata H (1996) Effects of irradiation on terminal differentiation and cartilage matrix calcification on rabbit growth plate chondrocytes in culture. Bone 18(3):233–238
167. Hiranuma H, Jikko A, Maeda T, Matsumura S, Deguchi A, Hayami A, Iwamoto K, Kurisu K, Asada A, Fuchihata H (1996) Changes in the irradiation sensitivity of cultured growth plate chondrocytes during cytodifferentiation. Oral Radiol 12(1):19–25
168. Horton JA, Margulies BS, Strauss JA, Bariteau JT, Dameron TA, Spadaro JA, Farnum CE (2006) Restoration of growth plate function following radiotherapy is driven by increase proliferation and synthetic activity of expansion of chondrocytic clones. J Orthop Res 24(10):1945–1956
169. Kember NF (1967) Cell survival and radiation damage in growth cartilage. Br J Radiol 40:496–505
170. Langenskiöld A (1988) Growth plate regeneration. In: Uhthoff HK, Wiley JJ (eds) Behavior of the growth plate. Raven Press, New York, pp 47–50
171. Langenskiöld A, Edgren W (1950) Imitation of chondrodysplasia by localized roentgen ray injury. Acta Chir Scand 99:353–373
172. Langenskiöld A, Edgren W (1949) The growth mechanism of the epiphyseal cartilage in the light of experimental observations. Acta Orthop Scand 19(1):19–24
173. Langenskiöld A, Heikel HVA, Nevalainen T, Österman K, Videman T (1989) Regeneration of the growth plate. Acta Anat 134:113–123
174. Melanotte PL, Follis RH (1961) Early effects of x-irradiation on cartilage and bone. Am J Pathol 39(1):1–7
175. Meng QF (1987) Radiation damage of growth bone in rabbits [Chinese]. Chinese J Path 16(4):298–300
176. Rissanen P, Rokkanen P, Paatsama S (1969) The effect of Co^{60} irradiation on bone in dogs. Strahlentherapie 137(3):344–354

Oxygen Effect

177. Morita K, Ishigaki T (1971) Comparison of the effect of hyperbaric oxygen with that of mixed gas (95% O2 + 5% CO2) on the developmental retardation of the tibiae of young mice after irradiation. Strahlentherapie 142(6):695–698
178. Olerud B, Olerud S (1971) Effect of hypoxia on x-ray radiation damage to the growth zone of the radius in rabbits. Acta Soc Med Ups 76(2):1–9
179. Wang X, Ding I, Xie H, Wu T, Wersto N, Huang K, Okunieff P (1998) Hyperbaric oxygen and basic fibroblast growth factor promote growth of irradiated bone. Int J Radiat Oncol Biol Phys 40(1):189–196
180. Wright EA, Howard-Flanders P (1957) The influence of oxygen on the radiosensitivity of mammalian tissues. Acta Radiol 48:26–32

Local Hormonal Effect

181. Bakker B, Van Der Eerden BCJ, Koppenaal DW, Karperien M, Wit JM (2003) Effect of X-irradiation on growth and the expression of parathyroid hormone-related peptide and Indian hedgehog in the tibial growth plate of the rat. Horm Res 59(1):35–41
182. Wang Y, Zhang M, Middleton FA, Horton JA, Pritchard M, Spadaro JA, Farnum CE, Damron TA (2007) Connective tissue growth factor and insulin-like growth factor 2 show upregulation in early growth plate radiorecovery response following irradiation. Cells Tissues Organs 186(3):192–203

Abscopal Effect

183. Carroll HW, Phillips RD, Kimeldorf DF (1966) Effects of irradiation on bone-growth of rats during protracted parabiosis. Int J Radiat Biol Relat Stud Phys Chem Med 11(3):205–208
184. Pappas AM, Cohen J (1963) The abscopal effect of X-irradiation on bone growth in rats. J Bone Joint Surg 45A:765–772

Compensatory Overgrowth

185. Dawson A, Kember NF (1974) Compensatory growth in the rat. Cell Tissue Kinet 7:285–291
186. Hall-Craggs ECB (1968) The effect of experimental epiphysiodesis on growth in length of the rabbit's tibia. J Bone Joint Surg 50B(2):392–400

Targeted Radiotherapy

187. Essman SC, Lewis MR, Miller WH (2005) Intraorgan biodistribution and dosimetry of 153Sm-ethylenediaminetetramethylene phosphonate in juvenile rabbit tibia: Implications for targeted radiotherapy of osteosarcoma. J Nucl Med 46(12):2076–2082
188. Olson NC, Carrig CB, Brinker WO (1979) Asynchronous growth of the canine radius and ulna: effects of retardation of longitudinal growth of the radius. Am J Vet Res 40(3):351–355

Intraarticular Radiotherapy

189. Rebut-Bonneton C, Roucayrol JC, Delbarre F (1975) Effect of intra-articular injection of radioactive colloids of erbium and yttrium on the growth of rabbit legs. Ann Rheum Dis 34(6):529–533

Radioprotectants

190. Damron TA, Horton JA, Naqvi A, Loomis RM, Margulies B, Strauss J, Farnum CE, Spadaro JA (2006) Combination radioprotectors maintain proliferation better than single agents by decreasing early parathyroid hormone-related protein changes after growth plate irradiation. Radiat Res 165(3):350–358
191. Damron TA, Margulies B, Biskup D, Spadaro JA (2001) Amifostine before fractionated irradiation protects bone growth in rats better than fractionation alone. Int J Radiat Oncol Biol Phys 50:479–483
192. Damron TA, Margulies BS, Strauss JA, O'Hara K, Spadaro JA, Farnum CE (2003) Sequential histomorphometric analysis of the growth plate following irradiation with and without radioprotection. J Bone Joint Surg 85A:1302–1313
193. Damron TA, Mathur S, Horton JA, Strauss J, Bargulies B, Grant W, Farnum CE, Spadaro JA (2004) Temporal changes in PTHrP, Bcl-2, Bax, Caspase, TGF-β, and FGF-2 expression following growth plate irradiation with or without radioprotectant. J Histochem Cytochem 52(2):157–167
194. Damron TA, Spadaro JA, Horton JA, Margulies BS, Strauss JA, Farnum CE (2004) Combinations of radioprotectants spare radiation-induced damage to the physis. Clin Orthop 426:110–116
195. Damron TA, Spadaro JA, Horton JA, Margulies BS, Strauss JA, Farnum CE (2004) Novel radioprotectant drugs for sparing radiation-induced damage to the physis. Int J Radiat Biol 80:217–228
196. Damron TA, Spadaro JA, Margulies B, Damron LA (2000) Dose response of amifostine in protection of growth plate function from irradiation effects. Int J Cancer 90:73–79
197. Damron TA, Spadaro JA, Tamurian RM, Damron LA (2000) Sparing of radiation-induced damage to the physis: fractionation alone compared to amifostine pretreatment. Int J Radiat Oncol Biol Phys 47(4):1067–1071
198. Hicks DJ, O'Keefe RJ, Teot LA, Constine LS, Puzas JE, Reynolds PR, Roseier RN (1998) Molecular mechanisms in radiation injury to the growth plate: suppression of autocrine mitogenic stimuli. In: 44th annual meeting of the orthopaedic research society, New Orleans, March 1998
199. Horvath F, Horvath J (1968) Studies on decreasing radiation injuries of the ossification zones in growing rabbits by administration of Durabolin, vitamin D2 and egg shell powder. Strahlentherapie 135(1):38–47

200. Pateder DB, Elixeev RA, O'Keefe RJ, Schwarz EM, Okunieff P, Constine LS, Puzas JE, Rosier RN (2001) The role of autocrine growth factors in radiation damage to the epiphyseal growth plate. Radiat Res 155:847–857
201. Pateder DB, Sheu TJ, O'Keefe RJ, Puzas JE, Schwarz EM, Constine LS, Okunieff P, Rosier RN (2002) Role of pentoxifyline in preventing radiation damage to epiphyseal growth plate chondrocytes. Radiat Res 157(1):62–68
202. Spadaro JA, Baesl MT, Conta AC, Margulies BM, Damron TA (2003) Effects of irradiation on the appositional and longitudinal growth of the tibia and fibula of the rat with and without radioprotectant. J Pediatr Orthop 23:35–40
203. Spadaro JA, Horton JA, Margulies BS, Luther J, Strauss JA, Farnum CE, Damron TA (2005) Radioprotectant combinations spare radiation-induced damage to the physis more than fractionation alone. Int J Radiat Biol 81(10): 759–765
204. Tamurian RM, Damron TA, Spadaro JA (1999) Sparing radiation-induced damage to the physis by radioprotectant drugs: laboratory analysis in a rat model. J Orthop Res 17:286–292
205. Visser E, Krenning P, De Jong M (2003) The addition of DTPA to [^{177}LuDOTA^{0}Tyr^{3}]octreotate prior to administration reduces rat skeleton uptake of radioactivity. Eur J Nucl Med Mol Imaging 30(2):312–315
206. Yaruz MN, Yavuz AA, Ulku C, Sener M, Yaris E, Kosucu P, Karslioglu I (2003) Protective effect of melatonin against fractionated irradiation-induced epiphyseal injury in a weaning rat model. J Pineal Res 35(4):288–294

Experimental Irradiation; Head, Neck and Trunk

207. Arkin AM, Simon N (1950) Radiation scoliosis; an experimental study. J Bone Joint Surg 32A:396–401
208. Arkin A, Simon N, Siffert R (1948) Asymmetrical suppression of vertebral epiphyseal growth with ionizing radiation. Proc Soc Exp Biol Med 69:171–173
209. Dixon B (1969) The effect of radiation on the growth of vertebrae in the tails of rats. II. Split doses of x-rays and the effect of oxygen. Int J Radiat Biol 15(3):215–226
210. Engel D (1939) Experiments on the production of spinal deformities by radium. Part I. Am J Roentgenol 42(2):217–234
211. Engel D (1986) Can juvenile scoliosis be corrected by circumscribed radium-irradiation of the spine? Med Hypotheses 19(2):161–168
212. Mosier HD Jr, Jansons RA (1967) Stunted growth in rats following x-irradiation of the head. Growth 31:139–148

Light Waves

14.1 Phototherapy

Phototherapy is the treatment of disease by the influence of light, especially by various concentrations of light waves. Phototherapy (up to 40 MW/cm^2/nm) is a photodynamic stress and induces lipid peroxidation [2, 3]. A common use is in the treatment of neonatal hyperbilirubinemia. Phototherapy administered to newborns with jaundice is effective in lowering serum bilirubin levels and may reduce the need for exchange transfusion. There are numerous reports of the use of phototherapy in infants. The usual follow-up reports are relatively short and no mention of physeal damage is recorded. The treatment of hyperbilirubinemia with phototherapy has always been believed to be safe; so much so that the safety has been taken for granted [3].

However, because of findings in rats a little caution is warranted, especially in the use of intensive phototherapy [3]. Phototherapy exposing newborn rats to a bank of two white and two blue lights with wave lengths of 400–500 nm, resulted in early impairment of growth plate structure [2]. There was a dramatic reduction in the proliferative activity of the physis and marked loss of cellularity in 1 week [2]. The inhibitive effect of phototherapy on physeal cellularity appears to be temporarily related to the elevation of oxidative stress [2]. A relatively low dose of pentoxifylline was found to reduce the effect of phototherapy on the physes of neonatal rats [1].

14.2 Ultraviolet

Ultraviolet light emitted by the sun is beneficial for some hard-to-treat skin problems and certain medical conditions. The main forms of ultraviolet light that reach us from the sun are called ultraviolet A (UVA) and ultraviolet B (UVB). UVA is the predominant type of ultraviolet light that comes from tanning beds. It penetrates the skin more deeply and sets the stage for skin cancer development. UVB rays are those responsible for sunburn. UV light and has been found useful in conditions such as psoriasis, vitiligo, eczema, pruritis, cutaneous T cell lymphoma, and graft-versus-host disease, which is a complication associated with blood and bone marrow transplants. Ultraviolet light therapy is usually initiated in a medical clinic. Therapy sessions commonly last from a few seconds to an hour and may take place for 2–7 days a week for dozens of sessions. No problems relative to the physis have been noted.

In one group of immature mice exposed to UV light to study its effect on immunization, the columns of cartilage in the physis were shorter than the control group [4].

14.3 Laser

LASER is an acronym for "light amplification by stimulated emission of radiation". Laser beams are strong beams of light produced by electrically stimulating a particular material (solid, liquid, or gas). Lasers are generally named for the active medium that produces the light, for example carbon dioxide and argon.

The combination of the intensity of the light and the ability to focus it on a small area gives lasers their useful role in medicine. Lasers can be used to cut or destroy tissue that is abnormal or diseased, shrink or destroy tumors or lesions, burn off or vaporize tissue, sculpt tissue, and seal bleeding blood vessels. The depth of penetration is determined by the wavelength of the light, and is controlled by adjusting the light's intensity.

Laser therapy has been used clinically for some 35 years, most often in dermatology to treat birthmarks, portwine stains, spider-veins, warts, and to destroy abnormal blood vessels. It is also used often in ophthalmology, cardiology, gastroenterology, ENT, urology, and dentistry. In orthopedics laser has been used to relieve nerve tissue impinged by herniated disks, to trim tissues in the knee, and to tighten ligaments around the shoulder. The discussion which follows is limited to the effect of lasers on the physis, about which little is known.

14.3.1 Human Involvement

A single case report documents premature partial arrest of two distal phalangeal physes as a sequela of laser beam injury [7]. This resulted in progressive angular deformity and relative shortening of the digits, requiring multiple osteotomies for correction.

A 5 year 5 month old girl underwent aggressive laser ablation of warts on the adjacent sides of the dominant left ring and long fingers at the level of the distal interphalangeal (DIP) joints. Unfortunately the type of laser and intensity used is unknown. The parents reported that bone was visible at the base of the vaporized site. The soft tissue wounds took 3 months to heal by secondary intent. There was no gross infection. Finger motion gradually returned, aided by physical therapy. Progressive angulatory deformity of the digits developed.

When first seen at our institution 6 months after the laser exposure, at age 6 years 0 months, there was full extension and flexion of 40° in the DIP joint of the long finger, and 25° in the DIP joint of the ring finger. There was no crepitus on motion. There was active control of both flexion and extension. Roentgenographs revealed partial destruction of the distal end of the middle phalanx with an open physis at the base of the distal phalanx of each finger (Fig. 14.1a). Corrective closing wedge osteotomies were performed on the distal ends of the middle phalanges from the side of each finger opposite the site of laser therapy (i.e., the radial side of the long finger and the ulnar side of the ring finger) (Fig. 14.1b).

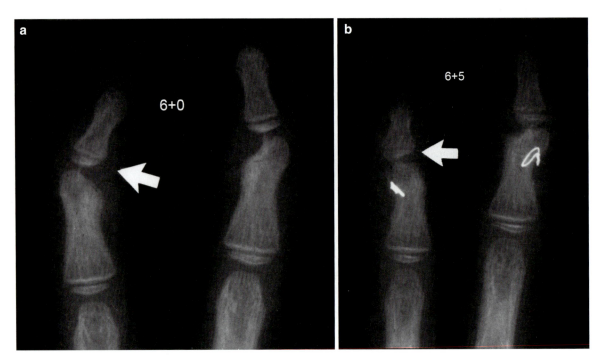

Fig. 14.1 Premature physeal closure following laser therapy. (**a**) Patient at age 6 years, 0 months. There is absence of the distal articular condyle of the middle phalanx on the ulnar side of the long finger and on the radial side of the ring finger. The distal phalanx of the middle finger and its physis and epiphysis appear normal. The distal phalanx of the ring finger shows indistinct physis and diminished development of the epiphysis on the radial side (*arrow*). (**b**) Age 6 years, 5 months. Two months after closing wedge osteotomies of the distal end of both middle phalanges. The fingers are relatively straight. The radial side of the distal phalanx of the ring finger shows peripheral bar formation of the physis and an incompletely formed epiphysis (*arrow*). (**c**) Age 10 years, 9 months. The middle phalanges have retained normal longitudinal alignment and growth. The distal phalanx of the long finger shows ulnar deviation with premature partial closure of the physis on the ulnar side (*arrow*). The distal phalanx of the ring finger shows radial angulation, relative shortening, and premature complete closure of its physis (compare with D). (**d**) Age 10 years 9 months. Normal right long and ring fingers for comparison. (**e**) Clinical photograph of both hands at age 11 years, 4 months shows angular deformities and relative shortening of the distal phalanges of the left ring and long fingers (From Peterson and Wood [7], with permission)

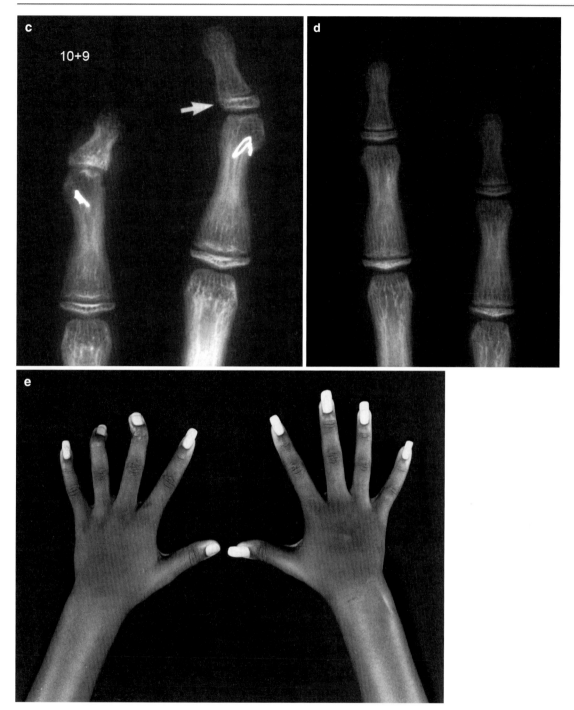

Fig. 14.1 (continued)

At the time of surgery, the articular surfaces of the respective DIP joints were not visualized, nor was there known exposure or injury to the respective distal phalangeal physes. There was no sign of infection. The osteotomy sites healed uneventfully, but gradual and progressive recurrence of deformities of the fingers followed.

At age 10 years 9 months, there was 30° ulnar deviation of the long finger DIP joint and 35° of the ring finger. There was no crepitus on motion. Roentgenographs showed complete physeal closure of the distal phalanx on the ring finger with relative shortening of the phalanx (Fig. 14.1c, d). On the long finger, the physis was partially closed along the ulnar side but open on the radial side. The phalanx was only minimally short.

At age 11 years 4 months, functional problems included interference with ability to use the hand for fine activities such as keyboarding (Fig. 14.1e). It was elected to allow the patient to finish growing, with repeat corrective osteotomies planned at the completion of growth.

14.3.2 Animal Research

Orthopedic animal research using laser beams has been directed primarily toward bone promotion and bone repair. The results of limited research on the physis are mixed. Morein, et al. [6] in 1978 reported that laser-induced defects in the growth cartilage of the distal femur of rabbits led to premature physeal arrest and disappearance of the physis. The "Sharplan 791" CO_2 laser apparatus was used with an output of 7–10 W. The authors commented that "when a low power laser beam is applied directly to epiphyseal cartilage it damages the cartilage selectively without affecting the adjacent bone". On the other hand, Cheetham, et al. [5] in 1992 reported that a low level light of wavelength 820 mm and energy density 5 J cm^{-2} had no significant effect on healthy growth plates of the rat knee. These disparate findings might be explained by the different animals and techniques used.

14.4 Author's Perspective

From the evidence collected so far it appears that light waves have little effect on the physis. If the correct wave length is used, risk to the physis is minimal. Since only one case of physeal damage due to laser has been reported in a human, and since its use in this case produced an open wound requiring a long time to heal, we can assume the laser dose was excessive. It is also possible that the physeal closures in this case were the result of reduced blood flow caused by bone and soft tissue scarring, rather than by direct physeal injury from the laser. Nevertheless, this case and the research by Morein, et al. [6] suggest that care must be exercised when using lasers near physes in growing children.

References

Phototherapy

1. Atabek ME, Pirgon O, Esen HH (2007) Protective effect of pentoxifyline on growth plate in neonatal rats following long-term phototherapy. Pediatr Res 62(2):163–166
2. Atabek ME, Pirgon O, Kurtoglu S, Tavli L, Esen HH, Koylu O, Erkul I (2006) Effects of phototherapy on the growth plate in newborn rats. J Pediatr Orthop 26(1):144–147
3. Gathwala G, Sharma S (2000) Oxidative stress, phototherapy and the neonate. Indian J Pediatr 67(11):805–808

Ultraviolet

4. Qiu SC (1985) Ultraviolet radiation (UR) of living room sunlight [Chinese]. Zhonghua Yu Fang Yi Xue Za Zhi 19(6):329–332

Laser

5. Cheetham MJ, Young SR, Dyson M (1992) Histological effects of 820 mm laser irradiation on the healthy growth plate of the rat. Laser Therapy 4(2):59–63
6. Morein G, Gassner S, Kaplan I (1978) Bone growth alternation resulting from application of CO_2 laser beam to the epiphyseal growth plates. An experimental study in rabbits. Acta Orthop Scand 49:244
7. Peterson HA, Wood MB (2001) Physeal arrest due to laser beam damage in a growing child. J Pediatr Orthop 21(3):335–337

Sound Waves

Sound is the effect produced on the organ of hearing and its central connections by the vibrations of air or other media. Sound is mechanical radiant energy, the motion of particles of the material medium through which it travels (gas, liquid, or solid) being longitudinal along the line of transmission. This energy, of frequency between 8 and 20,000 cycles per second (hertz), provides the subjective sensation of hearing in humans.

Ultrasonic waves are those in the acoustic spectrum which are beyond the range of the human ear. Ultrasound (US) is mechanical radiant energy with a frequency greater than 20,000 Hz. Ultrasonography, also called ultrasound or sonography, combines high-frequency sound waves with computer processing and uses no radiation. No other agent heats bone so effectively.

Diagnostic ultrasonography, as well as echocardiography or echoencephalography, utilizes a range of 1 million to 10 million hertz, or 1–10 MHz. Such sound waves are transmissible only in liquids and solids. Diagnostic US visualizes deep structures of the body by recording the reflections (echoes) of pulses of ultrasonic waves directed into the tissues. It is especially good for providing information about the size, shape, texture and make-up of tumors and cysts. High resolution US scanning probes facilitate studies of cartilaginous joint structures and growth plate in young children, which cannot be seen directly on plain roentgenographs [3]. Its use for bone and joint injuries avoids the shortcomings of ionizing radiation, contralateral joints can be examined for comparison, dynamic functional studies can be obtained easily, and the examination can be done in the presence of the parents [3–5]. It can replace roentgenographs in some situations [5]. No physeal damage has been recorded in humans by the use of diagnostic ultrasound.

Therapeutic ultrasonography typically uses a wavelength of 1.5 MHz. It is often used by physical therapists to decrease joint stiffness, reduce muscle spasm and pain, to improve muscle mobility, to improve outcomes of fracture healing. No physeal damage has been reported from the use of therapeutic ultrasound [2].

Experimentally, an early (1953) study on dogs and rabbits found that US had a destructive effect on the physis [1]. The percentages of animals that had widening of the physis, slipping (displacement) of the epiphysis, and premature closure of the physis varied with the dose. Widening of the physis with subsequent premature closure was associated with lower doses of US, while slipping was associated with higher doses. Although the US was applied to the upper tibial physis, similar less marked changes were found in the distal femoral physis. Perhaps more troubling was the conclusion that there was great variability in the reaction to US, causing the degree of destruction of the physis caused by any dose to be unpredictable.

In more recent studies, therapeutic levels of US on rabbits have produced no difference in the mean growth rate of US exposed physes compared with controls, and no evidence of premature partial or complete physeal closure [2, 6]. The researchers concluded that the use of pulsed therapeutic US at the intensities used was not harmful to physes [2]. However, higher doses of US had a marked toxic and profound pathologic effect in growing bone [2]. Histological results showed disordered arrays of the cartilaginous cells in the proliferative zone with the physes flattened and indistinct [2].

Although diagnostic and therapeutic US have not produced impairment of physeal growth in humans, some researchers caution "its use around the joints of children with open physes remains controversial" [2].

References

1. DeForest RE, Herrick JF, Janes JM, Krusen FH (1953) Effects of ultrasound on growing bone: an experimental study. Arch Phys Med Rehabil 34:21–31
2. Lyon R, Liu XC, Meier J (2003) The effects of therapeutic vs. high-intensity ultrasound on the rabbit growth plate. J Orthop Res 21:865–871
3. Mayr J, Gretchenig W, Peicha G, Tesch NP (2002) Sonographic anatomy of pediatric joints. Orthopade 31(2):135–142
4. Ogurtan Z, Celik I, Izci C, Boydak M, Alkan F, Yilmaz K (2002) Effect of experimental therapeutic ultrasound on the distal antebrachial growth plates in one-month-old rabbits. Vet J 164:280–287
5. Rathfelder FJ, Paar O (1995) Ultrasound as an alternative diagnostic measure for fractures during the growth phase. Unfallchirurg 98(12):645–649
6. Vaughen JL, Bender LF (1959) Effects of ultrasound on growing bone. Arch Phys Med Rehabil 40:158–160

Shock Waves

A shock wave is a single-pressure impulse which is created by a high voltage spark discharged under water causing an explosive evaporation of water. These waves enter the human body because the body has acoustic characteristics similar to water. Shock waves can be focused and concentrated on small areas by the construction of various semi-ellipsoids [4]. Protocols in clinical use differ with respect to the number of shock wave pulses, pulse frequency and the applied shock wave energy [2]. These variables make comparison of data difficult.

Extracorporeal shock wave lithotripsy (ESWL) is commonly used in pediatric urology to break kidney stones into tiny pieces that can be more easily passed naturally. In orthopedics, ESWL has been used to treat calcifying tendonitis, epicondylitis, plantar heel spurs, delayed unions, non-unions, bone tumors, bone infection, and infected pseudarthrosis [2, 5]. In the treatment of fracture delayed union and non-union, the extra corporeal high energy shock waves break up the sclerotic bone ends, producing microfissures which enhance blood supply. The production of numerous small detached, or partly attached, fragments of bone exerts a stimulating effect on osteogenesis which leads to union of the fracture.

Side effect usually occurs in alveolar tissue, where high energy shock waves cause hemorrhage through disruptions at the border to neighboring water-soluble tissues. The lower levels of ESWL applied to non bone sites are not associated with severe side effects [2]. In general, when applied to bone the energy levels are higher and more prone to produce side effects.

Four animal studies with reference to the physis are worth noting. One found that shock wave treatment in rats caused focal growth plate dysplasia in eight out of 18 (44%) treated bones [8]. There was no effect on growth unless a large dysplastic lesion was produced, which occurred in three out of 18 (17%) rats. Physes with small lesions functioned normally, whereas physes with large lesions ultimately fused early. The reason for the varied lesion severity was not determined. It was noted, however, that the shock wave energy levels used were higher than those used for ESWL in children in clinical practice and that there is little soft tissue surrounding the rat tibia, which is also relatively small [8]. A second study concluded that extracorporeal shock waves do not adversely affect rabbit bone growth, making treatment of pediatric patients with ESWL appear safe in regard to the parameters used. [7] A third report also found no damage to rabbit epiphyses when applying conditions comparable to those used in human shock wave therapy [1]. A fourth study noted both increases in bone mineral content and overgrowth in length and width of immature male rabbits femora subjected to extracorporeal shock waves [3].

Numerous reports of the use of ESWL in children in the urology literature make no mention of growth arrest. Most of these reports do not follow the patients long enough or do not evaluate the physis to determine a physeal problem. Two studies concerning longitudinal growth in children following ESWL are worth noting. In one, 12 children treated for ureteral calculi were followed 74–238 weeks (average 149 weeks) [6]. The author's concluded "there was no evidence of retardation of linear growth (body height) in these patients following ESWL." A study of 276 patients who received 542 lithotripsy's for orthopedic diseases included 190 patients treated for calcifying tendonitis, epicondylitis, and plantar head spurs [5]. The authors concluded that in these patients lithotripsy had only minor complications when the shock wave was used properly. However, using higher energy lithotripsy in children for bone tumors, bone infection, or infected pseudarthrosis in the area of a physis is "an absolute contraindication" [5].

16.1 Author's Perspective

More clinical research focused on the physis and with longer follow-up is needed to determine which parameters of ESWL are safe or not safe to use in children in areas containing a physis. More animal research regarding the mechanism of growth arrest using high levels of ESWL would also be of interest.

References

1. Nassenstein K, Nassenstein I, Schleberger R (2005) Effects of high-energy shock waves on the structure of the immature epiphysis – a histomorphological study [German]. Z Orthop Ihre Grenzgeb 143(6):652–655
2. Refior HJ (2002) Extracorporeal shock waves in orthopedics: benefits and risks. Orthopedics Today 22(3):4
3. Saisu T, Takahashi K, Kamegaya M, Mitsuhashi S, Wada Y, Moriya H (2004) Effects of extracorporeal shock waves on immature rabbit femurs. J Pediatr Orthop B 13(3):176–183
4. Schleberger R, Senge T (1992) Non-invasive treatment of long-bone pseudarthrosis by shock waves (ESWL^R). Arch Orthop Trauma Surg 111:224–227
5. Sistermann R, Katthagen BD (1998) Complications, side-effects and contraindications in the use of medium an high-energy extracorporeal shock waves in orthopedics [German]. Z Orthop Ihre Grenzgeb 136(2):175–181
6. Thomas R, Frentz JM, Harmon E, Frentz GD (1992) Effect of extracorporeal shock wave lithotripsy on renal function and body height in pediatric patients. J Urol 148:1064–1066
7. Van Arsdalen K, Kurzweil S, Smith J, Levin RM (1991) Effect of lithotripsy on immature rabbit bone and kidney development. J Urol 146:213–216
8. Yeaman LD, Jerome CP, McCullough DL (1989) Effects of shock waves on the structure and growth of the immature rat epiphysis. J Urol 141:670–674

Atmospheric Pressure

17.1 Decreased Atmospheric Pressure

There are numerous recent reports on bone metabolism in animals subjected to weightlessness or hypogravity. A few of these reports concern bone growth. Rat tibial growth plate activity was significantly reduced after 7 days of space flight [4]. Twelve hours post landing there was a rebound response to preserve/restore growth. In similar studies, the diminished growth of the proximal tibial and humeral physes at the end of a 2 weeks suspension period [6], was fully recovered after 2 weeks of subsequent activity [5]. These studies demonstrate that the physes of growing rats are capable of rapid recovery from the effects of weightlessness of moderate duration. Immature rats suspended by their tail for 304 weeks had growth suppression only in weight bearing bones [1], and greater inhibition in male than female [2]. Immature rats suspended in space had decreased longitudinal growth irrespective of being fed space food or standard pellet food [7]. However, when central nervous system stimulators (ephedrine and strychnine) were used, suspension-induced inhibition of physeal growth was prevented [3].

17.2 Increased Atmospheric Pressure

Children with open growth plates are exposed to increased atmospheric pressure when diving underwater as well as during treatment in a hyperbaric chamber for conditions such as osteomyelitis, gas gangrene, CO_2 poisoning, and for improving viability of skin grafts. No physeal impairment has been recorded.

Immature rats exposed to raised atmospheric pressures in hyperbaric chambers for different periods of time showed no differences in growth compared with control animals [9]. No roentgenographs or histologic differences were observed. The authors speculated that this would also be true for the human growth plate [9]. However, hypergravity provided by centrifuging immature rats has caused reduced enchondral bone formation and a decrease in the width of tibial and humeral physes [8].

17.3 Author's Perspective

No case of human physeal abnormality has been recorded with either decreased or increased atmospheric pressure. Short exposure times could be a factor. However, the animal reports noted here might have implications concerning space travel for children.

References

Decreased Atmospheric Pressure

1. Cao XS, Yang LJ, Wu XY, Wu H, Zhang LN, Zhang LF (2003) Changes of bone morphogenesis proteins and transforming growth factor-beta in hind-limb bones of 21 day trial-suspended rats [Chinese]. Space Med Med Eng (Beijing) 16(4):269–271
2. Durnova GN, Kaplanskii AS (2003) Comparative histomorphometric studies of shin bones of male and female rats following tail suspension [Russian]. Aviakosm Ekolog Med 37(4):29–32
3. Durnova GN, Kaplanskii AS (1998) Effect of ephedrine and support loads on development of osteopenia and growth shin bones in suspended rats [Russian]. Aviakosm Ekolog Med 32(2):27–31
4. Montufar-Solis D, Duke PJ, Morey-Holton E (2001) The Spacelab 3 simulation: basis for a model of growth plate response in microgravity in the rat. J Gravit Physiol 8(2):67–76

5. Wronski TJ, Morey ER (1983) Recovery of the rat skeleton from the adverse effects of simulated weightlessness. Metab Bone Dis Relat Res 4(6):347–352
6. Wronski TJ, Morey ER (1982) Skeletal abnormalities in rats induced by simulated weightlessness. Metab Bone Dis Relat Res 4(1):69–75
7. Zerath E, Holy X, Andre C, Renault S (2002) Effects of space food bar feeding on bone mass and metabolism in normal and unloaded rats. Nutr Res 22(11):1309–1318

Increased Atmospheric Pressure

8. Vico LO, Barou O, Laroche N, Alexandre C, Lafage-Proust MH (1999) Effects of centrifuging at 2g on rat long bone metaphyses. Eur J Appl Physiol Occup Physiol 80(4):360–366
9. Walker P, Bates EH, Chung W, Walsh WR, Leicester A (1997) Effect of hyperbaric pressure on growth plates of rats. J Bone Joint Surg 79B(Suppl IV):400

Oxygen

The amount of available oxygen plays a major role in determining cellular behavior and has been called the "oxygen factor" [4]. The physis is extremely sensitive to the prevailing oxygen tension [1, 4, 5]. The most sensitive index to increased oxygen tensions is an initial, transitory increase in length of the zones of hypertrophy and calcification [1, 5]. In higher oxygen tensions the physis narrows, associated with a progressive loss of acid mucopolysaccharide stainability, eventual loss of the zone of hypertrophic cells, and an accumulation of neutral mucopolysaccharide or glycomucoprotein at its base [1]. In one study a 2% increase of the rate of growth of the rabbit tibia was noted during pure oxygen breathing for three 2 h sessions in a single 24 h period, with an interval of 1–2 h between the 2 h sessions [3]. The increase in rate of growth during the actual 6 h of treatment implies that rate of growth exceeded 2% assuming that growth proceeded at a normal rate during the intervals between the intermittent exposures. However, this was followed by a 7% deceleration of growth the day after the oxygen treatment.

Neonates with severe, reversible respiratory failure are sometimes treated with extracorporeal membrane oxygenation (ECMO). Hypoxia is corrected by reinfusing well-oxygenated blood into the systemic circulation. Known complications from ECMO include intracranial bleeding and thrombosis. ECMO activates the platelets and the clotting mechanism requiring systemic anticoagulation to prevent these complications. Physeal growth disturbance in a few neonates has been suspected of being another complication of ECMO [2]. The exact mechanism of growth arrest was undetermined and no mention was made of there being too little oxygen initially, too much oxygen with the treatment, or a bleeding or coagulation problem.

In the treatment of bone and soft tissue tumors by radiation therapy a change in radiosensitivity of the physis due to an increase or decrease of oxygen is known as the "oxygen effect" (Sect. 13.9.3). Radiosensitivity of the physis is increased by administration of hyperbaric oxygen, and decreased by ischemia.

References

1. Brighton CT, Ray RD, Soble LW, Kuettner KE (1969) In vitro epiphyseal-plate growth in various oxygen tensions. J Bone Joint Surg 51A(7):1383–1396
2. DiFazio RL, Kocher MS, Berven S, Kasser J (2003) Coxa vara with proximal femoral growth arrest in patients who had neonatal extracorporeal membrane oxygenation. J Pediatr Orthop 23(1):20–26
3. Persson BM (1967) Effect of hyperbaric oxygenation on longitudinal growth of bones. Acta Orthop Scand 38:23–34
4. Persson BM (1968) Growth in length of bones in change of oxygen and carbon dioxide tensions. Acta Orthop Scand Suppl 117:1–99
5. Shaw JL, Bassett CAL (1967) The effects of varying oxygen concentrations on osteogenesis and embryonic cartilage in vitro. J Bone Joint Surg 49A(1):73–80

Developmental

19

19.1 Introduction

Developmental physeal injuries are ones not present at birth, develop gradually, have no proven underlying cause, involve random physeal sites, and are sometimes associated with nearby otherwise unrelated conditions. The developmental physeal injuries recorded here occur frequently enough to have a sizable amount of references. Diseases which effect growth at all physeal sites in the body and might be thought of as being developmental, such as osteogenic imperfecta, achondroplasia, Morquio's disease, etc. [2] are not physeal "injuries" in the context discussed in this text.

Traditionally the most commonly mentioned developmental physeal injuries that effect only one physeal site are the conditions of Blount, Madelung, Osgood-Schlatter, Sever, and Scheuermann, developmental humerus varus, ankle valgus associated with distal fibular deficiency, and wrist ulnar deviation associated with distal ulnar deficiency. By the criteria stated above many other conditions, such as disuse, scoliosis, kyphosis, slipped capital femoral epiphysis (SCFE), physeal widening and separation associated with meningomyelocele, developmental dislocation of the hip (DDH), and Perthes disease, could also be called "developmental." There are probably more, less frequent and less commonly reported developmental injuries, for example those which are reported as "Unknown" in Chap. 21.

Blount disease is discussed in Sect. 19.2 of this chapter. Madelung's deformity is now generally accepted to be secondary to tethering of the distal radial physis by an abnormal radial-lunate ligament, and is therefore discussed in Sect. 10.2. Osgood-Schlatter and Sever lesions are apophyseal injuries not discussed in this text. Scheuermann's thoracic kyphosis is frequently called an osteochondrosis. The deformities of kyphosis and scoliosis are generally thought to be due to asymmetric pressure on the physes of vertebral bodies and are discussed in Sect. 10.2. Developmental humerus varus is an extreme varus angulation of the proximal humeral epiphysis with relative shortening of the humerus due to early premature closure of the medial portion of the physis. It is most often the residual of neonatal septic arthritis and therefore is discussed and illustrated in Sect. 3.9, Shoulder. It may also be found as a consequence of birth separation of the epiphysis, hematologic disorders such as thalassemia (Sect. 1.4, Thalassemia), bone infection, metabolic and neuromuscular disorders such as cerebral palsy and Erb's palsy (Chaps. 3, 5 and 6), and pathologic fracture through some benign tumors (Sect. 4.2) [1]. In many cases so much time has elapsed between the initial insult and the discovery of the deformity that it is just called "developmental humerus varus." [1] Ankle valgus associated with fibular deficiency is discussed in Sect. 19.3, and wrist ulnar deviation associated with ulnar deficiency in Sect. 19.4, of this chapter. Disuse is discussed in Chap. 2. Slipped capital femoral epiphysis is discussed in this text in multiple places according to suspected etiology and treatment (see Index). Physeal abnormality associated with spinal cord developmental injury (meningomyelocele) is discussed in Sect. 6.3 and with developmental dislocation of the hip (DDH) and Perthes disease in Sect. 1.3.

19.2 Knee

Blount disease is an idiopathic developmental condition characterized by disordered enchondral ossification of the medial proximal tibial physis. The disease is not

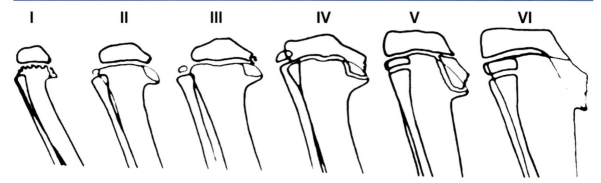

Fig. 19.1 Diagram of roentgenographic changes seen in the infantile type of tibia vara and their development with increasing age (From Langenskiöld and Riska [6] with permission)

present at birth. Clinically it appears gradually as a localized varus deformity of the proximal tibia associated with internal rotation of the tibia. There are two forms of the disease, infantile and adolescent, which are different in several respects, but have tibia vara in common.

The pathogenesis is theoretical and involves both mechanical and biologic factors. Genetic predisposition, environmental factors, and mechanics of the knee during childhood are frequently mentioned [5]. Exactly how much each factor contributes to either the infantile or adolescent deformity is unknown. No tether on the medial side of the tibia (as found in the distal radius in Madelung's deformity, Sect. 10.2) has been identified. Blount disease could also be recorded in this text in Chap. 21, Unknown, and possibly in Chap. 10, Compression. If left untreated a physeal bar will eventually develop in the medial portion of the physis (Fig. 19.1). The literature on Blount disease is voluminous. For the purpose of categorizing Blount disease as developmental condition, the essence of the disease and its treatment can be found in five articles [3–7].

19.3 Ankle

Developmental growth problems of the ankle are primarily associated with length deficiency of the fibula. An intact normally growing fibula during early childhood is essential to the normal growth and development of the ankle. In the absence of a normally growing fibula, the physis of the secondary center of ossification (Fig. 1.2) of the distal tibial epiphysis grows more slowly on the lateral side than the medial side causing the epiphysis to become wedge-shaped, resulting in ankle valgus (Fig. 19.2). The valgus angulation is greatest when the entire lateral malleolus is absent,

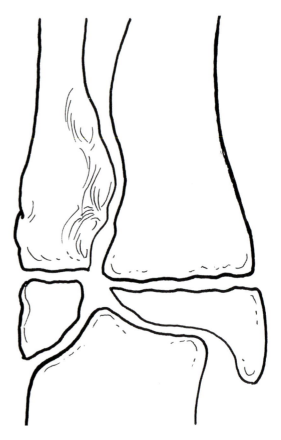

Fig. 19.2 Osteochondroma of the distal fibula characteristically results in some degree of relative fibular shortening and tibiofibular diastasis, both contributing to developmental tapering of the lateral tibial epiphysis and ankle valgus. The width and angle of the distal tibial physis changes little, if at all (From Snearly and Peterson [41] with permission)

less when the fibular deficiency is metaphyseal, and least when the deficiency is diaphyseal or proximal.

Fibular deficiency occurs with a variety of clinical conditions, most consistently with congenital pseudarthrosis of the fibula, acquired pseudarthrosis of the fibula (following resection of a fibular segment for infection, tumor, or for use as a bone graft), multiple hereditary osteochondromatosis of the distal fibula, neurologic conditions, and traumatic loss of the distal fibula. Developmental ankle valgus also occurs with tibial overgrowth (creating a relative fibular deficiency), for example after removing cortical bone grafts from the tibia.

In normal growing children the distal tibia and fibula have an ongoing changing relationship [8, 46]. In the first 4 years of life the distal fibular physis is 2–3 mm proximal to the plane of the tibiotalar joint; at 4–8 years of age, at the same level; and in children > 8 years of age, 2–3 mm distal to the ankle joint. A relative shortening of < 10 mm from normal can be considered mild shortening, but any shortening > 10 mm is clinically significant [46]. The tibiotalar joint is in slight valgus up to about age 10. After age 10 the plane of the joint remains horizontal in spite of the rather complicated growth patterns of the tibia and fibula [33].

The pathophysiologic mechanism producing of the ankle valgus is subjective. The speculated causes of gradual valgus deformity are increased weight bearing laterally and the tethering effect of contracted soft tissue lateral to the distal tibia, each of which might cause diminished growth of the lateral part of the distal tibial epiphysis due to uneven axial overloading [22, 29]. Normally the lateral malleolus provides ankle stability and aids in bearing weight, estimated from 6% to 16% by different authors [23, 24]. Resection of the proximal fibula results in a significant reduction of load through the distal fibular remnant [23]. In cadaver specimens, longitudinal weight pressures on the tibial articular surfaces became more compressive after partial fibulectomy [31]. Relative shortening of the fibula or absence of the lateral malleolus may allow the talus to tilt or sublux laterally enough to allow weight to be shifted disproportionately to the lateral portion of the tibial epiphysis [26, 51]. This theory is supported by the development of hypertrophy of the lateral cortex of the tibial diaphysis which occurs in some cases [24, 26]. If this is indeed the mechanism that inhibits development of the lateral tibial epiphysis, or if there is a tether, the injury could also be reported as a compression injury (Sect. 10.2). However, the same ankle valgus deformity occurs in patients who are not weight bearing (for example those with meningomyelocele), and a similar phenomenon occurs with the distal radius with deficiency of the distal ulna (Sect. 19.4), neither of which can be attributed to weight bearing or compression. In addition, if it is due to weight bearing the "compression" would be intermittent rather than continuous. Since neither a tether nor compression has been proven, the ankle valgus in these is condition is considered to be "developmental."

The point to be emphasized is that the ankle valgus deformity is due to wedging of the lateral aspect of the distal tibial *epiphysis* (Fig. 19.2). This means that lack of development of the physis of the secondary center of ossification of the epiphysis (Fig. 1.2) is the major cause of deformity, rather than slow growth or arrest of the lateral side of the primary physis. Only one article has recorded premature closure of the lateral side of the primary physis of the distal tibia [29]. It is also worth emphasizing that prophylactic surgery carried out *before* development of significant epiphyseal wedge deformity is the best way to prevent subsequent osteoarthritis of the ankle joint [29].

Diminished growth of the tibia from any cause accompanied by normal growth (relative overgrowth) of the fibula results in ankle valgus (Fig. 4.20g). This developmental ankle varus is less common than ankle valgus due to undergrowth of the fibula, and does not appear to be associated with asymmetric growth of the distal tibial epiphysis.

19.3.1 Congenital Pseudarthrosis of the Fibula

Isolated congenital pseudarthrosis of the fibula (ICPF) is an uncommon entity. Some 40 cases have been reported in the literature [14]. Approximately 50% of these are associated with neurofibromatosis, though the pathogenic relationship between these two conditions is unknown [14]. Anterolateral bow of the otherwise normal tibia and varus of the ankle is frequently present in infancy [10, 11, 13, 16, 17, 19]. In many patients fibular pseudarthrosis is first noted later when the child begins to walk and sustains a fracture [12, 13, 18–20], or following corrective tibial osteotomy in infancy (Fig. 19.3) [16]. In either case the initial ankle varus noted in infancy gradually reverses into a valgus deformity as the fibular pseudarthrosis becomes established and weight bearing has begun. The level of pseudarthrosis (the more distal, the more likely the development of deformity) and the type of pseudarthrosis (amount of gap, and shape and quality of fibular ends) influence the development of the valgus deformity [14].

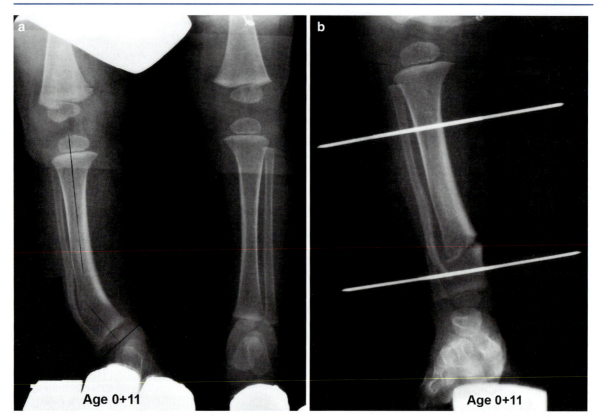

Fig. 19.3 Developmental ankle valgus secondary to isolated congenital pseudarthrosis of the fibula (*ICPF*). This boy was born with bilateral internal tibial bowing. The left lower leg corrected spontaneously, but the right did not. There was no anterior tibial dimple and no café au lait skin markings. (**a**) At age 11 months the right 35° medial angulation had not improved. The right fibula was thin at the site of maximal angulation. The epiphyses and physes of both knees and ankles appeared normal and the physes were perpendicular to the longitudinal alignment of the metaphyses. Clinically the tibial bowing and ankle varus were interfering with attempts to walk. A single café au lait spot had appeared. (**b**) Steinmann pins were placed transversely in the proximal and distal metaphyses at an angle of 35° to each other. Osteotomies were performed across each bone through separate incisions at the site of maximal deformity. The pins were made parallel, creating an open wedge osteotomy, and incorporated into a long leg cast with the foot in neutral position. (**c**) At age 1 year 8 months, 9 months postoperative, the tibia was well healed. The fibula had developed pseudarthrosis at the site of osteotomy and the distal fibular fragment had migrated proximally. The distal tibial epiphysis had developed a triangular tapered shape, as compared with preoperatively and with the normal left tibial epiphysis. (**d**) Photographs taken 11 months post operative, age 1 year 10 months, showed significant right ankle valgus, sufficient to impair function and cause abnormal shoe wear. One year postoperatively, age 1 year 11 months, surgery at the site of the fibular nonunion revealed a large mass of fibrous tissue having the gross appearance of a typical congenital pseudarthrosis. The fibrous tissue was more massive than expected from scar tissue following osteotomy on a normal bone. The abnormal tissue was removed. Histologic analysis revealed noninflammatory fibrous tissue with synovium, consistent with pseudarthrosis. Iliac corticocancellous grafts were placed across the fibular defect. A long leg cast with the foot in slight varus was worn for 3 months. (**e**) At age 6 years 4 months the patient was running and playing normally with a plantagrade foot. The ankle had normal motion. AP, lateral, and oblique roentgenograms showed a thin united fibula without an intramedullary cavity distally, but with improved length compared with the tibia. The distal tibial physis is normally oriented, but the distal tibial epiphysis remains mildly tapered. *Note*: This case is typical of ICPF in that at birth the leg had varus deformity, followed by ankle valgus after the fibular pseudarthrosis became manifest. The case demonstrates developmental ankle valgus due to tapering of the distal tibial epiphysis as a consequence of the proximal position of the distal fibula relative to the tibia. The distal tibial physis remained normally aligned at all times (Reproduced from Markel and Peterson [16] with permission)

19.3 Ankle

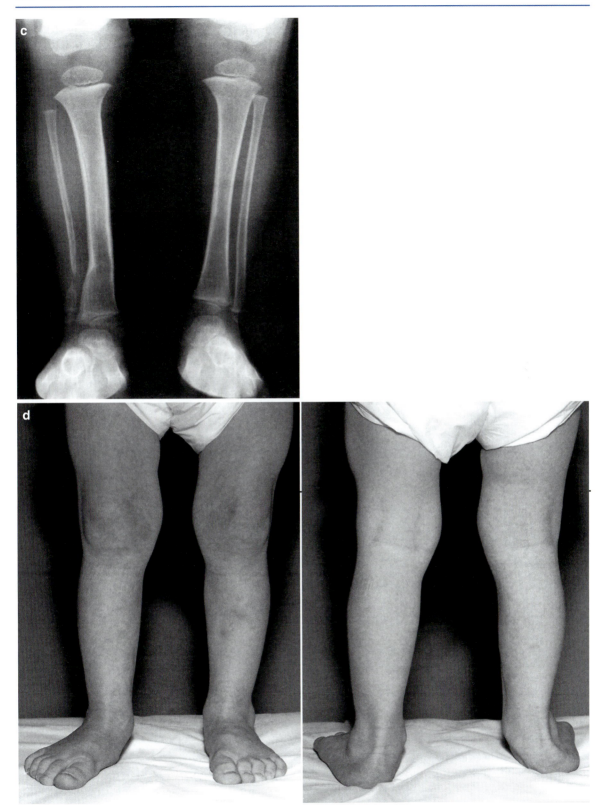

Fig. 19.3 (continued)

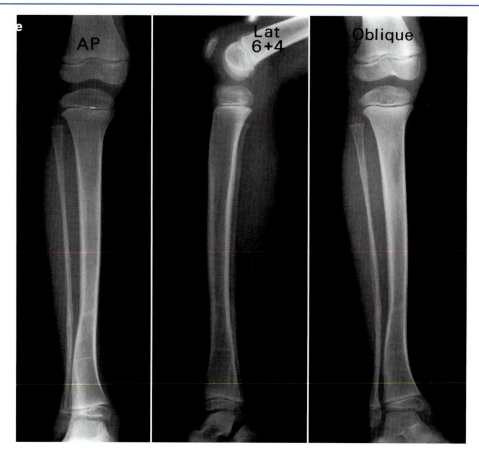

Fig. 19.3 (continued)

Treatment of ICPF is dependent on several factors. The patient's age, amount of ankle deformity, and degree of functional disability are all important. Bracing beginning at an early age and continuing until skeletal maturity has been used, but corrective tibial osteotomy was required at maturity [12, 17]. When progressive ankle valgus occurs more aggressive measures are required [12].

When ankle alignment is neutral and the fibular pseudarthrosis gap is small with large and long fibular fragments, the pseudarthrosis can be excised, filled with bone grafts, and the bone ends internally fixed [10, 14]. Even though fibular osteosynthesis using autogenous bone grafts alone has been successful [16, 19], it has failed when used with plate fixation [11] or an intramedullary nail [13, 14].

In most cases, however, the ankle will be in valgus and distal tibial osteotomy is necessary. Corrective tibial osteotomy combined with excision of the fibular pseudarthrosis and insertion of iliac corticocancellous bone grafts, without internal fixation has been successful (Fig. 19.3). [16] Fibular union and correction of deformity was achieved in an 11 year old boy using a long freeze-dried interposition allograft, iliac crest bone grafts, and two plates and screws to fill the fibular defect, accompanied by staples over the medial tibial physis to correct the valgus deformity [12]. Another case treated by diaphyseal bone transport using an Ilizarov frame followed by internal splinting with a metal plate and cancellous bone grafting was also successful in achieving union and improving the distal tibial-fibular relationship [18].

When fibular osteosynthesis is not feasible or has been unsuccessful, distal tibio-fibular surgical synostosis is an effective alternative to prevent progression of, or to reverse, the ankle valgus in growing children [11, 13–15, 19]. Once skeletal maturity is reached closing wedge osteotomy of any remaining distal tibia valgus is appropriate [17].

In summary, resection of the pseudarthrotic tissue in conjunction with fibular osteosynthesis or distal tibial-fibular fusion provide the least chance of developmental ankle valgus and the best results [13, 14].

Congenital pseudarthrosis involving both the tibia and the fibula is much more common than ICPF. Surgical attainment of union in the tibia, but not the fibula, may also result in developmental ankle valgus [9].

19.3.2 Acquired Pseudarthrosis of the Fibula

Loss of integrity of the diaphysis of the fibula from any cause will result in proximal migration of the lateral malleolus relative to the tibia, and subsequent ankle valgus [25, 26]. The most common cause of acquired fibular pseudarthrosis is iatrogenic surgical removal of a portion of the fibula for bone graft [21, 22, 24–27, 31–33], for tumor [30, 32, 34], or for osteomyelitis [29, 32]. In one study 24 cases had resection of fibular diaphyseal segments of 2 cm or more for grafting purposes [24]. Nonunion resulted in 58% (14 of 24 cases), proximal migration of the lateral malleolus in 55%, distal tibial articular valgus tilt in 45%, and diaphyseal valgus bowing of the tibia with hypertrophy of the lateral cortex in 20%. The same deformities may occur after fracture nonunion of the fibula [29, 32], or with absence of the distal fibula from trauma [29]. Clinically the deformity occurs gradually and can become significant prior to detection by the patient or parents. Functional impairment and pain may be minor or absent.

The mechanism of developing ankle deformity due to fibular nonunion is the same as that discussed in the beginning of this section. The level of resection and age of the patient are important factors. Twenty of 28 low fibular resections developed pseudarthrosis, whereas only 1 of 9 mid fibular resections developed pseudarthrosis [26]. All of these pseudarthroses resulted in proximal migration of the lateral malleolus together with valgus tilting of the talus. In one study the fibula failed to regenerate fully in all patients older than 10 years [26]. Between the ages of 6 and 9 years, the fibula failed to regenerate in less than half the patients. However, ankle valgus becomes pronounced only when the pseudarthrosis is present from an early age [33]. If the patient is over the age of 10 or 12 years at the time of acquired distal fibular deficiency, ankle stability and function may not be altered and valgus deformity is unlikely [30, 32–34].

Whenever a portion of the fibular diaphysis is surgically removed an effort should be made at that time to maintain the normal length of the fibula. The periosteum should be preserved whenever possible [24]. However, the periosteum of the fibular diaphysis is not a strong structure, and maintaining it for bone regeneration is not always possible. Other methods to prevent proximal migration of the distal fibula include fibular reconstruction with a tibial autograft, or insertion of a distal tibiofibular syndesmotic wire or screw [22].

Once fibular nonunion is established, treatment by autogenous bone grafting has been successful in achieving growth of the distal fibula in excess of the distal tibia, as well as regeneration of the wedged tibial epiphysis [25]. The amount of regeneration of the tapered tibial epiphysis is directly proportional to the amount of growth remaining [25]. Thus the earlier the pseudarthrosis is treated, the more complete the regeneration will be. Surgical reconstructive osteosynthesis of fibular nonunion has been achieved using sliding fibular grafts [21], by fibular transport using an Ilizarov device [18], and by tibial autograft [22].

If fibular osteosynthesis is not successful, distal tibiofibular synostosis is an effective alternative to prevent ankle valgus in older children [10, 11, 14, 15, 22, 24, 29, 32, 33]. However, in younger children (3 years or less) tibio-fibular synostosis only lessens the final tibio-fibular length discrepancy because of the differences in the tibia and fibula growth rates [27]. If residual distal tibial valgus is significant (greater than 10°), and the patient is ambulatory, physeal arrest of the medial tibial physis or closing wedge varus supramalleolar tibial osteotomy becomes necessary [11, 22, 28, 49].

19.3.3 Multiple Hereditary Osteochondromatosis

The effects of bones with MHO on adjacent bones are discussed here. The effects of osteochondromas directly on the physis are discussed and referenced in Sect. 4.2 Tumor, Osteochondroma.

Multiple hereditary osteochondromatosis (MHO) is a disorder of enchondral bone growth manifest by abnormal metaphyseal bone prominences capped with cartilage and accompanied by defective metaphyseal remodeling and asymmetric retardation of bone growth. The cause of bone growth retardation is unknown, but the exostosis appears to have direct influence on growth of the physis. The disordered exuberant growth of cartilage cells in the osteochondroma in the metaphysis seems to detract from the normal longitudinal growth of cartilage cells in the physis. One of the most common sites of involvement is the distal fibula. The lack of growth of the distal fibula is invariably accompanied by developmental ankle valgus [37, 39–41]. Obliquity of the distal tibial epiphyseal surface was markedly abnormal in 54% of

24 patients in one series [40]. The ankle deformity is due to lack of growth of the lateral side of the tibial epiphysis, and not of the lateral portion of the physis (Fig. 19.2). The distal tibial physis remains perpendicular to the long axis of the tibia [40–42]. Severe tibio-talar obliquity is accompanied by lateral subluxation of the talus in some patients [40].

Early excision of fibular osteochondromas prior to the onset of deformity is the only way to prevent the deformity. This is rarely done because there are usually dozens of lesions in the body, and in the absence of deformity or functional impairment parents are reluctant to submit the child to surgery (Fig. 4.12). Once tibio-talar valgus is established, excision of the fibular osteochondromas alone will not alter the tibio-fibular length discrepancy or tibio-talar inclination [41]. Correction can be achieved by excision of the fibular osteochondroma along with tibial medial hemiphyseal surface arrest [35, 36], Phemister arrest (Sect. 20.2), or retardation by staples or eight plates (Sect. 10.2), combined with fibular

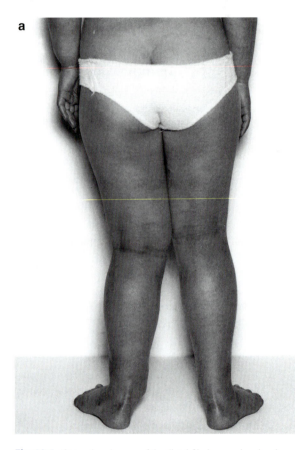
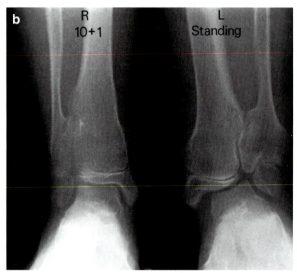

Fig. 19.4 Osteochondromas of the distal fibulae causing developmental ankle valgus. This 10 year 1 month old girl was brought for evaluation of left "knock-knee" deformity. (**a**)There is moderate left genu valgum and significant left ankle valgus. A scanogram showed the left tibia was 1.9 cm shorter than the right (note the level of the popliteal creases). (**b**) There were osteochondromas on both distal fibulae. The largest, on the left was associated with relative fibular shortening, distal tibia-fibula diastasis, lateral tapering deformity of the distal tibial epiphysis, and 30° valgus tilt of the talus. The left tibial physis was basically transverse, curving slightly upward laterally. (**c**) At age 10 years 4 months osteochondromas were removed from the left distal medial fibula, staples were placed over the medial tibial physes proximally and distally, and the fibula was lengthened 12 mm by step-cut osteotomy. Resuture of the anterior tibiofibular ligament did not reduce the diastasis intraoperatively. (**d**) At age 12 years 4 months the left ankle valgus and tibia-fibula diastasis were significantly improved. However, the tapering deformity of the epiphysis is unchanged, possibly aided by residual fibular shortening. The staples were removed at age 12 years 6 months.(**e**) At age 16 years 2 months the left ankle was clinically normal, the right ankle in mild valgus. The left popliteal crease is now higher than the right (compare with **a**), due more to limb realignment (aided by the staples placed over the proximal medial tibial physis) than to mild (3 mm) improvement of tibial length discrepancy. Symptomatic osteochondromas were removed from the right ankle at age 16 years 10 months. (**f**) At age 17 years 8 months her only complaint was mild discomfort at the distal tip of the right fibula with activities. No surgery had been done in this area. The symptoms were judged to be due to fibula-talus impingement, but were not sufficient to warrant treatment. Both ankles functioned normally and the gait was normal. Standing roentgenographs showed 10° residual ankle valgus on the left, which could become symptomatic in the future (Reprinted from Peterson [39] with permission and additional follow-up)

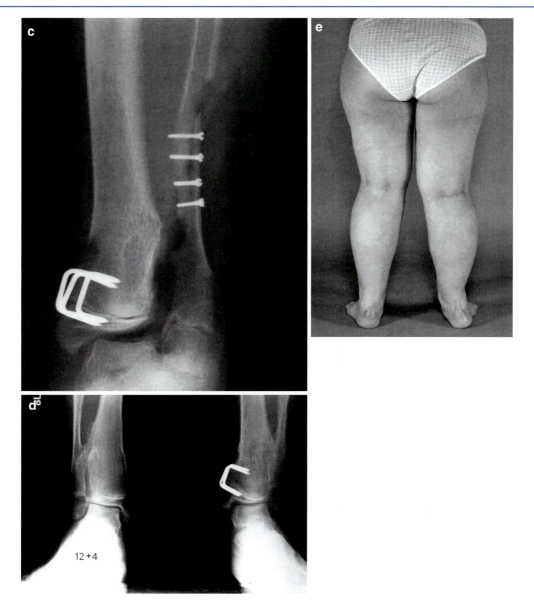

Fig. 19.4 (continued)

Fig. 19.4 (continued)

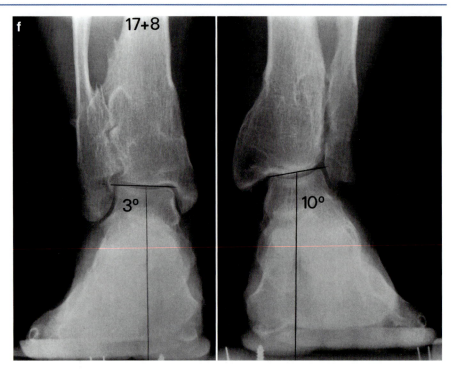

lengthening if necessary (Fig. 19.4) [39, 41]. To help prevent secondary ankle arthritis prophylactic and corrective treatment ideally should be carried out before the development of ankle valgus [38].

Residual ankle valgus persisting into adulthood significantly predisposes the ankle to arthritic changes and diminished ankle motion (Fig. 4.12). A study of 38 subjects with MHO followed for an average of 42 years found an average of 9° ankle valgus [38]. Fourteen ankles (18%) had demonstrable degenerative joint changes. Of the 38 patients, 12 (32%) were limited in recreational sports, seven (18%) had pain in at least one ankle on a weekly basis, and three (8%) indicated their ankle involvement affected their vocation.

19.3.4 Neurologic Conditions

Paralytic conditions of the lower extremities often result in relative undergrowth of the fibula compared with the tibia. The conditions most frequently reported are meningomyelocele [43–46, 48, 49], poliomyelitis [46, 47, 50], and cerebral palsy [46]. The two most important factors affecting normal fibular growth are anatomic continuity of the fibula and muscle strength [44, 46]. Any degree of muscular paralysis, especially affecting the soleus, will slow fibular growth leading to relative shortening [45, 46]. Decreased soleus strength is found in meningomyelocele, poliomyelitis, and cerebral palsy [46]. In poliomyelitis the degree of relative fibular shortening is most evident in flail lower limbs. Children with early age of onset of paralysis have delay in the appearance of the distal fibular epiphyseal secondary center of ossification which contributes to the fibular shortening [47].

As in the previous sections the relative fibula shortening is accompanied with lateral tapering of the epiphysis [45, 50] (rather than diminished growth of the lateral portion of the physis). The resulting wedge shaped epiphysis is responsible for the valgus of the tibio-talar joint [48]. The distal tibial physis typically remains perpendicular to the longitudinal axis of the tibia (as in Fig. 19.2) [48].

Once ankle valgus is present, bracing will not correct the valgus deformity [44]. Braces are frequently worn for the muscle deficit [44], but no author has reported correction of ankle deformity by the use of braces. Operations performed below the ankle, such as extra-articular subtalar arthrodesis (the Grice procedure), triple arthrodesis, osteotomy of the calcaneus (Dwyer procedure), and talectomy have all been ineffective. [44, 48] Soft tissue tenodesis of the Achilles tendon to the fibula has corrected the paralytic pes calcaneus of polio patients, as well as the associated ankle valgus associated with a relatively short fibula and tapered distal fibular epiphysis [50]. However, most authors prefer osseous correction above the ankle by medial tibial physeal arrest if the patient is young and the physis is open, or by supramalleolar osteotomy if the patient is over age 8 years or if the physis is closed [43, 44, 48, 49]. Supramalleolar osteotomy is effective in correcting the ankle valgus, but has more complications than hemiphyseal arrest at an earlier age. [44] In one series the best results were obtained when the tibiotalar angle was corrected to 5° varus [43].

19.3.5 Scleroderma

Scleroderma confined to the lateral aspect of the lower leg can be accompanied by muscle and soft tissue atrophy, tight tendons, and progressive relative shortening of the fibula. These combined may cause ankle valgus associated with lateral tapering of the distal tibial physis (Fig. 19.5). Speculated causes could be soft tissue tethering of the lateral side of the leg and/or decreased blood supply to support normal fibular growth.

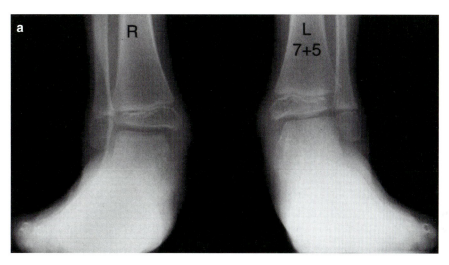

Fig. 19.5 Developmental right distal fibular relative shortening and tapering of the lateral portion of the distal tibial epiphysis associated with scleroderma. This boy had linear scleroderma on the lateral side of the right lower extremity, present at birth. At age six and a half years the parents noted a mild limp and mild right heel valgus. At age 7 years 5 months he had a normal gait and could walk on his heels and toes without difficulty. The left lower leg circumference was less than the right, and the peroneal tendons were tight. Mild right heel valgus was correctible passively with the foot in equinus. (**a**) A standing roentgenogram showed mild bilateral foot eversion. The distal end of the right fibula was relatively short compared with the left. (**b**) At age 14 years 1 month the right foot was pronated (*left view*) and ankle valgus was marked (*right view*). There is atrophy of the left calf and the patellae and popliteal creases are at different levels. A scanogram showed the right femur 11 mm longer, the right tibia 10 mm shorter than the left, for a 1 mm leg length difference. (**c**) At age 15 years 3 months the relative shortening of the right fibula and lateral tapering of the tibial epiphysis had progressed. The distal tibial physis remained perpendicular to the diaphysis. (**d**) A right tibial closing wedge varus osteotomy was combined with osteotomy of the fibula, triple arthrodesis of the foot, and Z lengthenings of the peroneus longus and brevis tendons. (**e**) At age 15 years 8 months the feet were plantigrade (*left*) and the heels in normal mild valgus (*right*). (**f**) A standing roentgenogram showed satisfactory ankle joint alignment and diminished height of the right foot compared with the left. *Note*: Would surgical lengthening of the fibula at an early age have made a difference?

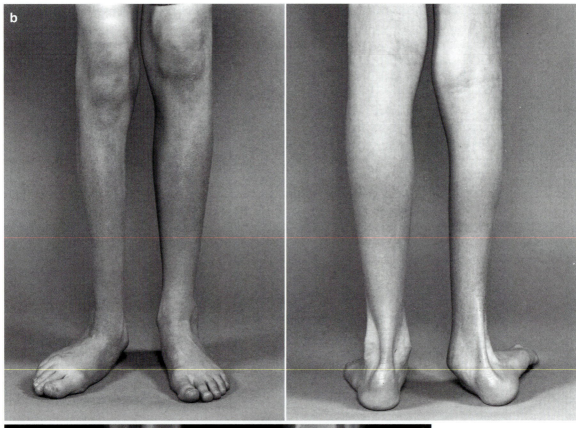
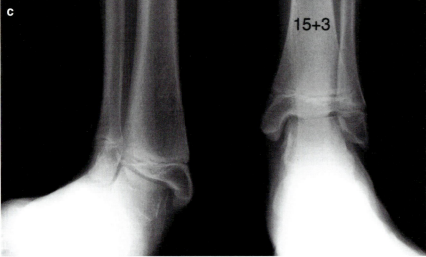

Fig. 19.5 (continued)

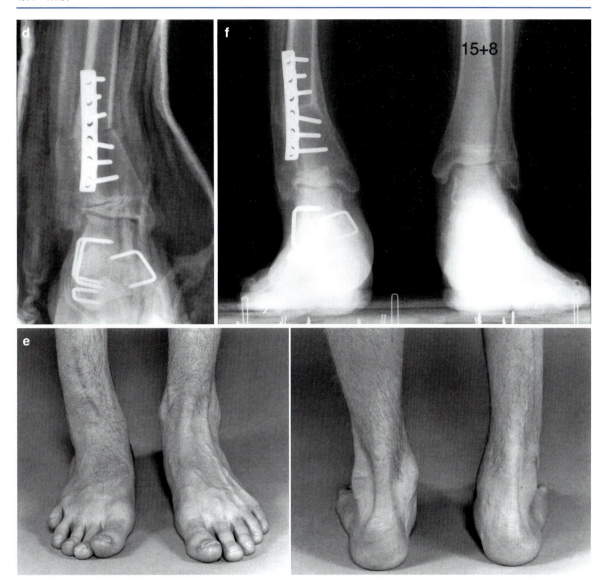

Fig. 19.5 (continued)

19.3.6 Tibial Relative Overgrowth Compared to the Fibula

Removal of bone from the tibia for grafting purposes may stimulate overgrowth of the tibia relative to the fibula. If the fibula is already short relative to the tibia, for example in paralytic limbs, the stimulatory effect of removing bone from the tibia may exaggerate the ankle valgus sufficiently to require treatment, such as staple arrest of the medial tibial physis [51].

19.4 Wrist

Developmental ulnar angulation of the distal radius associated with ulnar deficiency is similar to ankle valgus associated with fibular deficiency (Sect. 19.3) in four ways: (a) deficiency of distal ulnar length, (b) distal radial articular angle increase, primarily due to asymmetric narrowing of the epiphysis, rather than increased inclination of the physis, (c) ulnarward translocation of the carpus, (d) and bowing of the radial diaphysis [53, 55]. It differs from fibular deficiency in two ways: (a) weight bearing is not a potential etiologic factor, and (b) if the ulnar deficiency is significant, the proximal radial head can subluxate or dislocate (Fig. 4.5) [42, 52]. If untreated the natural history of these deformities is progression [52].

Animal studies have confirmed the process. Premature closure of the ulnar physis in puppies produced distal radial medial bowing, valgus deviation of the fore paw, carpal subluxation, and osteoarthritis [56]. An excellent histologic study in rabbits showed that removal of the distal ulna physis caused gradual combined increased chondrogenesis and decreased osteogenesis on the radial side of the radial physis (the physis widened) and decreased chondrogenesis and increased osteogenesis (the physis narrowed) on the ulnar side [58]. As the angular deformity increased cracks appeared in the physis concomitant with tilting of the epiphysis.

The ulnar minus deficiency in humans is most often a product of traumatic premature closure of the distal ulnar physis (Fig. 19.6) [53–55, 57, 62], or tumors of the ulna such as MHO [52, 59, 63]. Ulnar deficiency also occurs in a variety of conditions, such as congenital defects and pseudarthrosis of the ulna [20]. A distal ulnar physeal fracture is often overlooked or minimally treated because of more obvious injury to the distal radius. In 51 patients with forearm exostoses 30% had relative shortening of the ulna, 19% had increased radial articular angulation, and 14% had radial head subluxation or dislocation (Fig. 4.7). [52] Since the ulna is an uncommon donor site for bone graft, iatrogenic deficiency from segmental removal of portions of the ulna is rare.

The ulnar deformity occurs gradually with either previous fracture or osteochondroma and can become significant prior to detection by the parent or patient.

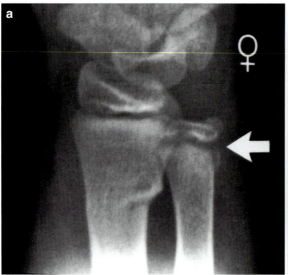
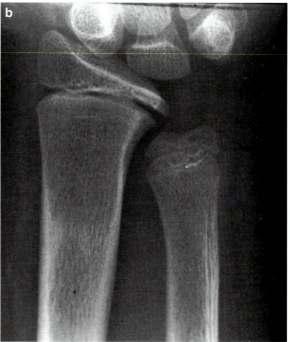

Fig. 19.6 Developmental deformity of the radius associated with ulnar deficiency, treated with ulnar lengthening. This 7 year 11 month old girl fell on her outstretched left hand. (**a**) An oblique roentgenogram of the wrist shows a buckle fracture of the distal radial metaphysis and a Peterson type 5 fracture of the distal ulnar physis (*arrow*). A short arm cast was worn 6 weeks. (**b**) One year post injury the distal ulna is short relative to the radius and its physis was indistinct. A distal ulnar physeal bar was excised at age 9 years 10 months. (**c**) Seventeen months post bar excision, age 11 years 7 months, scanograms showed recurrent bar formation, no increase in length between the metal markers inserted in the ulna at time of bar excision, increasing ulnar minus deformity, mild bowing of the radius, and mild increased angulation of the distal radial articular angle. (**d**) Step cut ulnar lengthening was begun at age 11 years 9 months and achieved 28 mm of length in 28 days. The length was secured with two screws and the fixator removed. The screws were later removed. (**e**) At age 17 years 8 months the patient was normally active, asymptomatic, and had full range of wrist and forearm motion. There is a 1 mm negative ulnar variance. The ulnar lengthening was successful, but did not improve the radial bowing and the distal radial articular angle increased. Hemiepiphysiodesis on the radial side of the distal radial physis may have improved these findings (see Fig. 19.7) (Reproduced from Peterson [60] with permission)

Fig. 19.6 (continued)

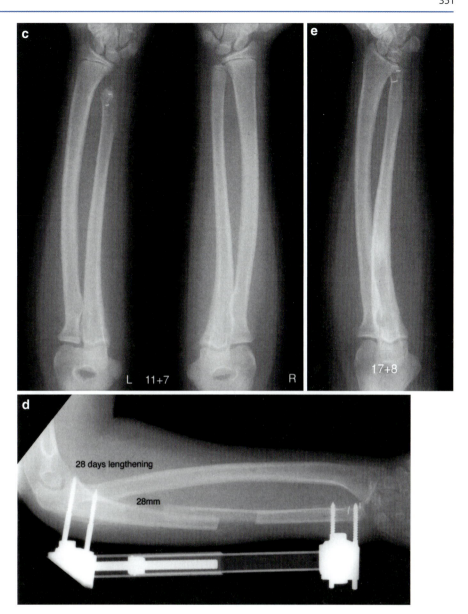

Cosmetic appearance is the most common complaint [53]. Functional impairment and pain are rarely present. No patient has developed Kienbock's disease despite up to 30 mm relative shortening of the ulna [53].

Treatment is variable. Corrective surgery is often refused by the patient and parents because the cosmetic deformity is initially mild, asymptomatic, and without functional impairment (Fig. 4.4) [53]. Surgical intervention is indicated for progressive cosmetic deformity, pain, restricted wrist motion, ulnar subluxation of the carpus, and beginning radial head subluxation [53–55]. Ulnar lengthening alone may correct the ulnar variance, but will not correct the increased radial articular angle or bowing of the radius (Fig. 19.6), or the radial head dislocation (Fig. 4.9). The best results are achieved with physeal arrest of the radial side of the distal radius with staples [52, 55, 63], combined with ulnar lengthening (Fig. 19.7) [39, 52, 59]. If inadequate growth remains for the use of staples, the options include closing wedge distal radial osteotomy [54, 55, 62], ulnar bone lengthening [53–55], and the Kapandji procedure [62]. In one case of congenital pseudarthrosis of the ulna, union was achieved by the application of a compression plate, but subsequent fracture at the site of the most distal screw developed permanent non-union [20]. Resection of an abnormal

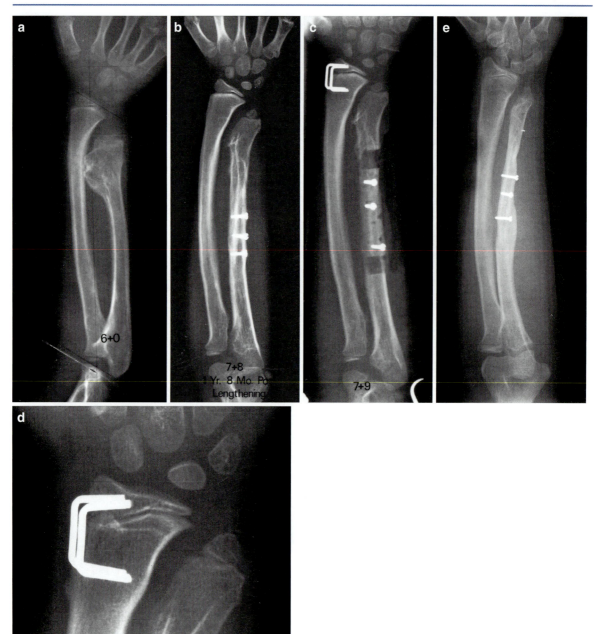

Fig. 19.7 Wrist ulnar angulation associated with MHO treated by distal radial staples and ulnar lengthening. (**a**) Osteochondroma of the distal ulna in a 6 year old girl with accompanying relative shortening of the ulna, bowing of the distal radius, increased radial articular angle (*RAA*), increased carpal slip, and ulnar deviation of the hand. The osteochondroma was excised and the ulna lengthened 1 cm by a one-stage step-cut osteotomy. (**b**) At age 7 years 8 months, 1 year 8 months post surgery, relative ulnar shortening was improved; the radial bowing, RAA, and carpal slip were unchanged. (**c**) One month later, age 7 years 9 months, insertion of two staples over the radial sided of the distal radial physis was accompanied by a second 1 cm step-cut ulnar lengthening. (**d**) At age 8 years 7 months, 10 months after stapling, only the ulnar side of the distal radial physis had grown (note growth arrest line). The radial bowing, RAA, and carpal slip were all improved. The staples were removed 2 months later. (**e**) At age 12 years 6 months, the patient had normal forearm function. The distal radial physis remained open, the RAA and carpal slip were normal, and the radial head remained reduced. There was residual mild negative ulnar variance. The patient was last seen at age 23 years 9 months following an injury to an ankle. There were no complaints about the forearms and no roentgenograms were taken. Ulnar lengthening with a distracting device (as in Fig. 19.6d) may have achieved a better distal radial and ulnar length relationship (Reprinted from Peterson [59] with permission and additional follow-up)

impinging distal ulna or a remnant of the triangular fibrocartilage complex acting as soft tissue tethers have also been done [53]. If the ulnar deficiency is severe and results in radial head dislocation at a young age, the creation of a one bone forearm may be the best solution (Fig. 4.8) [59, 61].

A more complete discussion and list of references for osteochondroma as it affects the physis directly are found in Sect. 4.2 Tumor, Osteochondroma.

References

Introduction

1. Ogden JA, Weil UH, Hempton RF (1976) Developmental humerus varus. Clin Orthop 116:158–166
2. Siffert RS (1966) The growth plate and its affections. J Bone Joint Surg 48A(3):546–563

Knee

3. Bathfield CA, Beighton PH (1978) Blount disease. A review of etiological factors in 110 patients. Clin Orthop 135:29–33
4. Blount WP (1937) Tibia vara: osteochondritis deformans tibiae. J Bone Joint Surg 19:1–29
5. Bradway JK, Klassen RA, Peterson HA (1987) Blount disease: a review of the English literature. J Pediatr Orthop 7(4):472–480
6. Langenskiöld A, Riska EB (1964) Tibia vara (osteochondrosis deformans tibiae). A survey of seventy-one cases. J Bone Joint Surg 46A(7):1405–1420
7. Schoenecker PL, Meade WC, Pierron RL, Sheridan JJ, Capelli AM (1985) Blount's disease: a retrospective review and recommendations for treatment. J Pediatr Orthop 5(2):181–186

Ankle

8. Beals RK, Skyhar M (1984) Growth and development of the tibia, fibula, and ankle joint. Clin Orthop 182:289–292

Congenital Pseudarthrosis of the Fibula

9. Boyd HB (1941) Congenital pseudarthrosis. Treatment by dual bone grafts. J Bone Joint Surg 23(3):497–515
10. Cho TJ, Choi IH, Chung CY, Yoo WJ, Lee SY, Lee SY, Suh SW (2006) Isolated congenital pseudarthrosis of the fibula. Clinical course and optimal treatment. J Pediatr Orthop 26(4):449–454
11. Dal Monte A, Donzelli O, Sudanese A, Baldini N (1987) Congenital pseudarthrosis of the fibula. J Pediatr Orthop 7(1):14–18
12. DiGiovanni CW, Ehrlich MG (1998) Treatment of congenital pseudarthrosis of the fibula with interposition allograft. Orthopedics 21(11):1225–1228
13. Dooley BJ, Menelaus MB, Paterson DC (1974) Congenital pseudarthrosis and bowing of the fibula. J Bone Joint Surg 56B(4):739–743
14. Lampasi M, Antonioli D, Di Gennaro GL, Magnani M, Donzelli O (2008) Congenital pseudarthrosis of the fibula and valgus deformity of the ankle in young children. J Pediatr Orthop B 17(6):315–321
15. Langenskiöld A (1967) Pseudarthrosis of the fibula and progressive valgus deformity of the ankle in children: treatment by fusion of the distal tibial and fibular metaphyses. Review of three cases. J Bone Joint Surg 49A(3):462–470
16. Merkel KD, Peterson HA (1984) Isolated congenital pseudarthrosis of the fibula: report of a case and review of the literature. J Pediatr Orthop 4(1):100–104
17. Narasimhan RR, Banta JV (2001) Congenital pseudarthrosis of the fibula. Case report. Orthopedics 24(5):499–500
18. Ng BKW, Saleh M (2001) Fibula pseudarthrosis revisited treatment with Ilizarov apparatus: case report and review of literature. J Pediatr Orthop B 10(3):234–237
19. Yang KY, Lee EH (2002) Isolated congenital pseudoarthrosis of the fibula. J Pediatr Orthop B 11(4):298–301
20. Younge D, Arford C (1991) Congenital pseudarthrosis of the forearm and fibula. A case report. Clin Orthop 265:277–279

Acquired Pseudarthrosis of the Fibula

21. Babhulkar SS, Pande KC, Babhulkar S (1995) Ankle instability after fibular resection. J Bone Joint Surg 77B(2):258–261
22. Fragniére B, Wicart P, Mascard E, Dubousset J (2003) Prevention of ankle valgus after vascularized fibular grafts in children. Clin Orthop 408:245–251
23. Goh JCH, Mech AMI, Lee EH, Ang EJ, Eng B, Bayon P, Pho RWH (1992) Biomechanical study on the load-bearing characteristics of the fibula and the effects of fibular resection. Clin Orthop 279:223–227
24. González-Herranz P, del Río A, Burgos J, López-Mondejar JA, Rapariz JM (2003) Valgus deformity after fibular resection in children. J Pediatr Orthop 23(1):55–59
25. Hsu LCS, O'Brien JP, Hodgson AR (1974) Valgus deformity of the ankle in children with fibular pseudarthrosis. J Bone Joint Surg 56A(3):503–510
26. Hsu LCS, Yau ACMC, O'Brien JP, Hodgson AR (1972) Valgus deformity of the ankle resulting from fibular resection for a graft in subtalar fusion in children. J Bone Joint Surg 54A(3):585–594
27. Kanaya K, Wada T, Kura H, Yamashita T, Usui M, Ishii S (2002) Valgus deformity of the ankle following harvesting of a vascularized fibular graft in children. J Reconstr Microsurg 18(2):91–96
28. Lubicky JP, Altiok H (2001) Transphyseal osteotomy of the distal tibia for correction of valgus/varus deformities of the ankle. J Pediatr Orthop 21(1):80–88
29. Moon MS, Rhee SK, Lee HD, Ju IT, Nam SH (1997) Valgus ankle secondary to acquired fibular pseudarthrosis in children. Long-term results of the Langenskiold operation. Bull Hosp Jt Dis 56(3):149–153

30. Shoji H, Koshino T, Marcove RC, Thompson TC (1970) Subperiosteal resection of the distal portion of the fibula for aneurysmal bone cyst. Report of two cases. J Bone Joint Surg 52A(7):1472–1476
31. Thomas KA, Harris MB, Willis MC, Lu Y, MacEwen GD (1995) The effects of the interosseous membrane and partial fibulectomy on loading of the tibia: a biomechanical study. Orthopedics 18(4):373–383
32. Wiltse LL (1972) Valgus deformity of the ankle. A sequel to acquired or congenital abnormalities of the fibula. J Bone Joint Surg 54A(3):595–606
33. Wiltse LL (1968) Valgus of the ankle after removing a segment of the fibula in children. (Abstr). J Bone Joint Surg 50A(4):829
34. Yadav SS (1981) Ankle stability after resection of the distal third of the fibula for giant-cell lesions: report of two cases. Clin Orthop 155:105–107

Multiple Hereditary Osteochondroma

35. Beals RK (1991) The treatment of ankle valgus by surface epiphysiodesis. Clin Orthop 266:162–169
36. Beals RK, Shea M (2005) Correlation of chronological age and bone age with the correction of ankle valgus by surface epiphysiodesis of the distal medial tibial physis. J Pediatr Orthop B 14(6):436–438
37. Jahss MH, Olives R (1980) The foot and ankle in multiple hereditary exostoses. Foot Ankle 1(3):128–142
38. Noonan KJ, Feinberg JR, Levenda A, Snead J, Wurtz LD (2002) Natural history of multiple hereditary osteochondromatosis of the lower extremity and ankle. J Pediatr Orthop 22(1):120–124
39. Peterson HA (1989) Multiple hereditary osteochondromata. Clin Orthop 239:222–230
40. Shapiro F, Simon S, Glimcher MJ (1979) Hereditary multiple exostoses. Anthropometric, roentgenographic, and clinical aspects. J Bone Joint Surg 61A(6):815–824
41. Snearly WN, Peterson HA (1989) Management of ankle deformities in multiple hereditary osteochondromata. J Pediatr Orthop 9(4):427–432
42. Solomon L (1961) Bone growth in diaphyseal aclasis. J Bone Joint Surg 43B(4):700–716

Neurologic Conditions

43. Abraham E, Lubicky JP, Songer MN, Millar EA (1996) Supramalleolar osteotomy for ankle valgus in myelomeningocele. J Pediatr Orthop 16(6):774–781
44. Burkus JK, Moore DW, Raycroft JF (1983) Valgus deformity of the ankle in myelodysplastic patients. Correction by stapling of the medial part of the distal tibial physis. J Bone Joint Surg 65A(8):1157–1162
45. Dias LS (1978) Ankle valgus in children with meningomyelocele. Dev Med Child Neurol 20:627–633
46. Dias LS (1985) Valgus deformity of the ankle joint: pathogenesis of fibular shortening. J Pediatr Orthop 5(2):176–180
47. Makin M (1965) Tibio-fibular relationship in paralysed limbs. J Bone Joint Surg 47B(3):5005–5006
48. Malhotra K, Puri R, Owen R (1984) Valgus deformity of the ankle in children with spina bifida aperta. J Bone Joint Surg 66B(3):381–385
49. Sharrard WJW, Webb J (1974) Supra-malleolar wedge osteotomy of the tibia in children with myelomeningocele. J Bone Joint Surg 56B(3):458–461
50. Westin GW, Dingeman RD, Gausewitz SH (1988) The results of tenodesis of the tendo achillis to the fibula for paralytic pes calcaneus. J Bone Joint Surg 70A(3):320–328

Tibial Relative Overgrowth Compared to the Fibula

51. Paluska DJ, Blount WP (1968) Ankle valgus after the grice subtalar stabilization: the late evaluation of a personal series with a modified technic. Clin Orthop 59:137–146

Wrist

52. Fogel GR, McElfresh ED, Peterson MA, Wicklund PT (1984) Management of deformities of the forearm in multiple hereditary osteochondromas. J Bone Joint Surg 66A(5):670–680
53. Golz RJ, Grogan DP, Greene TL, Belsole RJ, Ogden JA (1991) Distal ulnar physeal injury. J Pediatr Orthop 11(3):318–326
54. Kaempffe FA (1999) Biplane osteotomy and epiphysiodesis of the distal radius for correction of wrist deformity due to distal ulnar growth arrest. Orthopedics 22:84–86
55. Nelson OA, Buchanan JR, Harrison CS (1984) Distal ulnar growth arrest. J Hand Surg 9A(2):164–171
56. O'Brien TR (1971) Development deformities due to arrested epiphyseal growth. Vet Clin North Am 1(3):441–454
57. Paul AS, Kay PR, Haines JF (1992) Distal ulnar growth plate arrest following a diaphyseal fracture. J R Coll Surg Edinb 37:347–348
58. Peinado A (1979) Distal radial epiphyseal displacement after impaired distal ulnar growth. An experimental study in rabbits. J Bone Joint Surg 61A(1):88–92
59. Peterson HA (1994) Deformities and problems of the forearm in children with multiple hereditary osteochondromata. J Pediatr Orthop 14(1):92–100
60. Peterson HA (2007) Epiphyseal growth plate fractures. Springer, Heidelberg
61. Peterson HA (2008) The ulnius: a one-bone forearm in children. J Pediatr Orthop B 17:95–101
62. Ray TD, Tessler RH, Dell PC (1996) Traumatic ulnar physeal arrest after distal forearm fractures in children. J Pediatr Orthop 16(2):195–200
63. Siffert RS, Levy RN (1965) Correction of wrist deformity in diaphyseal aclasis by stapling. Report of a case. J Bone Joint Surg 47A(7):1378–1380

Surgical

20.1 Introduction

Surgical injury of the physis is iatrogenic and can be either *intentional* or *unintentional*. The word *iatrogenic* denotes any condition generated by a physician or surgeon. The result may be positive or negative, as seen in this chapter. Examples of intentional surgical physeal arrest already reported in this text include the removal of physes during the treatment of benign and malignant bone tumors (Sects. 4.2 and 4.3), as well as when using compression to curtail growth (Sect. 10.2). Distraction of the physis (Sect. 11.2) results in physeal arrest so often that many orthopedists regard the arrest to be intentional, and plan accordingly. Surgery on physeal bars or bridges, including those due to injuries other than fracture, was reported in depth in Epiphyseal Growth Plate Fractures [228].

20.2 Intentional Physeal Arrest – Humans

Intentional surgical physeal arrest (*epiphysiodesis*, or perhaps more appropriately *physiodesis*), may be performed (1) to curtail slipping of an epiphysis, (2) to arrest longitudinal bone growth, or (3) to improve or prevent angular bone deformity. The physeal arrest may be designed to be *immediate and irreversible*, or *temporary and reversible*. The following is a brief chronological saga of intentional surgical physeal arrest.

20.2.1 Physeal Arrest to Curtail Slipping of an Epiphysis (1931)

Slipping of the capital femoral epiphysis, *epiphysiolisthesis*, first described by Paré in 1572 [1, 47, 89], is the most common disorder of the hip in adolescents. The etiology remains unknown. Its origin does not depend upon trauma and it is not a fracture [86]. Untreated cases often develop deformity and relative shortening of the affected femur, and subsequent arthrosis of the hip joint. Following Roentgen's discovery of X-rays in 1895, slipped capital femoral epiphysis (SCFE) became more accurately diagnosed, and was treated by bed rest, traction, cast or bracing. In the 1920s the favored treatment was protection without interference, immobilization in plaster, traction, or manipulative reduction [1, 2]. Advanced chronic cases were treated by open reduction "freeing the head from the neck with a chisel" replacing the head on the neck, followed by a cast [2, 3]. The ensuing physeal arrest was a complication of the procedure, rather than an intended outcome.

The discussion which follows is focused on surgical treatments designed to intentionally close the physes of hips with SCFE, and not on the controversies over etiology, pathology, imaging, classification, grades and duration of slips, indications for accompanying closed reduction, prophylactic pinning the opposite normal hip, etc.

20.2.1.1 Transphyseal Bone Graft Physiodesis

In an effort to stabilize the epiphysis and to promote physeal arrest in patients with SCFE, bone "slivers" or "pegs" were inserted into the femoral capital epiphysis through drill holes starting in the femoral neck. The first operation was done in 1928 [7]. The first report in 1931, included 15 cases and noted that "the operation to hasten ossification [closure of the physis] is better and safer than long periods of bed rest or brace treatment" [7]. "This was the first operation for closure of any physis" [14]. Drilling across the physis without inserting the bone pegs had little or no effect on the course of SCFE [16, 17].

The operation initially used an anterior ileofemoral Smith–Petersen approach to the hip, which gave good access to the antero-superior portion of the femoral neck as well as to the lateral side of the ileum [16, 24]. After 1985 the anterolateral approach similar to that used in total hip surgery became more common [22]. Both incisions allow good visualization of the head–neck junction to assess the head position, stability, and mobility. The superior limb of both incisions facilitates removal of cortico-cancellous strips or pegs of bone from the outer surface of the ileum, which are placed across the capital physis through a trough in the antero-superior portion of the femoral neck [22, 24]. Any bony prominence on the antero-lateral neck as a result of the displaced epiphysis, which is obstructing motion in any plane, can easily be removed at the same time [9, 10, 18, 22]. Any residual deformity restricting motion maybe treated later by osteotomy of the femoral neck, or of the intertrochanteric or subtrochanteric areas [6, 15].

The primary goals of bone pegging the physis are stabilization and fusion of the epiphysis to the metaphysis. Since SCFE usually occurs in teenagers with little growth remaining, and since the proximal femoral physis provides very little longitudinal growth at this age, the resulting femoral relative shortening is usually minor and of little clinical concern. The maximum limb length discrepancy rarely exceeds one half inch [10]. Occasionally contralateral distal femoral physeal arrest at the appropriate time may be necessary to equalize limb lengths at skeletal maturity [6].

The main advantage of bone grafting is that it is a single operative procedure without need for hardware removal [25]. In the first reported series with good follow-up data, grafting achieved fusion and a good result in all 17 cases [11]. When successful it prevented further displacement and eliminated the physeal barrier of the medullary blood supply to the head of the femur [10].

The main disadvantages of bone pegging are that it does not produce immediate mechanical stability or physeal arrest. This results in lengthy hospitalization and post operative activity restrictions. Patients are usually treated postoperatively by some combination of bed rest, balanced suspension, non-weight bearing, or hip spica cast for 3–4 weeks [8], or until the physis is fused on roentgenograms [92]. In one study the average time for fusion was 2.3 months (range 4 weeks to 4.5 months) [11]. The average time between operation and partial weight bearing was 10 weeks; full weight was allowed at 18 weeks [11]. If physeal closure does not progress as expected, a repeat grafting procedure, with or without supplemental in situ pinning, may be considered [18].

Follow-up studies from the beginning reported favorable results with high percentages of success (prompt physeal arrest) and few complications [4, 8–14, 16–18, 25]. A 1966 article proclaimed "There are no adverse effects, except for slight restriction of growth of the femur" [14]. As time went on some investigators felt the long term results were "at least as good as multiple pin fixation" [25]. However, in large recent series (1990–2003) the bone pegs resulted in an unacceptable rate of additional slipping due to "graft insufficiency," meaning resorption or fracture of the graft, resulting in a high likelihood that physeal fusion would not occur and in further displacement of the femoral head [5, 21]. Attempts to improve stability and still promote physeal closure used fibular diaphyseal allografts [5], and freeze-dried irradiated cortical allografts [20]. Complications in a 1996 study of 64 cases of bone peg epiphysiodeses included 4 avascular necroses, 3 chondrolyses, 3 infections, 4 delayed wound healings, 7 transient thigh hypoesthesias, and 44 hips with heterotopic ossification [19]. These authors concluded that "the morbidity associated with open bone peg epiphysiodesis seems unacceptable when compared with the complications seen with internal fixation and hardware removal, and the extensive surgery and prolonged hospitalization become prohibitive considerations in today's health care economies."

20.2.1.2 Transphyseal Metallic Pin

In 1894 Sturrock [83] reported the insertion of a metal pin to stabilize a slipped capital femoral epiphysis. The pin was smooth, but was removed 2 days later because of infection. This was followed in the early 1930s by the tri-flanged (trifin) Smith–Petersen (SP) nail, commonly used in the treatment of adult hip fractures. When the SP nail was applied to SCFE some good results were obtained when nailing mild slips in situ [58, 59, 86, 88], after reduction of displaced femoral heads [12], as well as nailing after osteotomy or wedge ostectomy through the physis [58, 69, 89]. However, the large size of the nail was difficult to accurately position, sometimes resulted in further displacement or fracture of the femoral head, had a high incidence of avascular necrosis and degenerative changes of the femoral head, and did not promote bone formation or physeal closure [9, 16, 34, 45, 47, 53, 54, 62, 71, 89]. Modifications of the Smith-Petersen nail included the triflanged nails of Johansson, Nyström, and the Vitalium nail. The results using these slimmer nails were slightly better despite continued problems of driving the epiphysis off the metaphysis, the head growing off the nail, fracture at the nail insertion site, and necrosis of the femoral head [87].

Beginning in the late 1930s a variety of threaded solid pins (i.e., Lippman, Steinmann, Knowles, Moore, Neuman, Hagie, Gouffon, Zimmer, Tachdjian, Lloyd–Collison lag screw, and ASIF cancellous screws, etc.) were devised in an effort to improve insertion, produce a compressive effect across the physis, and reduce complications [36, 47]. The pin achieving the best compression was possibly the A-O screw [90].

Acute and chronic slips with less than 1/3 head displacement were fixed in situ with two or more pins without reduction [32–34, 42, 72, 79]. Acute slips greater than 1/3 head displacement were often treated by closed manipulation and pinning with multiple pins [32, 48]. Postoperatively, no cast was used. In one study of 75 hips with SCFE the average physeal fusion time with Knowles pins was 9.4 months, for Hagie or Tachdjian pins was 3.7 months, and for bone pegging was 4.8 months [54]. In another study using Steinmann and Knowles pins, the mean time to physeal closure was 5.4 months with a single pin, 5.5 months with two pins, and 6.4 months with three or more pins [30].

Chronic moderate or severe slips were sometimes treated with open separation of the head from the metaphysis, removal of the physis with a gouge, and fixing the head to the neck with a screw (Dunn's operation) [38, 45, 46], or by excision of a wedge of bone (cuneiform osteotomy) from high on the neck including the physis, or lower on the neck, and internal fixation with pins [27, 29, 34, 37, 42, 47, 49–51, 57, 61, 69, 75, 79]. Post operatively, a hip spica cast was often used. The potential risks of vascular impairment of the femoral head with intraarticular realignment osteotomies are high [35, 50, 53]. The risks of vascular impairment of the head with extraarticular biplane intertrochanteric or subtrochanteric realignment osteotomies are low [35, 40, 53, 55, 74, 76, 82, 89]. However, some investigators found that even moderate and severe slips had better long term results after in situ pinning alone, than after manipulative reduction or corrective osteotomy combined with pinning [35, 39].

The problem of unsuspected pin penetration into the hip joint causing chondrolysis was prevalent with all types of solid pins [66, 70]. In the early 1980s internal fixation of all types and degrees of slips was facilitated by the development of intraoperative fluoroscopy and of a cannulated screw with larger diameter and larger threads than the solid screws [60, 65, 66]. In addition to greater strength of a hollow screw, reducing the need for only one screw, the cannulation allowed the insertion of contrast material through the screw to document roentgenographically penetration or non-penetration of the screw into the joint. The wider threads of the cannulated screws also promoted physeal fusion. In one study the epiphysis "grew off" the pins in 9 of 49 (18%) hips pinned with Knowles pins, 4 of 14 (29%) pinned with Steinmann pins, and 0 of 14 (0%) hips pinned with cannulated screws [64]. No hips with cannulated screws continued to grow after surgery.

Hip motion returns quite well following in situ fixation despite often minimal remodeling [81]. Remodeling of the femoral head-neck angle in SCFE has been noted to occur with both in situ pinning [41, 73, 91] as well as with immobilization in a spica cast [2, 41]. The mechanism of the restoration or correction of the slip is unknown [41]. One study using pinning with a single cannulated screw found an average of 11.7° remodeling of the displaced head on the neck in 5% of mild slips, 20% of moderate slips, and 100% of all 11 severe slips [91]. The authors advised waiting at least 2 years after pinning before considering realignment osteotomy.

In the early 1990s it was recognized that stabilization of SCFE without fusion of the femoral capital physis would be desirable in young children [80]. This could be accomplished by an entirely smooth pin without threads, which would allow continuing growth of the head and neck, avoiding the problems of relative overgrowth of greater trochanter, coxa vara, and relative femoral shortening. A second option is a long cannulated screw with only 10 mm of threads [63]. All of the threads could be contained within the femoral capital epiphysis without impinging the physis. The base of the screw was allowed to protrude laterally 15–20 mm from the lateral side of the femur. As the femoral neck grew in length the base of the screw was drawn into the femoral neck. Thus stability was achieved yet allowing growth of the proximal femoral physis and normal hip development to continue.

The advantages of pin fixation in the treatment of SCFE are that the method is relatively simple, blood loss is minimal, the hip joint is not opened, and the pins are usually easily removed [68]. The duration of anesthesia, hospitalization time, complications, and surgical scars are also less with pins than with the bone pegging procedures. The main disadvantages are difficulty of pin insertion in severe chronic slips [68] and lack of prompt physeal arrest due to small threads of some pins [14].

Complications of the pinning operation included pin joint penetration, metal failure, fracture at the site of pin entry, fracture of the femoral neck, failure of physeal arrest allowing the epiphysis to "grow off" the pin, chondrolysis, avascular necrosis of the epiphysis, and wound infection [4, 28, 36, 41, 52, 56, 67, 68, 77, 78]. The degree of the initial slip is directly correlated with worsening of results [31]. Complications of pin removal included difficulties with pin removal and fracture at the site of pin removal [36, 52, 60, 68, 85]. Small diameter non-cannulated and titanium pins have the highest failure of removal because of pin breakage or stripping of the pin heads [85]. Although most of the complications were "minor," they were sufficient to question prophylactic pinning of the contralateral normal hip, and to reconsider alternative procedures such as bone pegging physiodesis [52].

Commentary

Many articles extol the virtues of either bone-pegging or metallic pinning for SCFE, only a portion of which are reported here. An aura of competition developed between proponents of the two methods [23, 44]. Comparison of results is made difficult by the influence of multiple factors such as age, gender, and race of the patients, duration of the slip (acute or chronic), degree of slip, attempt of reduction (manipulation), the type of bone pegs used, and the number and types of pins used. The bone-grafting method has the advantage of earlier fusion of the physis, but the disadvantage of requiring a larger incision, and more patient care and protection while waiting for the physis to fuse [29].

Neither the bone grafting nor the pinning in situ guarantees certain closure of the physis [18]. Pinning in situ resulted in 1+% further slipping in two reports combined [89, 92]. Bone graft resorption resulted in 3% further slipping in two reports combined [14, 18]. The factors responsible for the bone graft failures were thought to be resorption of the graft or failure of the graft to cross the physis [18].

In 1963 one of the originators of the bone pegging operation felt that acute slips should be reduced and internally fixed with pins; pre-slipping and slight to moderate slipping (up to ¾ in.) should be treated with bone pegging [15]. In 1989 a strong proponent of bone-pegging concluded that in cases of minimal slipping, metallic fixation and bone-graft physiodesis both seem justified on the basis of studies of complications, but that in moderate or severe slipping bone-graft physiodesis is strongly recommended [22]. Another study that compared results of pinning in 65 hips and open physiodesis in 33 hips concluded that "pinning in-situ is the treatment of choice in hips with slippage up to 55°, and that patients with slippage of greater than 55° are best treated by subtrochanteric osteotomy" [92]. There is no method of restoring the normal anatomy without considerable risk of damaging the femoral head [43].

The advent of better fracture tables, intraoperative radiographic imaging, cannulated screws with larger threads, improvements in implant technology, and the advent of managed care affecting the length of hospital stay, have resulted in the majority of cases of SCFE being treated today with a single cannulated screw across the physis [26, 44]. Pinning "eliminates the danger of further displacement, promotes fusion of the epiphyseal plate and allows the patient to return to full activity within 1 month, thus avoiding joint stiffness, muscle atrophy, osteoporosis, and interference with growth at other sites" [71]. "This gives results equal to bone peg epiphysiodesis, in a perioperative setting that is superior" [44]. In 1984 an article proclaimed "pinning in-situ is the treatment of choice. It is more predictable, has fewer complications, and provides better long term results" [92]. A 1991 article declared "regardless of severity of the slip, pinning in situ provided the best long-term function and delay of degenerative arthritis, with a low risk of complications" [39]. An internet communication from the Pediatric Orthopedic Society of North American on 14 February, 2011, stated that the "Gold standard method for the treatment of slipped capital femoral epiphysis is still "in situ fixation"" [84].

Author's Perspective

Today metallic pining is used more commonly than bone grafting because the majority of slips are diagnosed earlier and are therefore often mild and easier to pin, and because of factors listed in the previous paragraph. I was unable to identify a report or assign a date to the first metallic pinning to intentionally achieve physeal arrest for SCFE or other conditions.

20.2.2 Immediate Irreversible Physeal Arrest (1933)

20.2.2.1 Introduction

The purpose of this section is to discuss the surgical methods and techniques by which physeal growth can be intentionally curtailed to improve bone length discrepancy and angular deformity. No attempt is made to evaluate the relative worth of the multiple measuring techniques, or of tables, atlases, charts, mathematical and calculating methods used in determining the timing or follow-up of the arresting procedure. None of the calculating methods takes into account qualitative factors often used by clinicians, such as secondary sexual characteristics, menarche, parent or sibling height, or surgical factors. Current methods of determining timing of physiodesis are of similar accuracy, with no clear advantage to any method [98]. The available charts of prediction are a guide in deciding the timing of arrest, but do not supersede clinical judgment [95]. It is inadvisable to recommend any surgical procedure based on mathematical calculation alone.

Intentional surgical physeal arrest is the most frequently performed lower limb length equalization procedure [99]. Lower limb length inequality of one-half to three-quarters of an inch ordinarily causes no clinical impairment or morbidity. Physiodesis is generally performed for discrepancies predicted to be between 2 and 5 cm at maturity [96, 97]. Greater differences become an increasing problem, more or less in proportion to the amount of discrepancy, and are often treated by lengthening and shortening operations, and if severe occasionally by amputation [94, 96, 97]. In these cases of greater discrepancy, physiodesis may be used as a supplementary procedure to reduce the magnitude of the lengthening or shortening surgery. Physiodesis has also been used after amputation on the stump physis to negate the problem of stump overgrowth [100].

Procedures to surgically arrest longitudinal growth are usually done on the *normal* longer extremity, but can be done on an *abnormal* longer extremity, for example for overgrowth in cases of congenital hemihypertrophy, arteriovenous aneurysm, hemangioma, and neurofibromatosis, following inflammatory processes such as osteomyelitis, and following diaphyseal fractures, particularly of the femur [95].

Surgical physeal arrest of the distal femur or proximal tibia often results with the knees at different levels. This is a small price to pay for equal leg lengths, and causes little if any morbidity. Since most surgical physeal arrests are done after mid-teen years the amount of total height lost is usually of little concern. Children who have physeal arrest must be observed regularly until their growth is completed. Any untoward factors that might arise can thus be promptly corrected.

Knowledge of the underlying physeal anatomy and the relationship of structures overlying the physis are vital in preparing for precise surgical arrest [93]. The relative technical ease of physiodesis, the short post-surgical recovery period, and its reliability, compared to alternative surgical procedures of bone length equalization and deformity correction, have contributed to its popularity. Intentional surgical physeal arrest is accomplished by one of four methods.

The Block Method

In 1933 Phemister reported the removal of a rectangular block of metaphyseal and diaphyseal bone including the physis [119]. The depth of the block was typically 1.5–2.5 cm. Additional physis was removed under direct vision with a curette, drill, or cautery. Rotating the block 180° and reinserting it resulted in immediate physeal arrest. Phemister termed the procedure "epiphyseodiaphyseal fusion" [119]. A cylinder cast postoperatively for 3 weeks allowed weight bearing on crutches [120].

In 1938 White and Warner [129] improved the method by using a four sided one-half inch square mortising chisel with a hollow center to remove of a square block of bone containing the physis. The square bone block is removed more quickly and is rotated only 90° for reinsertion. This gives better stability and bone to bone contact for fusion than the Phemister rectangular shaped bone. The incision is slightly smaller than with the Phemister technique. White published two more papers reporting this chisel [127, 128].

Typically the Block Method is performed medially and laterally on two sides of a physis to achieve total arrest and reduce limb length discrepancy. The procedure has also been used bilaterally on both knees in "unacceptably tall" boys to reduce anticipated total body height [120]. The Block Method has also been used on only one side of the physis to correct angular deformity [107]. Careful planning and timing is necessary to avoid over or undercorrection [104, 111]. A recent modification of the Block Method to correct angular deformity is surface physiodesis, which is the removal of a cortical strip 1 cm wide, 2 cm long, and only 0.5 cm deep, placing an intact piece of bone across the physis without removal of additional physis [101, 102].

Results using the Block Method improved with experience and date of report [93, 103, 105, 106, 108, 109, 111, 113, 114, 116, 117, 120, 121, 123–125, 130, 151, 153]. In a 1994 MRI study, a mature bridge of bone was seen at the operative site 8 months after the operation, but no growth recovery lines were observed, evidence that the arrest was immediate [126]. A high percentage of patients (50–90%) achieved length discrepancy reduction to within ½ to 1 in. in most studies. Phemister reasoned that it is better to under correct and accept a difference of 1–2 cm in limb length, than risk having the short limb become the longer one as a result of overzealous attempts to obtain perfectly equal lengths. In addition, unilateral paralytic lower limbs function better with slight shortening compared with the normal side.

The complication rate of the Block Method is 5–10% [151]. Several authors stated that the serious drawbacks are the many ugly scars. However, the failure of closure on one side of the physis, but not the other, resulting in angular deformity requiring repeat arrest [116] or corrective osteotomy [99, 112, 118, 122, 123, 130], is much more serious. The Block Method of physeal arrest was a significant addition to surgical techniques of leg length equalization available at the time (bone shortening, bone lengthening, and sympathectomy), and is still in use today in some treatment centers.

The Trough Method

In a 1960 attempt to improve idiopathic scoliosis, a trough of bone was excised from the convex side of three or four vertebral bodies at the apex of the convexity of the curve [132]. The trough was filled with a section of rib. Progression of the curve was not altered in 4 patients followed for 2½ to 3 years.

Fluoroscopic Assisted Physeal Ablation

The advent of intraoperative image intensification in the late 1970s introduced a completely new concept of physeal arrest by immediate ablation with relatively little disturbance of the metaphysis or epiphysis.

Physeal Curettement

In 1984 Bowen and Johnson [136] reported advancing a 3 mm curette into the medial one-third of the physis through a 3 mm skin incision using image intensification. This was the first report of using fluoroscopy to guide the surgeon in removing the physeal cartilage. The curette was swept anterior and posterior in the physis to ablate one-third of the physis. The procedure was then repeated on the lateral side. The middle one-third of the physis was left intact to preserve some stability. This method has also been used on only one side of the physis to correct angular deformity [111, 143]. The advantages are the small incisions and scars, short operating time, little post operative pain, no hardware to remove, and results comparable with other methods. Several follow-up articles using curettement attest to its success [111, 141, 143, 145, 150, 151, 155]. Complications include hemarthrosis, asymmetric closure of the physis requiring repeat physiodesis, overcorrection, and undercorrection [107, 145].

Although this procedure and the numerous similar procedures that followed emphasize the "percutaneous" benefit, the advent of image intensification was the real impetus driving this advancement.

Intraphyseal Drilling

In 1986 Canale et al. [138], guided by image intensification, inserted a smooth Kirschner wire half way into one side of the physis through a 5 mm incision. A 4 mm diameter cannulated reamer was placed over the K-wire. Pneumatically driven drills, reamers, and burrs of various design and sizes up to 3 mm in diameter were then used to completely obliterate the physis anteriorly to posteriorly. The procedure was then repeated on the other side of the physis. The medial and lateral physeal disruptions may be connected, but removal of all the physis was deemed unnecessary [137]. Introduction of contrast material may help visualize adequate physeal excision [152].

Advantages of drilling are the short operating, hospitalization, and rehabilitation times, the small scars, reliable physeal arrest, and low incidence of complications [137, 142]. Numerous authors have reported successful results [133–135, 137, 139, 142, 144, 149], including three groups that ablated the entire physis from only one side [140, 150, 153]. However, the unilateral approach to intraphyseal drilling may contribute to partial failure of arrest with subsequent angular deformity [153].

Complications in addition to failure of arrest, angular deformity, etc., include burning of the skin from the drill, postoperative effusion or hematoma, and deep peroneal palsy [96, 137, 142]. In one study no tourniquet was used allowing the blood to lubricate the interface between the drill and the soft tissues and also to help extrude the physeal material [150]. Low speed drills are preferred over high speed drills which generate unacceptable heat in contact with soft tissue, and seize more easily in bone [150]. A guard over the shaft of the drill or reamer is also helpful in reducing skin necrosis [137].

Cannulated Tubesaw

In 1997 Macnicol and Gupta [147] inserted a guidewire from one side completely across the physis under image intensification control. A hollow tube saw was placed over the guide wire to remove a 1 cm core of cancellous bone and physis. After curettage of additional anterior and posterior physis through the tunnel, the cylinder of bone was replaced. This reduced bleeding from the tunnel and augmented growth arrest. No patient series has been reported.

Commentary

The amount of irradiation absorbed by the patient or the surgical team has not been reported in any of these studies of fluoroscopic assisted methods. Magnetic resonance-imaging studies following fluoroscopic assisted physeal ablation have shown no growth recovery lines confirming that growth arrest is immediate [154]. A mature bone bridge or bar is visible in the non-ablated area approximately 8 months after the surgery [154]. A 2004 article reporting on immediate irreversible hemiphysiodesis of 125 angular deformities at the knee noted a "trend" suggesting that fluoroscopic assisted ablation was not as consistent in correcting deformities as the Block Method, which was noted to be "consistent and reliable" [107].

Endoscopic Assisted Physeal Ablation

An arthroscope in the knee has been used to directly observe ablation of the medial aspect of the distal femoral physis to correct angular deformity [156]. A $1 \times 1 \times 2$ cm defect containing primarily physis was removed by a motorized burr inserted percutaneously. The cavity was irrigated and the incision closed. Three girls with idiopathic genu valgum, ages between 12 and 13 years were successfully treated by this method of hemiphysiodesis. The authors speculated that the procedure would also be applicable to the lateral side of the distal femoral physis, but not to the proximal tibial physes or other extra articular physes. The advantages are direct vision of the ablation and less irradiation.

The latest advancement in surgical physeal arrest was reported by Gamble et al. [157], in 2010 to achieve complete physiodesis. Single medial and lateral 9 mm diameter drill holes made percutaneously into the physis under brief image intensifier control are connected in the middle. An endoscope with inflow is placed in one side and a drill in the other. Multiple drilling fans out in the physis anteriorly and posteriorly from the original peripheral position, with the tip of the drill always within site of the scope inserted from the opposite side. The endoscope and drill switch sides to complete the physiodesis. Only the periphery of the physis is left undrilled. Complete physiodesis was accomplished on both the distal femoral and proximal tibial physes. The major advantages over drilling under fluoroscopy are the constant video visualization of the drills, the precise ablation of the physeal tissue, and much less radiation exposure to the patient and the surgical team. The equipment and monetary charges are the same as that for routine knee arthroscopy.

20.2.3 Temporary Reversible Physeal Arrest (1945)

The only method to accomplish temporary reversible physeal arrest of a random physis at the present time is by passive compression. These procedures are reported in more detail in Sect. 10.2. Only a brief chronologic outline is presented here.

The physis is not initially affected by passive compression. With time, as the physis grows it compresses itself by the confines of the implant, causing gradual slow down of growth with the maximal effect being reached in 6 months. Timely and careful removal of the implant will allow the physis to resume growing. Implants left in place over 2 years often result in permanent physeal arrest, and if left more than 4 years *always* result in permanent arrest. Thus, these same reversible techniques may be used to intentionally achieve permanent irreversible physeal arrest. This is done mostly in older children.

Temporary reversible techniques are particularly useful in correcting angular deformity by inserting a device, such as 1–3 staples, on only one side of the physis (*hemiphysiodesis*). Less commonly a wire loop encompassing the physis or the placement of staples on two sides of the physis are used to gradually slow down longitudinal growth (*physiodesis*). In both cases the implants may be used in younger children with less reliance on the timing of the procedure since there is potential for growth to resume after implant removal. However, care must be taken with both implant insertion and removal to ensure that no permanent damage occurs to the physis preventing its resumption of growth.

20.2.3.1 Wire Loop

In 1945 Haas [160] reported insertion of a wire loop through the metaphysis and epiphysis around the physis. As the physis grows it becomes compressed by the wire. Subsequent timely release of the wire has the potential to allow resumption of growth. Breakage of the wire was a frequent problem (Fig. 10.4).

Staples

Blount and Clarke [159] in 1949 reported insertion of the two tines of rigid stainless steel staples into the metaphysis and epiphysis. As the physis grows it becomes compressed by the staples. Growth slowdown occurs gradually before complete arrest. The method is commonly used only on one side of the physis to correct angular deformity (hemiphysiodesis) (Figs. 4.13, 19.2, 19.5), but is also used on two sides of the physis to correct length inequality (Fig. 10.5a, b). Resumption of growth following staple removal relies upon preservation of the perichondral ring and epiphyseal vessels and is not always predictable (Fig. 10.5c–k). Staple loosening and breakage are other occasional problems.

Transphyseal Screws

In 1992 Belle and Stevens [158] reported the insertion of a cannulated threaded screw percutaneously perpendicularly (more or less) across the distal tibial medial malleolar physis to correct ankle valgus deformity. Experiments on rabbits by Green, reported in 1950, had shown that transphyseal screws produced enough anchorage on the two sides of the plate to exert compression upon it and thus gradually inhibit growth [188]. Forty years transpired before the screws were used in humans. The method has been used successfully at the tibial medial malleolus to correct ankle valgus deformity, as well as at the distal femur and proximal tibia to correct both angular deformity and leg length discrepancy.

Tension Band Plate (Eight Plate)

In 2006 Stevens and Pease [161] reported the use of single screws inserted transversely in the metaphysis and epiphysis, connected by an extraperiosteal two hole plate (which looks like an 8). This method is used most advantageously on only one side to achieve "guided growth" of angular deformity, but may be used on two sides of the physis to control longitudinal growth. Timely removal of the plate allows resumption of growth. Recurrent angular deformity can be treated with repeat application of the 8 plate.

Commentary

Each of the methods of intentional physeal arrest for limb discrepancy and angular deformity has advantages and disadvantages. The advantages of complete immediate irreversible physiodesis are its low risk, a high probability of arrest, and ease of performance [99]. The main disadvantage is that it is usually performed on a normal extremity, an almost exclusively rare surgical occurrence other than for obtaining bone or other tissue for analysis or transfer. The advantage of temporary growth slowdown over immediate arrest is that it can be done at younger ages followed by resumption of growth, obviating the necessity of relying as heavily on predetermined calculations of growth expectancy, which may not fit every patient. When performed on one side of the physis to correct angular deformity the surgery is done on the abnormal bone.

All methods of intentional physeal arrest now use intraoperative roentgenography or image intensification to insure proper location of the surgery, the implant, or the position of the device used in the ablation of the physis. Calculation of the amount of radiation exposure has not been reported in any of these studies. The amount of irradiation received by the patient is probably inconsequential, but if surgical teams are performing these operations frequently their radiation exposure could be substantial.

All the strategies of physiodesis are done more commonly for patients with non-traumatic conditions than following trauma [95, 103, 107, 109, 111, 113–116, 121–125, 129, 131, 133, 140, 142, 149–151, 156–158]. Selection of the site or sites depends on the bone or bones involved in the relative shortening or angular deformity. The most common sites subjected to physiodesis are the distal femur and proximal tibia. Less common sites are the distal tibia, distal radius, and distal ulna. Fibular arrest needs to be considered when either tibial physis is arrested, particularly if several years of growth remain [99, 148].

The timing of immediate irreversible physeal arrest is critical [97, 98, 103]. Generally, immediate permanent physiodesis is preferred when the discrepancy does not exceed 5 cm and there is sufficient anticipated growth remaining in the contralateral shorter limb so that gradual correction of the length inequality can be expected after surgery [150]. The average age at time of surgery for immediate arrest of either the Block Method or the Fluoroscopic Assisted Method is approximately 13 years 6 months for boys and 12 years 4 months for girls [146, 155]. Careful clinical and roentgenographic measuring to monitor growth and the pattern of discrepancy or angular deformity, both preoperatively and postoperatively compared to appropriate charts of normal growth over time, achieve the best results [99, 105, 131]. Use of chronologic age alone is not reliable and skeletal age should be determined [94, 97, 110, 115, 116].

The timing of temporary reversible methods is less critical. The wire loops, staples, screws, and tension band plates all utilize *passive* compression and are reported in more detail in Sect. 10.2.

Most methods have been followed by subsequent articles reporting results of the technique. Results and complication rates between the Block Method and the Fluoroscopic Assisted Method are similar [146, 151]. The advantages of using the Fluoroscopic method compared to the Block method are the shorter hospital stay, less postoperative joint stiffness, and smaller scars [146, 151].

Complications are inevitable regardless of the method or the technique, and most involve undercorrection or overcorrection of the length discrepancy or angular deformity. Failures beyond the control of the physician include late discovery or referral resulting in undercorrection, the vagaries of the growth pattern in each individual child [106, 131], patient associated medical comorbidities preventing metal removal at the appropriate time, and failure of the patient to return resulting in overcorrection. Failures within the control of the physician (iatrogenic) include errors in timing surgery due to incomplete data collection, incorrect use of growth prediction tables, discrepancies in interpreting bone age roentgenographs, incomplete surgical physiodesis, lack of appreciation of the primary underlying cause, and damage of the physis at time of implant removal (Fig 10.5).

Patients who undergo physeal arrest must be observed regularly until growth is complete. Any untoward factors that might arise should be promptly corrected.

Author's Perspective

From a historical perspective it is sometimes difficult to look back to assign credit for discoveries and innovations. Nevertheless, it appears that the Bone Graft Method of physiodesis first reported by Ferguson and Howorth in 1931, set in motion ongoing interest and innovation in the field of intentional surgical physeal arrest. Their report was quickly followed by Phemister in 1933 (the Block Method), and subsequently by Haas in 1945 and Blount and Clarke in 1949 (the Compression Method). All three methods were used extensively for 50 years with generally favorable results. SCFE is now treated primarily with a single cannulated screw. Immediate permanent arrest to improve bone length discrepancy is now more commonly accomplished by direct ablation of the physis aided by image intensification. The endoscopic assisted physiodesis method shows promise to achieve immediate permanent growth arrest using less radiation. Angular deformity in a growing child is still most reliably corrected by the Compression Method. The recently introduced tension band plate replacing staples is rapidly gaining popularity for achieving unilateral temporary growth slowdown.

20.3 Intentional Physeal Arrest – Animal Experiments

The effects of physeal injury caused by surgically produced incisions, defects, or implants have been observed in numerous animal experimental investigations. Ollier, in 1867, showed that deep linear incisions across the physis caused retardation of growth. Jahn, in 1892 noted that physeal cartilage columns were unable to reproduce themselves following removal of transversely oriented discs from the physis. Hass in 1917 and 1919 analyzed growth disturbances following incisions, crushing, and curettement of the physis. After World War II (1945) the investigations became more scientifically detailed and relevant.

The amount of growth slowdown and arrest of the operated physis and the compensatory overgrowth on the unoperated physis at the other end of the bone can only be determined accurately by inserting metal markers in both the operated and the contralateral unoperated bones. This is rarely done in animal experiments or in humans.

Intentional physeal arrest in animals by compression, for example by staples, threaded screws, crossed smooth wires, biodegradable implants, and tensioned soft tissue grafts, is discussed in Sect. 10.3.

20.3.1 Resection of the Periphery of the Physis

Resection of the periphery of the physis and adjoining epiphysis and metaphysis in immature dogs resulted in an osseous bridge at the site of ostectomy in all cases [162]. The physeal cells adjacent to the bridge were clumped and irregular in arrangement with marked distortion of the columns. This was the experimental validation for including the Type 6 physeal fracture in the Peterson classification [165, 166]. Excision of one half of the third metacarpal of dogs resulted in minimal growth of the remaining physis postoperatively [163]. Elevation of a flap of metaphyseal bone and epiphyseal cartilage in rabbit femora resulted in "some interference" of growth with angular deformity and moderate relative shortening of the femur [164].

20.3.2 Osteotomy Across the Physis

Osteotomies across the epiphysis perpendicular to the physis and into the metaphysis of dogs caused growth retardation in most cases, and if excentrally placed caused angulation [162]. Osteotomy alone [167], or osteotomy with wedge-resection of the acetabular roof [168] in rabbits caused acetabular dysplasia with subsequent femoral head subluxation and dislocation. The practical conclusion is to avoid injury to the triradiate cartilage when performing periacetabuler osteotomies in young children.

20.3.3 Curettement

Curettement of the lateral half of the distal femoral physis in rabbits caused marked valgus and relative shortening [164, 171]. Curettement of the medial portion of the proximal tibial physis in rabbits caused "gross" varus deformity [191]. The curetted defect "was never repaired by proliferation of epiphyseal cartilage cells, but rather repaired by bone." Curettement of both the medial and lateral proximal tibial physis in rabbits caused a marked decrease in the width of the central uninjured physis by the 2nd week postoperative, and a mature bone bar in the areas of the curettement in 3–4 weeks [172]. This study suggests that growth arrest starts before bone bar formation. Curettement of the femoral capital physis in goats resulted in a short femoral neck, coxa vara, and shortening of the femur measured from the head to the distal end [169]. Circumferential curettement of the periphery of the distal femoral physis caused relative shortening and angular deformity in "some" dogs [170], suggesting the curettement was incomplete in those dogs without shortening and deformity.

20.3.4 Burring

A dental burr used medially and laterally to destroy the tibial physes of rabbits resulted in relative shortening [173]. In another group of rabbits, physeal closure of the proximal tibia was slower with percutaneous burring than with the Block Method or stapling due to a lesser amount of physis ablated [174].

20.3.5 Intraphyseal Drilling

Using image intensification multiple reamer penetrations transversely within the physis made through one incision, followed by cutting with a burr, achieved virtually total ablation of the distal femur and proximal tibial physes in rabbits and dogs [138, 175].

20.3.6 Transphyseal Drilling

Drilling holes perpendicularly across the physes of animals has produced mixed results. A single drill hole (3 mm in rabbits and 5 mm in dogs) perpendicularly across the proximal tibial physis was followed by normal growth, "entirely or almost unchanged." [183]. In another rabbit study a single 7/16 in. drill hole (estimated to be one-ninth or 11% of the area of the physis) was placed across the center of the distal femoral physis [193]. "Microscopic sections at various times after surgery showed considerable new bone growth through the defects. Despite this, in the majority of cases a microscopic defect developed in the new bone and epiphyseal growth continued. These bone defects or stress fractures are shown to be accompanied by an intense cellular reaction." In a third group of rabbits a single 1/8 in. hole drilled across the center of the distal femoral physis and filled with Gelfoam or bone wax caused no growth retardation [164, 170]. In a fourth study in 22 rabbits, a 1.3 mm drill hole across the proximal tibial physis produced no shortening [184]. In a fifth rabbit study 2 mm diameter tunnels across the distal femoral physis filled with semitendenosis tendon caused 11% damage to the physis on the frontal plane and 3% of its cross-section area, but no alteration of growth [178]. In the proximal tibial physis the 2 mm in diameter tunnels caused 12% damage to the physis in the frontal plane and 4% of the cross-sectional area: two tibiae developed valgus deformities and one was shortened. A thin lamella of bone between the graft and the physis is usually present histologically, but is usually discontinuous [178]. The distracting forces of growth are usually able to break these minor tunnel wall bone bridges [178]. In two studies in dogs, no growth retardation occurred when 8–10 holes measuring 0.45 mm in diameter were drilled perpendicularly across femoral, tibial, and radial physes [162, 180]. One of these experiments was used to justify the use of intramedullary nails crossing the physis in children without risk to the growth of the bone [180].

However, drilling across the physis in animals has also caused arrest. A one-sixteenth diameter drill passed through the femoral capital physis 5–6 times in goats, "uniformly" caused growth arrest resulting in a short femoral neck, coxa vara, and functional shortening of the femur [169]. A single 3.2 mm drilling followed by a 4.5 mm tap across the femoral greater trochanteric physis of rabbits caused a bone bridge in all cases [177]. A single hole ¼ of an inch in diameter across the center of the distal radial and femoral physis of dogs rapidly filled with cancellous bone, causing marked growth retardation [162]. A 1 mm wide drill hole across the center of the distal femoral physis of rats consistently produced a bridge of bone insufficient to alter overall bone growth [176]. The authors cautioned that "with multiple passes of the pin during attempted fracture fixation, the sum of these passes may become clinically significant and create a subsequent growth deformity, even though a single pass will not." An identical experiment in rats using a 1 mm drill found that drilling alone did not influence growth at 7 weeks post operative, but significantly retarded growth when the animals were sacrificed at 14 weeks [186]. Drilling of the femoral capital physis through the neck of goats caused arrest with a short femoral neck and coxa vara deformity similar to that caused by curettement, except that the drill arrest took longer [169].

Perhaps the most definitive studies are those which determine the percentage of physis destroyed. One study used 2 and 3 mm drill holes across the distal femoral physes of rabbits [182]. The 2 mm drill hole caused destruction of 3% of the physis and no disturbance of growth, whereas the 3 mm hole caused destruction of 7% of the cross-sectional area of the physis permanent growth disturbance and shortening of the femur. A second study on rats showed that "growth retardation occurs in drill injuries destroying 7–9% of the distal femoral physis, but no retardation is seen with injuries of 4–5%" [181]. These authors cautioned that "the size of physeal injury causing growth retardation in humans is still unknown." In a study assessing ACL repair in rabbits tunnels of various sizes were made across both the distal femoral and proximal tibial physes and filled with tensioned tendon graft [179]. Eight of the ten animals had growth arrest of one or both physes. The tendon transplant had no protective effect against the formation of a physeal bar, "and may have contributed to it by tethering the physis." The authors recommended that tunnels involving more than 1% of the area of the physis be avoided in children.

Thus, the amount of growth retardation appears to be proportional to the amount or percentage of physeal destruction, and whether anything is placed in the drill hole to retard the inflow of blood. If there is nothing to obstruct the ingrowth of tissue the hole is filled with undifferentiated mesenchymal tissue which later forms a cancellous bone bridge. If the bridge is small, growth of the physis may be able to break it.

20.3.7 Longitudinal Smooth Metallic Pins, Wires, and Nails

Smooth metallic pins, wires, and nails of small diameter inserted perpendicularly across the center of large physes typically cause little or no growth retardation in animals. This observation was apparently first recorded by Siffert in 1956 [191]. A 5/64 in. smooth Kirschner wire passed perpendicularly across the center of the proximal tibial physis of rabbits caused no interference with growth at the time of animal sacrifice 2, 4, and 6 weeks later. As the physis grew, leaving the wire in the metaphysis, the path of the wire was replaced with a small transphyseal plug of bone which was insufficient to curtail growth [191]. Additional animal experimentation corroborated these results [162, 164, 185, 187, 190, 223]. A "small" vitallium nail placed across the distal femoral physis of rabbits and left in situ caused no growth disturbance [164]. A single 5/32 in. smooth Steinmann pin placed longitudinally across the distal femoral physis of dogs caused "minimal" growth retardation, while five 0.045 cm Kirschner pins caused variable retardation (none to minimal) [162]. A study using smooth nails of different metals (copper, steel, brass, and nickel-plated, of unspecified diameter) perpendicularly across the center of the distal femoral physis of rabbits and left 5–6 months, showed neither retardation nor stimulation of growth [187]. When two nails (one steel and one brass) were placed perpendicularly across each condyle of the physis and left 3 months there was mild growth retardation (0.1–0.6 cm) in 7 of 10 rabbits. The extensible telescoping rod ultimately used in fragile bone in young children, which crossed the physes at both ends of the bone, was first tested in dogs [185]. The authors found no growth arrest when the nails crossed the center of the physis. A metallic needle placed longitudinally across the distal femoral and humeral physes of young rabbits, and allowed to remain 10, 20 and 30 days, showed no changes in the amount of bone growth [190].

Two exceptions to the above exist. One or two small pins placed longitudinally across the distal radial physis of rabbits, caused a "definite retardation in growth in both instances" [189]. Intramedullar nailing through the distal femoral physis of rats results in "significant retardation of longitudinal growth" [186].

20.3.8 Bone Grafts Across the Physis

A 7/64 in. drill hole (estimated to be one-ninth of the area of the physis) placed perpendicularly across the center of the distal femoral physis of rabbits was completely filled with a section of fibula [193]. The grafts "fused by new bone to the epiphysis and metaphysis. Despite this, in the majority of cases a microscopic defect developed in the bone and epiphyseal growth continued."

Insertion of 5/32 in. thick cortical homogenous bone graft across the distal femoral physis of dogs caused arrest in all 8 cases [162]. Cancellous homologous bone placed across the pelvic triradiate cartilage as an onlay graft in rabbits resulted in premature fusion, thickening of the medial wall of the acetabulum, and subluxation of the femoral head [192].

20.3.9 Staples

See Compression, Sect. 10.3.

20.3.10 Transphyseal Threaded Metallic Screws and Pins

See Compression, Sect. 10.3.

20.3.11 Crossed Smooth Metallic Pins

See Compression, Sect. 10.3

20.3.12 Biodegradable Pins, Screws, and Filaments

See Compression, Sect. 10.3.

20.3.13 Tensioned Soft Tissue Grafts

See Compression, Sect. 10.3.

20.3.13.1 Author's Perspective

The amount of physeal arrest caused by metallic devices placed across the physis depends on their size, number, and location within the physis (peripheral vs. central), angle relative to the physis, presence or absence and size of threads, duration of retention, and possibly the type of metal (e.g. titanium) and the age of the patient. The amount of physeal arrest caused by drilling holes across the physis depends on their size, number, position within the physis (peripheral vs. central), and whether the hole is filled with a substance to prevent accumulation of blood and subsequent bone. In the future, biodegradable screws with large threads and longer degradation periods might find use to temporarily slow down or completely arrest physeal growth in children (Sect. 10.3). Further investigation is needed.

20.4 Unintentional Physeal Arrest – Human Involvement

It is tempting to suspect that unintentional surgical physeal arrest is underreported because surgeons may be reluctant to report poor outcomes of an iatrogenic nature. Unintentional physeal arrest associated with compression, for example cases of bone lengthening or the use of staples, are reported in Sect. 10.2. Unintentional injuries to the apophysis, for example genu recurvatum following skeletal traction by means of a pin in the anterior tibial tubercle, are not reported in this book. Unintentional physeal arrest associated with reimplantation of bone containing the physis is reported in the text Epiphyseal Growth Plate Fractures, Peterson HA, Springer, Heidelberg, 2007, chap. 35.

20.4.1 Smooth Nails, Rods, and Prosthetic Stems

Single, smooth metallic nails, rods, and prosthetic stems of pencil size or larger, placed perpendicularly across the center of a physis *usually* cause little detrimental effect on the longitudinal growth of the involved physis. The nails and rods reported in this section are mainly those of Kuntscher, Rush, large Steinmann, Hansen-Street, Ender, Schneider, Bailey-Dubow, and Sheffield.

Sofield and Millar first used intramedullary rod fixation to stabilize correction of osteotomized deformities of long bones in children in 1948. The first report was in 1959 [216]. By necessity, insertion of the rod required crossing the physis at one end of the long bone. Children often outgrew these rods of fixed length, requiring additional operations to implant longer rods.

Extensible telescoping rods, first used in 1962 [194, 195], reduced the frequency of revisions [211], or negated replacement altogether, despite usually crossing physes at both ends of the bone. Normal growth has been noted in nearly all cases (sometimes even with permanent retention of these devices across the physes) involving the proximal tibia [194, 200, 201, 205, 206, 208, 210, 212, 214, 215, 217], distal femur [194, 197, 201, 205, 206, 208, 210, 212, 214, 217], and proximal humerus [201, 210, 214]. Interestingly, in some cases the anchoring T part of the elongating nail in the epiphysis was overgrown by the physis so that the T portion ended up in the metaphysis [205, 206].

Intramedullar rods of various types are frequently used in children to secure and maintain alignment of diaphyseal femoral fractures, following femoral osteotomy, and during femoral lengthening. When the rod is placed through the piriformis fossa proximally there is the potential for physeal arrest of the proximal femoral trochanterocervical area or greater trochanter producing coxa valga [202, 213]. This is usually regarded as being due to direct physeal injury. An alternative theory for the arrest is occlusion of the lateral epiphyseal branch of the circumflex artery which lies close to the piriformis fossa, rather than direct damage to the physis [204]. In one study arrest occurred in 30% of patients, mostly in those under age 13 years, and was sufficient to warrant corrective proximal femoral varus osteotomy in some cases [202]. The nail size and duration of retention did not influence the result. However, in another study the size of the nail did make a difference: three of eight femoral fractures fixed with Kuntscher nails after reaming the proximal femoral physis developed arrest, whereas none of nine femoral fractures fixed with smaller Rush rods without reaming the physis developed arrest [218]. These authors concluded that reaming of the proximal femoral physis should be avoided in a growing child. But was the arrest found with Kuntscher nails due to the reaming, or the larger size of the hole?

Other authors have had more favorable results treating femoral shaft fractures. Kuntschner rods, interlocking nails, and Ender nails have all been inserted proximally through the piriformis fossa or greater trochanter with no subsequent growth arrest [203]. Despite these generally good results there was enough concern of growth arrest that it was recommended that flexible intramedullary Ender nails be inserted in the metaphysis away from the physis to stabilize long bone fractures [209]. The absence of growth disturbance is the important benefit of this technique.

Physeal growth has also continued in the presence of permanent prosthetic stems (cemented or uncemented, with or without a polyethylene sleeve) placed across the proximal tibial or distal femoral physis [196, 198–200, 207, 215]. The amount of growth with the use of uncemented stems with a polyethylene sleeve has varied from 43 to 100% compared with the normal side [198].

Continued growth from all types of transphyseal implants is more likely to occur if the device is in the center of the physis and when the diameter of the device is small relative to the area of the physis. These cases demonstrate that the physis is a formidable biological structure capable of overcoming partial ablation and considerable tethering forces in order to continue growth [215]. An example of growth continuing despite significant tethering force is shown in Fig. 10.7.

20.4.2 Smooth Wires and Pins

Wires and pins of small diameter, such as those of Kirschner and Steinmann, are commonly placed obliquely across the physis to temporarily stabilize (fix) both physeal and metaphyseal fractures. Less commonly these small diameter pins and wires are also placed perpendicularly across some physes. In most instances smooth wires of small diameter, few in number, and left across a physis only a short time (e.g., 3–4 weeks), do not disturb physeal growth [223]. However, as early as 1958 physeal fractures were noted to "hardly ever" develop disturbed growth, "unless metal was introduced near the cartilage" [234]. One author stated that "perforation of an epiphyseal cartilage was dangerous, except at the lower end of the humerus, which can be nailed with impunity" [237]. Crossed wires used to control distal femoral metaphyseal and physeal fractures inserted proximally and advance distally into the epiphysis avoids intra-articular placement of wires, but increases risk to femoral vessels medially [233]. A report of 49 physeal fractures at three different sites, recorded 100% premature closure of the three cases in which K-wire internal fixation had traversed the physis (proximal humerus, distal humerus, and distal femur) [219]. The authors commented that "it is probable that reduction could have been maintained in all of them without use of direct fixation." If physeal arrest occurs following the pinning of a physeal fracture, the surgeon often attributes the arrest to the fracture, rather than the pin, and the case goes unreported.

20.4.2.1 Finger Phalanges

Hand phalanges are the most common site of physeal fracture [228]. Eighty-three percent are Peterson type 2 and 3 (Salter-Harris types 1 and 2) [228]. Despite significant displacement these fractures are usually stable after reduction and can be successfully managed with splints and cast without internal fixation. If necessary for stabilization the pin should be single, of small diameter, and pass through the center of the physis (Fig. 20.1). The chances of maintaining an open physis is greater without internal fixation.

20.4.2.2 Distal Radius

The distal radius is the second most frequent site of physeal fracture [228]. Only occasionally is a distal radial physeal fracture so unstable that internal fixation obliquely across the physis is necessary. Small diameter pins placed across the physis usually cause no growth arrest [221, 223, 230]. However, physeal arrest has been reported [220, 224]. There may be several potential causes for the arrest other than the pin, and the incidence is unknown. An example is shown in Fig. 20.2.

Fractures of the mid-radius and distal radial metaphysis in children are sometimes treated with longitudinal Kirschner wires, or flexible or rigid intramedullary rods, inserted retrograde beginning in the distal radial epiphysis. One hundred ninety-two patients in three studies have been treated with retrograde K-wires crossing the physis without a single case of premature physeal closure [221, 232, 239]. The pins were removed in 3–6 weeks. Despite this lack of physeal injury, starting the entry point proximal to the distal radial physis enhances three point fixation and obviates potential physeal problems [232].

20.4 Unintentional Physeal Arrest – Human Involvement

Larger flexible intramedullary rods may, however, cause arrest (Fig. 20.3). When possible, these larger rods should be inserted retrogradely beginning in the distal radial metaphysis and passed proximally into the diaphysis [238].

20.4.2.3 Distal Tibia

The distal tibial is the third most common site of physeal fracture, and a relatively high percentage are treated surgically (16.5%) [228]. Smooth pins or wires are frequently used to stabilize these fractures. The incidence of physeal arrest in cases where the wire crosses the physis is unknown. It can occur following fractures in which the epiphysis is displaced (Fig. 20.4) or undisplaced (Fig. 20.5). Techniques for open visualization and reduction of distal tibial physeal fractures with separate percutaneous fixation not crossing the physis have been described (Fig. 20.6) [226, 228, 229]. Of 13 cases treated by this technique, only one had growth derangement, and since the pin did not cross the physis the pin could not be implicated [226].

20.4.2.4 Distal Humerus

A 1958 report stated that perforation of an epiphyseal cartilage was dangerous, except at the lower end of the humerus, which can be nailed with impunity [237]. Smooth pins crossing the physis obliquely are used more commonly to secure fractures of the distal humerus than at any other site. Complications, including premature partial and complete physeal arrest, are

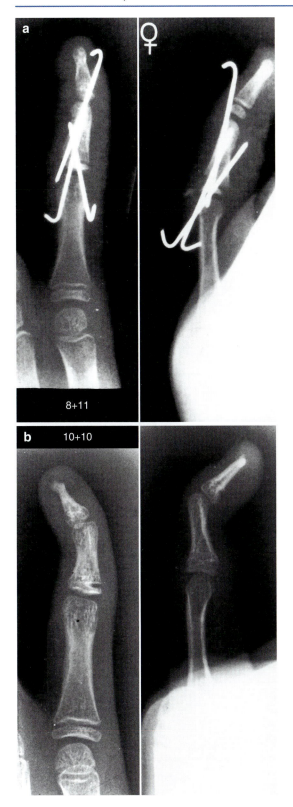

Fig. 20.1 Distal and middle phalangeal arrest associated with smooth Kirschner wires. This girl was 8 years 11 months old when her left little finger was caught in an automobile door, displacing the middle phalangeal epiphysis. (**a**) The epiphysis was reduced and stabilized with 3 Kirschner wires. There was no injury to the distal phalanx, but the retrograde distal wire crossed its physis. Duration of the K-wire retention is unknown. (**b**) Twenty-three months later there was partial premature physeal closure of the middle phalangeal physis without deformity, and complete closure of the distal phalangeal physis with deformity. (*Note*: The middle phalangeal physeal arrest may be associated with the epiphyseal displacement, but corresponds in location with the position of the three relatively large pins. The distal phalangeal closure with deformity has no explanation other than the single more distal excentric K-wire caused a peripheral bar, angular deformity, and subsequent complete physeal closure)

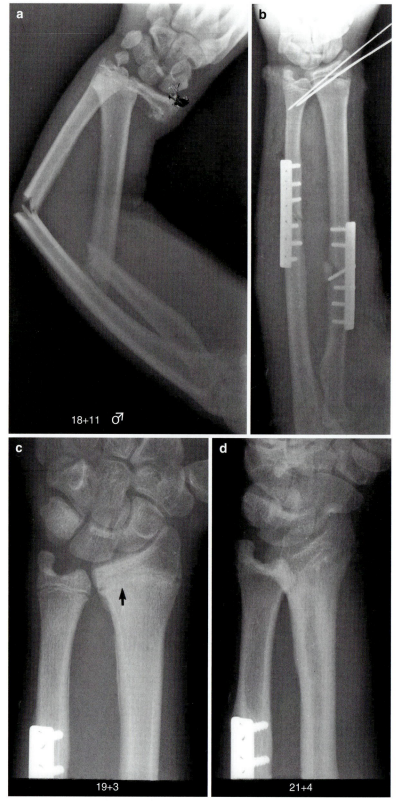

Fig. 20.2 Distal radial partial physeal arrest associated with oblique Kirschner wires. (**a**) This boy was 18 years 11 months old when he sustained complete displacement of the right radial epiphysis, fracture of the ulnar styloid, and radial and ulnar midshaft fractures. (**b**) Treatment included open reduction of the distal radial epiphysis and fixation with two oblique kirschner wires, and of the radius and ulna with plates and screws. The K-wires were removed 44 days later and the final cast 10 weeks post fracture. (**c**) Four months post fracture, age 19 years 3 months, forearm and wrist motion was improving. The distal radial physis was indistinct and abnormal at the site of the previous pins (*arrow*). Two years 5 months post fracture, age 21 years 4 months, wrist flexion, extension, radial and ulnar deviation, and forearm rotation were all slightly less than the left, but grip strength was 45 kg on the right and 35 kg on the left. There was relative overgrowth of the radial side of the radial epiphysis. The patient was seen 2½ years later with an ankle injury; there was no mention of wrist difficulty.(*Note*: The premature partial physeal arrest in this case could be associated with the displaced epiphysis, but is located suspiciously close to the site of the physeal penetration by the wires)

Fig. 20.3 Distal radius partial physeal arrest associated with a perpendicular transphyseal metal rod. (**a**) This girl was 9 years 8 months old when she fell off a bunk bed sustaining fractures of the mid left radius and ulna. (**b**) Titanium flexible intramedullary rods were inserted percutaneously the same day. The pin in the radius was inserted through the radial styloid crossing the distal radial physis. (**c**) The pin in the ulna was inserted at the elbow crossing the center of the proximal ulnar physis. The duration of pin retention was 3 months. (**d**) At age 12 years 5 months the patient noted reduction of wrist strength and motion, with pain when lifting more than 10 lbs. The roentgenogram shows premature partial physeal closure at the site of the radial pin, radial angulation of the distal radial epiphysis, and relative overgrowth of the ulna. The bar was excised and the defect filled with fat from the antecubital fossa. The bar excision was unsuccessful. At age 13 years 8 months physeal arrests were performed on the distal ulna and the ulnar side of the distal radius. The ulna was later shortened. (**e**) At age 17 years 3 months there was residual radial angulation of the distal radial articular surface. (*Note:* The radial pin did not need to cross the physis, was large, excentric, and was retained too long. Did the fact that the pin was Titanium play any role in the arrest? An identical case recorded in the literature did not result in physeal arrest despite Rush rod retention for one year (type of metal not specified) [Pritchett 230])

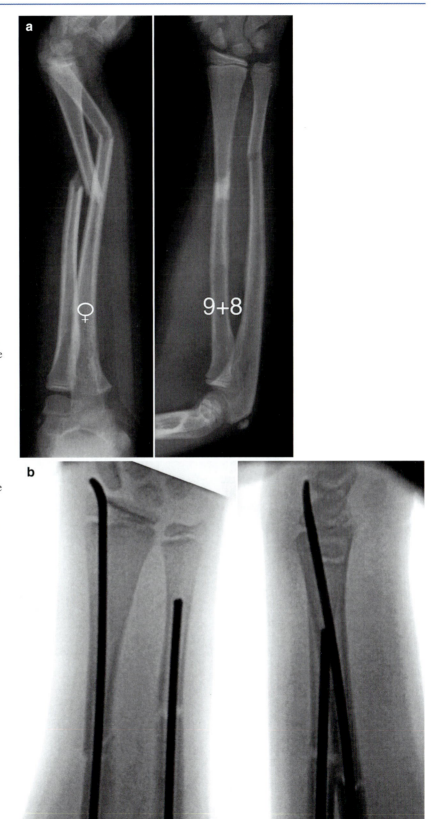

Fig. 20.3 (continued)

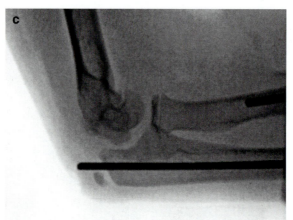
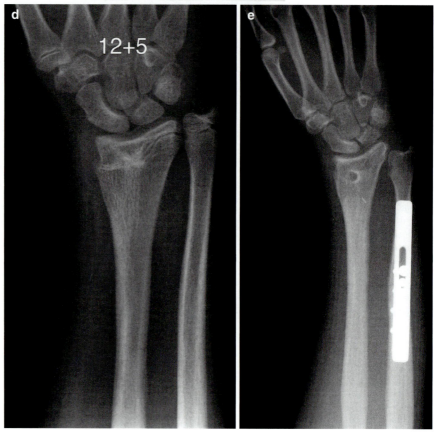

20.4 Unintentional Physeal Arrest – Human Involvement

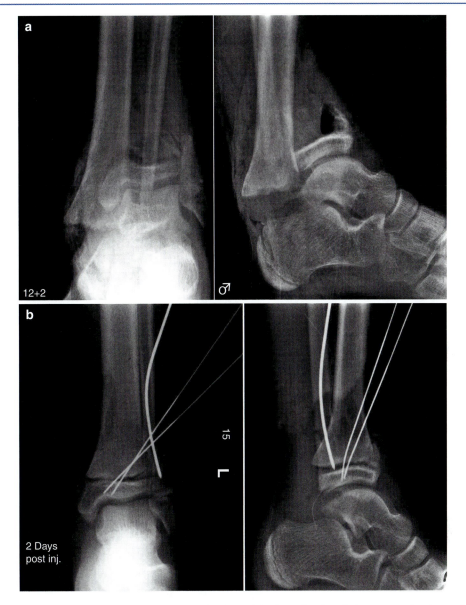

Fig. 20.4 Distal tibial premature physeal closure associated with transphyseal pins. This 12 year 2 month old boy sustained an open fracture when 10–12 sheets of sheetrock fell on his left ankle. (**a**) There is complete displacement of the distal tibial epiphysis (type 2) and a fracture of the distal fibular metaphysis. (**b**) Open reduction included two small k-wires crossing the center of the distal tibial physis obliquely. The pins were removed 5½ weeks post injury. The final cast was removed 7 weeks post injury. (**c**) Six months later, age 12 years 8 months, MRI showed an intact physis "except for an area approximately 1 cm in diameter located centrally," comprising 6% of the area of the physis, and contiguous with abnormalities in the metaphysis and epiphysis at the site of pin transgression (*arrows*). (**d**) At age 14 years 2 months, the distal tibial physis was completely closed and the left tibia was 15 mm shorter than the right. Surgical physeal arrests were performed on the proximal right tibia and fibula and left distal fibula, using the Block Method and a White osteotome on the tibia. (**e**) At age 16 years 1 month the patient was normally active and asymptomatic. The left tibia was 14 mm shorter than the right. (*Note*: Was this physeal arrest a product of the displaced epiphysis or of the pins? The slow development of the bar, its initial location and size, and the MRI abnormalities adjacent to the early arrest (Fig. 20.4c) favor the pins)

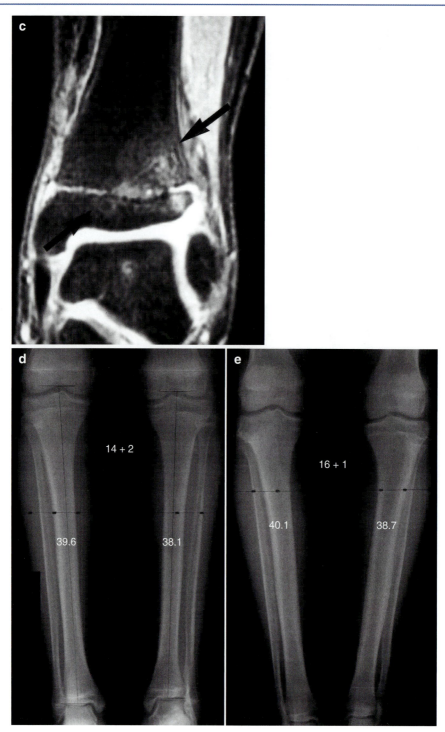

Fig. 20.4 (continued)

20.4 Unintentional Physeal Arrest – Human Involvement

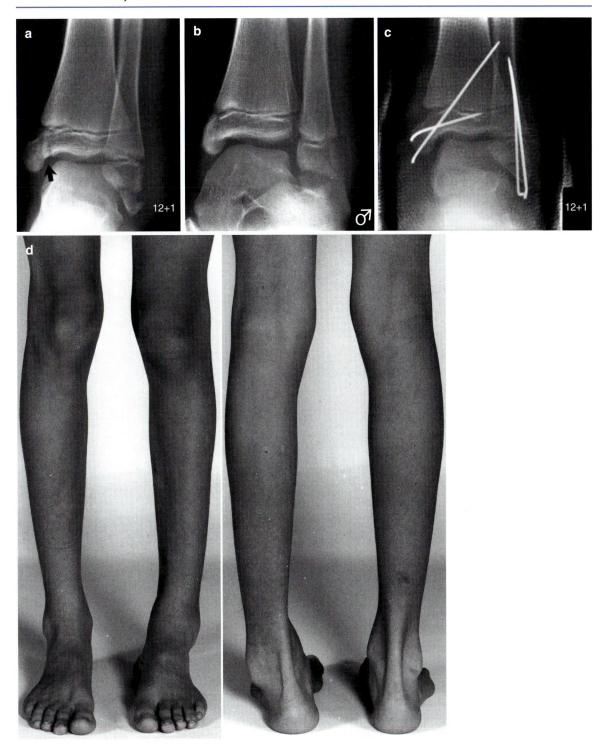

Fig. 20.5 Distal tibial partial physeal arrest associated with a single oblique smooth transphyseal pin. This boy sustained an inversion injury to his left ankle while jumping on a trampoline at age 12 years 1 month. (**a**) There is a fracture of the medial malleolus (*arrow*) which does not appear to involve the physis, and a displaced fracture of the tip of the distal fibular epiphysis. (**b**) A mortise view shows the tibial fracture may involve the peripheral edge of the physis medially, but not the metaphysis. (Peterson type 4 physeal fracture). (**c**) Treatment included open reduction and internal fixation of both fractures using Kirschner wires, one of which crossed the distal tibial physis obliquely. The pins were removed 8 weeks postoperatively. (**d**) At age 14 years 5 months, 2 years 4 months post fracture, ankle varus was obvious both from in front (*left*) and behind (*right*).

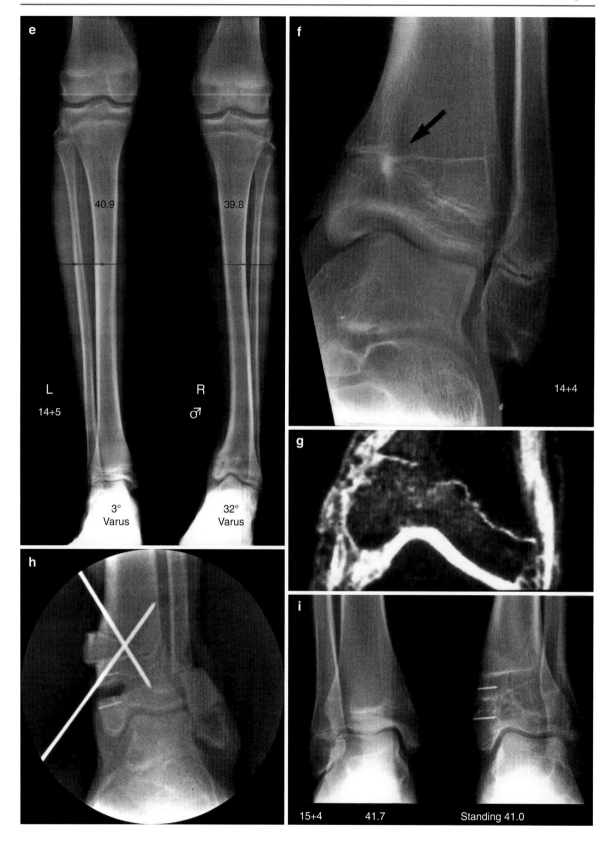

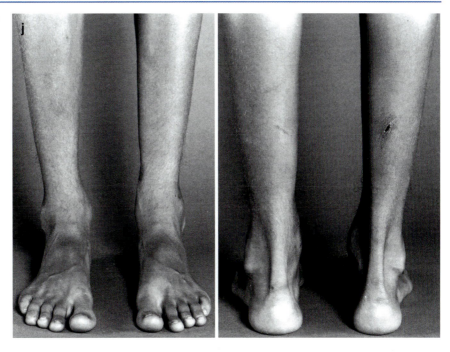

Fig. 20.5 (continued) (**j**) The mild left tibio-talar varus noted roentgenographically on figure **i**. was not noticeable clinically. (*Note*: This fracture could have been treated with one or two pins in the two epiphyseal fragments without the pin crossing the physis)

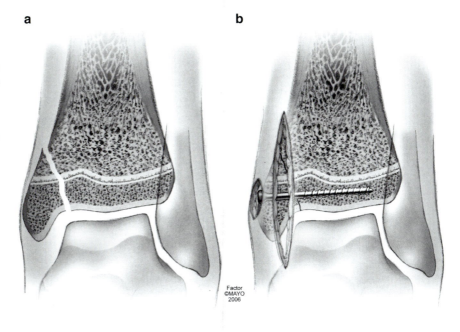

Fig. 20.6 Distal tibial medial malleolus fracture. (**a**) Displaced fragment. (**b**) An anterior incision is used to clean the fracture site of any debris and to visualize anatomic reduction. The screw is inserted percutaneously without crossing the physis (From Peterson [210], with permission)

Fig. 20.5 (continued) (**e**) The left tibia was 11 mm shorter than the right and the tibio-talar varus angle was 32°. (**f**) A close up view of the ankle showed premature partial physeal closure at the site of the traversing pin (*arrows*), not at the periphery which might occur with a peripheral physeal fracture. The lateral side of the distal tibial physis and the distal fibular physis are growing normally, causing ankle varus. (**g**) An MRI confirmed a physeal bar at the pin site. The bar measured 14% of the entire physis on MRI projection technique. (**h**) The bar was excised from the periphery and filled with fat. An osteotomy was held open with iliac crest bone and fixed with crossed Steinmann pins [213]. The fibular closing wedge osteotomy was not internally fixed. At age 14 years 11 months the osteotomies were healed, the metal markers were only 2 mm farther apart and there was mild recurrent ankle varus. Surgical arrests were performed on the distal physes of both fibulae, the right tibia, and the lateral side of the left tibia. (**i**) At age 15 years 4 months all ankle physes were closed. The left tibia was 7 mm shorter than the right and there was mild left tibio-talar varus.

common. The exact cause of the arrest is usually almost impossible to determine and is rarely attributed to the pins. The duration of pin retention is sometimes cited as a factor. One study found that 3 weeks of Kirschner wire fixation was associated with union in 103 of 104 displaced lateral condyle fractures treated by open reduction [236]. At late review (mean 6 years) 28 of 66 of these children (44%) had an abnormally shaped elbow. The value of this report is confirmation that pin retention for 3 weeks was sufficient to achieve union. However, the etiology of the 44% "abnormally shaped elbows" was not specified.

20.4.2.5 Metatarsal

Metatarsal osteotomies are frequently done for foot deformities secondary to clubfoot, skewfoot, and metatarsus adductus. Osteotomy of the proximal base of the first metatarsal is often stabilized with a single longitudinal smooth wire crossing the proximal physis. Premature closure of the physis with significant relative shortening of the great toe may occur, despite the single pin being in the center of the physis (Fig. 20.7) [222, 225, 227, 235]. This may be a problem of the small area of the physis relative to the diameter of the pin. Performing the osteotomy of the first ray only

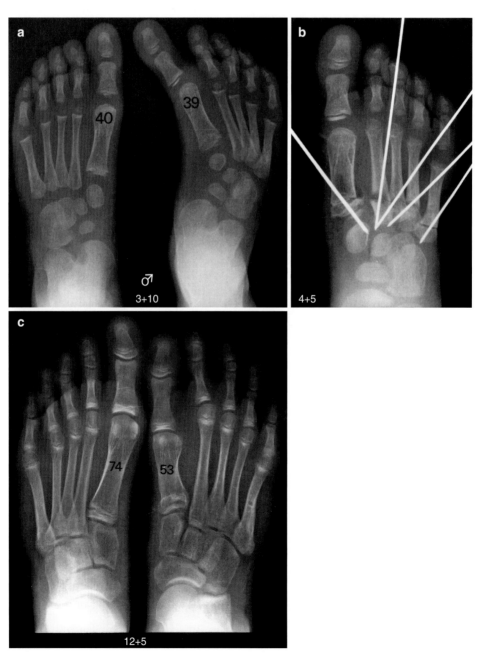

after ossification of the epiphysis at age 5 years or so and the use of a smaller pin may reduce this complication [222]. The relative shortening may be sufficient to warrant metatarsal surgical lengthening [227, 235].

20.4.3 Threaded Pins and Screws

The use of threaded metallic pins and screws to intentionally arrest the physis is discussed in Chap. 10. Threaded implants across the physis are rarely used in trauma care because of their likelihood to cause physeal arrest. Threaded screws which cross the proximal tibial physis to internally fix avulsion fractures of the anterior cruciate ligament have been noted to cause premature partial arrest and genu recurvatum [240, 241].

Proximal femoral derotation osteotomy is used frequently in the treatment of developmental dislocation of the hip (DDH) in young children. Growth disturbance (coxa valga) is common if the top screw of the fixation plate violates the cartilaginous precursor of the greater trochanter [243].

Threaded Steinmann pins used to stabilize a dislocated joint during soft tissue repair should also be avoided (Fig. 20.8) [242].

20.4.4 Cortical Bone Grafts

A single strut of cortical bone taken from the anterior tibial metaphysis and placed across the center of the distal femoral, proximal and distal tibial physes to achieve arthrodesis, did not cause any physis to fuse in two reports [244, 245]. One author concluded that "growth arrest does not occur from a graft passing through the epiphyseal plates at or near the *central area*" [244].

20.4.5 Osteotomy Across the Physis

Multiple types of innominate osteotomies are used in the treatment of developmental dislocation of the hip (DDH). These periacetabuler osteotomies are eponymous and include those of Pemberton, Salter, Chiari, Steele, Ganz, etc. None intend to injure the acetabular physis, but in young children this sometimes occurs leading to premature physeal closure, with subsequent widening of the acetabular wall, a shallow acetabulum, and hip subluxation or dislocation [246–248]. Premature closure is even more likely to occur if the bone graft used to maintain fragment displacement crosses the triradiate cartilage [247]. The extent of deformity depends on the patient's age at injury and the specific triradiate cartilage area involved [247].

Acetabular development and formation of its cup shape and size depends upon the triradiate and acetabular cartilages, the apophyseal rim cartilage, and the pressure of the femoral head [228]. Although the triradiate cartilage does not close until the 15th–18th year, the acetabulum is sufficiently developed by the 11th or 12th year that injury to any of these physes after these ages is unlikely to cause a shallow acetabulum sufficient to result in hip subluxation.

20.4.6 Drilling Across the Physis

Drilling a hole or tunnel across a physis had mixed results regarding damage to the physis in animals (Section 20.3), and had little or no need or use in children until the proliferation of anterior cruciate

Fig. 20.7 First metatarsal complete physeal arrest associated with a perpendicular transphyseal pin. This boy was 3 years 10 months old when he presented with mild toeing in and occasional ache in the right foot. (**a**) There is a typical right skewfoot which was passively correctable. An out flare shoe was worn day and night for 6 months without improvement. The right 1st metatarsal is 1 mm shorter than the left. (**b**) At age 4 years 5 months closing wedge metatarsal osteotomies were performed on the lateral four metatarsals. The 1st metatarsal was treated by an opening wedge osteotomy (bone taken from a closing wedge osteotomy of a lesser metatarsal) and fixed with a 0.062 cm Kirschner wire through the center of the proximal physis. The physis was not exposed or visualized at the time of surgery. The pins were removed 7 weeks post op and the final cast 11 weeks post op. At age 12 years 5 months the patient was normally active and asymptomatic. There was a prominence with thickened skin beneath the right second metatarsal head. There was premature closure of the proximal physis of the right 1st metatarsal which was 21 mm shorter than the left. The physis closed despite the pin being smooth, single, and traversing the physis perpendicularly in its center. Was the size of the pin relative to the area of the physis too great, or did the pin remain in place too long? (*Note*: The position and alignment of mid and hind foot bones is improved)

Fig. 20.8 Physeal arrest associated with a transphyseal threaded Steinmann pin. The left knee of this 2 year 3 month old boy was severely lacerated by a lawn mower. There was disruption of the patellar tendon, joint capsule, and collateral and cruciate ligaments, and comminution of the patella, resulting in complete knee dislocation, but no other bone or cartilage injury. (**a**) The patellar fragments were removed, the ligaments repaired, and joint stability was supplemented by a single longitudinal threaded Steinmann pin. Duration of the Steinmann pin retention is unknown. (**b**) Three years 2 months later, age 5 years 6 months, there was a distal femoral physeal bar at the site of pin penetration (*arrow*) and angular growth of the physis. A proximal tibial physeal bar was developing more slowly (*arrow*). The distal femoral bar was excised at age 5 years 8 months. (**c**) At age 11 years 4 months there was significant leg length inequality, primarily femoral. On scanogram the left leg was 5.2 cm shorter than the right. Treatment included bar excision of the distal left femoral physis, and subsequent femoral lengthening followed by tendon lengthening and skin grafting procedures. (**d**) Photograph at age 14 years 4 months shows improved body alignment and pelvic tilt with persistent leg length discrepancy due to continuing growth of the right leg. (**e**) A scanogram shows a total leg discrepancy of 6.4 cm. A second femoral lengthening was combined with physeal arrest of the distal right femur. The proximal right tibial physis was arrested at age 15 years 7 months. A scanogram at age 17 years 6 months showed the left femur 3 mm longer and the left tibia 3.8 mm shorter than the right, for a combined 3.5 cm limb length discrepancy, treated by shoe lift. Gradual painful degenerative arthritis led to surgical arthrodesis of the knee at age 34 years 11 months. (**f**) At age 37 years 7 months a motorcycle fell on his left leg causing discomfort prompting a visit to the emergency department. A standing roentgenographs showed a well-healed knee fusion with no alteration of the massive metal supports. There are degenerative changes in the left hip and right knee. (**g**) Lateral view at same time as **f**. (*Note*: The initial transphyseal threaded pin (Fig. 20.8a) provided good stability at a time before external fixators were available, facilitating reconstructive soft tissue procedures, (tendon/ligament repair, skin grafting and scar revisions), but caused significant growth impairment. Would a smooth pin have made a difference? Knee instability requiring fusion was probably inevitable, but earlier right femoral and tibial physeal arrests would have helped reduce the final leg length discrepancy. The lesson learned is to avoid placing threaded pins across the physis (From Peterson [223], with permission and additional follow-up))

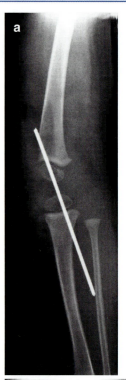

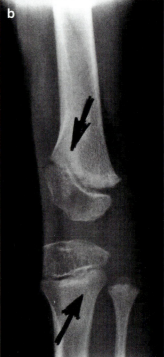

20.4 Unintentional Physeal Arrest – Human Involvement

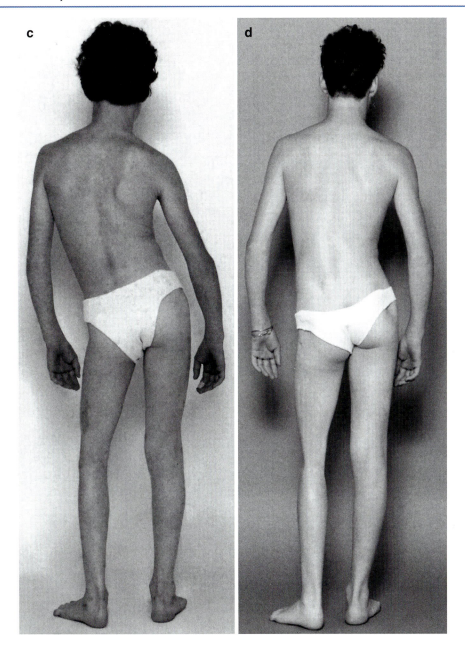

Fig. 20.8 (continued)

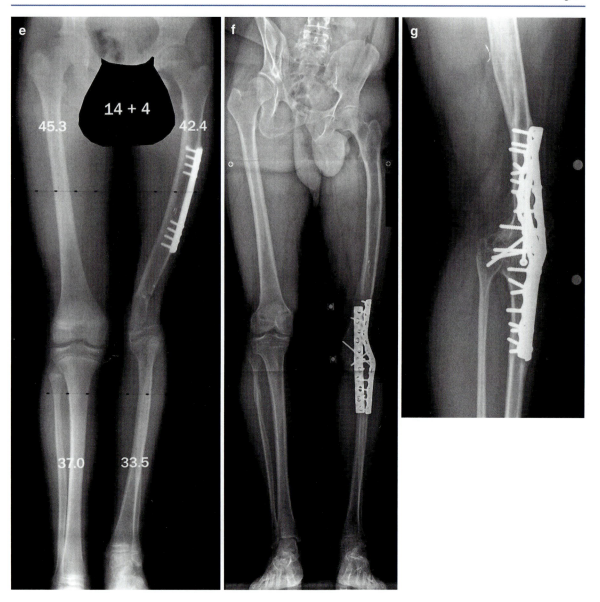

Fig. 20.8 (continued)

ligament (ACL) injuries beginning in the mid 1970s. An increasing number of both young boys and girls participating in more vigorous sports, along with improved clinical examination, diagnostic imaging, and arthroscopy have contributed to a greater awareness of the ACL injury [264, 278, 282, 292, 294, 295, 297]. Although there are no official or complete numbers, orthopedists at leading medical centers estimated in 2008 that several thousand children and young adolescents sustain ACL tears each year, with the numbers increasing recently [278]. Centers that used to see a few cases each year may now see several each week. Girls are more prone to the injury than boys [278, 292, 300]. More than 2,000 articles were written on the ACL in the decade 1993–2003, yet the incidence in the skeletally immature patient population is unknown [259, 297, 300]. A 2002 multi institutional survey found 15 cases of growth arrests producing knee angular deformities and leg length discrepancies due to ACL reconstruction [277]. Based on this data a "guarded approach to ACL reconstruction in the skeletally immature patient" was recommended, with careful attention to technique and follow-up [277].

ACL disruption in children may be due to a midsubstance tear, or to a detachment at either end. A tibial intercondylar eminence fracture with an intact ligament is the most common [270, 272, 273, 281, 285] while avulsion of the ligament from its attachment to the distal femoral epiphysis is rare [260]. One dissenting article recorded many more midsubstance tears than tibial eminence fractures [294]. Fracture of the tibial eminence treated with a screw across the physis results in premature closure of the anterior half of the proximal tibial physis and genu recurvatum [240, 241]. It is best to treat a tibial eminence fracture with a small screw [253, 295, 297] by transosseous suture fixation [253, 264] or by crossed pins [303], all confined within the anterior portion of the tibial epiphysis avoiding the physis. Avulsion of the ACL from its femoral attachment is exceedingly rare. In one 7 year old girl the ACL was successfully reattached to the femoral epiphysis using drill holes and suture entirely within the epiphysis [260]. A similar case in a 3 year old was treated with two 1.8 mm drill holes across the distal femoral epiphysis, physis and metaphysis to secure the avulsed proximal end of the ACL with 0.5 mm looped stainless steel wire [273]. The wire was removed 5 months later. The distal femur grew normally over the next 13 years.

Midsubstance tears of the ACL have been found in children as young as 3 years of age [298], and are rarely amenable to primary repair at any age. Those treated non-operatively frequently develop impaired knee function, giving way episodes, recurrent meniscal tears, and early onset of degenerative arthrosis [249–251, 256, 264, 275, 285, 287, 294, 299]. Long term results are worse in children than in adults [250, 281]. Extra articular reconstructions of ACL midsubstance tears avoid the physis, but have little value in preventing ACL instability or meniscal damage and are of historical interest only [300]. The result of midsubstance ligament repair in children is also poor [263, 264, 270, 282, 295, 297], and generally as poor as they are in adults [253, 263, 264, 272, 285]. Consequently, the primary goal of surgical treatment in adults, restoration of the ACL, is even more important in children [250]. Treatment outcomes have steadily improved with advances in diagnosis, operative techniques, stronger graft fixation, and accelerated rehabilitation. Nevertheless, management of ACL injuries in skeletally immature patients remains a subject of controversy [253, 256, 257, 259, 264, 266, 275, 280, 290, 297, 301], primarily because of the presence of the physes.

In adults the most effective treatment of the symptomatic ACL deficient knee is the anatomic replacement of the ligament with autogenous or allograft tendon or ligament, or with a similar foreign substance. Placement and fixation of the graft in the most anatomical position is achieved by an oblique drill hole beginning in the proximal medial tibial metaphysis extending through the center of the proximal tibial epiphysis, the joint, the distal femoral epiphysis, and exiting in the distal lateral femoral metaphysis. This allows the graft passing through the joint to exit the tibia and enter the femur at the normal sites of attachment of the original ACL. The diameter of the drill hole is usually 8–10 mm. This anatomic replacement provides the best long term stability and is generally successful in adults. However, in a skeletally immature individual the drill hole of this procedure crosses both the distal femur and proximal tibial physes, creating the risk of physeal arrest with subsequent leg length discrepancy or angular deformities.

Reconstruction of the midsubstance ACL disruption in skeletally immature patients has therefore developed into a variety of methods which may be grouped as follows: (a) delay repair until the physis is nearly closed, (b) the femoral *and* tibial transphyseal method, (c) the femoral *or* tibial transphyseal (partial physeal sparing) method, and (d) the complete physeal sparing method. Each method has a variety of technical options. The graft material used as a substitute for ACL reconstruction in children is usually autogenous fascia lata, iliotibial band, or semi tendinosis, gracilis, hamstring, patellar, or Achilles tendon.

20.4.6.1 Delay Repair Until the Physis Is Nearly Closed

This risk of iatrogenic surgical bone growth disturbance causes many pediatric orthopedists to advocate non-operative treatment with bracing and activity modification, postponing the surgical repair until at least 13 years of age in females or 14 years of age in males, or shortly before or after physeal closure [255, 256, 259, 264, 266, 271, 272, 288, 295, 301, 302]. This is feasible only when the patient and parents are willing to forgo athletic pursuits until the physes is closed. Absolute activity restriction is key to decreasing the risk of additional knee injuries [301]. However, low patient adherence to activity modification and bracing at this age leads to increased risk of ACL instability, meniscal and chondral injury and premature degenerative arthritis [256, 266, 272, 280, 282, 285, 294, 295].

20.4.6.2 Tibial *and* Femoral Transphyseal Method

The transarticular grafting method (used in adults, above) in children crosses both the distal femoral and proximal tibial physes. Case reports [277, 279] and animal studies [267, 289] showing iatrogenic growth disturbance after drilling and repair through both physes discouraged surgeons from universal acceptance of this method in younger skeletally immature patients. Graphs have even been developed to predict the amount of shortening and angular deformity to expect after repair [299]. Nevertheless, this method has been used successfully in older children without causing physeal arrest (Fig. 20.9) [249, 261, 285, 290, 293, 294], even in children as young as 9 years [265]. One study of 10 patients with mean age 14 years 6 months, showed narrowing of the growth plates, corticalization around the graft, early closure of the physis, but no limb length discrepancies or angular deformities [270]. Another study of 8 patients with average age of 14 years 9 months had hamstring tendon placed through 7–9 mm drill holes with no identifiable premature physeal arrest [284]. There have been no clinical trials reporting the incidence or sequelae of transphyseal ACL reconstructions in patients with bone age of 10 years or less, who would have significant growth remaining.

Two animal studies address the use of transphyseal ligament reconstruction and the issue of a transphyseal tunnel filled with a graft. In one study 5/32 in. drill holes across the distal femoral and proximal tibial physes of dogs resulted in a bony bridge as early as 2 weeks [296]. However, if the tunnels were completely filled with fascia lata no bone bridge developed and growth continued normally. In a second study in rabbits, drill holes across the distal femoral physis filled with tendon developed tubular bone bridges surrounding the tendon [181]. The size of the bridge varied from a peripheral rim of bone surrounding the graft, to bone bridges occupying two thirds of the width of the drill tunnel [181]. This suggests that the diameter of the bone tunnel was larger than that of the graft.

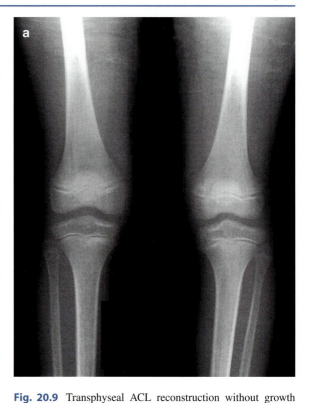

Fig. 20.9 Transphyseal ACL reconstruction without growth arrest. This 11 year 0 month old boy injured his right knee playing kickball. Knee swelling gradually resided but giving way (subluxation) persisted. He was of small stature and had 3+ Lachman, 2+ pivot shift, and positive drawer tests. (**a**) Knee roentgenograms were normal. The treating physician felt the risk of physeal arrest with surgical treatment was less than the risk of additional knee damage with subluxation episodes. (**b**) At age 11 years 1 month endoscopic semitendinosis-gracilis ACL reconstruction was performed. A 7 mm diameter drill hole crossing the center of the proximal tibial (*left*) and distal femoral physis (*right*), was combined with medial meniscus repair and partial menisectomy of a lateral discoid meniscus. The *arrows* mark the physes. The semitendinosis and gracilis tendons measuring 26 cm in length were harvested, doubled, sutured together, and easily fit through a 7 mm sizing cylinder before placing it through the tunnels. The graft was tensioned to 20 lb as it was secured at both ends with metallic devices. (**c**) Arthroscopic visualization of the graft entering the femoral tunnel. Tension on the graft was excellent when tested with a probe. A more snug fit of the graft within the tunnel would reduce the chance of physeal bar formation. (**d**) Three weeks after surgery, age 11 years 2 months, a baseline scanogram showed the right lower extremity 4 mm longer than the left. (**e**) One year post operative, age 12 years 1 month, both the distal femoral physes are open and have grown as shown by the growth arrest lines. There is no physeal bar. The distance between the metallic anchoring devices was increased and the graft in the tunnel has not turned to bone. Assuming the graft is still intact within the bone and has not increased in length, will growth of the physes cause sufficient increased tension on the graft to compress the physis and impair growth?

20.4 Unintentional Physeal Arrest – Human Involvement

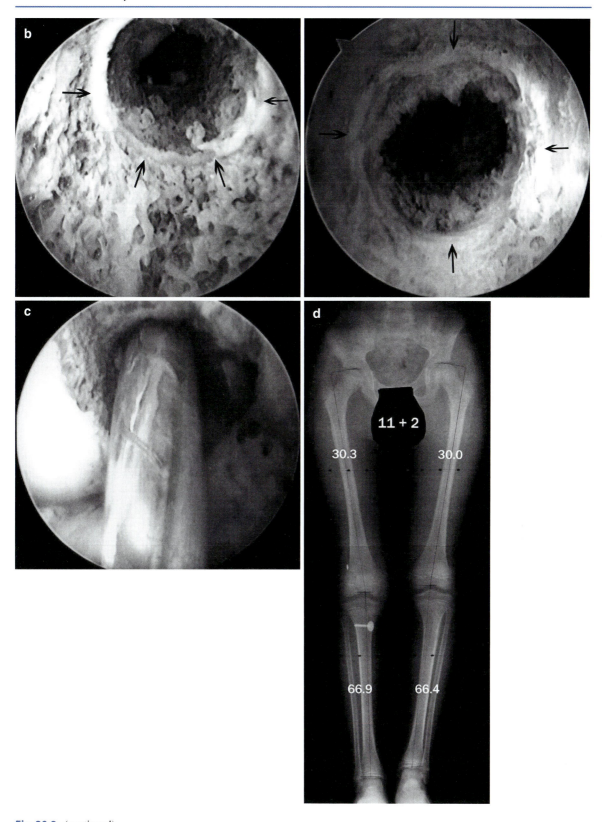

Fig. 20.9 (continued)

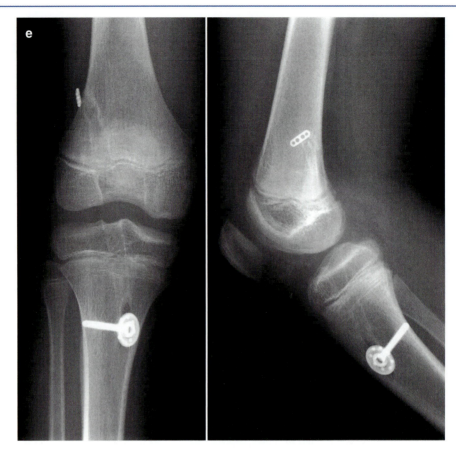

Fig. 20.9 (continued)

20.4.6.3 Tibial *or* Femoral Transphyseal Method (Partial Physeal Sparing)

Partial physeal sparing is accomplished by routing the graft through a tunnel crossing the tibial metaphysis, physis, and epiphysis, but coursing the graft obliquely proximally and posteriorly between the femoral condyles to attach to the distal femoral metaphysis posteriorly (sparing the distal femoral physis) [253, 258, 259, 281–283, 297, 302], or by routing the graft through the tibial epiphysis (sparing the proximal tibial physis) and the physis of the femur [268]. Physeal arrest should be less common with femoral *or* tibial transphyseal techniques than with femoral *and* tibial transphyseal techniques.

Careful attention to technical details during ACL reconstruction in children is essential. During femoral over the top placement or tunnel placement, dissection, notching or aggressive notch-plasty around the posterolateral aspect of the physis should be avoided [276]. On the tibial side care should be taken to avoid injury to the tibial tubercle apophysis. Any fixation device must not involve the physis.

With any transphyseal technique, factors influencing potential physeal closure include tunnel location (central vs. peripheral), tunnel size relative to the cross-sectional area of the physis (<5% of cross-sectional area of the physis is better), tunnel inclination across the physis (perpendicular is better than oblique), and perhaps most important is to have the graft completely fill the tunnel. If blood can be excluded from the tunnel the likelihood of developing a physeal bar is essentially eliminated. A tight fitting graft acts like an interposition material used during physeal bar excision.

Another potential cause of physeal injury in a young child is excessive tension by the graft across the physis. As the physes grows increasing tension on the graft could theoretically produce compression of the physes and cause growth arrest. Significant valgus deformity of the distal femur and varus deformity of the proximal tibia were found in dogs with no radiographic or histologic evidence of physeal bar formation [262]. The observed deformities were felt to be a result of reduced physeal growth tethered by the tensioned graft, rather than premature physeal closure. Could the tension of an ACL graft in a young child gradually increase due to growth sufficiently to compress the physis and cause deformity (Fig. 20.9)?

20.4.6.4 Complete Physeal Sparing Method

Complete physeal sparing was first accomplished by routing medial hamstring or semitendinosis tendons still attached distally to the proximal tibial metaphysis, anterior to the proximal tibial epiphysis, obliquely and proximally through the joint, coursing between the femoral condyles posteriorly, and attached to the distal femoral metaphysis. Thus, the graft passes anterior to the proximal tibial physis and posterior to the distal femoral physis [253, 257, 259, 282, 295, 297]. Care should be taken to avoid dissection or notching of the physis (anterior tibial or posterior femoral) during graft placement to avoid injury to the perichondral ring and subsequent deformity [277]. Or the graft can be placed through a tunnel in the proximal tibial epiphysis avoiding the physis and posterior to the distal femoral physis attaching to the distal femoral metaphysis [271, 281, 288, 295]. Another variation imbedded the graft into the proximal tibial epiphysis with a screw avoiding the physis [274]. The graft was then attached to the distal femoral metaphysis posteriorly. Still another variation routed the iliotibial band around the lateral side of the lateral femoral condyle and back anteriorly through the femoral notch, over the top of the tibial physis anteriorly to attach medial to the tibial tubercle [275, 286].

Both the partial and the complete physeal sparing methods (c and d, above) have been successful in avoiding physeal arrest most of the time [253, 269, 286, 302]. Unfortunately neither of these methods provide anatomic isometry [250, 297], and the long term results are marginal to poor.

This resulted in the development of a complete physeal sparing technique with tunnels in both the proximal tibial and distal femoral epiphyses, neither of which cross the physis [250, 251]. The position of the graft within the joint is anatomic and attaches to both the distal femoral and the proximal tibial epiphyses at their normal sites within the joint. However, this technique is technically demanding, has a 0–2 mm margin of error for growth plate contact, and should be performed only by accomplished knee surgeons [250, 291]. The smallest appropriate drill is used over guide wires to achieve a tight fit of the graft. The position of the intraepiphyseal tunnels is critical in avoiding intraarticular graft impingement and physeal arrest [252, 254]. Precise tunnel placement is enhanced by arthroscopy and intraoperative fluoroscopic imaging, 3-D imaging and navigation, or a dedicated pediatric guide set to counteract this small margin of error. This technique has been performed in prepubescent patients with efficacy and relative safety [250]. An alternative is to route the graft through a tunnel in the proximal tibial epiphysis (avoiding the physis) attaching to the distal femoral epiphysis with a staple [268]. Staples must be placed well away from the physis [283].

20.4.6.5 Author's Perspective

Since nonsurgical treatment of ACL disruption in children is prone to increasing instability and degenerative changes, treatment predicated on assessment of maturity is indicated. The ideal treatment for young children, for example girls under age 13 years and boys under age 14 years, is the complete physeal sparing method with drill holes in both the femoral and tibial epiphyses, neither of which cross the physis [250–252]. This gives the most anatomic repair without risk of premature physeal closure. This technique requires precision and ideally would be done by someone who has had special training in the technique and uses it often. After age 13 in girls and 14 in boys, anatomic reconstruction of the ACL crossing the physes is unlikely to cause a significant growth problem, particularly if the size of the tunnel and the graft are equal. No technique placing screws or bone plugs across the physis should be used.

20.5 Unintentional Physeal Arrest – Animal Involvement

Although I did not search the veterinary literature diligently, two disparate articles came to my attention. Distal femoral physeal fractures in 21 dogs and cats treated with intramedullary transphyseal smooth Steinmann pins all had physeal arrest irrespective of the technique or the animals' age [304]. However, proximal tibial type 2 physeal fractures in three horses all less than 3 weeks old treated with transphyseal screws removed 50–60 days later, did not develop physeal arrest [305].

References

Intentional Irreversible Physeal Arrest – Humans

1. Howorth B (1966) Slipping of the capital femoral epiphysis. History. Clin Orthop Relat Res 48:11–32
2. Key JA (1926) Epiphyseal coxa vara or displacement of the capital epiphysis of the femur in adolescence. J Bone Joint Surg 8:53–117
3. Wilson PD (1924) Displacement of upper epiphysis of femur treated by open reduction. JAMA 83(22):1749–1756

Physeal Arrest to Curtail Slipping of an Epiphysis: Transphyseal Bone Graft Physiodesis

4. Aadalen RJ, Weiner DS, Hoyt W, Herndon CH (1974) Acute slipped capital femoral epiphysis. J Bone Joint Surg 56A(7): 1473–1487
5. Adamczyk MJ, Weiner DS, Hawk D (2003) A 50-year experience with bone graft epiphysiodesis in the treatment of slipped capital femoral epiphysis. J Pediatr Orthop 23(5): 578–583
6. Crawford AH (1989) The role of osteotomy in the treatment of slipped capital femoral epiphysis, Chapter 22. AAOS Instructional Course Lectures 38:281–290
7. Ferguson AB, Howorth MB (1931) Slipping of the upper femoral epiphysis: a study of seventy cases. J Am Med Assn 97(25):1867–1872
8. Herndon CH (1972) Treatment of minimally slipped upper femoral epiphysis, Chapter 19. AAOS Instructional Course Lectures 21 : 188–196
9. Herndon CH (1972) Treatment of severely slipped upper femoral epiphysis by means of osteoplasty and epiphyseodesis, Chapter 22. AAOS Instructional Course Lectures 21: 214–221
10. Herndon CH, Heyman CH, Bell DM (1963) Treatment of slipped capital femoral epiphysis by epiphyseodesis and osteoplasty of the femoral neck: a report of further experiences. J Bone Joint Surg 45A(5):999–1012
11. Heyman CH, Herndon CH (1954) Epiphyseodesis for early slipping of the upper femoral epiphysis. J Bone Joint Surg 36A(3):539–555
12. Howorth B (1951) Slipping of the upper femoral epiphysis, Chapter 19. AAOS Instructional Course Lectures 8:306–317
13. Howorth B: Slipping of the upper femoral epiphysis, (Chap 15). Clin Orthop 10 : 148–173, 1957.
14. Howorth B (1966) The bone-pegging operation: for slipping of the capital femoral epiphysis. Clin Orthop 48:79–87
15. Howorth MB (1963) Slipping of the capital femoral epiphysis. J Bone Joint Surg 45A(8):1776
16. Howorth MB (1949) Slipping of the upper femoral epiphysis. J Bone Joint Surg 31A(4):734–747
17. Howorth MB (1941) Slipping of the upper femoral epiphysis. Surg Gynecol Obstet 73:723–732
18. Melby A, Hoyt WA Jr, Weiner DS (1980) Treatment of chronic slipped capital femoral epiphysis by bone-graft epiphyseodesis. J Bone Joint Surg 62A(1):119–125
19. Rao SB, Crawford AH, Burger RR, Roy DR (1996) Open bone peg epiphysiodesis for slipped capital femoral epiphysis. J Pediatr Orthop 16(1):37–48
20. Schmidt TL, Cimino WG, Seidel FG (1996) Allograft epiphysiodesis for slipped capital femoral epiphysis. Clin Orthop 322:61–76
21. Ward WT, Wood K (1990) Open bone graft epiphyseodesis for slipped capital femoral epiphysis. J Pediatr Orthop 10(1): 14–20
22. Weiner DS (1989) Bone graft epiphysiodesis in the treatment of slipped capital femoral epiphysis, Chapter 21. AAOS Instructional Course Lectures 38 : 263–272
23. Weiner DS (1998) Bone-peg epiphysiodesis: letters to the Editors. J Pediatr Orthop 18(1):136
24. Weiner DS, Weiner SD, Melby A (1988) Anterolateral approach to the hip for bone graft epiphysiodesis in the treatment of slipped capital femoral epiphysis. J Pediatr Orthop 8(3):349–352
25. Weiner DS, Weiner S, Melby A, Hoyt WA Jr (1984) A 30-year experience with bone graft epiphysiodesis in the treatment of slipped capital femoral epiphysis. J Pediatr Orthop 4(2):145–152

Transphyseal Metal Pins

26. Aronson DD, Carlson WE (1985) Single screw fixation for slipped capital femoral epiphysis. Orthop Trans 9:497
27. Badgley CE, Isaacson AS, Wolgamot JC, Miller JW (1948) Operative therapy for slipped upper femoral epiphysis: an end-result study. J Bone Joint Surg 30A(1):19–30
28. Baynham GC, Lucie RS, Cummings RJ (1992) Femoral neck fracture secondary to in situ pinning of slipped capital femoral epiphysis: a previously unreported complication. J Pediatr Orthop 11(2):187–190
29. Bianco AJ (1966) Treatment of slipping of the capital femoral epiphysis. Clin Orthop 48:103–110
30. Blanco JS, Taylor B, Johnston CE II (1992) Comparison of single pin versus multiple pin fixation in treatment of slipped capital femoral epiphysis. J Pediatr Orthop 12(3):384–389
31. Boero S, Brunenghi GM, Carbone M, Stella G, Calevo MG (2003) Pinning in slipped capital femoral epiphysis: long-term follow-up study. J Pediatr Orthop B 12(6): 372–379

References

32. Boyd HB (1972): Treatment of acute slipped upper femoral epiphysis, Chapter 23. AAOS Instructional Course Lectures 21: 222–223
33. Boyd HB (1972) Treatment of minimally slipped upper femoral epiphysis, Chapter 18. AAOS Instructional Course Lectures 21: 186–187
34. Boyd HB, Ingram AJ, Bourkard HO (1949) The treatment of slipped femoral epiphysis. South Med J 42(7):551–560
35. Boyer DW, Mickelson MR, Ponseti IV (1981) Slipped capital femoral epiphysis: long-term follow-up study of one hundred and twenty-one patients. J Bone Joint Surg 63A(1):85–95
36. Cameron HU, Wang M, Koreska J (1978) Internal fixation of slipped femoral capital epiphyses. Clin Orthop 137:148–153
37. Canale, TS (1989) Problems and complications of slipped capital femoral epiphysis, Chapter 23. AAOS Instructional Course Lectures 38: 281–290
38. Carlioz H, Vogt JC, Barba L, Doursounian L (1984) Treatment of slipped upper femoral epiphysis: 80 cases operated on over 10 years (1968–1978). J Pediatr Orthop 4(2):153–161
39. Carney BT, Weinstein SL, Noble J (1991) Long-term follow-up of slipped capital femoral epiphysis. J Bone Joint Surg 73A(5):667–674
40. Clark CR, Southwick WO, Ogden JA (1980) Anatomic aspects of slipped capital femoral epiphysis and correction by biplane osteotomy, Part 4. AAOS Instructional Course Lectures 27: 90–100
41. Clarke NMP, Harrison MHM (1986) Slipped upper femoral epiphysis: a potential for spontaneous recovery. J Bone Joint Surg 68B(4):541–544
42. Compere CL (1950) Correction of deformity and prevention of aseptic necrosis in late cases of slipped femoral epiphysis. J Bone Joint Surg 32A(5):351–362
43. Crawford AH (1988) Slipped capital femoral epiphysis: current concepts review. J Bone Joint Surg 70A(9):1422–1427
44. Crawford AH, Rao SG, Roy DR (1998) Bone –peg epiphysiodesis: letter to the editors. J Pediatr Orthop 18(1):136–137
45. Dunn DM (1964) The treatment of adolescent slipping of the upper femoral epiphysis. J Bone Joint Surg 46B(4):621–629
46. Dunn DM, Angel JC (1978) Replacement of the femoral head by open operation in severe adolescent slipping of the upper femoral epiphysis. J Bone Joint Surg 60B(3):394–403
47. Durbin FC (1960) Treatment of slipped upper femoral epiphysis. J Bone Joint Surg 42B(2):289–302
48. Fahey JJ, O'Brien ET (1965) Acute slipped capital femoral epiphysis: review of the literature and report of ten cases. J Bone Joint Surg 57A(6):1105–1127
49. Fish JB (1984) Cuneiform osteotomy of the femoral neck in the treatment of slipped capital femoral epiphysis. J Bone Joint Surg 66A(8):1153–1168
50. Gage JR, Sundberg AB, Nolan DR, Sletten RG, Winter RB (1978) Complications after cuneiform osteotomy for moderately or severely slipped capital femoral epiphysis. J Bone Joint Surg 60A(2):157–165
51. Ghormley RK, Fairchild RD (1940) The diagnosis and treatment of slipped epiphyses. JAMA 114(3):229–235
52. Greenough CG, Bromage JD, Jackson AM (1985) Pinning of the slipped upper femoral epiphysis – a trouble-free procedure? J Pediatr Orthop 5(6):657–660
53. Hall JE (1957) The results of treatment of slipped femoral epiphysis. J Bone Joint Surg 39B(4):659–673
54. Irani RN, Rosenzweig AH, Cotler HB, Schwentker EP (1985) Epiphysiodesis in slipped capital femoral epiphysis: a comparison of various surgical modalities. J Pediatr Orthop 5(6):661–664
55. Ireland J, Newman PH (1978) Triplane osteotomy for severely slipped upper femoral epiphysis. J Bone Joint Surg 60B(3):390–393
56. Jacobs B (1972) Chondrolysis after epiphyseolysis, Chapter 24. AAOS Instructional Course Lectures 21: 224–226
57. Jacobs B (1972) Treatment of severly slipped upper femoral epiphysis by wedge osteotomy, Chapter 20. AAOS Instructional Course Lectures 21: 197–199
58. Klein A, Joplin RJ, Reidy JA, Hanelin J (1949) Roentgenographic changes in nailed slipped capital femoral epiphysis. J Bone Joint Surg 31A(1):1–22
59. Klein A, Joplin RJ, Reidy JA, Hanelin J (1952) Slipped capital femoral epiphysis: early diagnosis and treatment facilitated by "normal" roentgenograms. J Bone Joint Surg 34A(1):233–239
60. Koval KJ, Lehman WB, Rose D, Koval RP, Grant A, Strongwater A (1989) Treatment of slipped capital femoral epiphysis with a cannulated-screw technique. J Bone Joint Surg 71A(9):1370–1377
61. Kramer WG, Craig WA, Noel S (1976) Compensating osteotomy at the base of the femoral neck for slipped capital femoral epiphysis. J Bone Joint Surg 58A(6):796–800
62. Kulick RG (1982) A retrospective study of 125 cases of slipped capital femoral epiphysis. Clin Orthop 162:87–90
63. Kumm DA, Lee SH, Hackenbroch MH, Rütt J (2001) Slipped capital femoral epiphysis: a prospective study of dynamic screw fixation. Clin Orthop 384:198–207
64. Laplaza FJ, Burke SW (1995) Epiphyseal growth after pinning of slipped capital femoral epiphysis. J Pediatr Orthop 15(3):357–361
65. Lehman WB, Grant A, Rose D, Pugh J, Norman A (1984) A method of evaluating possible pin penetration in slipped capital femoral epiphysis using a cannulated internal fixation device. Clin Orthop 186:65–70
66. Lehman WB, Menche D, Grant A, Norman A, Pugh J (1982) The problem of in situ pinning of slipped capital femoral epiphysis. Orthop Trans 6(3):380
67. Lehman WB, Menche D, Grant A, Norman A, Pugh J (1984) The problem of evaluating in situ pinning of slipped capital femoral epiphysis: an experimental model and a review of 63 consecutive case. J Pediatr Orthop 4(3):297–303
68. MacEwen GD (1948) Advantages and disadvantages of pin fixation in slipped capital femoral epiphysis, Part III. AAOS Instructional Course Lectures 29: 86–90.
69. Martin PH (1948) Slipped epiphysis in the adolescent hip: a reconsideration of open reduction. J Bone Joint Surg 30A(1):9–19

70. Moss J, Zuelzer W, Nogi J (1982) Slipped capital femoral epiphysis: a review of treatment and complications. Orthop Trans 6(3):380
71. Newman PH (1960) The surgical treatment of slipping of the upper femoral epiphysis. J Bone Joint Surg 42B(2): 280–288
72. O'Beirne J, McLoughlin R, Dowling F, Fogarty E, Regan B (1989) Slipped upper femoral epiphysis: internal fixation using single central pins. J Pediatr Orthop 9(3):304–307
73. O'Brien ET, Fahey JJ (1977) Remodeling of the femoral neck after in situ pinning for slipped capital femoral epiphysis. J Bone Joint Surg 59A(1):62–68
74. Parsch K, Zehender H, Bühl T, Weller S (1999) Intertrochanteric corrective osteotomy for moderate and severe chronic slipped capital femoral epiphysis. J Pediatr Orthop 8(3):223–230, Part B
75. Pearl AJ, Woodward B, Kelly RP (1961) Cuneiform osteotomy in the treatment of slipped capital femoral epiphysis. J Bone Joint Surg 43A(7):947–954
76. Rao JP, Francis AM, Siwek CW (1984) The treatment of chronic slipped capital femoral epiphysis by biplane osteotomy. J Bone Joint Surg 66A(8):1169–1174
77. Riley PM, Weiner DS, Gillespie R, Weiner SC (1990) Hazards of internal fixation in the treatment of slipped capital femoral epiphysis. J Bone Joint Surg 72A(10):1500–1509
78. Schmidt R, Gregg JR (1985) Subtrochanteric fractures complicating pin fixation of slipped capital femoral epiphysis. Orthop Trans 9:497
79. Schnute WJ (1958) Slipped capital femoral epiphysis. Clin Orthop 11:63–80
80. Segal LS, Davidson RS, Robertson WW Jr, Drummond DS (1991) Growth disturbances of the proximal femur after pinning of juvenile slipped capital femoral epiphysis. J Pediatr Orthop 11(5):631–637
81. Siegel DB, Kasser JR, Sponseller P, Gelberman RH (1991) Slipped capital femoral epiphysis: a quantitative analysis of motion, gait, and femoral remodeling after insitu fixation. J Bone Joint Surg 73A(5):659–666
82. Southwick WO (1967) Osteotomy through the lesser trochanter for slipped capital femoral epiphysis. J Bone Joint Surg 49A(5):807–835
83. Sturrock CA (1894) The after results of simple separation of epiphyses. Edinburg Hosp Rep 2:598–604
84. Thawrani D, Feldman D (February 4, 2011) Current practice in the management of slipped capital femoral epiphysis. POSNA e-mail
85. Vresilovic EJ, Spingler KP, Robertson WW Jr, Davidson RS, Drummond DS (1990) Failures of pin removal after in situ pinning of slipped capital femoral epiphyses: a comparison of different pin types. J Pediatr Orthop 10(6):764–768
86. Waldenström H (1940) Slipping of the upper femoral epiphysis. Surg Gynecol Obstet 71:198–210
87. Wiberg G (1959) Considerations on the surgical treatment of slipped epiphysis with special reference to nail fixation. J Bone Joint Surg 41A(2):253–261
88. Wilson PD (1938) The treatment of slipping of the upper femoral epiphysis with minimal displacement. J Bone Joint Surg 20(2):379–397
89. Wilson PD, Jacobs B, Schecter L (1965) Slipped femoral capital epiphysis: an end-result study. J Bone joint Surg 47(6):1128–1145
90. Wojciechowski P, Tokarowski A, Kusz D, Pasierbek M (1996) Growth disturbances after A-O cancellous screw head-neck transfixation for slipped femoral epiphysis [Polish]. Chir Narzadow Ruchu I Ortopedia Polska 61(4): 379–384
91. Wong-Chung J, Strong ML (1991) Physeal remodeling after internal fixation of slipped capital femoral epiphyses. J Pediatr Orthop 11(1):2–5
92. Zahrawi FB, Stephens TL, Spencer GE Jr, Clough JM (1983) Comparative study of pinning in situ and open epiphysiodesis in 105 patients with slipped capital femoral epiphyses. Clin Orthop 177:160–168

Immediate Irreversible Physeal Arrest
Introduction

93. Birch JG, Herring JA, Wenger DR (1984) Surgical anatomy of selected physes. J Pediatr Orthop 4(2):224–231
94. Blount WP (1960) Unequal leg length. AAOS Instructional Course Lectures 17: 218–245
95. Green WT, Anderson M (1951) Discrepancy in length of the lower extremities, Chapter 18. AAOS Instructional Course Lectures 8: 294–305
96. Guille JT, Yamazaki A, Bowen JR (1997) Physeal surgery: indications and operative treatment. Am J Orthop 26(5): 323–332
97. Johnston II CE, Bueche MJ, Williamson B, Birch JG (1992) Epiphysiodesis for management of lower limb deformities, Chapter 50. AAOS Instructional Course Lectures 41:: 437–444
98. Little DG, Nigo L, Aiona MC (1996) Deficiencies of current methods for the timing of epiphysiodesis. J Pediatr Orthop 16(2):173–179
99. Siffert RS (1987) Lower limb-length discrepancy: current concepts review. J Bone Joint Surg 69A(7): 1100–1106
100. Vom Saal F (1939) Epiphysiodesis combined with amputation. J Bone Joint Surg 21(2):442–443

The Block Method

101. Beals RK (1991) The treatment of ankle valgus by surface epiphysiodesis. Clin Orthop 266:162–169
102. Beals RK, Shea M (2005) Correlation of chronological age and bone age with correction of ankle valgus by surface epiphysiodesis of the distal medial tibial physis. J Pediatr Orthop B 14(6):436–438
103. Blair VP III, Walker SJ, Sheridan JJ, Schoenecker PL (1982) Epiphysiodesis: a problem of timing. J Pediatr Orthop 2(3):281–284
104. Bowen JR, Leahey JL, Zhang Z, MacEwen GD (1985) Partial epiphysiodesis at the knee to correct angular deformity. Clin Orthop 198:184–190

105. Bowen JR, Torres RR, Forlin E (1992) Partial epiphysiodesis to address genu varum or genu valgum. J Pediatr Orthop 12(3):359–364
106. Eckardt A, Karbowski A, Schwitalle M (1997) Epiphysiodesis as a procedure for correcting leg length discrepancy (abstr). J Bone Joint Surg 79B(Supp II):264
107. Ferrick MR, Birch JG, Albright M (2004) Correction of non-Blount's angular knee deformity by permanent hemiepiphysiodesis. J Pediatr Orthop 24(4):397–404
108. Green WT, Anderson M (1957) Epiphyseal arrest for the correction of discrepancies in length of the lower extremities. J Bone Joint Surg 39A(4):853–872
109. Green WT, Anderson M (1947) Experiences with epiphyseal arrest in correcting discrepancies in length of the lower extremities in infantile paralysis. J Bone Joint Surg 29(3):659–674
110. Green WT, Anderson M (1960): Skeletal age and the control of bone growth. AAOS Instructional Course Lectures 17:119–217
111. Henderson RC, Kemp GJ, Greene WB (1992) Adolescent tibia vara: alternatives for operative treatment. J Bone Joint Surg 74A(3):342–350
112. Hodgen JT, Frantz CH (1946) Arrest of growth of the epiphyses. Arch Surg 53(6):664–674
113. Högberg N, Lidström A (1957) Aspects of epiphyseodesis. Acta Orthop Scandinav 27(1):69–77
114. Karaharju EO, Raunio PV (1970) Clinical experience of epiphyeal arrest of the lower extremities. Acta Orthop Scand 41:565–571
115. Mayhall WST (1978) Leg length discrepancy treated by epiphyseodesis: a 37-year experience. Orthop Rev 7(4): 41–44
116. Menelaus MB (1966) Correction of leg length discrepancy by epiphysial arrest. J Bone Joint Surg 48B(2):336–339
117. Menelaus MB (1981) The growth plate: proceedings and reports of universities, colleges, councils and associations. J Bone Joint Surg 63B(3):475
118. Nordentoft EL (1964) Radiological assessment of the function of the epiphyseal plates (abstr). J Bone Joint Surg 46B(3):572–573
119. Phemister DF (1933) Operative arrestment of longitudinal growth of bones in the treatment of deformities. J Bone Joint Surg 15(1):1–15
120. Plaschaert VFP, van der Eijken JW, Odink RJH, Delemarre HA, Caron JJ (1997) Bilateral epiphysiodesis around the knee as treatment for excessive height in boys. J Pediatr Orthop B 6(2):212–214
121. Porat S, Peyser A, Robin GC (1991) Equalization of lower limbs by epiphysiodesis: results in treatment. J Pediatr Orthop 11(4):442–448
122. Regan JM, Chatterton CC (1946) Deformities following surgical epiphyseal arrest. J Bone Joint Surg 28(20): 265–272
123. Stamp WG, Lansche WE (1960) Treatment of discrepancy in leg length. South Med J 53:764–774
124. Stephens DC, Herrick W, MacEwen GD (1978) Epiphysiodesis for limb length inequality: results and indications. Clin Orthop 136:41–48
125. Straub LR, Thompson TC, Wilson PD (1945) The results of epiphyseodesis and femoral shortening in relation to equalization of limb length. J Bone Joint Surg 27(2):254–266
126. Synder M, Harcke HT, Bowen JR, Caro PA (1994) Evaluation of physeal behavior in response to epiphyseodesis with the use of serial magnetic resonance imaging. J Bone Joint Surg 76A(2):224–229
127. White JW (1949) Leg – length discrepancy. In: AAOS Instr Course Lecturer, VI, CV Mosby Co., St. Louis, pp 201-211.
128. White JW, Stubbins SG Jr (1944) Growth arrest for equalizing leg lengths. JAMA 126(18):1146–1149
129. White JW, Warner WP (1938) Experiences with metaphyseal growth arrests. South Med J 31(4):411–414
130. Wilson PD, Thompson TC (1939) A clinical consideration of the methods of equalizing leg length. Ann Surg 110(6):992–1015
131. Zimbler S, Nehme AE, Raimondo L, Stephen LL, Chorney GS, Craig CL (1988) Correction of leg length discrepancy: Use of epiphysiodesis (Tufts experience). In: Uhthoff HK, Wiley JJ (eds) Behavior growth plate. Raven, New York, pp 223–232

The Trough Method

132. McCarroll HR, Costen W (1960) Attempted treatment of scoliosis by unilateral vertebral epiphyseal arrest. J Bone Joint Surg 42A:965–978

Fluoroscopic Assisted Physeal Ablation

133. Atar D, Lehman WB, Grant AD, Strongwater A (1990) A simplified method for percutaneous epiphysiodesis. Orthop Rev 19(4):358–359
134. Atar D, Lehman WB, Grant AD, Strongwater A (1991) Percutaneous epiphysiodesis. J Bone Joint Surg 73B(1):173
135. Bernard RSJ, Craviari T, Muller C (1997) The treatment of inequality of lower limb length by percutaneous epiphysiodesis: a review of 64 cases (abstr). J Bone Joint Surg 79B(Supp IV):30
136. Bowen JR, Johnson WJ (1984) Percutaneous epiphysiodesis. Clin Orthop 190:170–173
137. Canale ST, Christian CA (1990) Techniques for epiphysiodesis about the knee. Clin Orthop 255:81–85
138. Canale ST, Russell TA, Holcomb RL (1986) Percutaneous epiphysiodesis: experimental study and preliminary clinical results. J Pediatr Orthop 6(2):150–156
139. Craviari T, Bérard J, Willemen L, Kohler R (1998) Percutaneous epiphysiodesis: a study on 60 skeletally mature patients (abstr). Rev Chir Orthop 84:172–179
140. Gabriel KR, Crawford AH, Roy DR, True MS, Sauntry S (1994) Percutaneous epiphyseodesis. J Pediatr Orthop 14(3):358–362
141. Givon U, Bowen JR (1998) Physeal surgery for the treatment of lower limb length discrepancy, Chapter 27. In: de Pablos J (ed) Surgery of the growth plate. Ediciones Ergon, S.A, Madrid, pp 229–237

142. Horton GA, Olney BW (1996) Epiphysiodesis of the lower extremity: results of the percutaneous technique. J Pediatr Orthop 16(2):180–182
143. Inan M, Chan G, Bowen JR (2006) Correction of angular deformities of the knee by percutaneous hemiepiphysiodesis. Clin Orthop 456:164–169
144. Jones (1985) Percutaneous epiphysiodesis: meeting highlights. J Pediatr Orthop 5(6):745–746
145. Kemnitz S, Moens P, Fabry G (2003) Percutaneous epiphysiodesis for leg length discrepancy. J Pediatr Orthop B 12(1):69–71
146. Liotta FJ, Ambrose TA II, Eilert RE (1992) Fluoroscopic technique versus Phemister technique for epiphysiodesis. J Pediatr Orthop 12(2):248–251
147. Macnicol MF, Gupta MS (1997) Epiphysiodesis using a cannulated tubesaw. J Bone Joint Surg 79B(2):307–309
148. McCarthy JJ, Burke T, McCarthy MC (2003) Need for concomitant proximal fibular epiphysiodesis when performing a proximal tibial epiphysiodesis. J Pediatr Orthop 23(1):52–54
149. Menelaus MB (1991) Growth plate arrest. In: Menelaus MB (ed) The management of limb inequality. Churchill Livingstone, London, pp 71–94, Chap 6
150. Ogilvie JW, King K (1990) Epiphysiodesis: two-year clinical results using a new technique. J Pediatr Orthop 10(6):809–811
151. Scott AC, Urquhart BA, Cain TE (1996) Percutaneous vs. modified phemister epiphysiodesis of the lower extremity. Orthopedics 19(10):857–861
152. Stanitski DF (1999) Limb-length inequality: assessment and treatment options. J Am Acad Orthop Surg 7(3):143–153
153. Surdan JW, Morris CD, DeWeese JD, Drvaric DM (2003) Leg length inequality and epiphysiodesis: review of 96 cases. J Pediatr Orthop 23(3):381–384
154. Synder M, Harcke HT, Bowen JR, Caro PA (1994) Evaluation of physeal behavior in response to epiphyseodesis with the use of serial magnetic resonance imaging. J Bone Joint Surg 76A:224–229
155. Timparlake RW, Bowen JR, Guille JT, Choi IH (1991) Prospective evaluation of fifty-three consecutive percutaneous epiphysiodeses of the distal femur and proximal tibia and fibula. J Pediatr Orthop 11(3):350–357

Endoscopic Assisted Physeal Ablation

156. de Pablos J, Capdevila R, Bruguera JA (1998) Arthroscopic hemiepiphysiodesis: preliminary results in the correction of idiopathic genu valgum in adolescents, Chapter 34. In: de Pablos J (ed) Surgery of the growth plate. Ediciones Ergon, S.A, Madrid, pp 281–285
157. Gamble JG, Imrie M, Rinsky LA (2010) Endoscopic assisted percutaneous epiphyseodes. In: Western Orthopaedic Assn Annual Meeting, Monterey CA, Program, August 2010, pp 70–71.

Temporary Reversible Physeal Arrest: Compression Method

158. Belle RM, Stevens PM (1992) Medial malleolar screw epiphysiodesis for ankle valgus. Orthop Trans 16:655
159. Blount WP, Clarke GR (1949) Control of bone growth by epiphyseal stapling: a preliminary report. J Bone Joint Surg 31A(3):464–478
160. Haas SH (1945) Retardation of bone growth by a wire loop. J Bone Joint Surg 27A:25–36
161. Stevens PM, Pease F (2006) Hemiepiphysiodesis for post traumatic tibial valgus. J Pediatr Orthop 26(3):385–392

Intentional Physeal Arrest – Animal Experiments: Resection of the Periphery of the Physis

162. Campbell CJ, Grisolia A, Zanconato G (1959) The effects produced in the cartilaginous epiphyseal plate of immature dogs by experimental surgical traumata. J Bone Joint Surg 41A(7):1221–1242
163. Haas SL (1919) The changes produced in the growing bone after injury to the epiphyseal cartilage plate. J Orthop Surg 1:67–99
164. Key A, Ford LT (1958) A study of experimental trauma to the distal femoral epiphysis in rabbits – II. J Bone Joint Surg 40A(4):887–896
165. Peterson HA (1994) Physeal fractures: part 3. Classification. J Pediatr Orthop 14:439–448
166. Peterson HA (1994) Physeal fractures: part 2. Two previously unclassified types. J Pediatr Orthop 14:431–438

Osteotomy Across the Physis

167. Leet AI, Mackenzie WG, Szoke G, Harcke HT (1999) Injury to the growth plate after Pemberton osteotomy. J Bone Joint Surg 81A:169–176
168. Soini J, Ritsilä V (1984) Experimentally produced growth disturbance of the acetabulum in young rabbits. Acta Orthop Scand 55:14–17

Currettment

169. Compere EL, Garisson M, Fahey JJ (1940) Deformities of the femur resulting from arrestment of growth of the capital and greater trochanteric epiphyses. J Bone Joint Surg 22(4):909–915
170. Ford LT, Key JA (1956) A study of experimental trauma to the distal femoral epiphysis in rabbits. J Bone Joint Surg 38A(1):84–92
171. Friedenberg ZB (1957) Reaction of the epiphysis to partial surgical resection. J Bone Joint Surg 30A(2):332–340
172. Synder M, Harcke HT, Conard K, Bowen JR (2001) Experimental epiphysiodesis: magnetic resonance imaging evaluation with histopathologic correlation. Int Orthop (SICOT) 25:337–342

Burring

173. Hall-Craggs ECB (1968) The effect of experimental epiphysiodesis on growth in length of the rabbit's tibia. J Bone Joint Surg 50B(2):392–400

174. Ross TK, Zionts LE (1997) Comparision of different methods used to inhibit physeal growth in a rabbit model. Clin Orthop 340:236–243

Intraphyseal Drilling

175. Ogilvie JW (1986) Epiphysiodesis: evaluation of a new technique. J Pediatr Orthop 6(2):147–149

Transphyseal Drilling

176. Garcés GL, Mugica-Garay I, López-González Coviella N, Guerado E (1994) Growth-plate modifications after drilling. J Pediatr Orthop 14(2):225–228
177. Gil-Albarova J, Fini M, Gil-Albarova R, Melgosa M, Aldini-Nicolo N, Giardino R, Seral F (1998) Absorbable screws through the greater trochanter do not disturb physeal growth: rabbit experiments. Acta Orthop Scand 69(3):273–276
178. Guzzanti V, Falciglia F, Gigante A, Fabriciani C (1994) The effect of intra-articular ACL reconstruction on the growth plates of rabbits. J Bone Joint Surg 76B(6):960–963
179. Houle JB, Letts M, Yang J (2001) Effects of a tensioned tendon graft in a bone tunnel across the rabbit physis. Clin Orthop 391:275–281
180. Imbert MR (1951) Experimental pathology of the epiphyseal disc of the long bones: therapeutic deductions [French]. Marseille Chirurgical 3(5):581–599
181. Janarv PM, Wikström B, Hirsch G (1998) The influence of transphyseal drilling and tendon grafting on bone growth: an experimental study in the rabbit. J Pediatr Orthop 18(2):149–154
182. Mäkelä A, Vainiopää S, Vihtonen K, Mero M, Rokkanen P (1988) The effect of trauma to the lower femoral epiphyseal plate: an experimental study in rabbits. J Bone Joint Surg 70B:187–191
183. Nordentoft EL (1969) Experimental epiphyseal injuries: grading of traumas and attempts at treatment traumatic epiphyseal arrest in animals. Acta Orthop Scand 40(2):176–192
184. Otsuka NY, Mah JY, Orr FW, Martin RF (1992) Biodegradation of polydioxanone in bone tissue: effect on the epiphyseal plate in immature rabbits. J Pediatr Orthop 12(2):177–180

Longitudinal Smooth Metallic Pins, Wires, and Nails

185. Bailey RW, Dubow HI (1981) Evolution of the concept of an extensible nail accommodating to normal longitudinal bone growth: clinical considerations and implications. Clin Orthop 159:157–170
186. Bjerkreim I, Langård Ø (1983) Effect upon longitudinal growth of femur by intramedullary nailing in rats. Acta Orthop Scand 54:363–365
187. Ford LT, Canales GM (1960) A study of experimental trauma and attempts to stimulate growth of the lower femoral epiphysis in rabbits – III. J Bone Joint Surg 42A(3):439–446
188. Green WT (1950) Restriction of bone growth: discussion. J Bone Joint Surg 32A:350
189. Haas SL (1950) Restriction of bone growth by pins through the epiphyseal cartilaginous plate. J Bone Joint Surg 32A(2):338–343
190. Kolesnikov YP (1967) The effect of injury to proliferating epiphyseal cartilage on bone growth in length (experimental studies) [Russian]. Orthopedia travmatologia I protezirovanie 28(8):46–50
191. Siffert RS (1956) The effect of staples and longitudinal wires on epiphyseal growth: an experimental study. J Bone Joint Surg 38A(5):1077–1088. doi:5

Bone Grafts Across the Physis

192. Hallel T, Salvati EA (1977) Premature closure of the triradiate cartilage: a case report and animal experiment. Clin Orthop 124:278–281
193. Johnson JTH, Southwick WO (1960) Growth following transepiphyseal bone grafts: an experimental study to explain continued growth following certain fusion operations. J Bone Joint Surg 42A(8):1381–1395

Unintentional Physeal Arrest – Human Involvement: Smooth Nails, Rods, and Prosthetic Stems

194. Bailey RW (1981) Further clinical experience with the extensible nail. Clin Orthop 159:171–176
195. Bailey RW, Dubow HI (1965) Experimental and clinical studies of longitudinal bone growth – utilizing a new method of internal fixation crossing the epiphyseal plate (Abstr). J Bone Joint Surg 47A(8):1669
196. Blunn GW, Wait ME (1991) Remodelling of bone around intramedullary stems in growing patients. J Orthop Res 9(6):809–819
197. Chockalingam S, Bell MJ (2002) Technique of exchange of Sheffield telescopic rod system. J Pediatr Orthop 22(1):117–119
198. Cool WP, Carter SR, Grimer RJ, Tillman RM, Walker PS (1997) Growth after extendible endoprosthetic replacement of the distal femur. J Bone Joint Surg 79B(6):938–942
199. Cool WP, Grimer RJ, Carter SR, Sneath RS, Walker PS (1995) Passive growth at the sliding component following endoprosthetic replacement in skeletally immature children with a primary bone tumour around the knee. J Bone Joint Surg 78B(Supp I):33
200. Eckardt JJ, Kabo JM, Kelley CM, Ward WG Sr, Asavamongkolkul A, Wirganowicz PZ et al (2000) Expandable endoprosthesis reconstruction in skeletally immature patients with tumors. Clin Orthop 373:51–61
201. Gamble JG, Strudwick WJ, Rinsky LA, Bleck EE (1988) Complications of intramedullary rods in osteogenesis

imperfecta: Bailey-Dubow rods versus nonelongating rods. J Pediatr Orthop 8(6):645–649
202. Gönzalez-Herranz P, Burgos-Flores J, Rapariz JM, Lopez-Mondejar JA, Ocete JG, Amaya S (1995) Intramedullary nailing of the femur in children: effects on its proximal end. J Bone Joint Surg 77B(2):262–266
203. Herndon WA, Mahnken RF, Yngve DA, Sullivan JA (1989) Management of femoral shaft fractures in the adolescent. J Pediatr Orthop 9(1):29–32
204. Hosny GA, Moens P, Fabry G (1999) Complications of Küntscher intramedullary nailing in a child: a case report. J Pediatr Orthop B 8:100–102
205. Janus GJM, Vanpaemel LADM, Engelbert RHH, Pruijs HEH (1999) Complications of the Bailey-Dubow elongating nail in osteogenesis imperfecta: 34 children with 110 nails. J Pediatr Orthop B 8(3):203–207
206. Jerosch J, Mazzotti I, Tomasevic M (1998) Complications after treatment of patients with osteogenic imperfecta with a Bailey-Dubow rod. Arch Orthop Trauma Surg 117:240–245
207. Inglis AE Jr, Walker PS, Sneath RS, Grimer R, Scales JT (1992) Uncemented intramedullary fixation of implants using polyethylene sleeves: a roentgenographic study. Clin Orthop 284:208–214
208. Lang-Stevenson AI, Sharrard WJW (1984) Intramedullary rodding with Bailey-Dubow extensible rods in osteogenesis imperfecta. J Bone Joint Surg 66B(2):227–232
209. Mann DC, Weddington J, Davenport K (1986) Closed Ender nailing of femoral shaft fractures in adolescents. J Pediatr Orthop 6(6):651–655
210. Marafioti RL, Westin GW (1977) Elongating intramedullary rods in the treatment of osteogenesis imperfecta. J Bone Joint Surg 59A(4):467–472
211. Marafioti RL, Westin GW (1975) Twenty years experience with multiple osteotomies and intramedullary fixation in osteogenesis imperfecta (including the Bailey expandable rod) at the Shriner's Hospital, Los Angeles, California. J Bone Joint Surg 57A:136
212. Mulpuri K, Joseph B (2000) Intramedullary rodding in osteogenesis imperfecta. J Pediatr Orthop 20(2):267–273
213. Raney EM, Ogden JA, Grogan DP (1993) Premature greater trochanteric epiphysiodesis secondary to intramedullary femoral rodding. J Pediatr Orthop 13(4):516–520
214. Rodriguez RP (1976) Report of multiple osteotomies and intramedullary fixation by an extensible intramedullary device in children with osteogenesis imperfecta (Abstr). Clin Orthop 116:261
215. Safran MR, Eckardt JJ, Kabo JM, Oppenheim WL (1992) Continued growth of the proximal part of the tibia after prosthetic reconstruction of the skeletally immature knee. J Bone Joint Surg 74A(8):1172–1179
216. Sofield HA, Millar EA (1959) Fragmentation, realignment, and intramedullary rod fixation of deformities of the long bones in children: a ten-year appraisal. J Bone Joint Surg 41A(8):1374–1391
217. Zionts LE, Ebramzadeh E, Stott NS (1998) Complications in the use of the Bailey-Dubow extensible nail. Clin Orthop 348:186–195
218. Ziv I, Blackburn N, Rang M (1984) Femoral intramedullary nailing in the growing child. J Trauma 24(5):432–434

Smooth Wires and Pins

219. Bisgard JE, Martenson L (1937) Fractures in children. Surg Gynec Obst 65:464–474
220. Boyden EM, Peterson HA (1991) Partial premature closure of the distal radial physis associated with Kirschner wire fixation. Orthopedics 14(5):585–588
221. Choi KY, Chan WS, Lam TP, Cheng JCY (1995) Percutaneous Kirschner-wire pinning for severly displaced distal radial fractures in children: a report of 157 cases. J Bone Joint Surg 77B:797–801
222. Gamble JG, Decker S, Abrams RC (1982) Short first ray as a complication of multiple metatarsal osteotomies. Clin Orthop 164:241–244
223. Harsha WN (1957) Effects of trauma upon epiphyses. Clin Orthop 10:140–147
224. Hernandez J Jr, Peterson HA (1986) Fracture of the distal radial physis complicated by compartment syndrome and premature physeal closure. J Pediatr Orthop 6(5):627–630
225. Holden D, Siff S, Butler J, Cain T (1984) Shortening of the first metatarsal as a complication of metatarsal osteotomies. J Bone Joint Surg 66A(4):582–587
226. Lintecum N, Blasier RD (1996) Direct reduction with indirect fixation of distal tibial physeal fractures: a report of a technique. J Pediatr Orthop 16(1):107–112
227. Peterson H (1994) Brachymetatarsia of the first metatarsal treated by surgical lengthening. In: Simons GW (ed) The clubfoot, the present and a view of the future, chapter 11. Springer-Verlag, New York, pp 360–369
228. Peterson HA (2007) Epiphyseal growth plate fractures. Springer, Heidelberg
229. Peterson HA (1995) Techniques of open reduction internal fixation of Salter-Harris type II, III, and IV fractures of the distal tibia in children. Oper Tech Orthop 5(2):164–170
230. Pritchett JW (1994) Does pinning cause distal radial growth plate arrest? Orthopedics 17:550–552
231. Scheffer MM, Peterson HA (1994) Opening-wedge osteotomy for angular deformities of long bones in children. J Bone Joint Surg 76A(3):325–334
232. Shoemaker SC, Comstock CP, Mubarak SJ, Wenger DR, Chambers HG (1999) Intramedullary Kirschner wire fixation of open or unstable forearm fractures in children. J Pediatr Orthop 19(3):329–337
233. Smith NC, Parker D, McNicol D (2001) Supracondylar fractures of the femur in children. J Pediatr Orthop 21(5):600–603
234. Sorrel E (1958) Physeal separation treated with metal (Abstr). J Bone Joint Surg 40B(1):155
235. Steedman JT Jr, Peterson HA (1992) Brachymetatarsia of the first metatarsal treated by surgical lengthening. J Pediatr Orthop 12(6):780–785

236. Thomas DP, Howard AW, Cole WG, Hedden DM (2001) Three weeks of Kirschner wire fixation for displaced lateral condylar fractures of the humerus in children. J Pediatr Orthop 21(5):565–569
237. Verbrugge J (1958) Perforation of epiphyseal cartilage: Proceedings and Reports of Councils and Associations. J Bone Joint Surg 40B(1):155
238. Wright J, Rang M (1989) Internal fixation for forearm fractures in children. Tech Orthop 4(3):44–47
239. Yung PSH, Lam CY, Ng BKW, Lam TP, Cheng JCY (2004) Percutaneous transphyseal intramedullary Kirschner wire pinning: a safe and effective procedure for treatment of displaced diaphyseal forearm fracture in children. J Pediatr Orthop 24(1):7–12

Threaded Wires and Screws

240. Berg EE (1995) Pediatric tibial eminence fractures: arthroscopic cannulated screw fixation. Arthroscopy 11(3):328–331
241. Mylle J, Reynders P, Broos P (1993) Transepiphysial fixation of anterior cruciate avulsion in a child: report of a complication and review of the literature. Arch Orthop Trauma Surg 112:101–103
242. Peterson HA (1984) Partial growth arrest and its treatment. J Pediatr Orthop 4:246–258
243. Schofield CM, Smibert JG (1990) Trochanteric growth disturbance after upper femoral osteotomy for congenital dislocation of the hip. J Bone Joint Surg 72B(1):32–36

Cortical Bone Grafts

244. Hatt RN (1940) The central bone graft in joint arthrodesis. J Bone Joint Surg 22(2):393–402
245. Van Gorder GW, Chen CM (1959) The central-graft operation for fusion of tuberculous knees, ankles, and elbows. J Bone Joint Surg 41A(6):1029–1046

Osteotomy Across the Physis

246. Makin M (1980) Closure of the epiphysis of the femoral head and of the triradiate cartilage of the acetabulum following surgery for congenital hip dislocation. Isr J Med Sci 16:307–310
247. Plaster RL, Schoenecker PL, Capelli AM (1991) Premature closure of the triradiate cartilage: a potential complication of pericapsular acetabuloplasty: case report. J Pediatr Orthop 11(5):676–678
248. Valdiserri L, Gasbarrini S, Fabbri N (1997) Complications in acetabuloplasty in the treatment of CHD during the growth age [Italian]. Chirurgia Degli Organi de Movimento 82(2):155–163

Drilling Across the Physis

249. Aichroth PM, Patel DV, Zorrilla P (2002) The natural history and treatment of rupture of the anterior cruciate ligament in children and adolescents. J Bone Joint Surg 84B(1):38–41
250. Anderson AF (2003) Transepiphyseal replacement of the anterior cruciate ligament in skeletally immature patients: a preliminary report. J Bone Joint Surg 85A(7):1255–1263
251. Anderson A, Anderson AF (2004) Transepiphyseal replacement of the anterior cruciate ligament using quadruple hamstring grafts in skeletally immature patients: surgical technique. J Bone Joint Surg 86A(Suppl 1):201–209, Part 2
252. Anderson AF (2003) Tunnel placement in anterior cruciate reconstruction: letters to the Editor. J Bone Joint Surg 85A(3):647–648
253. Andrish JT (2001) Anterior cruciate ligament injuries in the skeletally immature patient. Am J Orthop 30:103–110
254. Apel PJ, Shea KG (2003) Tunnel placement in anterior cruciate reconstruction: letters to the Editor. J Bone Joint Surg 85A(3):647
255. Aronowitz ER, Ganley TJ, Goode JR, Gregg JR, Meyer JS (2000) Anterior cruciate ligament reconstruction in adolescents with open physes. Am J Sports Med 28(2):168–175
256. Barber FA, Sanders JO, Clark R (2000) Anterior cruciate ligament reconstruction in the skeletally immature high-performance athlete: what to do and when to do it? Current controversies point counterpoint. J Arthroscopic and Relat Surg 16(4):391–394
257. Behr CT, Potter HG, Paletta GA Jr (2001) The relationship of the femoral origin of the anterior cruciate ligament and the distal femoral physeal plate in the skeletally immature knee: an anatomic study. Am J Sports Med 29(6):781–787
258. Bisson LJ, Wickiewicz T, Levinson M, Warren R (1998) ACL reconstruction in children with open physes. Orthopedics 21(6):659–663
259. Dorizas JA, Stanitski CL (2003) Anterior cruciate ligament injury in the skeletally immature. Orthop Clin N Am 34:355–363
260. Eady JL, Cardenas CD, Sopa D (1982) Avulsion of the femoral attachment of the anterior cruciate ligament in a seven-year-old child: a case report. J Bone Joint Surg 64A(9):1376–1378
261. Edwards PH, Grana WA (2001) Anterior cruciate ligament reconstruction in the immature athlete: long-term results of intra-articular reconstruction. Am J Knee Surg 14:232–237
262. Edwards TB, Greene CC, Baratta RV, Zieske A, Willis RB (2001) The effect of placing a tensioned graft across open growth plates. J Bone Joint Surg 83A(5):725–734
263. Engebretsen L, Svenningsen S, Benum P (1988) Poor results of anterior cruciate ligament repair in adolescence. Acta Orthop Scand 59(6):684–686
264. Fehnel DJ, Johnson R (2000) Anterior cruciate injuries in the skeletally immature athlete: a review of treatment and outcomes. Sports Med 29(1):51–63

265. Fuchs R (July 2000) ACL technique proves viable for skeletally immature patients. Reported by Hamm T. Orthopedics Today 15–16
266. Fuchs R, Wheatley W, Uribe JW, Hechtman KS, Zvijac JE, Schurhoff MR (2002) Intra-articular anterior cruciate ligament reconstruction using patellar tendon allograft in the skeletally immature patient. J Arthroscopic and Relat Surg 18(8):824–828
267. Guzzanti V, Falciglia F, Gigante A, Fabbriciani C (1994) The effect of intra-articular ACL reconstruction on the growth plates of rabbits. J Bone Joint Surg 76B(6): 960–963
268. Guzzanti V, Falciglia F, Stanitski CL (2003) Physeal-sparing intraarticular anterior cruciate ligament reconstruction in preadolescents. Am J Sports Med 31(6):949–953
269. Guzzanti V, Falciglia F, Stanitski CL (2003) Preoperative evaluation and anterior cruciate ligament reconstruction technique for skeletally immature patients in Tanner stages 2 and 3. Am J Sports Med 31(6):941–948
270. Higuchi T, Hara K, Tsuji Y, Kubo T (2009) Transepiphyseal reconstruction of the anterior cruciate ligament in skeletally immature athletes: an MRI evaluation for epiphyseal narrowing. J Pediatr Orthop B 18(6):330–334
271. Janarv P, Nyström A, Werner S, Hirsch G (1996) Anterior cruciate ligament injuries in skeletally immature patients. J Pediatr Orthop 16(5):673–677
272. Johnston DR, Ganley TJ, Flynn JM, Gregg JR (2002) Anterior cruciate ligament injuries in skeletally immature patients. Orthopedics 25:864–871
273. Kawate K, Fujisawa Y, Yajima H, Sugimoto K, Tomita Y, Takakura Y (2004) Avulsion of the cartilaginous femoral origin of the anterior cruciate ligament in a three-year-old child: a case report with a thirteen-year follow-up. J Bone Joint Surg 86A(8):1787–1792
274. Kim S, Ha K, Ahm J, Chang D (1999) Anterior cruciate ligament reconstruction in the young patient without violation of the epiphyseal plate: technical note. J Arthroscopic Surg 15(7):792–795
275. Kocher MS, Garg S, Micheli LJ (2006) Physeal sparing reconstruction of the anterior cruciate ligament in skeletally immature prepubescent children and adolescents: surgical technique. J Bone Joint Surg 86A(Suppl 1):283–293, Part 2
276. Kocher MS, Hovis WD, Curtin MJ, Hawkins RJ (2005) Anterior cruciate ligament reconstruction in skeletally immature knees: an anatomical study. Am J Orthop 34(6):285–290
277. Kocher MS, Saxon HS, Hovis WD, Hawkins RJ (2002) Management and complications of anterior cruciate ligament injuries in skeletally immature patients: survey of the Herodicus Society and the ACL Study Group. J Pediatr Orthop 22(4):452–457
278. Kolata G (18 Feb, 2008) A big-time injury striking little players' knees. New York Times
279. Koman JD, Sanders JO (1999) Valgus deformity after reconstruction of the anterior cruciate ligament in a skeletally immature patient: a case report. J Bone Joint Surg 81A(5):711–715
280. Kouyoumjian A, Barber FA (2001) Management of anterior cruciate ligament disruptions in skeletally immature patients: aspects of sports medicine. Am J Orthop 30(10):771–774
281. Lipscomb AB, Anderson AF (1986) Tears of the anterior cruciate ligament in adolescents. J Bone Joint Surg 68A(1):19–28
282. Lo IK, Bell DM, Fowler PJ (1998) Anterior cruciate ligament injuries in the skeletally immature patient. AAOS Inst Course Lect 47:351–359
283. Lo IK, Kirkley A, Fowler PJ, Miniaci A (1997) The outcome of operatively treated anterior cruciate ligament disruptions in the skeletally immature child. Arthroscopy 13(5):627–634
284. Matava JM, Siegel MG (1997) Arthroscopic reconstruction of the ACL with semitendinosis-gracilis autograft in skeletally immature adolescent patients. Am J Knee Surg 10(2):60–69
285. McCarroll JR, Shelbourne D, Patel DV (1995) Anterior cruciate ligament injuries in young athletes: recommendations for treatment and rehabilitation. Sports Med 20(2):117–127
286. Micheli LJ, Rask B, Gerberg L (1999) Anterior cruciate ligament reconstruction in patients who are prepubescent. Clin Orthop 364:40–47
287. Mizuta H, Kubota K, Shiraishi M, Otsuka Y, Nagamoto N, Takagi K (1995) The conservative treatment of complete tears of the anterior cruciate ligament in skeletally immature patients. J Bone Joint Surg 77B(6):890–894
288. Nakhostine M, Bollen SR, Cross MJ (1995) Reconstruction of mid-substance anterior cruciate rupture in adolescents with open physes. J Pediatr Orthop 15(3):286–287
289. Ono T, Wada Y, Takahashi K, Minamide M, Moriya H (1955) Tibial deformities and failures of anterior cruciate ligament reconstruction in immature rabbits. J Orthop Sci 3:150–155
290. Pressman AE, Letts RM, Jarvis JG (1997) Anterior cruciate ligament tears in children: an analysis of operative versus nonoperative treatment. J Pediatr Orthop 17(4):505–511
291. Sharma V, Wall EJ, Laor R (2008) Epiphyseal to epiphyseal ACL reconstruction: MRI evaluation of anatomical graft placement. Poster No. 37. In: POSNA Annual Meeting, Albuquerque, Apr 29-May 3, 2008.
292. Shea K (2001) ACL injuries in adolescent soccer players are increasing: reported by Pastorius D. Orthop Today 21(8): 12–13
293. Shelbourne KD, Gray T, Wiley BV (2004) Results of transphyseal anterior cruciate ligament reconstruction using patellar tendon autograft in Tanner stage 3 or 4 adolescents with clearly open growth plates. Am J Sports Med 32(5): 1218–1222
294. Shelbourne KD, Patel DV, McCarroll JR (1996) Management of anterior cruciate ligament injuries in skeletally immature adolescents. Knee Surg, Sports Traumatol, Arthroscopy 4:68–74
295. Simonian PT, Metcalf MH, Larson RV (1999) Anterior cruciate ligament injuries in the skeletally immature patient: a review paper. Am J Orthop 28(11):624–628

296. Stadelmaier DM, Arnoczky SP, Dodds J, Ross H (1995) The effect of drilling and soft tissue grafting across open growth plates: a histologic study. Am J Sports Med 23(4):431–435
297. Stanitski CL (1995) Anterior cruciate ligament injury in the skeletally immature patient: diagnosis and treatment. J Am Academy Orthop Surg 3(3):146–158
298. Waldrop JI, Broussard TS (1984) Disruption of the anterior cruciate ligament in a three-year-old child: a case report. J Bone Joint Surg 66A(7):113–114
299. Wester W, Canale ST, Dutkowsky JP, Warner WC, Beaty JH (1994) Prediction of angular deformity and leg-length discrepancy after anterior cruciate ligament reconstruction in skeletally immature patients. J Pediatr Orthop 14(4):516–521
300. Willis RB (2001) ACL injury in the patient with open physes. In: Mini symposium. POSNA Specialty Day, San Francisco, March 3, 2001
301. Woods GW, O'Connor DP (2004) Delayed anterior cruciate ligament reconstruction in adolescents with open physes. Am J Sports Med 32(1):201–210
302. Yiannakopoulos CK, Mowbray M (2003) Transepiphyseal replacement of the anterior cruciate ligament in skeletally immature patients: a preliminary report: letters to the Editor. J Bone Joint Surg Am 85A(3):648
303. Zaricznyj B (1977) Avulsion fracture of the tibial eminence: treatment by open reduction and pinning. J Bone Joint Surg 59A(8):1111–1114

Unintentional Physeal Arrest: Animal Involvement

304. Parker RB, Bloomberg MS (1984) Modified intramedullary pin technique for repair of distal femoral physeal fractures in the dog and cat. J Am Vet Med Assoc 184(10):1259–1265
305. Wagner PC, DeBowes RM, Grant BD, Kaneps AJ, Watrous BJ (1984) Cancellous bone screws for repair of proximal growth plate fractures of the tibia in foals. J Am Vet Med Assoc 184(6):688–691

Unknown

21.1 Introduction

Premature physeal arrest may occur in random physis with no apparent etiology. These idiopathic and unclassified physeal arrests have been reported at several sites, most commonly at the knee. Several examples are recorded here in which the treating physicians could find no cause for the arrest.

21.2 Knee

In 1947 Kestler documented three types of unclassified cessation of physeal growth about the knee [3]. The first group included growth cessation at the knee associated with infections of the hip, such as tuberculosis and *Staphylococcus aureus*. These are documented in this text in Chap. 2, Disuse. The second group included non-infectious disorders, such as congenital dislocation of the hip, causing knee physeal arrest on the same side. These are also documented in this text in Chap. 2, Disuse. The third group included patients with no hip lesions or other pathologic process. Kestler attributed the early growth cessation in these cases to impaired blood supply to the physis as noted in Chap. 1.

Premature closure of the physis of both the distal femur and proximal tibia have been noted with diaphyseal fractures of the femur and tibia. These physeal closures are recorded in detail in Sect. 10.4, and as noted there these arrests are not regarded as being due to compression of the physis. The cause of these arrests is unknown.

Pappas et al. reported six cases of premature asymmetrical closure of the proximal tibial physis with associated genu recurvatum deformity in which "no single etiological factor could be implicated," despite risk factors including trauma, prolonged immobilization, and tibial wire traction [4]. Siegling reported a patient with premature arrest of the proximal tibial physis without any accompanying suspicious factor [10]. An eleven and half year old girl had frequent attacks of pain medially in the left leg just below the knee for 2 years. There was no swelling, local heat or redness. Progressive tibial varus and 1 in. tibial shortening were found to be due to premature partial closure of the proximal tibial physis. Exploratory surgery revealed only the premature physeal arrest. Treatment consisted of corrective osteotomy and surgical closure of the lateral portion of the tibial physis along with the fibular physis and the contralateral proximal tibial and fibular physis.

Recorded here is a case of premature partial closure of a distal femoral physis (Fig. 21.1) and two cases of the proximal tibial physis (Figs. 21.2 and 21.3), all of which occurred without a direct link to trauma, traction, disuse, infection, vascular deprivation, hip pathology, or other obvious cause.

21.3 Ankle

A 5 month old boy had bilateral greater saphenous cutdowns at the ankle for treatment of meningitis [1]. There was no obvious infection of the ankles at any time. At age 5 years 11 months both distal tibial and fibular physis were closed and left ankle varus was noted. Corrective osteotomy was performed on the left distal tibia at age 11 years 4 months. At age 15 years 6 months function was normal bilaterally and the left tibia measured ¼ in. shorter than the right.

Recorded here is a case of bilateral distal tibial physeal and epiphyseal abnormalities of unknown etiology (Fig. 21.4).

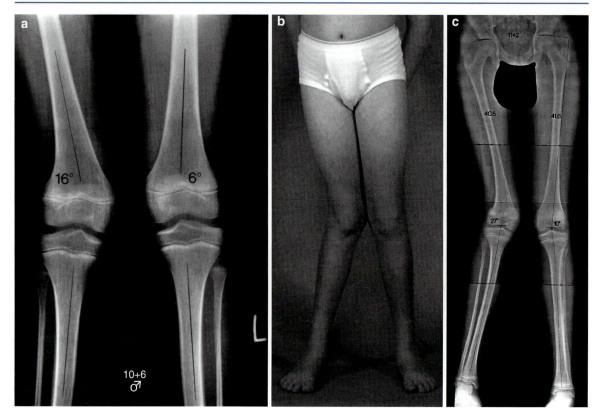

Fig. 21.1 Idiopathic partial physeal arrest of the distal femoral physis. At age 3 years this patient had meningococcemia and refused to bear weight on the right lower extremity. His illness was mild. No skin or soft tissue changes occurred as noted in the patient in Fig. 1.14a. His recovery was uneventful and he enjoyed normal unrestricted activities. (**a**) At age 10 years 6 months mild right knee valgus was noted. A standing roentgenogram of the legs showed mild right genu valgus. (**b**) Eight months later the genu valgum had increased. (**c**) Scanograms showed the genu valgum had increased to 27°, and the right femur was 11 mm shorter than the left. (**d**) Coronal (*left*) and sagittal (*right*) GRE MR images showed a small physeal bar located laterally. (**e**) A 3D rendered physeal map showed the location, size, and contour of the bar, which occupied 4.6% of the physis. (**f**) The bar occupied 3.8% of the physis on a 3D projection physeal map. (**g**) The bar was excised at age 11 years 2 months and the cavity filled with cranioplast. There was no sign of infection. The metal markers were placed 30 mm apart. (**h**) At age 12 years 4 months the right genu valgum had reduced to 13°, the metal markers were 48 mm apart, and both distal femur and tibia physis were growing well as judged from the growth arrest lines. The femoral length discrepancy measured 13 mm. His care was assumed by a Shriner's Hospital closer to his home. (**i**) At age 15 years 8 months the metal markers were 67 mm apart, but there was a recurrent bar and the genu valgum was increased. At age 16 years 1 month the femoral discrepancy was 3.6 cm. (**j**) At age 16 years 3 months, femoral lengthening and angular correction were carried out. No contralateral physeal arrests were done. The last correspondence, at age 23 years 8 months, reported that the patient was doing well and the leg lengths were clinically equal. *Note*: This premature physeal arrest is presented here as "unknown" etiology, because (**a**) there was no bone or joint abnormality present at the time of his meningococcal infection, (**b**) there was no skin or soft tissue deficit to cause diminished blood supply to the physis as noted in Sect. 1.4, and in Fig. 1.14a, (**c**) the long duration between the infection and onset of deformity (7 years), and (**d**) no sign of infection at the time of bar excision. It is difficult to conceptualize a connection between the meningococcemia and the development of a bar 7 years later in the absence of overt findings at the time of infection, at the time of bar development, or at the time of bar excision. Also note this bar was <5% of the physis and did not correct spontaneously. Case referred and followed by Dr. R.P. Lewallen, Billings, MT (Reproduced from Borsa et al. [2], with permission and additional follow-up)

21.3 Ankle

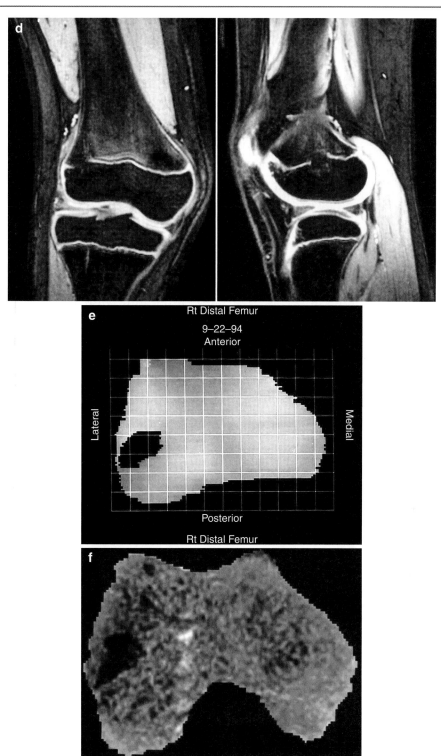

Fig. 21.1 (continued)

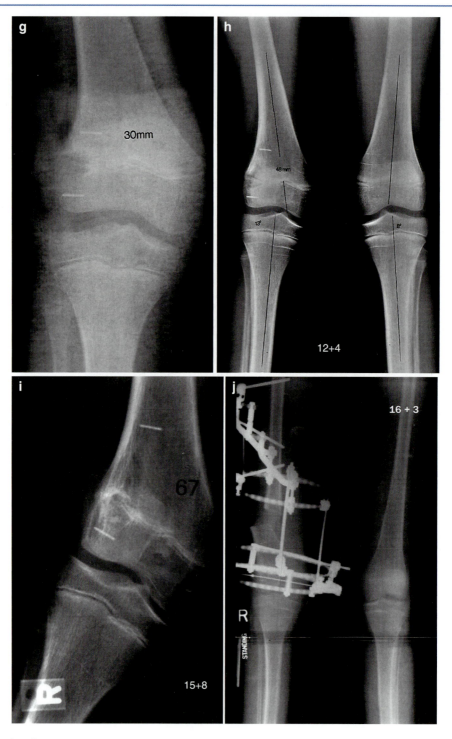

Fig. 21.1 (continued)

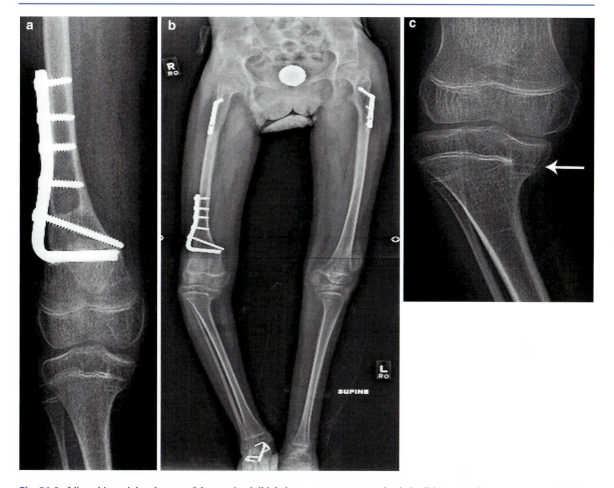

Fig. 21.2 Idiopathic peripheral arrest of the proximal tibial physis. This girl had spastic quadriparesis and severe seizure disorder since birth. Bilateral proximal femoral varus osteotomies at an early age were successful in keeping the hips reduced. She had little independent function and did not ambulate. At age 16 an extension osteotomy of the distal right femur was performed to straighten the knee for standing. (**a**) At age 17 years 2 months the osteotomy was healed, all knee physis were open, and the legs were clinically straight. (**b**) When she returned for reevaluation at age 19 years 2 months, right genu varus was noted. (**c**) There was premature partial arrest of the proximal tibial physis (*arrow*), etiology unknown. A bone age film indicated 2–3 years of growth remaining (Case contributed by Dr. F. Stig Jacobsen, Marshfield, WI, with permission)

Fig. 21.3 Idiopathic central arrest of the proximal tibial physis. This female had microcephaly, developmental delay, and seizures. Evaluation at two tertiary pediatric facilities resulted in no specific diagnosis. She was non-ambulatory. At age 4 she resisted weight bearing on the left leg when placed standing. There had been no observed trauma. (**a**) A roentgenogram at age 4 years 5 months revealed moderate cupping of the proximal tibial physis with mild relative overgrowth of the proximal fibula. (**b**) An MRI confirmed a central physeal bar (*arrow*). The bar was excised at age 4 years 9 months and the cavity filled with fat. (**c**) The most recent evaluation at age 7 years 3 months shows excellent growth, normal proximal tibio-fibular relationship, and an irregular proximal tibial physis without a bar (Case contributed by F. Stig Jacobsen, Marshfield, WI, with permission)

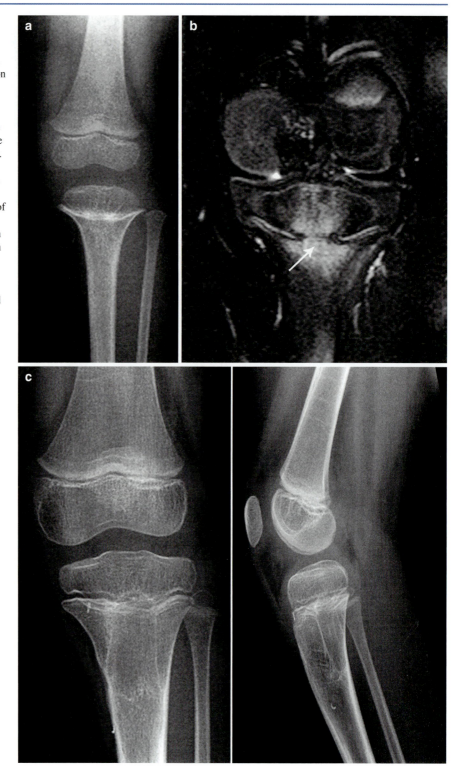

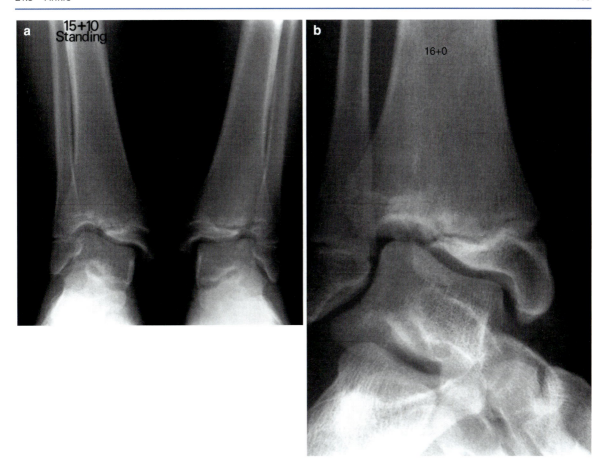

Fig. 21.4 Idiopathic bilateral distal tibial bipartite epiphyses. This boy first noted bilateral ankle stiffness at age 12 years. In the morning he exercised both ankles for 5 min while sitting. He then had no further trouble throughout the day, other than sports and work. He participated in junior high football and wrestling noting a mild ache in both ankles after running for 2–3 min and while working in a grocery store. The patient first presented for evaluation at age 15 years 10 months. Clinically both medial malleoli were prominent. Ankle dorsiflexion was 5° on the right, 15° on the left; plantar flexion was 25° on the right, 20° on the left. He was mildly obese and had thoracic kyphosis diagnosed as Scheuermann's osteochondrosis (treated successfully with a Milwaukee brace). (**a**) Roentgenograms of the ankles standing showed bilateral tapering of the lateral distal tibial epiphyses and ankle valgus, right greater than left. Fibular lengths were normal. Family history for similar problems was negative. (**b**) A right ankle mortise view at age 16 years 0 months showed a tapered distal tibial epiphysis and a possible lateral component of the epiphysis. (**c**) A tomogram confirmed a two part right distal tibial epiphysis, with premature partial arrest. (**d**) At age 16 years 0 months Phemister arrests were performed on the medial side of both distal tibial physes. Following removal of a 20° wedge of bone from the medial side of the distal right tibial metaphysis, the osteotomy could be closed only after an oblique osteotomy of the fibula. (**e**) The osteotomies were healing well at time of last cast removal 11 weeks lateral. (**f**) One year post operatively, age 17 years 1 month, the patient was ambulating normally without ankle stiffness or pain. The ankle mortises were parallel with the floor. There were no symptoms associated with the mild relative overgrowth of both fibulae distally. (**g**) At age 17 years 3 months mild left knee varus was noted. (**h**) A standing roentgenogram showed 3° left knee varus, compared with a normal 4° valgus on the right. All knee physis were open. Staples were placed over the left proximal tibial physis laterally, accompanied by Phemister arrest of the proximal fibular physis. (**i**) At age 17 years 11 months both knees are in 4° valgus; the left tibia was 10 mm longer, and the left femur 3 mm shorter than the right, for a 7 mm leg length difference. (**j**) At age 19 years 6 months the patient was doing well and was advised to gain no more weight

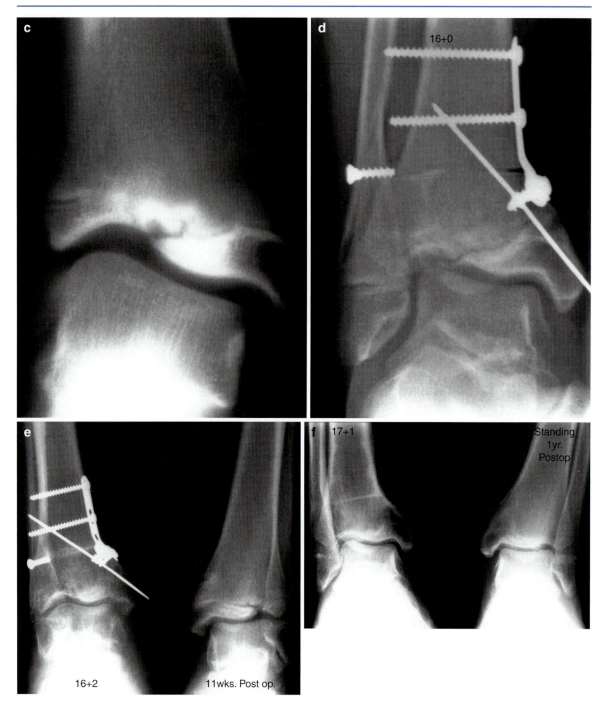

Fig. 21.4 (continued)

21.3 Ankle

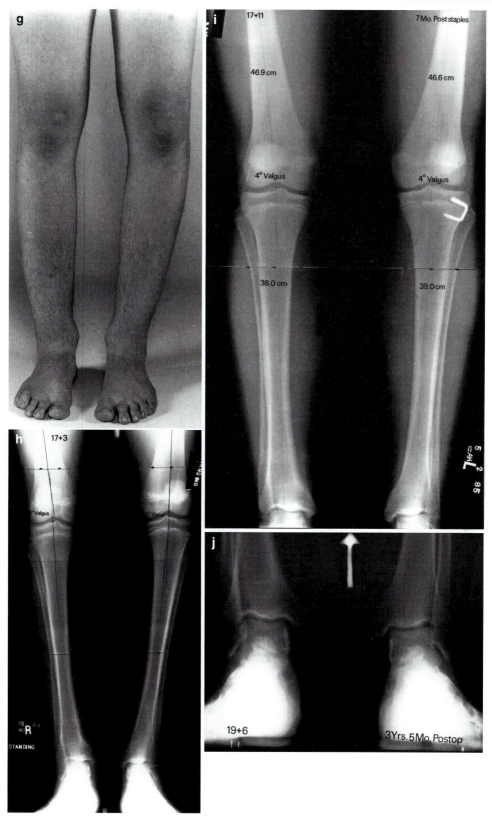

Fig. 21.4 (continued)

21.4 Knee and Ankle

Recorded here is a case of unilateral abnormality of the left distal femoral and proximal and distal left tibial physis with relative shortening of the extremity (Fig. 21.5).

21.5 Hand

Severance reported the case of a 10 year old girl with premature closure with significant relative shortening of several random metacarpals in both hands [9]. There was no history of injury, disease, mal-nutrition, or any other etiologic factor, including hereditary influence.

Pellise et al. reported premature closure of all physis in one hand of a 17 year old boy who at age 5 years had a physeal fracture of the distal radius with subsequent metacarpal and phalangeal physeal closures and relative finger shortening [5]. The authors determined that the premature metacarpal and phalangeal physeal closures on the injured side occurred more than 10 years after the original radius fracture. The authors reviewed multiple possible theories of premature physeal closure mentioned in the literature and concluded that none of them explained the closures in their patient.

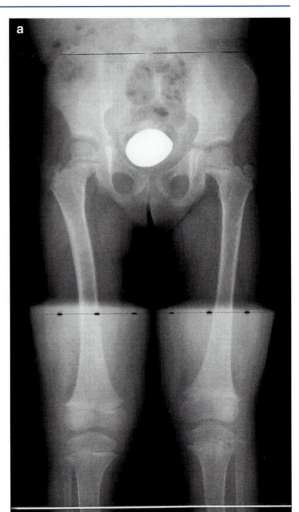

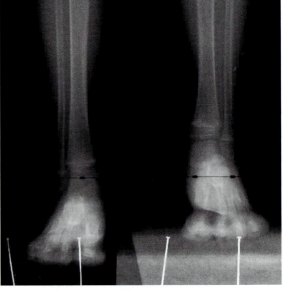

Fig. 21.5 Unilateral abnormal distal femoral and proximal and distal tibial physis of unknown origin. This young girl was born with pulmonary stenosis, syndactyly of some fingers, and foot deformities which were thought to be due to intrauterine malposition. (**a**) At age 3 years 8 months left lower limb relative shortening was associated with abnormal distal femoral and proximal and distal tibial physis. (**b**) Left distal femoral and proximal tibial irregular physis and sclerosis of the metaphyses. The left proximal fibular physis was normal and had relative overgrowth. (**c**) Mild cupping of the left distal tibial physis was accompanied by mild relative overgrowth of the normal distal fibular physis (*right*). The normal right ankle is shown for comparison (*left*). *Note*: Although this patient had some congenital abnormalities she did not fit into any known syndrome. Selective unilateral physeal abnormality would be unusual with any syndrome (Case contributed by Dr. F. Stig Jacobson, Marshfield, WI, with permission)

21.5 Hand

Fig. 21.5 (continued)

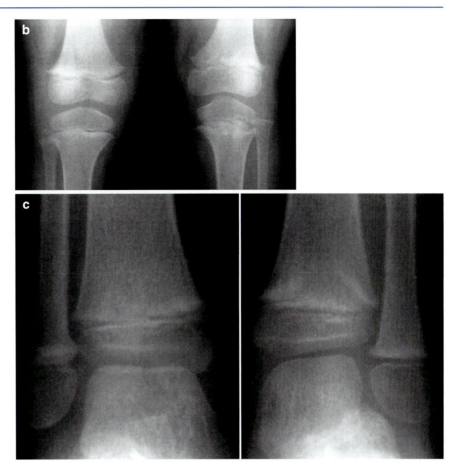

21.6 Wrist

Recorded here are two cases of idiopathic premature partial closure of the distal radial physis, cause unknown (Figs. 21.6 and 21.7).

21.7 Hip

Recorded here is a case of idiopathic premature partial closure of a proximal femoral capital physis, cause unknown (Fig. 21.9).

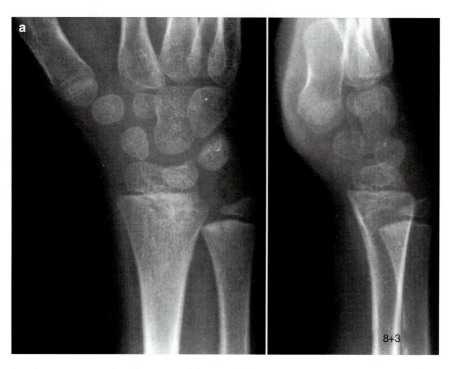

Fig. 21.6 Distal radius premature physeal arrest, etiology unknown. At age 3 years this boy fell down stairs fracturing his right humerus and distal right forearm. Treatment included traction for 18 days followed by a long arm cast. He regained normal form, function and growth. He was right hand dominant. (a) Five years later, at age 8 years 3 months, he complained of pain in the right forearm (*not wrist*). There was no history of injury. The plane of the AP roentgenogram (*left*), was perpendicular to the ulnar physis which was normal, but slightly oblique to the radial physis which is therefore blurred. The lateral view (*right*) is normal. There was no soft tissue swelling on either view and both were regarded normal. There was no treatment or follow-up visit. At approximately age 10 years a mild wrist deformity was noted. The patient was right hand dominant and noted pain in the wrist at the end of days after playing baseball. (b) At age 10 years 8 months the parents sought medical help again. There was significant deformity of the right distal radial physis and epiphysis, but no visible physeal bar (*right*). Normal left wrist for comparison (*left*). (c) At age 11 years 4 months the distal right radial deformities were markedly increased. Coronal cut tomograms confirmed significant irregularity of the physis and epiphysis on one cut (*left*) and a physeal bar on another cut (*right*). (d) Bar excision with cranioplast interposition was performed. (e) The bar excision provided no growth. (f) Twenty-two months later, age 13 years 2 months, the bar had reformed. The right forearm was 1 in. shorter than the left. (g) A step cut osteotomy lengthening of the radius was performed (*arrows*). (h) At age 13 years 11 months the radial lengthening was well healed and the ulna plus deformity was corrected. There was marked increase in the radial articular angle. (i) The patient had full wrist and elbow flexion and extension, but lacked 10° full supination and 50° full pronation. There was occasional wrist discomfort over the distal radial prominence. *Note*: It is difficult to find an association of the forearm diaphyseal fracture with the premature partial closure of the distal radial physis 7 years later. Surgical physeal closure of the radial side of the distal radius and the entire distal ulna after the failed bar excision would have resulted in more forearm length discrepancy, but would have prevented the radial articular angle from increasing, improved wrist medial and lateral wrist motion, and reduced the likelihood of future wrist degenerative changes (compare with Fig. 19C-2) (From Peterson [6], with permission and additional follow-up)

21.6 Hip

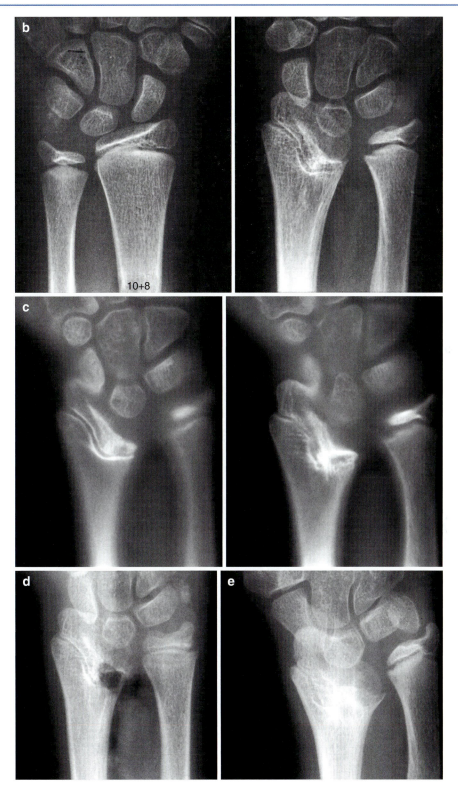

Fig. 21.6 (continued)

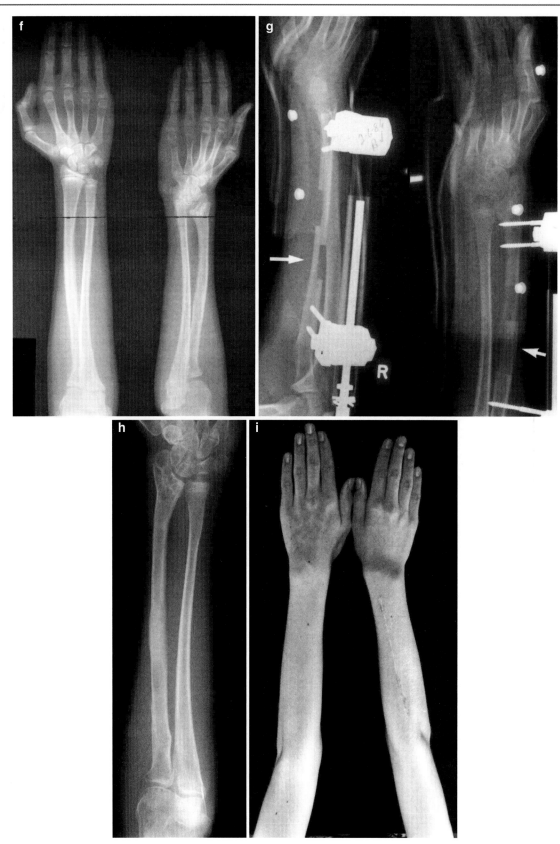

Fig. 21.6 (continued)

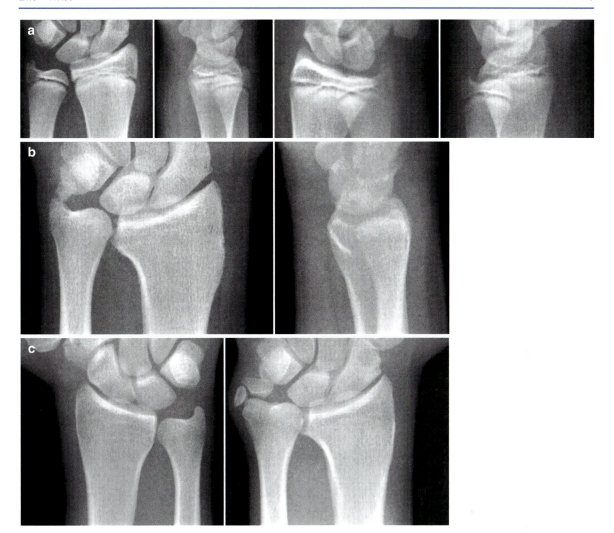

Fig. 21.7 Distal radius premature arrest, cause unknown. This 13 year 11 month old boy struck the dorsum of his right wrist against the helmet of another boy while playing football. He did not fall down and exited the playing field on his own power. The pain was sufficient to prevent him from returning to the game. (**a**) Multiple views of the wrist showed only an undisplaced fracture of the tip of the ulnar styloid on some views. A cock-up splint and ace bandage were worn for 6 days. (**b**) At age 16 years 7 months while being evaluated for a new unrelated shoulder injury the patient mentioned continuing discomfort and click in the area of the right ulnar styloid. There is now a well established non-union of an enlarged tip of the ulnar styloid with a mild ulnar plus deformity suggesting early premature closure of the distal radius. All physis are closed. Operative osteosynthesis of the ulnar styloid was undertaken. (**c**) At age 22 years 1 month the patient was recalled during a review in an attempt to find a Salter-Harris (*S-H*) type 5 fracture in Mayo Clinic files (no cases were found). He now had only occasional discomfort over the right ulnar styloid (*right*) which did not limit his employment or activities. *Left*: normal left wrist. *Right*: styloid fragments. The right radial articular surface was mildly tilted and was more proximal relative to the ulna than on the left wrist. *Note*: The cause of the premature partial closure of the distal radius is unknown. Since the blow was directly to the dorsum of the wrist this could be an example of a Rang type 6 injury (Fig. 21.8). Was the premature partial arrest due to direct physeal injury to the Ring of Ranvier or to ischemia?

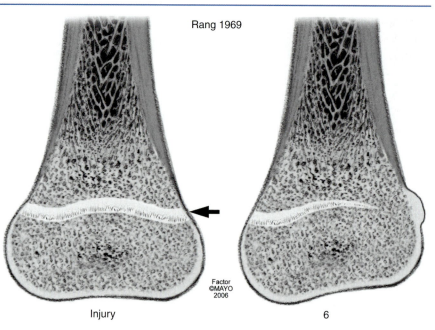

Fig. 21.8 Rang type 6 injury. In 1969 Salter's associate, Mercer Rang, described a physeal injury which became known as a Salter-Harris type 6 or a Rang physeal injury [8]. This was described as a rare injury produced by a direct blow to the periosteum or perichondral ring (*arrow*). Rang never illustrated a case or specified whether the subsequent partial arrest was produced by compression or ischemia of the peripheral physis. Neither Salter nor Rang included this injury in later publications classifying physeal injuries (From Peterson [7], with permission)

21.8 Author's Perspective

The etiology of physeal closure in each of these illustrated cases is undetermined, despite the fact that each patient had some other identifiable medical problem in his/her past or current history. It seems plausible to suspect that deficient vascular supply to the physis was a factor in each case (as demonstrated in Fig. 21.9), but the etiology of the deficiency remains unknown.

Fig. 21.9 Idiopathic premature partial physeal arrest of the proximal femoral capital physis. This female patient was referred from another tertiary medical center at age 6 years 10 months for evaluation of "poor weight gain." She was born with pyloric stenosis and within the first year had undergone pyloromyotomy, pyloroplasty, vagotomy, fundo plication, appendectomy, and hernia repair. A gastrostomy tube was in place from birth until age 3 years. She was a "picky eater." On examination there was mild relative shortening of the right lower extremity and mild limitation of right hip rotation and abduction, but no pain or limp. The gait was normal despite a positive Trendelenburg sign. Three cervical vertebrae were fused (presumably congenital in origin). (**a**) A scanogram at age 6 years 10 months revealed a short right femoral neck with a tilted physis, and moderate relative overgrowth of the greater trochanter. The right femur was 12 mm shorter than the left. (**b**) An MRI confirmed a peripheral physeal bar located laterally. (**c**) A projection MRI confirmed the posterolateral bar adjacent to the articular cartilage occupying 16% of the area of the physis. (**d**) Right hip arteriography at age 7 years 0 months was reported "Normal right common femoral, superficial femoral and deep femoral arteries. The artery supplying the head ascends on the medial aspect of the femoral neck and supplies the entirety of the femoral head. No other vessels are seen supplying the head." Left hip arteriography for comparison was not performed. (**e**) At age 7 years 2 months the physeal bar was excised through a Watson-Jones incision. The articular cartilage of the femoral head was normal. A tight heavy band of cartilage was found posterolaterally directly over the physeal bar continuous with the cartilage of the greater trochanter. It is interesting to speculate whether this was the primary cause or a secondary result of the premature closure. After excision of the bar the cavity was lined with a thin layer of bone wax and filled with cranioplast. Two halves of a titanium vascular clip were placed in the femoral head and neck 9 mm apart. The greater trochanteric physis was arrested by removing 80% of the physis with a curette. A single spica cast was worn for 3 weeks. (**f**) Three weeks later the markers were 13 mm apart. No further growth or change in the position of the markers occurred. At age 14 years 8 months arrest of the distal left femoral physis was accomplished by drilling under fluoroscopic guidance. (**g**) At age 17 years 3 months the patient was ambulating comfortably without limp. The right femur was 1.6 cm shorter than the left, and the right tibia 0.5 cm, for a total discrepancy of 2.1 cm. *Note*: This patient had multiple known congenital abnormalities. Congenital deficient vascular perfusion of the lateral aspect of the right femoral head could possibly be the etiology of this physeal bar

21.8 Author's Perspective

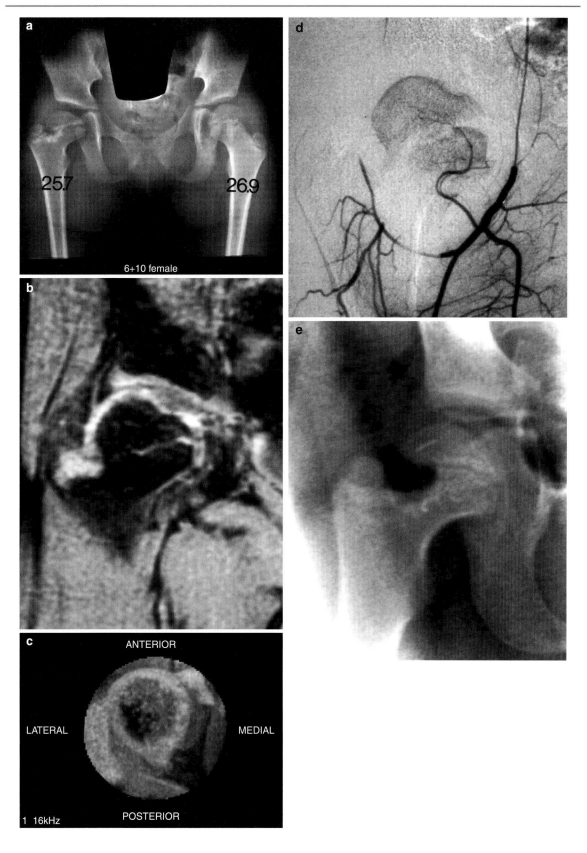

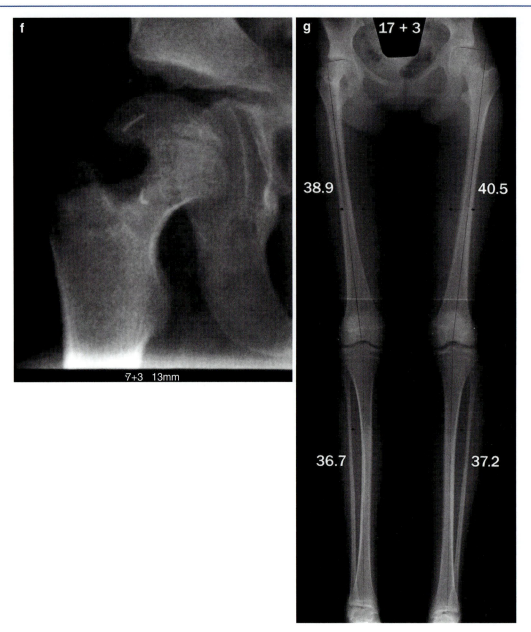

Fig. 21.9 (continued)

References

1. Ahstrom JP Jr (1965) Epiphyseal injuries of the lower extremity. Surg Clin North Am 1:119–134
2. Borsa JJ, Peterson HA, Ehman RL (1996) MR imaging of physeal bars. Pediatr Radiol 199(3):683–687
3. Kestler OC (1947) Unclassified premature cessation of epiphyseal growth about the knee joint. J Bone Joint Surg 29(3):788–797
4. Pappas AM, Anas P, Toczylowski HM Jr (1984) Asymmetrical arrest of the proximal tibial physis and genu recurvatum deformity. J Bone Joint Surg 66A(4):575–581
5. Pellise F, Aguirre M, Nardi J (1993) Premature monmomelic physeal closure. J Bone Joint Surg 75A(2):276–280
6. Peterson HA (1988) Scanning the bridge. In: Uhthoff HK, Wiley JJ (eds) Behavior of the growth plate. Raven, New York, pp 247–261
7. Peterson HA (2007) Epiphyseal growth plate fractures. Springer, Heidelberg
8. Rang M (1969) The growth plate and its disorders. Williams & Wilkins, Baltimore
9. Severance RD (1923) Bilateral asymmetrical cessation of growth of unknown etiology in epiphyses. J Bone Joint Surg 5:443–444
10. Siegling JA (1937) Lesions of the epiphyseal cartilages about the knee. Surg Clin North Am 17:373–379

Epilogue

Upon review of the information contained within this book one gains a greater appreciation of the function, strength, and resiliency of the physis, as long as it has a good blood supply. It appears that the small vessels which supply the physis are more fragile than the germinal chondrocytes of the physis, and that impairment of the vascular supply to the physis is the major factor in most of the injuries reported in this book.

Index

A
Abscopal effect *See* Irradiation, experimental
Acrophyses, 249
Active compression *See* Compression, active
Acute compression *See* Compression, acute
Allograft
 intercalary, 152
 osteoarticular, 157, 158
 reconstruction, 155, 158
Aminonucleoside, 181
Anatomy *See* Vascular anatomy
Aneurysmal bone cyst (ABC), 122–125
Angular deformity
 ankle valgus
  fibular deficiency, 339–349
  chronic renal failure, 188–189
 ankle varus
  congenital insensitivity to pain, 210–215
  cupping, 44–45
  due to pins, 371–374
  fibular overgrowth, 162–163
  meningococcemia, 32–40
  unknown, 405–407
 genu valgus, 72–76, 89, 188, 295, 400–402
 genu varus, 337, 403, 407
 surgical hemiphysiodesis, 361
 wrist, 127–136, 350–353, 370–372, 410–413
Ankle
 bilateral distal tibial physeal and epiphyseal abnormalities, 399, 405–407
 developmental injuries
  acquired fibula pseudarthrosis, 343
  isolated congenital pseudarthrosis of the fibula (ICPF), 339–343
  multiple hereditary osteochondromatosis (MHO), 343–346
  neurologic conditions, 346–347
  osteochondroma, distal fibula, 338
  pathophysiologic mechanism, 339
  scleroderma, 347–349
  tibial relative overgrowth *vs.* fibula, 349
 unilateral abnormal knee and distal tibia, 408–409
Anterior cruciate ligament repair, 379–383
Apophysis
 definition, 233, 281
 stress, 281
 unintentional injury, 367
Arterial catheterization, 14–17

Arterial deficiency *See* Vascular deficiency
Arterial disruption, 11–13
Arterial injection, 18
Arterial ligation, 14
Artery
 epiphyseal, 2
 intramedullary, 4
 metaphyseal, 4
 nutrient, 4, 46
 periosteal, 9
Arthrodesis, resection, 148
Atmospheric pressure, 333
Atomic bomb, 312
Autograft, frozen, 157
Avascular necrosis, 69

B
Bacteremia. 69
Benign bone tumors. *See* Tumor, benign bone
Biodegradable pins, 252
Binding of feet, 236
Bisphosphonates, 182
Blount disease, 337–338
Blount staples
 animals, 251
 humans, 240, 366
Blunt trauma, 69–71
Body height
 endocrine, 176
 chemotherapy, 188
 nuclear irradiation, 312
 nutrition, 173
 shock waves, 331
Bone
 length retardation (*see* Surgical injury)
  lengthening, 234, 253
 tumor (*see* Tumor)
Brachial plexus palsy, 196
Brain injury
 hemiplegia, 206
 quadriplegia, 207
Brodie's abscess, 94
Bryant's skin traction, 29
Burn injury
 physeal arrest, 225
 vascular deficiency, 42
2-Butoxyethenal, 182

C

Calcitriol, 182
Callotasis, of bone, 152, 157
Casts
    compression, 239
    vascular deficiency, 27
Catcher's knee, 283
Cerebral palsy, 206
cGy, 289
Chemotherapy, 187
Chemically induced immobilization, 62
Chondroblastoma, 141–142
Chondrodiatasis *See* Distraction of physis
Chondrosarcoma, 159
Chronic osteomyelitis, 95
Chronic recurrent multifocal osteomyelitis (CRMO), 95–96
Chronic renal failure (CRF), 188–190
    angular deformities, 189
        ankle valgus, 190
        genu valgus, 189
    slipped capital femoral epiphysis, 189
Classification
    cupping, 43
    physeal fracture, 262
Cold injury *See* Frostbite
Compartment syndrome, 18
Compression
    active compression, 234–236
        asymmetric pressure, 234
        bone lengthening, 234
        elastic compression, 234
        kyphosis, 235–236
        muscle pull, 234
        scoliosis, 235
        slipped capital femoral epiphysis, 236
    acute compression 253–278
        animal research, 262–263
            compression concept, support and refute of, 262–263
        human involvement, 253–261
            alternative mechanisms, 257–260
            articular surface abnormalities, 255–256
            Brashear, 254
            Cassidy, 253–254
            classification, 254
            clinical evidence against compression theory, 260–261
            clinical support for compression theory, 256–257
            compression theory challenged, 256
            concept 253–256
            crush injury, Salter–Harris type 5, 254–257
            epiphysis, roentgenogram, 255–256
            new classifications, 262
            physeal injury, Salter–Harris type 5, 254–256
            premature physeal closure, wastebasket, 263
    continuous compression
        animal research, 246–253
            absorbable filament, 253
            amount of, 250
            biodegradable screws and crossed pins, 252–253
            compensatory growth, 253
            crossed smooth metallic pins, 252
            direction of pressure applied, 250–251
            duration of, 250
            histologic studies, 250
            pathophysiologic mechanism of injury, 246, 250
            periosteal tether, 251
            spine fusion, 253
            staples, 251
            surgical bone lengthening, 253
            tensioned soft tissue grafts, 253
            transphyseal threaded screws and pins, 251–252
        human involvement, 233–246 (*see also* Compression, active; Compression, passive)
            pathophysiologic mechanism of injury, 233–234
    passive compression, 236–249
        casts, 239
        feet binding, 236
        metallic devices, 246
        oblique smooth pins, 245
        physis tethering, soft tissue, 236–239
        rigid containment, staple breaking, 246–249
        spine fusion, 245–246
        staples, 239–244
        tension band plate, 245
        transphyseal threaded screws, 245
        wire loops, 239
Cone epiphyses, 44, 46
Congenital insensitivity to pain (CIP), 208–215
Cooley's anemia *See* Thalassemia major
Copper deficiency, cupping, 46
Corticosteroids, 182–186
Cruciate ligament repair, 379–383
CRMO *See* Chronic recurrent multifocal osteomyelitis
Cupping
    arterial catheterization, 14–17
    arterial disruption, 11–13
    classification, 43
    congenital insensitivity to pain, 210
    copper deficiency, 46
    diphosphonate therapy, 46
    etiology, 43
    frostbite, 46, 220
    hypervitaminosis A, 46, 174
    irradiation, 46
    meningococcemia, 41
    osteomyelitis, 46
    pathogenesis, 43
    poliomyelitis, 46
    reduced vascular quality, 32
    rickets, 46, 175
    scurvy, 46, 175
    sickle cell anemia, 33
    tuberculosis, 46
    vascular deficiency, 42
    vitamin C deficiency, 46, 175
    vitamin D deficiency, 46, 175

D

DDH *See* Developmental dislocation of hip
Deferoxamine, 183
Denervation

brain injury, 206
    hemiplegia, 206
    quadriplegia, 207
  peripheral nerve injury, 195
    brachial plexus palsy, 196
    lumbar sympathetic ganglionectomy, 196
  spinal cord injury, 196
Developmental dislocation of the hip (DDH)
  developmental, 337
  disuse atrophy, 61
  vascular deficiency, 29–31
Developmental humerus varus, 337
Developmental injuries
  ankle
    acquired fibula pseudarthrosis, 343
    ankle valgus, 349
    cerebral palsy, 346
    congenital fibular pseudarthrosis, 339
    isolated congenital pseudarthrosis of the fibula (ICPF), 339–343
    meningococcemia, 202
    multiple hereditary osteochondromatosis (MHO), 343–346
    neurologic conditions, 346–347
    osteochondroma, distal fibula, 338
    pathophysiologic mechanism, 339
    poliomyelitis, 346
    scleroderma, 347–349
    tibial relative overgrowth *vs.* fibula, 349
  hip
    developmental dislocation of hip, 29, 61, 337
    Perthes disease, 31, 61, 337
    SCFE (*see* Slipped capital femoral epiphysis)
  knee, 337–338
  shoulder, 337
  spine
    kyphosis, 235, 337
    Scheuermann's kyphosis, 236, 237
    scoliosis, 235, 337
  wrist
    cosmetic appearance, 351
    Madelung's disease, 337
    osteochondroma, 350, 352
    ulnar lengthening, 351–352
    ulnar minus deficiency, 350–351
Diaphyseal fracture
  disuse atrophy, 57–61
  femoral and tibial, 27, 28
  proximal and distal tibia physes, premature arrest of, 18–22
  of tibial diaphysis, 18, 23–26
Diathermy, 231
Disphosponate therapy, 46
Direct chondrolysis, 67–69
Disseminated intravascular coagulopathy (DIC), 40
Distal ulnar osteochondromas, 128
Distraction of physis (chondrodiatasis)
  animal research, 276–278
  human involvement
    advantages and disadvantages, 273–274
    angular bending, 273–275

chondrodiatasis, 273
hemichondrodiatasis, 273
limb alignment, 272
physiolysis, 271
procedure, 271
psychological resistance, 272
results, 272
Steinmann pins, 271
tumor, 152
Distraction of bone (callotasis), 152, 157
Disuse injury
  chemically induced immobilization, 62
  developmental, 337
  DDH, 61
  diaphyseal fracture, 57–61
  osteomyelitis, 61
  Perthes disease, 61
  poliomyelitis, 54–57
  SCFE, 61–62
  tuberculosis, 53–54
  vascular deficiency, 42
Drilling across physis
  anterior cruciate ligament (ACL) injuries, 379, 382–383
  complete physeal sparing method, 387
  delay repair, 383–384
  partial physeal sparing, 386–387
  tibial and femoral transphyseal method, 384–386

E
Elastic compression, 234
Electrical burn, 231. *See also* Heat injury
Electrical injuries
  current
    clinical aspects, 229
    management, 230
    pathological mechanism, 229–230
    roentgenography, 229
  diathermy, 231
  lightning, 230–231
Enchondroma, 140–141
Endocrine disorders, 176
Ephedrine, 333
Epiphyseal arteries, 2–4, 31
Epiphyseal osteomyelitis
  acute, 83
  disappearance and regeneration, 84–89
  subacute, 84
Epiphyseal stress injury, 283
Epiphysiodesis. *See* Physiodesis
Epiphysiolysis. *See* Physiolysis
Erb's palsy, 196, 337
Etretinate, 183, 186
Exostosis. *See* Osteochondroma
Ewing sarcoma (ES), 158–159, 187
Extracorporeal membrane oxygenation (ECMO), 335
Extracorporeal shock wave lithotripsy (ESWL), 331

F

Femoral artery cannulation, 14–17
Femoral artery transection, 11–13
Femoral shaft fractures, 29
FFCD. *See* Focal fibrocartilaginous dysplasia
Fibrous dysplasia, of bone, 144–148
Fish vertebra deformity, 33
Fixation bandages, 27
Fluid extravasation, in soft tissues, 18
Focal fibrocartilaginous dysplasia (FFCD), 144
Fracture
    diaphyseal, 18–27
    vascular deficiency, 18
Frostbite
    animal research, 223
    cupping, 46
    definition, 219
    human involvement, 219–223
        clinical aspects, 219
        differential diagnosis, 220
        epidemiology, 220
        imaging evaluation, 219–222
        management, 223
        pathological mechanisms, 222–223
        vascular deficiency, 42
Frozen autograft reconstruction, 157

G

GCT *See* Giant cell tumor
Genu valgum, 138–140
Giant cell tumor (GCT), 142
Glantzman's platelet deficiency, 197
Gray (Gy), 289
Growth
    hormones, 176, 226
    stimulation due to infection, 80
Gymnast's wrist, 283

H

Heat injury
    animal research, 226–227
    human involvement
        clinical aspects, 225
        management, 226
        pathological mechanism, 225–226
        types of, 225
Hemangioma, interosseous, 149
Hemichondrodiatasis
    animals, 276
    definition, 271
    humans, 271
Hemiphysiodesis, 240, 362
Hemiplegia, 206
Hip
    idiopathic premature partial closure, 409, 410–414
    septic arthritis, 97–100
    SCFE (*see* Slipped capital femoral epiphysis)
Hormonal effect of radiation, 318
Hormones
    effect on burns, 226
    effect on growth, 176
Hueter–Volkmann law of growth modulation, 233
Humerus varus, 103–106, 337
Hypervitaminosis A, 46, 174
Hypocalcemia, 182
Hypoparathyroidism, 182

I

Immediate irreversible physeal arrest *See* Physeal arrest, intentional, humans
Immobilization
    chemically induced, 62
    developmental dislocation of hip, 61
    diaphyseal fracture, 57
    osteomyelitis, 61
    Perthes disease, 61
    poliomyelitis, 54
    slipped capital femoral epiphysis, 61
Infection
    chronic osteomyelitis, 95
    chronic recurrent multifocal osteomyelitis (CRMO), 95–96
    epiphyseal osteomyelitis
        acute, 83
        epiphyseal disappearance and regeneration, 84–89
        subacute, 84
    metaphyseal osteomyelitis
        bone involved, 77
        diagnosis, 77
        growth, stimulation of, 80
        organism, 65–66
        pathogenesis, 66–70
        pathologic anatomy, 70–77
        patient age, 66
        treatment, 77–80
    physeal chondritis, 86
    septic arthritis (*see* Septic arthritis)
    subacute osteomyelitis, 94
    transphyseal osteomyelitis, 86, 87, 90–94
Injury. *See* Physeal injury
Insensitivity to pain, 208–215
Intentional surgical physeal arrest. *See* Surgical injury
Intentional irradiation physeal arrest, 304
Intercalary allograft reconstruction, 155, 157
Interosseous hemangioma, 149–150
Interosseous infusion, 18
Intramedullary artery, 4
Irradiation
    complications, 290, 297
    cupping, 46
    definitions, 289
    diagnostic, 291
    effects, 289
    experimental
        abscopal effect, 315
        compensatory overgrowth, 315
        head, neck and trunk, 315–316
        histologic result, 314

intra-articular radiotherapy, 315
local hormonal effect, 315
oxygen effect, 314
radiation dose effect, fractionation, and age-animal 313–314
radioprotectants, 315
targeted radiotherapy, 315
intentional physeal arrest, 304
nuclear, 312–313
nuclear imaging, 313
radiation effects, 289–290
radiation terminology, 289
side effects and complications, 290–291
terminology, 289
therapeutic
dose and age effects, 296
Ewing's sarcoma, fibula, 292–295
extremity physes, intentional physeal retardation, 304
hand, 292
of head and neck, 304
management, 297–298
multimodal therapy, 297
osteochondroma, 299, 304
pathologic conditions, 291
physes involvement, 296–297
proton pencil beam, 316
side effects, 297
slipped epiphyses, 298–303
total body, 312
of trunk, 304–312
Ischemia
of metaphysis, 4
oxygen factor, 335
physis, center of, 42
widening of physis, 4–8
Isolated congenital pseudarthrosis of the fibula (ICPF)
developmental ankle valgus, 339–342
fibular union and deformity correction, 342
treatment of, 342
Isotretinon, 186

J
Joint
dislocation, 27
infection, 96–108
monoarticular, 97–106
multiarticular, 106–108

K
Kirner's deformity, 220
Knee
anterior cruciate repair, 379–383
Blount disease, 337, 338
catcher's knee, 283
developmental injuries, 337–338
genu valgus, 189
genu varus, 338
Osgood–Schlatter, 337
premature closure, 399–404
septic arthritis, 100–103
tumor, malignant, 151–158
unknown injury, 399–404

L
Langerhan's cell histiocytosis (LCH), 142–143
Laser
animal research, 328
definition, 325
human involvement, 326–328
therapy, 326
LCH. *See* Langerhan's cell histiocytosis
Ligament repair (anterior cruciate), 379–383
Lightning, 230–231
Light waves
laser, 325–328
animal research, 328
definition, 325
human involvement, 326–328
therapy, 326
phototherapy, 325
ultraviolet, 325
Lithotripsy, 331
Little leaguer's elbow, 281
Little leaguer's shoulder, 283
Lumbar sympathetic ganglionectomy, 196
Lymphoma, of bone, 159–161

M
Madelung's deformity
compression, 237
developmental, 337
stress, 287, 337
Maffucci syndrome, 140
Malignant bone tumors. *See* Tumor, malignant bone
Marked cupping, 14–17, 43–44
Medications
aminomucleoside, 181
biophosphonates, 182
2-butoxyethanol, 182
calcitrol, 182
corticosteroids, 183
deferoxamine, 183
etretinate, 184
isotretinon, 185
papain, 186
^{153}Sm-EDTMP, 186
tetracycline, 187
Meningococcemia, 32–41
Meningomyelocele
developmental, 337
neurologic 198–206
Metabolic injury
chemotherapy, 187–188
chronic renal failure, 188–189
angular deformities, 189, 190

Metabolic injury (Cont.)
    ankle valgus, 190
    genu valgus, 189
    slipped epiphyses (epiphysioloysis), 189
  endocrine, 176–182
    slipped capital femoral epiphysis, 176–182
  medications (*see* Medications)
  nutrition
    nutritional deprivation, 173–174
    vitamin A deficiency, 174
    vitamin A excess, 174
    vitamin C deficiency, 174–175
    vitamin D deficiency, 175
  slipped capital femoral epiphysis (SCFE)
    age, 176–177
    endocrine disorders, 176
    pinning, 177
    in young child, 178–181
Metaphyseal arteries, 3–8
Metaphyseal-equivalent osteomyelitis, 80–83
Metaphyseal osteomyelitis
  bone involvement, 77
  diagnosis, 77
  growth, stimulation of, 80
  organism, 65–66
  pathogenesis
    avascular necrosis, 69
    blunt trauma, 69–71
    direct chondrolysis, 67–69
    joint and epiphyseal vessels, spread to, 67, 69
    lateral extension, 69
    transphyseal vessels, 66–67
  pathologic anatomy, 70, 72–77
  patient age, 66
  treatment, 77–80
Microtrauma, 281–282
Microwave, 231
Mild cupping, 43–44
Moderate cupping, 12–13, 43–45
Motor paralysis, 55
Multiple hereditary osteochondromatosis (MHO)
  definition, 343
  distal fibula causing ankle valgus, 344–346
  distal ulna causing wrist ulnar deviation, 349–353
Muscle pull, 234

N
Neural injury
  brachial plexus injury, 196
  brain injury, 206
    hemiplegia, 206
    quadriplegia, 207
  congenital insensitivity to pain, 208–215
  meningomyelocele, 198–206
  peripheral nerve injury, 195
  spinal cord injury, 196
    nontraumatic, 198–206
    traumatic, 196–197
Nuclear injury
  imaging, 313
  irradiation, 312

Nutrient artery. *See* Intramedullary artery
Nutrition
  deprivation, 173
  nutritional deprivation, 173
  vitamin A deficiency, 174
  vitamin A excess, 46, 174
  vitamin C deficiency, 174, 208
  vitamin D deficiency, 175

O
Ollier's disease, 140
Osteoblastoma, 144
Osteochondroma
  distal forearm, 127
  distal lower leg, 137
  excision of, 128–129
  genu valgum, 138–140
  growth of, 126
  incidence of, 128
  one bone forearm creation, 130–132
  proximal ulna dislocation, 130–132
  radial head reduction, 134–136
  solitary sessile, 127
  treatment of, 126
  ulnar lengthening
    by callous distraction, 133–134
    by step-cut osteotomy, 353, 354
Osteoid osteoma, 143–144
Osteomyelitis
  chronic, 95
  CRMO, 95–96
  disuse atrophy, 61
  epiphyseal
    acute, 83
    epiphyseal disappearance and regeneration, 84–89
    subacute, 84
  metaphyseal
    bone involved, 77
    diagnosis, 77
    growth, stimulation of, 80
    organism, 65–66
    pathogenesis, 66–71
    pathologic anatomy, 70, 72–77
    patient age, 66
    physeal arrest, 61
    treatment, 77–80
  pathogenesis
    avascular necrosis, 69
    blunt trauma, 69–71
    direct chondrolysis, 67–69
    joint and epiphyseal vessels, spread to, 67, 69
    lateral extension, of epiphysis, 67, 69
    transphyseal vessels, 66–67
  physeal, 86
  subacute, 94
  transphyseal, 86, 87, 90–94
Osteoporosis, disuse, 53
Osteosarcoma, malignant bone tumors, 151–158

Index

Oxygen
    injury, 335
    effect, 335
    effect of radiation, 314
    factor, 335
    radiosensitivity, 335
    tension, 335

P
Pain insensitivity. *See* Congenital insensitivity to pain
Palsy
    brachial plexus (Erb's), 196
    cerebral, 206
        hemiplegia, 206–207
        quadriplegia, 207–208
Papain, 186
Paré, 355
Passive compression. *See* Compression, passive
Peaking, 42
Periosteal arteries, 9
Periosteal stripping, 27
Peripheral nerve injury
    brachial plexus birth palsy (BPBP), 196
    denervation
        limb paralysis, 195
        sciatic neuropathy, 195–196
    lumbar sympathetic ganglionectomy, 196
Perthes disease
    developmental, 337
    disuse atrophy, 61
    vascular deficiency, 31
Phemister physeal arrest, 359–360
Physeal arrest
    intentional, irreversible, animal experiments, 364–366
        biodegradable pins, screws & filaments, 252–253, 366
        bone grafts, 366
        burring, 364
        crossed smooth pins, 252, 366
        curettement, 364
        intraphyseal drilling, 364
        longitudinal pins, 366
        osteotomy across physis, 364
        periosteal tether, 251
        peripheral resection of physis, 364
        screws, 251–252
        spine fusion, 253
        staples, 251, 366
        tensioned soft tissue grafts, 253, 366
        transphyseal drilling, 365
        transphyseal screws, 251–252, 366
    intentional irreversible (physiodesis), humans, 355–361
        for SCFE, 355–359
            bone graft, 356
            metallic pinning, 356–359
        for length discrepancy, 359
            block method, 359–360
            cannulated tubesaw, 361
            commentary, 361
            curettement, 360
            endoscopic, 361
            fluoroscopic, 360

        intraphyseal drilling, 360–361
        trough method, 360
    intentional reversible, humans, 361–363
        for angular deformity (hemiphysiodesis), 361–362
            screws, 362
            staples, 362
            tension band plate (8 plate), 362
            wire loop, 362
        for length discrepancy, 244–247, 361–362
    unintentional arrest, animals, 387–388
    for length discrepancy, 244–247, 361-362
    unintentional arrest, humans, 367–388
        bone grafts, 379
        drilling, 379, 382–387
            anterior cruciate ligament repair, 379–387
            delay repair, 383–384
            transphyseal repair, 384–386
            complete physeal sparing, 387
            partial physeal sparing, 386–387
        osteotomy, 379
        nails, rods & prosthetic stems, 367–368
        smooth wires and pins, 368–379
            distal humerus, 369, 378
            distal radius, 368–372
            distal tibia, 369, 373–377
            metatarsals, 378–379
            phalanges, 368, 369
        threaded pins and screws, 379–382
Physeal chondritis, 86
Physeal cupping *See* Cupping
Physeal closure, normal, 9
Physeal growth, normal, 9
Physeal injury
    atmospheric pressure, 333–334
    cold (frostbite), 219–224
    compression, 233–270
    developmental, 337–354
    distraction, 271–280
    disuse, 53–63
    electric, 229–232
    heat (burn), 225–227
    infection, 65–114
    irradiation, 289–323
    light waves, 325–328
    metabolic, 173–193
    neural, 195–217
    oxygen, 335–336
    shock waves, 331–332
    sound waves, 329–330
    stress, 281–288
    surgical, 355–397
    tumor, 115–172
    unknown, 399–416
    vascular, 1–51
Physeal widening
    meningomyelocele, 198–206
    rickets, 175
    scurvy, 174–175
    ultrasound, 329
    vascular, 4–8
    vitamin D deficiency, 175
Physiolysis, 271

Physis
    normal closure, 9, 10
    normal growth, 9
    premature closure, 10
Poliomyelitis, disuse atrophy, 54–57
Prednisone, 182–186
Premature physeal closure, 10
Proton pencil beam therapy, 316
Pseudo-bar, 90, 100–102
Pseudorickets, 283
Purpura fulminans, 41–42

Q
Quadriparesis, 207–208

R
Rad, 289
Radiation *See* Irradiation
Rang physeal injury, 413–414
Renal failure *See* Chronic renal failure
Retinoic acid, 186
Rickets
    cupping, 46, 175
    physeal widening, 175
    tumor induced, 161–163
    vascular deficiency, 42
    vitamin D deficiency, 175

S
Salter and Harris (S–H) compression theory, 254–256
    animal evidence against, 262–263
    animal support for, 262
    clinical support for, 256–257
    concept, 256–258
    concept challenged, 258
    human evidence against, 260–261
    human support for, 256–257
Salter and Harris (S–H)
Satoyoshi's syndrome, 234
Scheuermann
    disease, 337
    kyphosis, 236
SCFE. *See* Slipped capital femoral epiphysis
Sciatic nerve injury, 196–197
Scleroderma, 347–349
Scoliosis
    due to compression, 275
    due to irradiation, 305–310
Scurvy, 174–175
Secondary center of ossification (SCO), 3–4
Septic arthritis
    causes, 96
    of hip, 97–100
    knee, 85–89, 100–103
    monoarticular, 97
    multiarticular, 106–108
    prognostic factors, 97
    shoulder, 103–106
    wrist, 103
Septicemia, 106–108
Shock waves
    definition, 331
    extracorporeal (lithotripsy), 331–332
Shoulder varus
    developmental, 337
    malignant tumor, 158
    septic arthritis, 103–106
Sickle cell anemia, 33, 40
Slipped capital femoral epiphysis (SCFE)
    age, 176–177
    etiology
        benign tumor (solitary cyst), 118
        chronic renal failure, 189
        compression, 236
        developmental, 337
        disuse atrophy, 61–62
        endocrine disorders, 176–181
        irradiation 298–303
        total body irradiation, 312
        vitamin C deficiency, 175
    pinning, 177
    surgical treatment, 355–359
    transphyseal bone graft physiodesis, 356
    transphyseal metallic pin, 356–359
    in young child, 178–181
Slipped epiphysis other than hip
    costochondral junction
        vitamin C deficiency (scurvy), 175
    distal femur
        vitamin C deficiency (scurvy), 175
        meningomyelocele, 198–202
    distal tibia
        vitamin C deficiency (scurvy), 175
        meningomyelocele, 198, 202–205
    distraction physiolysis, 271
    proximal humerus
        developmental, 337
        septic arthritis, 103–106
        vitamin C deficiency (scurvy), 175
    proximal tibia
        sound waves, 329
[153]Sm-ethylenediaminetetramethylene phosphonate, 186
Soft tissue tumors, 159, 161
Solitary bone cyst, 115–122
Sound waves, definition , 329
Spinal cord injury
    nontraumatic
        healing of, 202
        meningomyelocele, bilateral premature closure, 198–202
        physeal widening and dysfunction, 206
        treatment of, 198
    traumatic, 196, 198
Spine deformity
    conditions, axial skeleton, 305, 306
    correction of, 312

etiology and natural history, 306–310
fusion, 245–246, 253
incidence of, 310
irradiation, 305
Spontaneous physeal disruption. *See*
Slipped epiphysis
Staphylococcus aureus
acute primary osteomyelitis, 83
metaphyseal osteomyelitis, 65
physeal chondritis, 86
septic arthritis, 96
subacute osteomyelitis, 94
Staples
animals, 251
humans, 239–244
complete permanent arrest, 197, 241
hemiphysiodesis, 240, 346, 352
temporary reversible arrest, 241
Steroid induced physeal closure
prednisone, 182–186
Stress injury
complications, 286, 287
evaluation, 283–284
management, 287
mechanism of
distractive forces, 282
microtrauma, provisional calcification, 281–282
repetitive subfracture loading, 281
Salter–Harris type 1, forme fruste, 283
unilateral/bilateral lesions, 283
traction apophysitis, 281
Strychnine, 333
Subacute osteomyelitis, 94
Surgical injury
intentional physeal arrest (*see* Physeal arrest, intentional)
unintentional physeal arrest (*see* Physeal arrest, unintentional)
Sympathetic lumbar ganglionectomy, 196
Sympathectomy, 55

T
Temporary reversible physeal arrest, 361–363
Tension band plate, 245
Tenting, 42
Tethering of physis
Madelung's deformity, 237–238
soft tissue, 236–239
Tetracycline, 186–187
Thalassemia major, 24–25, 40, 183, 337
Therapeutic irradiation, trunk
osteochondroma, 312
prophylaxis, 310–311
soft tissues, 297, 304–305
spine deformity, 305–310, 312
stature loss, 305
treatment, 311
Therapeutic ultrasonography, 329
Thiemann's disease, 220

Traction, extremity, vascular deficiency, 27
Transphyseal aneurysmal bone cysts, 125
Transphyseal osteomyelitis, 86, 87, 90–94
Transphyseal solitary bone cysts, 122
Transphyseal vessels, 66–67
Transplantation of physis, 32
Transverse metaphysitis, 65
Tuberculosis
cupping, 46
disuse atrophy, 53–54
Tumor
benign bone
aneurysmal bone cyst (ABC), 122–125
chondroblastoma, 141–142
enchondroma, 140–141
focal fibrocartilaginous dysplasia (FFCD), 144
fibrous dysplasia, of bone, 144–148
giant cell tumor (GCT), 142
interosseous hemangioma, 149–150
Langerhan's cell histiocytosis (LCH), 142–143
osteochondroma, 125–140
osteoid osteoma and osteoblastoma, 143–144
solitary bone cyst, 115–122
malignant bone
chondrosarcoma, 159
Ewing sarcoma (ES), 158–159
lymphoma, of bone, 159–161
osteosarcoma, 151–158
distal fibula, 158
distal radius, 158
distal tibia, 158
knee, 152–158
shoulder, 158
transphyseal, 152
soft tissue, 159, 161
tumor induced rickets, 161–163

U
Ulnar deficiency, 338, 349–353
Ultrasonic waves, 329
Ultrasonography, 329
Umbilical artery catheter, 100–102
Unintentional physeal arrest. *See* Physeal arrest, unintentional
Unknown injury, 399–416
ankle, 399, 405–407
hand, 408
hip, 410–414
knee, 399–404
knee and ankle, 408–409
wrist, 410–414
Uremia, 188

V
Van Nes rotation plasty
burn, 226
tumor, 158, 162–163

Vascular anatomy of physis
    epiphyseal arteries, 2–4
    metaphyseal and intramedullary arteries, 3–8
    normal physeal growth, 9
    normal physiologic physeal closure, 9–10
    periosteal arteries, 9
    premature physeal closure, 10

Vascular deficiency
    due to reduced quality
        collagen vascular disorders, 42
        Cooley's anemia, 40
        meningococcemia, 32–41
        metabolic disease, 42
        purpura fulminous, 41–42
        sickle cell anemia, 33, 40
        thalassemia major, 40
    due to reduced quantity
        arterial catheterization, 14–17
        arterial disruption, 11–13
        arterial injection, 18
        arterial ligation, 14
        arteriovenous fistula, 14
        burns, 42, 225
        collagen disorders, 42
        compartment syndrome, 18
        congenital, 414–416
        cupping (*see* Cupping)
        DDH, 29–31
        diaphyseal fracture (*see* Diaphyseal fracture)
        disuse, 42, 53
        extremity traction, 27
        fixation bandages, 27
        fluid extravasation, in soft tissues, 18
        freezing, 42, 222
        immobilization, 42
        interosseous infusion, 18
        irradiation, 42, 290, 316
        joint dislocation, 27
        metabolic disease, 42
        osteomyelitis, 42
        periosteal stripping, 27
        Perthes disease, 31
        rickets, 42, 175
        scurvy, 42, 174–175
        septic arthritis, 42
        transplantation, of physis, 32

Vitamin A, 174
Vitamin C deficiency, 174–175
Vitamin D deficiency, 175
Volkmann's ischemia, 220

W

White physiodesis, 359–360
Wilm's tumor, 306–309
Wire loops, 234, 362
Wrist
    aneurysmal bone cyst, 122–124
    developmental injuries, 349–353
    idiopathic premature partial closure, 410–414
    osteochondroma, 128–136
    osteomyelitis, 70
    septic arthritis, 103

Z

Zone of Ranvier, 9

Printing and Binding: Stürtz GmbH, Würzburg